Squire's
Basic Pharmacology
for Nurses

Squire's
Basic Pharmacology
for Nurses EIGHTH EDITION

Bruce D. Clayton, B.S., Pharm. D.
ASSOCIATE PROFESSOR AND VICE-CHAIRMAN
DEPARTMENT OF PHARMACY PRACTICE
COLLEGE OF PHARMACY
UNIVERSITY OF NEBRASKA MEDICAL CENTER
OMAHA, NEBRASKA

Yvonne N. Stock, R.N., B.S.N., M.S.
COORDINATOR OF NURSING EDUCATION AND SURGICAL TECHNOLOGY
HEALTH OCCUPATIONS DEPARTMENT
IOWA WESTERN COMMUNITY COLLEGE
COUNCIL BLUFFS, IOWA

Jessie E. Squire, R.N., B.A., M.Ed.
PROFESSOR EMERITUS
DE ANZA COLLEGE SCHOOL OF NURSING
CUPERTINO, CALIFORNIA

Illustrated by Lana Carter Maher, R.N., B.S.N., B.F.A.
INSTRUCTOR IN NURSING
IOWA WESTERN COMMUNITY COLLEGE
COUNCIL BLUFFS, IOWA

with 194 illustrations

THE C. V. MOSBY COMPANY • St. Louis • Toronto • Princeton

MOSBY

A TRADITION OF PUBLISHING EXCELLENCE

The authors and publisher have made a conscientious effort to ensure that the information on the use of drugs in this book is accurate and in accordance with accepted standards of practice at the time of publication. However, pharmacology is a rapidly changing science, so readers are advised, before administering a drug, to check the package insert provided by the manufacturer for the recommended dose, for contraindications for administration, and for new warnings and precautions.

Eighth Edition

Previous editions copyrighted 1957, 1961, 1965, 1969, 1973, 1977, 1981

Printed in the United States of America

The C.V. Mosby Company
11830 Westline Industrial Drive, St. Louis, Missouri 63146

Library of Congress Cataloging in Publication Data

Squire, Jessie E.
    Squire's Basic pharmacology for nurses.

    Rev. ed. of: Basic pharmacology for nurses.
    Bibliography: p.
    Includes index.
    1. Pharmacology. 2. Nursing. I. Clayton, Bruce D.
1947-   . II. Stock, Yvonne Washburn. III. Title.
IV. Title: Basic pharmacology for nurses. [DNLM:
1. Pharmacology—nurses' instruction. QV 4 S777b]
RM300.S67 1985   615'.1   85-345
ISBN 0-8016-1260-8

H/VH/VH 9 8 7 6 5 4 3 2 1   03/C/314

Preface

Purpose

The original purpose of this text, first published in 1957, was to motivate the learner to administer medication with concern for safety, precision, and attention to important physiologic factors. We have done our utmost to maintain standards that have been synonymous with this book for the past 28 years. To accomplish this, we conducted extensive discussions and reviews with students, practitioners, and faculty at hospitals and schools of nursing concerning changes in goals, scope, and depth of content and educational format. We offer our gratitude and sincere appreciation for this assistance.

It became apparent very early in our discussions that first and foremost, the original purpose of the book should not change. The information required to maintain this purpose would correlate pharmacologic response to nursing actions (i.e., if a medication causes a certain side effect, how should the nurse respond to it?). A second major request of practitioners and faculty was to place the role of pharmacology in perspective with the individual patient and the disease entity being treated. Practitioners recognize that therapy is only as good as the patient's willingness to accept and follow a treatment regimen. We have therefore identified and correlated items of importance in the overall treatment plan that the nurse must know to integrate patient education about medications into the patient's complete treatment plan.

New Organization and Coverage

Every chapter in this edition has been thoroughly revised and updated and instructional objectives that state expected learning outcomes have been added to each. In addition, the book has been reorganized into 21 chapters in four units with new appendixes, glossary, and index.

Unit I, Principles of Pharmacology, provides introductory discussions of pharmacology, drug nomenclature, drug and patient information sources, and legal standards. Chapter 2 is a foundational chapter on understanding drug actions, monitoring parameters, patient variables, and drug interactions.

Unit II, Administration of Medications, is almost completely new. Chapter 3 reviews mathematics to assist students in dosage calculations. Chapter 4 is a new chapter on drug distribution systems, the patient chart, and, most important, the principles of nursing responsibilities and ethics, the 5 RIGHTS of Medication Administration plus the new RIGHT of Documentation, application of the nursing process to the administration of medications, and patient teaching. Chapters 5 through 7 are new chapters that have very comprehensive, illustrated sections on dosage forms, administration sites, and techniques of administration.

Unit III, Drugs Affecting Body Systems, and Unit IV, Other Pharmacologic Agents, are organized to facilitate arrangement of content and health assessment. We have developed a standardized format that emphasizes helping the nurse make knowledgeable assessments of the effects of drugs and patient teaching.

The new format in these units includes four sections. General Nursing Considerations for patients with particular diseases provides health care personnel with a brief, accurate synopsis of psychosocial, physiological, and nutritional assessment factors, health care measures, and patient teaching variables, together with associated nursing interventions to complete the overview of nursing responsibilities in relation to pathophysiology. This affords the practitioner a solid foundation upon which to base an evaluation of specific drug effects on individual patients. The patient teaching section compliments and fosters the expanded role of the nurse as a patient educator. Patient teaching variables can easily be extracted from this reference by the nurse for preparing teaching plans for patients based upon their specific medication regimen. Examples of written records that may be developed to help patients monitor therapy between visits are given. Specific drug monographs provide a pronunciation guide, actions and uses, side effects, availability, dosage and administration, and drug interactions.

Finally, every aspect of the nursing intervention is considered, including examples and suggestions for assessing and eliciting a desired response in the patient (e.g., ways to detect ototoxicity, descriptions of palpitations, securing patient and family cooperation with I/O, etc.). Moreover, the interventions are substantiated with sound, succinctly stated rationales that foster credibility and increased professional compliance.

The appendixes list common medical abbreviations, prescription abbreviations, mathematical conversions, temperature conversion tables, weight conversion tables, formulas for pediatric doses, sodium and potassium content of selected foods, nomograms for estimating body surface area, and a table of normal values for commonly used laboratory tests. Also included is a template for developing written records, like those in the text, for patients to monitor their own therapy between visits.

The revised eighth edition reflects the nurse's responsibility to provide sound, knowledgeable care in the area of medication administration. We have tried to clarify content and reinforce learning throughout the text. We have also placed emphasis on assisting the patient to improve his or her health by providing appropriate physical care, emotional and social support, and information necessary for self-care. It is our hope that this revision will meet the needs of nurses for a book "to motivate the learner to administer medication with concern for safety, precision, and attention to important physiologic factors," and to teach and assist them in providing the best possible nursing care to their patients.

Acknowledgments

We are indebted to Bess Arends, developmental editor, and Megan Thomas, assistant editor at The C. V. Mosby Company, whose encouragement and assistance helped bring this revision to completion. Linda Beckius deserves recognition for her excellent secretarial assistance.

BRUCE D. CLAYTON
YVONNE N. STOCK
JESSIE E. SQUIRE

Contents

UNIT IV. OTHER PHARMACOLOGIC AGENTS

APPENDIXES

Unit I

*Principles
of
Pharmacology*

Chapter 1

Definitions, Names, Informational Sources, and Standards

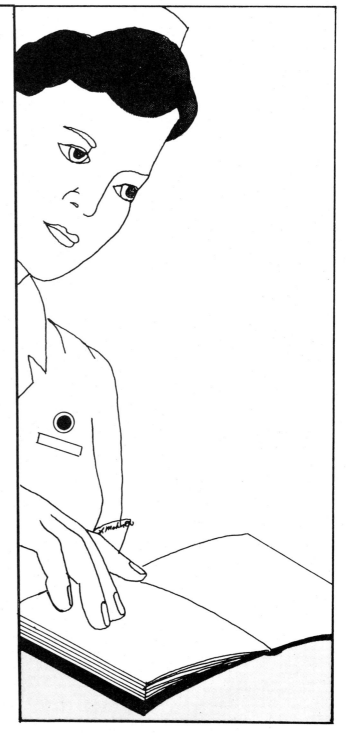

Objectives

After completing this chapter, the student should be able to do the following:

1. State the origin and definition of the word *pharmacology.*
2. Explain the meaning of "therapeutic methods."
3. Explain the differences between the chemical names, generic names, official names, and brand names of drugs.
4. List official sources of drug standards.
5. State how drugs are named.
6. List important literature resources for researching prescription and nonprescription drugs.
7. List important literature resources for researching drug interactions and drug compatibilities.
8. List important literature resources for reviewing information to be given to the patient.
9. Prepare a list of legislative acts controlling drug distribution and use.

Definitions

Pharmacology

Pharmacology (Greek *pharmakon*, "drugs" and *logos*, "science") deals with the study of drugs and their actions on living organisms.

Therapeutic Methods

Diseases may be treated in several different ways. The approaches to therapy are called *therapeutic methods*. Most illnesses require a combination of therapeutic methods for successful treatment. The following are some examples of therapeutic methods:

- Drug therapy—treatment with drugs.
- Diet therapy—treatment with diet, such as a low-salt diet for patients with cardiovascular disease.
- Physiotherapy—treatment with natural physical forces such as water, light, and heat.
- Psychological therapy—identification of stressors and methods to reduce or eliminate stress and/or the use of drugs.

Drugs

Drugs (Dutch *droog*, 'dry') are chemical substances that have an effect on living organisms. Therapeutic drugs are those drugs used in the prevention of treatment of diseases, and are often called *medicines*. Up until a few decades ago, dried plants were the greatest source of medicines, thus the word *drug* was applied to them.

Drug Names

Many drugs have a variety of names. This may cause confusion to the patient, physician, and nurse, so care must be taken in obtaining the exact name and spelling for a particular drug. When administering the prescribed drug, the *exact spelling* on the drug package must correspond exactly to the spelling of the drug ordered.

Chemical Name

The chemical name is most meaningful to the chemist. By means of the chemical name, the chemist understands an exact description of the chemical con-stitution of the drug and the exact placing of its atoms or molecular groupings.

Generic Name (Nonproprietary Name)

Before a drug becomes official, it is given a generic name or common name. A generic name is simpler than the chemical name. It may be used in all countries, by any manufacturer. It is not capitalized.

Generic names are provided by the United States Adopted Names (USAN) Council, an organization sponsored by the United States Pharmacopeial Convention, the American Medical Association, and the American Pharmaceutical Association.

Official Name

The official name is the name under which the drug is listed by the United States Food and Drug Administration (FDA). The FDA is empowered by federal law to name drugs for human use in the United States.

Trademark or Brand Name

A trademark or brand name has the symbol ® following the name. This indicates that the name is registered and its use is restricted to the owner of the drug, who is usually the manufacturer of the product. Some drug companies place their official drugs on the market under trade or proprietary names instead of official names. The trade names are deliberately made easier to pronounce, spell, and remember. The first letter of the trade name is capitalized.

EXAMPLE: Chemical name: 4-dimethylamino-1,4,4a,5,5a,6,11,12a-octahydro-3,6,10,12,12a-pentahydroxy-6-methyl-1,11, dioxo-2-naphthacenecarboxamide
Generic name: tetracycline.
Official name: Tetracycline, USP
Brand names: Achromycin, Panmycin, Tetracyn

Fig. 1.1. *Tetracycline, an antibiotic.*

4

Sources of Drug Standards

Standardization is needed to ensure uniformity of purity and potency of drug products between manufacturers and between batches made by one manufacturer. Before 1820 many drugs were manufactured in different parts of the United States with varying degrees of purity. This problem was solved by the establishment of an authoritative book that set forth required standards of purity for drugs as well as methods to determine purity. It is called the *Pharmacopeia–National Formulary of the United States of America.*

The United States Pharmacopeia (USP), 20th Revision, and The National Formulary (NF), 15th Revision

The USP and NF are now published as a single volume by the United States Pharmacopeial Convention, a nonprofit, nongovernmental corporation. The latest edition, published in 1980, represents the first time these two established reference books have been combined into one volume. This book is revised every 5 years. Supplements are published more frequently to keep it up to date.

The primary purpose of this volume is to provide standards for identity, quality, strength, and purity of substances used in the practice of health care. The standards set forth in the USP–NF have been adopted by the Food and Drug Administration as "official" standards for the manufacture and quality control of medicines produced in the United States.

USAN and the USP Dictionary of Drug Names

The USP dictionary is a compilation of over 11,000 drug names. Each drug monograph contains the United States Adopted Name (USAN), a pronunciation guide, the molecular and graphic formula, chemical and brand name, manufacturer, and therapeutic category. It also contains the Chemical Abstracts Service registry numbers for drugs.

Manufacturers submit a proposal for a name to the USAN Council in which they announce that a certain chemical compound has therapeutic potential and that they plan to run investigations on its use in human beings. The Council studies the chemical name, applies a series of nomenclature guidelines, and then selects the USAN (generic name). It is now customary for the Food and Drug Administraction to accept the adopted generic name as the FDA "official name" for a chemical compound.

Sources of Drug Information

American Drug Index

The *American Drug Index* is edited annually by Norman F. Billups, Ph.D., and is published by J. B. Lippincott Company of Philadelphia. It is an index of all drugs available in the United States.

Drugs in the *Index* are listed alphabetically by generic name and brand name. The generic name monographs indicate that the drug is recognized in the *United States Pharmacopeia–National Formulary* or *United States Adopted Names*, and give the chemical name, use, and cross-references to brand names. Each brand name monograph lists the manufacturer, composition and strength, pharmaceutical forms available, package size, dosage, and use. Other features of this reference book include a list of common medical abbreviations; tables of weights, measures, and conversion factors; a glossary to aid in interpretation of the monographs; a labeler code index to identify drug products; and a list of manufacturers' addresses. The book is useful for quickly comparing brand names and generic names and the availability of strengths and dosage forms.

American Hospital Formulary Service

The American Hospital Formulary Service is a comprehensive reference book published annually by the American Society of Hospital Pharmacists in Bethesda, Maryland. It is updated with four supplements yearly. This volume contains monographs on virtually every single-drug entity available in the United States. The monographs emphasize rational therapeutic use of drugs. Each monograph is subdivided into sections on chemistry and stability, pharmacology, pharmacokinetics, uses, cautions, toxicity, drug interactions, dosage and administration, and available products. The index is cross-referenced by both generic and brand names.

The *American Hospital Formulary Service* has been adopted as an official reference by the U.S. Public Health Service and the Veterans Administration. It has also been approved for use by the American Hospital Association, the Catholic Health Care Association of the United States, the National Association of Boards of Pharmacy, and the American Pharmaceutical Association and is included as a required or recommended standard reference in pharmacies in many states.

Drug Interaction Facts

Drug Interaction Facts is a new source on drug interactions published by the Facts and Comparisons Division (St. Louis) of J. B. Lippincott Company of Philadelphia.

This three-ring, loose-leaf, 600-page book, first published in 1983, is currently the most comprehensive book available on the subject of drug interactions. The format is somewhat different from that of most other books: the index is in the front, and the book is not subdivided into chapters. Drugs are arranged alphabetically, and the book is then subdivided every 100 pages by a plastic tab sheet. Each page is a single monograph describing a drug interaction. Each monograph is subdivided into a table that lists the onset and severity of the drug interaction, expected outcomes, a statement on the expected effects, the proposed mechanism, and how to manage the interaction. A short discussion (with references) follows on the relevance of the interaction.

One of the most meaningful, although not obvious, benefits is the source of information used to develop this book. All the information reviewed is from the MEDIPHOR Group of the Stanford University School of Medicine. This internationally renowned group of physicians and pharmacists has the personnel, clinical experience, scientific background, library, and computer resources to collect, collate, review, and evaluate the scientific accuracy of descriptions of drug interactions from the world literature. Thus, it is an extremely reliable source of information. The book is updated four times a year.

Facts and Comparisons

Facts and Comparisons is a large, loose-leaf compendium published by the Facts and Comparisons Division of J. B. Lippincott Company.

The loose-leaf book is divided into 12 chapters. At the beginning of each chapter is a detailed table of contents. All drugs within each chapter are subdivided by therapeutic classes. There is a monograph for each therapeutic class of drug that provides a brief description of drug action, pharmacokinetics, metabolism, uses, contraindications, warnings, precautions, adverse effects reported, treatment of overdosage, patient information in brief, and administration. The data base for the monographs is the most current FDA-approved package insert. The editors have reformatted the information and added additional information from the medical literature on investigational uses of the drugs.

At the end of each monograph are tables of all drugs in that therapeutic class. The tables are particularly valuable because they are designed to allow a comparison of similar products, brand names, manufacturers, cost index, and available dosage forms.

The index is quite comprehensive and is updated both monthly and quarterly. Within each chapter, there is an excellent cross-referencing system as well,

making it quite easy to gain information on drugs that may be categorized by more than one therapeutic class. Updated supplements for the entire book are provided monthly.

Handbook on Injectable Drugs

The *Handbook on Injectable Drugs*, the most comprehensive reference available on the topic of compatibility of injectable drugs, is written by Lawrence A. Trissel and published by the American Society of Hospital Pharmacists of Bethesda, Maryland. It is a collection of monographs on over 250 injectable drugs. Each monograph is subdivided into sections on availability of concentrations, stability, pH, dosage and rate of administration, compatibility information, and other useful information about the drug.

Handbook of Non-Prescription Drugs

This volume is prepared and published by the American Pharmaceutical Association, Washington, D.C. It is the most comprehensive text available on medications that may be purchased over the counter in the United States.

Chapters are divided by therapeutic activity, such as antacid products, cold and allergy products, nutritional supplements, mineral and vitamin products, and feminine hygiene products. Each chapter provides a brief review of anatomy and physiology, evaluation of the symptoms being treated, suggested treatments with appropriate dosages, and a listing of medications with their ingredients.

This book has three particular advantages for the health professional: (1) a list of questions to ask the patient to determine whether treatment should be recommended; (2) product selection guidelines for determining the most appropriate products; and (3) counseling to be conveyed to the patient on how to properly use the recommended product.

Martindale—The Extra Pharmacopoeia

This 2000-page volume is edited by James E. F. Reynolds and is published by The Pharmaceutical Press in London. It is one of the most comprehensive texts available for information on drugs in current use throughout the world. In addition to extensive referenced monographs (part 1) on the pharmacologic activity and side effects of 3990 medicinal agents, there are short monographs (part 2) on another 1120 agents that are either considered obsolete or too new for inclusion in part 1. Part 3 gives the composition and manufacturers of more than 900 over-the-counter pharmaceutical products.

The index contains more than 43,000 entries. Medicinal agents are indexed by official names, chemical names, synonyms, and proprietary names.

Medical Letter

The *Medical Letter*, published by Drug and Therapeutic Information, Inc., New York, is a semi-monthly periodical newsletter. It contains brief comments on newly released drug products and related topics by an independent board of competent authorities. The board relies upon the knowledge of specialists in various fields for their experience with certain drugs. The primary purpose of the newsletter is to report new data on drug action and comparative clinical efficacy. The *Medical Letter* presents timely and critical summaries of data on new drugs during their early period of promotion. Such appraisals must, necessarily, be tentative.

Package Inserts

Before a new drug is marketed, the manufacturer develops a comprehensive but concise description of the drug, indications and precautions in clinical use, recommendations for dosage, known adverse reactions, contraindications, and other pharmacologic information relating to the drug. Federal law requires that the insert be approved by the Food and Drug Administration before the product is released for marketing and that the insert accompany each package of the product.

Physicians' Desk Reference (PDR)

The *PDR* is published annually by Medical Economics, Inc. of Oradell, New Jersey. It lists approximately 2500 therapeutic agents in seven sections. Each section uses a different page color for easy access.

Section 1 (white), Manufacturers' Index—an alphabetic listing of each manufacturer, their addresses, emergency phone numbers, and a partial list of available products.
Section 2 (pink), Product Name Index—a comprehensive alphabetic listing of brand name products discussed in the Product Information section of the book.
Section 3 (blue), Product Classification Index—products are subdivided by therapeutic classes, such as analgesics, laxatives, oxytocics, and antibiotics.
Section 4 (yellow), Generic and Chemical Name Index—products are listed by their generic or chem-

ical names, with references to the Product Information section.
Section 5, Product Identification Section—each manufacturer has provided color pictures of the actual sizes of their tablets and capsules. This section is an invaluable aid in product identification.
Section 6 (white), Product Information Section—This section is a reprint of the package insert for the major products of manufacturers, with information on action, uses, administration, dosages, contraindications, composition, and how each drug is supplied.
Section 7 (green), Diagnostic Product Information—an alphabetic listing by manufacturer of many diagnostic tests used in hospital and office practice.

Sources of Patient Information

Over the past two decades, it has become evident that health care providers must do a better job of informing patients of what they must do to assume responsibility for their own health care. The following books are excellent sources of information for teaching patients how to use their medications properly.

Medication Guide for Patient Counseling

The *Medication Guide for Patient Counseling* is written by Dorothy L. Smith and published by Lea & Febiger of Philadelphia. This is an excellent resource book on the topic of patient counseling. It provides both a good discussion on *how* to counsel patients for health professionals and then provides a comprehensive set of medication instructions for almost all of the medications available in the United States and Canada. The medication instructions have been translated from medical terminology into language that most patients can understand. Each of the drug monographs contains the important information (including administration techniques) that should be conveyed to the patient.

United States Pharmacopeia Dispensing Information

USP DI is an annual publication written by the United States Pharmacopeial Convention, Inc. and distributed by the C. V. Mosby Company of St. Louis.
USP DI is a two-volume set supplemented with bimonthly updates. The first volume includes dispensing information for health care providers arranged in alphabetically ordered monographs. Each monograph is subdivided into sections on the individual drug's use, mechanism of action, precautions, side effects, patient

consultation information, general dosing information, and dosage forms available.

The second volume, *Advice for the Patient*, provides the layman's language for the patient consultation guidelines found in volume I. The second volume is designed to be used at the discretion of the health care provider as an aid to counseling the patient if written information is to be given to the patient. The publisher permits all health care practitioners to reproduce the pages of advice for their patients receiving the prescribed drug. Generic and brand names are cross-referenced in the index of *Advice for the Patient*.

Drug Legislation

Drug legislation protects the consumer and patient. The need for such protection is great because manufacturers and advertising agents may make unfounded claims about the benefits of their products.

Federal Food, Drug, and Cosmetic Act, June 25, 1938 (Amended 1952, 1962)

The 1938 act authorizes the federal Food and Drug Administration of the Department of Health and Human Services to determine the safety of drugs before marketing and to assure that certain labeling specifications and standards in advertising are met while marketing a product. Manufacturers are required to submit new drug applications to the FDA for review of safety studies before products can be released for sale.

The Durham-Humphrey Amendment in 1952 tightened control by restricting the refilling of prescriptions.

The Kefauver-Harris Drug Amendment in 1962 was brought about by the thalidomide tragedy. Thalidomide was an incompletely tested drug approved for use as a sedative-hypnotic during pregnancy. Infants exposed to thalidomide were born with serious birth defects. This amendment provides greater control and surveillance of the distribution and clinical testing of investigational drugs and requires that a product be proven to be both safe and effective before release for sale.

Harrison Narcotic Act, 1914

The Harrison Narcotic Act regulated the importation, manufacture, sale, and use of opium, cocaine, and all their compounds and derivatives. Its purpose was to limit the indiscriminate use of such drugs and to prevent the spread of the drug habit. The act was

amended many times. However, the law has been repealed and replaced by the Controlled Substances Act of 1970.

Controlled Substances Act, 1970

The Comprehensive Drug Abuse Prevention and Control Act was passed by Congress in 1970. This new statute, commonly referred to as the "Controlled Substances Act," repealed almost 50 other laws written since 1914 that relate to the control of drugs. The new composite law is designed to improve the administration and regulation of manufacturing, distributing, and dispensing of drugs found necessary to be controlled.

The Drug Enforcement Administration (DEA) was organized to enforce the Controlled Substances Act, to gather intelligence, and to train and conduct research in the area of dangerous drugs and drug abuse. The DEA is a bureau of the Department of Justice. The director of the DEA reports to the Attorney General of the United States.

The basic structure of the Controlled Substances Act consists of five classifications or "schedules" of controlled substances. The degree of control, the conditions of record keeping, the particular order forms required, and other regulations depend on these classifications. The five schedules, their criteria, and examples of drugs within each schedule are listed below:

Schedule I ℂ drugs

1. A high potential for abuse
2. No currently accepted medical use in the United States
3. A lack of accepted safety for use under medical supervision

EXAMPLES: LSD, marijuana, peyote, STP, heroin, hashish

Schedule II ℂ drugs

1. A high potential for abuse
2. A currently accepted medical use in the United States
3. An abuse potential that may lead to severe psychologic or physical dependence

EXAMPLES: secobarbital, pentobarbital, amphetamines, morphine, meperidine, methadone, methoqualone, Percodan

Schedule III ℂ drugs

1. A high potential for abuse, but less so than drugs in schedules I and II

2. A currently accepted medical use in the United States
3. An abuse potential that may lead to moderate or low physical dependence or high psychologic dependence

EXAMPLES: Empirin with codeine, Doriden, Fiorinal, paregoric, Noludar, Tylenol with codeine

Schedule IV Ⓒ drugs

1. A low potential for abuse, relative to those in schedule III
2. A currently accepted medical use in the United States
3. An abuse potential that may lead to limited physical or psychologic dependence, relative to drugs in schedule III

EXAMPLES: phenobarbital, Equanil, chloral hydrate, paraldehyde, Librium, Valium, Dalmane, Tranxene.

Schedule V Ⓒ drugs

1. A low potential for abuse, relative to those in schedule IV
2. A currently accepted medical use in the United States
3. An abuse potential of limited physical or psychologic dependence liability, relative to drugs in schedule IV

EXAMPLES: terpin hydrate with codeine, Lomotil, Robitussin A-C

The Attorney General, after public hearings, has authority to reschedule a drug, bring an unscheduled drug under control, or remove controls on scheduled drugs.

Every manufacturer, physician, dentist, pharmacy, and hospital that manufactures, prescribes, or dispenses any of the drugs listed in the five schedules must register annually with the Drug Enforcement Administration.

A physician's prescription for substances named in this law must contain the physician's name, address, DEA registration number and signature, the patient's name and address, and the date of issue. The pharmacist cannot refill such prescriptions without the approval of the physician.

All controlled substances for ward stock must be ordered on special hospital forms that are used to help maintain inventory and dispersion control records of the schedule drugs. When a nurse administers a schedule II drug, under a physician's order, the following information must be entered on the controlled substances record: name of the patient, date of administration, drug administered, and drug dosage.

Possession of Controlled Substances

Federal and state laws make the possession of controlled substances a crime, except in specifically exempted cases. The law makes no distinction between professional and practical nurses in regard to possession of controlled drugs. Nurses may give controlled substances only under the direction of a physician or dentist who has been licensed to prescribe or dispense these agents. Nurses may not have controlled substances in their possession unless they are giving them to a patient under a doctor's order, or the nurse is a patient for whom a doctor has prescribed schedule drugs, or the nurse is the official custodian of a limited supply of controlled substances on a ward or department of the hospital. Controlled substances ordered but not used for patients must be returned to the source from which they were obtained (the doctor or the pharmacy). Violation or failure to comply with the Controlled Substances Act is punishable by fine, imprisonment, or both.

Effectiveness of Legislation of Drugs

Effectiveness of legislation depends on the interest and determination used to enforce these laws, the appropriation by Congress of adequate funds for enforcement, the vigor used by proper authorities in enforcement, the interest and cooperation of professional people and the public, and the education of the public concerning the dangers of unwise and indiscriminate use of drugs in general. Many organizations help in this education, including the National Coordinating Council on Patient Information and Education, American Medical Association, American Dental Association, American Pharmaceutical Association, the American Society of Hospital Pharmacists, and local, state, and county health departments.

Chapter 2

Principles of Drug Action and Drug Interactions

Objectives

After completing this chapter, the student should be able to do the following:

1. Identify five basic principles of drug action.
2. Explain nursing assessments and/or interventions that enhance drug absorption.
3. List the three categories of drug administration and state the routes of administration for each category.
4. Describe drug distribution mechanisms and differentiate between general and selective types.
5. Name the process that inactivates drugs.
6. Name the primary routes of drug excretion from the body.
7. Identify the meaning and significance to the nurse of the term *half-life* when used in relation to drug therapy.
8. Compare and contrast the following terms: *reaction, side effects, adverse effects, allergic reactions,* and *idiosyncratic reactions.*
9. State the factors that cause variation in absorption, metabolism, distribution, and excretion of drugs.
10. State the mechanisms by which drug interactions may occur.

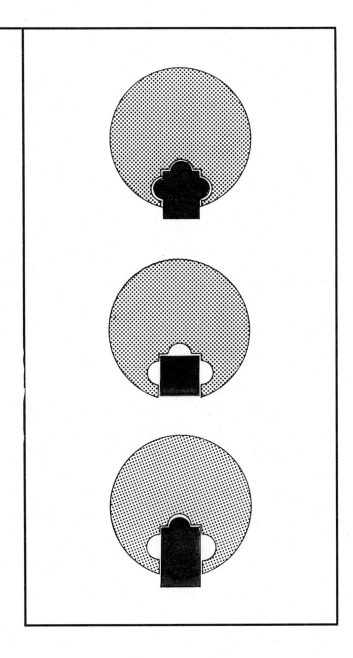

Basic Principles

How do drugs act in the body? A few key facts to remember are:

1. Drugs do not create new responses, but alter existing physiological activity. Thus, drug response must be stated in relation to what the physiological activity was before the response to drug therapy (e.g., an antihypertensive agent is successful if the blood pressure is lower during therapy than before therapy). Therefore, it is important to perform a thorough nursing assessment to identify the baseline data. Thereafter, regular assessments are performed by the nurse and compared to the baseline data by the physician, the nurse, and the pharmacist, in order to evaluate the effectiveness of the drug therapy.
2. Drugs interact with the body in several different ways. The most common way in which drugs act is by forming chemical bonds with specific sites called *receptors* within the body. Bonding occurs only if the drug and its receptor have similar shapes. An example of the relationship between a drug and a receptor is like a key and a lock (see Fig. 2.1a).
3. Most drugs have several different atoms within the molecule that interlock into several locations on the receptor. The better the "fit" between the receptor and the drug, the better the response.
4. Drugs that interact with a receptor to stimulate a response are known as *agonists* (see Fig. 2.1b). Drugs that attach to a receptor but do not stimulate a response are called *antagonists* (see Fig. 2.1c). Drugs that interact with a receptor to stimulate a response, but inhibit other responses are called *partial agonists* (see Fig. 2.1d).
5. Once administered, all drugs go through four stages: absorption, distribution, metabolism, and excretion (ADME). Each drug has its own unique ADME characteristics.

Absorption

Absorption is the process by which a drug is made available to the body fluids for distribution. It is the way in which a drug is transferred from its site of entry into the body to the circulating fluids of the body, the blood, and the lymphatic system. The rate at which this occurs depends on the route of administration, the blood flow through the tissue where it is administered, and the solubility of the drug. Therefore, it is important to administer oral drugs with an adequate amount of fluid, and to give parenteral forms properly so that they are deposited in the correct tissue for enhanced absorption. When administering drugs that are to be reconstituted or diluted, use only the diluent recommended by the manufacturer (in the package literature) so that drug solubility is not impaired. Equally important are nursing assessments that imply poor absorption (e.g., if insulin is administered subcutaneously and a "lump" remains at the site of injection 2-3 hours later, absorption from that site may be impaired).

The routes of drug administration are classified into three categories: enteral, parenteral, and percutaneous. The *enteral* route refers to administration directly into the gastrointestinal tract by oral, rectal, or nasogastric means. *Parenteral* routes of administration bypass the gastrointestinal tract and include subcutaneous, intramuscular, or intravenous injection. Methods of *percutaneous* administration include inhalation, sublingual, or topical administration. Absorption of topical drugs applied to the skin can be influenced by drug concentration, length of contact time, size of the affected area, thickness of the skin surface, tissue hydration, and degree of skin disruption. Inhalation of drugs and their absorption can be influenced by depth of respirations, size of the droplet particles, available surface area of mucous membrane, contact time, hydration state, blood supply to the area, and concentration of the drug itself.

The rate of absorption by parenteral routes is partially dependent upon the rate of blood flow through the tissues. (Therefore, the nurse should not give an injection where circulation is known to be impaired; another site on the rotation schedule should be used.) Subcutaneous injections have the slowest absorption rate, particularly if peripheral circulation is impaired. Intramuscular injections are more rapidly absorbed because of greater blood flow per unit weight of muscle. Depositing the medication into the muscle belly is important. Nurses must carefully assess individual patients for the correct needle length to be sure that this

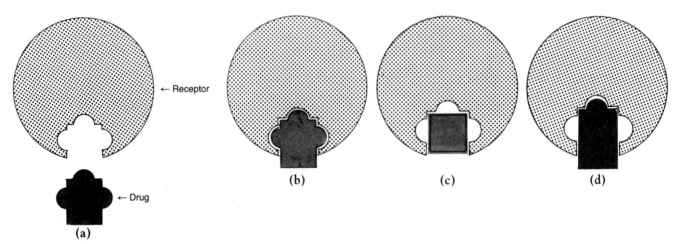

Fig. 2.1. (a) *Drugs act by forming a chemical bond with specific receptor sites, similar to a key and lock,* (b) *The better the "fit" the better the response. Those with complete attachment and response are called "agonists."* (c) *Drugs that attach but do not elicit a response are called "antagonists."* (d) *Drugs that attach, elicit a small response, but also block other responses are called "partial agonists."*

occurs. Cooling an area of injection will slow the rate of absorption while heat or massage will hasten the rate of absorption. When administered intravenously, the drug is dispersed throughout the body most rapidly. (Nurses must be thoroughly educated regarding the responsibilities and techniques associated with administering IV medications. Once the drug enters the bloodstream, it cannot be retrieved.)

Regardless of the route of administration, a drug must be dissolved in body fluids before it can be absorbed into body tissues. For example, before a solid drug, taken orally, can be absorbed into the bloodstream for transport to the site of action, it must disintegrate and dissolve in the gastrointestinal fluids and be transported across the stomach or intestinal lining into the blood. The process of converting the drug into a soluble form can be partially controlled by the pharmaceutical dosage form used (e.g., solution, suspension, capsule, or tablets with various coatings) or can be influenced by the time of administration in relation to the presence or absence of food in the stomach.

Distribution

The term *distribution* refers to the ways in which drugs are transported by the circulating body fluids to the sites of action (receptors), as well as to their metabolism and excretion. Drug distribution means transport throughout the entire body by the blood and lymphatic systems, and transport from the circulating fluids into and out of the fluids that bathe the receptor sites. Organs having the most extensive blood supply, such as the heart, liver, kidneys, and brain receive the distributing drug most rapidly. Areas with less extensive blood supply, such as muscle, skin, and fat receive the drug more slowly. However, drugs tend to stay in these tissues longer, due to lower circulation rate.

Distribution may be general or selective. Some drugs cannot pass certain types of cell membranes such as the central nervous system (the blood–brain barrier) or the placenta (placental barrier), while other drugs will very readily pass into these tissues. The distribution process is a very important one because the amount of drug that actually gets to the receptor sites determines the extent of pharmacological activity. If very little drug actually reaches and binds to the receptor sites, there will only be a minimal response.

Metabolism

Metabolism, also called *biotransformation*, is the process by which the body inactivates drugs. The enzyme systems of the liver are the primary site of metabolism of drugs, but other tissues and organs metabolize certain drugs, to a minor extent.

Excretion

Metabolites of drugs and, in some cases, the active drug itself, are eventually excreted from the body. The primary routes are through the gastrointestinal tract to the feces and through the renal tubules into the urine. Other routes of excretion include evaporation through the skin, exhalation from the lungs, and secretion into the saliva and mother's milk.

Figure 2.2 is a schematic review of the absorption, distribution, metabolism, and excretion process of an oral medication. It is important to note how little of the active ingredient actually gets to the receptor sites for action.

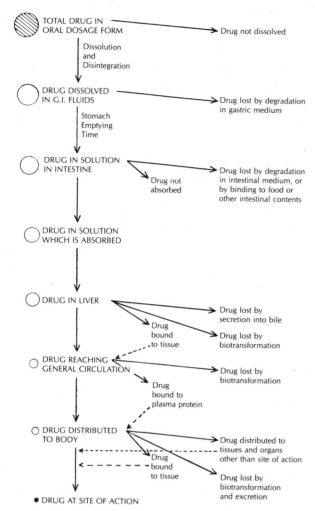

Fig. 2.2. *Factors modifying the quantity of drug reaching a site of action after a single oral dose. (From Levine, R. R.: Pharmacology, Drug Actions, and Reactions, Boston, 1973, Little, Brown & Co.)*

Half-life

Elimination of drugs occurs by metabolism and excretion. A measure of the time required for elimination is the half-life. The *half-life* is defined as the amount of time required for 50% of the drug to be eliminated from the body. For example, if a patient were given 100 mg of a drug that had a half-life of 12 hours, the following would be observed:

TIME (HR)	HALF-LIFE	DRUG REMAINING IN BODY
0	—	100 mg (100%)
12	1	50 mg (50%)
24	2	25 mg (25%)
36	3	12.5 mg (12.5%)
48	4	6.25 mg (6.25%)
60	5	3.12 mg (3.12%)

Note that as each 12 hours (one half-life) passes, the amount remaining is 50% of what was there the previous 12 hours. After six half-lives, over 98% of the drug is eliminated from the body.

The half-life is determined by an individual's ability to metabolize and excrete a particular drug. Since most patients metabolize and excrete the same drug at about the same rate, the approximate half-lives of most drugs are now known. When the half-life of a drug is known, dosages and frequency of administration can be calculated. Drugs with a long half-life, such as digoxin at 36 hours, need to be administered only once daily, while drugs with a short half-life, such as aspirin at 5 hours, need to be administered every 4 to 6 hours to maintain therapeutic activity. In patients who have impaired hepatic or renal function, the half-life may become considerably longer due to the inability to metabolize or excrete the drug. An example is digoxin with a half-life of about 36 hours in a patient with normal renal function, but a half-life of about 105 hours in a patient in complete renal failure. Monitoring diagnostic tests that measure renal or hepatic function are important. Whenever laboratory data is received that reflects impairment of either function, the nurse should notify the physician.

Drug Action

No drug has a single action. When a drug enters a patient and is absorbed and distributed, we usually see the *desired action*, the expected response. All drugs, however, have the potential to affect more than one body system at the same time, producing reactions known as *side effects* or *adverse effects*. Most of these side effects are predictable, and patients should be monitored for these side effects so that dosages can be adjusted to allow the maximum therapeutic benefit with a minimum of side effects. As described in Units 3 and 4 of this text, each drug has a series of *parameters* (therapeutic action to expect, side effects to expect, adverse effects to report, and probable drug interactions) that should be monitored by the nurse, physician, pharmacist, and the patient in order to optimize therapy, while reducing the possibility of serious adverse effects.

There are two other types of drug action that are much more unpredictable. These are idiosyncratic reactions and allergic reactions. An *idiosyncratic reaction* occurs when something unusual or abnormal happens when a drug is first administered. The patient usually shows an *over-response* to the action of the drug. This type of reaction is usually due to a patient's inability to metabolize a drug due to a genetic deficiency of certain enzymes. Fortunately, this type of reaction is fairly rare.

Allergic reactions, also known as hypersensitivity reactions, occur in about 6% to 10% of patients taking medications. Allergic reactions occur in patients who have previously been exposed to a drug and have developed antibodies from their immune systems to it. Upon reexposure, the antibodies cause a reaction, most commonly seen as raised, irregular shaped patches on the skin with severe itching, known as *urticaria* or *hives*. Occasionally, a patient will have a severe, life threatening reaction that causes respiratory distress and cardiovascular collapse, known as an *anaphylactic reaction*. This condition is a medical emergency and must be treated immediately. Fortunately, anaphylactic reactions occur much less frequently than the more mild urticarial reactions. If a patient has a mild reaction, it should be taken as a warning not to take the medication again. The patient is much more likely to have an anaphylactic reaction at the next exposure to the drug. Patients should receive information regarding the drug name and be told to tell health care professionals (i.e., nurses, physicians, pharmacists, and dentists) that they have had a reaction and must not receive the drug again. In addition, patients should wear an identification bracelet or necklace explaining the allergy.

Variable Factors Influencing Drug Action

Many times we have heard patients complain, saying "That drug really knocked me out!" or, "That drug didn't touch the pain!" In some patients the effects of drugs are unexpectedly potent while other patients show little response to the same dose. In addition, some patients will react differently to the same dose of a drug administered at different times. Due to individual patient variation, exact responses to drug therapy are extremely difficult to predict. Following are factors that have been identified as contributors to a variable response to drugs:

1. Age—Infants and the very elderly tend to be the most sensitive to the response of drugs, due to a reduced ability to metabolize and excrete drugs. The liver and kidneys of infants are not fully developed at birth, while elderly patients are more likely to have chronic illnesses that reduce liver and kidney function.
2. Body Weight—In general, considerably overweight patients will require an increase in dosage to attain the same therapeutic response. Conversely, patients that are underweight (compared with the general population) tend to require lower doses for the same therapeutic response. Most pediatric doses are calculated by milligrams of drug per kilogram of body weight to adjust for rate of growth.
3. Metabolic Rate—Patients with a higher metabolic rate tend to metabolize drugs more rapidly, thus requiring either larger doses or more frequent administration. The converse is true for those with lower metabolic rates.
4. Illness—Pathologic conditions may alter the rate of absorption, distribution, metabolism, and excretion. For example: patients in shock will have reduced peripheral vascular circulation and will absorb drugs injected intramuscularly or subcutaneously very slowly; vomiting patients may not be able to keep a medication in the stomach long enough for dissolution and absorption; diseases such as nephrotic syndrome or malnutrition may reduce the amount of serum proteins in the blood necessary for adequate distribution of drugs; patients with kidney failure must have significant reductions in the dosages of those medications that are excreted by the kidneys.
5. Psychological Aspects—Attitudes and expectations play a major role in a patient's response to therapy and the willingness to take the therapy as prescribed. Patients with diseases that have relatively rapid consequences for ignoring therapy (such as insulin-dependent diabetes), have a fairly good rate of compliance. Patients with "silent" illnesses, such as hypertension, tend to be much less compliant with the treatment regimen.

   Another psychological consideration is the "placebo effect." A *placebo* is a drug dosage form, such as a tablet or capsule, that has no pharmacological activity, since the dosage form has no active ingredients. When taken, the patient may report a therapeutic response. This response can be beneficial in patients being treated for such illnesses as anxiety, because the patient tends to take fewer, potentially habit forming, drugs.
6. Tolerance—*Tolerance* occurs when a person starts requiring higher dosages to produce the same effects that lower doses once provided. An example is the person who is addicted to heroin. After a few weeks of use, larger doses will be required to provide the same "high." Tolerance can be due to psychological dependence, or the body may metabolize a particular drug more rapidly than before, causing the effects of the drug to wear off more rapidly.
7. Dependence—*Drug dependence*, also known as "addiction" or "habituation," is the inability of a person to control the ingestion of drugs. The dependence may be physical, (in which the person develops withdrawal symptoms if the drug is withdrawn for a certain

period of time) or psychological (where the patient is emotionally attached to the drug). Drug dependence occurs most commonly with the use of schedule, or controlled, medications (see Drug Legislation) such as opiates and barbiturates.

8. Cumulative Effect—A drug may accumulate in the body if the next doses are administered before previously administered doses have been metabolized or excreted. Excessive accumulation of a drug may result in drug toxicity. An example of drug accumulation is the excessive ingestion of alcoholic beverages. A person becomes "drunk" or "inebriated" when the rate of consumption exceeds the rate of metabolism and excretion of the alcohol.

Drug Interactions

A *drug interaction* is said to occur when the action of one drug is altered by the action of another drug. Some drug interactions are beneficial, such as the use of caffeine, a central nervous system stimulant, with an antihistamine, a central nervous system depressant. The stimulatory effects of the caffeine counteract the drowsiness caused by the antihistamine without eliminating the antihistaminic effects.

The following terminology is used in describing drug interactions:

1. Additive Effect—Two drugs, with similar actions, are taken for a doubled effect.

EXAMPLE: propoxyphene + aspirin = added analgesic effect

2. Synergistic Effect—The combined effect of two drugs is greater than the sum of the effect of each drug given alone.

EXAMPLE: aspirin + codeine = much greater analgesic effect

3. Antagonistic Effect—One drug interferes with the action of another.

EXAMPLE: tetracycline + antacid = decreased absorption of the tetracycline

4. Displacement—The displacement of a drug by a second drug, increases the activity of the first drug.

EXAMPLE: warfarin + aspirin = increased anticoagulant effect

5. Interference—One drug inhibits the metabolism or excretion of a second drug, causing increased activity of the second drug.

EXAMPLE: probenecid + spectinomycin = prolonged antibacterial activity from spectinomycin due to blocking renal excretion by probenecid

6. Incompatibility—One drug is chemically incompatible with another drug (causing deterioration) when the two drugs are mixed in the same syringe or solution. Incompatible drugs should not be mixed together or administered at the same site together. Signs of incompatibility are haziness, a precipitate, or a change in color of the solution when drugs are mixed.

EXAMPLE: ampicillin + gentamicin = ampicillin inactivates gentimicin

Unit II

*Administration
of
Medications*

Chapter 3

A Review of Arithmetic

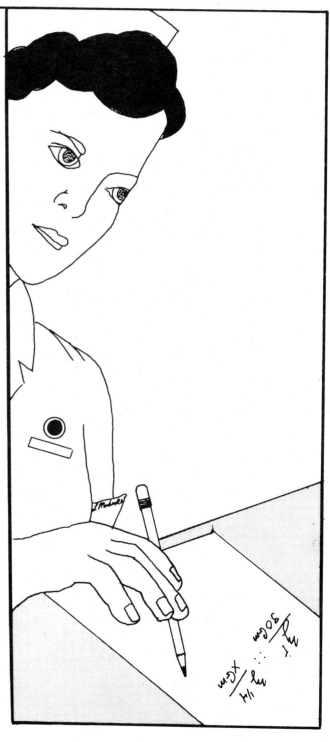

Although many hospitals are using the "unit dosage" system in dispensing drugs, it is still the nurse's responsibility to ascertain that the medication administered is exactly as prescribed by the physician. To give an accurate dosage, the nurse must have a working knowledge of basic mathematics. This review is offered so that individuals may determine areas in which improvement is needed.

Roman Numerals

Toward the end of the sixteenth century two systems of numbers emerged, Roman and Arabic. They are the basis for our communications in mathematics today, are used interchangeably, and are used by the physician in prescribing drugs. Roman numerals 1 through 100 are used frequently in medicine. Key symbols are

$$I = 1, V = 5, X = 10, L = 50,$$
$$C = 100, D = 500, M = 1000$$

Whenever a roman numeral is repeated, or when a smaller numeral follows, the numerals are added.

EXAMPLES

I = 1,	II = 2,	III = 3,	VI = 6,
(1+0=1)	(1+1=2)	(1+1+1=3)	(5+1=6)
VII = 7,	XI = 11,	XII = 12	
(5+1+1=7)	(10+1=11)	(10+1+1=12)	

Whenever a smaller Roman numeral appears before a larger Roman numeral, subtract the smaller numeral.

EXAMPLES

IV = 4,	IX = 9,	XC = 90
(5−1=4)	(10−1=9)	(100−10=90)

Whenever a smaller Roman numeral appears between two larger Roman numerals, subtract the smaller number from the numeral following it.

EXAMPLES

XIX = 19	XIV = 14	XCIX = 99
(10+10−1=19)	(10+5−1=14)	(100−10+10−1=99)

The most common Roman numerals associated with medication administration are ss = ½, i = 1, ii = 2, iii = 3, iv = 4, v = 5, vi = 6, vii = 7, viiss = 7½, viii = 8, ix = 9, x = 10, xv = 15.

Express the following in Roman numerals:

3 _____	20 _____	101 _____
9 _____	18 _____	499 _____
10 _____	49 _____	1979 _____

Express the following in Arabic numerals:

iv _____	xxxix _____	xix _____
vi _____	ix _____	xv _____

Fractions

Fractions are one or more of the separate parts of a substance, or less than a whole number or amount.

EXAMPLE: $1 - ½ = ½$

Common Fraction

A common fraction is part of a whole number. The numerator (dividend) is the number above the line. The denominator (divisor) is the number below the line. The line separating the numerator and denominator tells us to divide.

Numerator (Names how many parts are used)
_____
Denominator (Tabulates the pieces, or tells how many pieces the whole is divided into)

EXAMPLES

The denominator represents the number of parts or pieces the whole is divided into.

¼ means graphically that the whole circle is divided into four (4) parts; one (1) of the parts is being used.

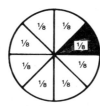

⅛ means graphically that the whole circle is divided into eight (8) parts; one (1) of the parts is being used.

From these two examples, ¼ and ⅛, you can see that the *larger* the *denominator* number, the *smaller* the *portion* is. (Each section in the ⅛ circle is smaller than each section in the ¼ circle.) This is an important concept to understand for persons who will calculate drug dosages. The drug ordered may be ¼ gr. and the drug source available on the shelf ½ gr. Before proceeding to do any formal calculations you should first decide if the dose you need to give is smaller or larger than the drug source available on the shelf.

EXAMPLES

Visualize:

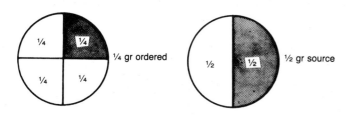

¼ gr ordered   ½ gr source

Decide: "Is what I need to administer to the patient a larger or smaller portion than the drug available on the shelf?"
Answer: ¼ is smaller; thus it would be less than one tablet.

Try a second example. ⅛ gr is ordered; the drug source on the shelf is ½ gr.

Visualize:

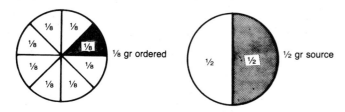

⅛ gr ordered   ½ gr source

Decide: "Is what I need to administer to the patient a larger or smaller portion than the drug available on the shelf?"
Answer: ⅛ is smaller than the drug source; thus it would be less than one tablet.

Types of Common Fractions

1. *Simple:* contains *one* numerator and *one* denominator: ¼, ¹⁄₂₀, ¹⁄₆₀, ¹⁄₁₀₀

2. *Complex:* may have a simple fraction in the numerator or denominator:

$$\frac{1}{2} \text{ over } 4 = \frac{\frac{1}{2}}{4}, \quad \frac{1}{2} \text{ over } \frac{1}{4} = \frac{\frac{1}{2}}{\frac{1}{4}}$$

3. *Proper:* numerator is smaller than denominator: ⅛, ⅖, ¹⁄₁₀₀
4. *Improper:* numerator is larger than denominator: 4/3, 6/4, ¹⁰⁰⁄₁₀
5. *Mixed number:* a whole number and a fraction: 4⅝, 6⅔, 1⁵⁄₁₀₀
6. *Decimal:* fractions written on the basis of a multiple of ten: 0.5 = ⁵⁄₁₀, 0.05 = ⁵⁄₁₀₀, 0.005 = ⁵⁄₁₀₀₀
7. *Equivalent:* fractions that have the same value: ⅓ and ²⁄₆

Working with Fractions

1. *Reducing to lowest terms.* Divide both the numerator and the denominator by a number that will divide into both evenly (a common denominator).

   EXAMPLE: $\dfrac{25}{125} \div \dfrac{25}{25} = \dfrac{1}{5}$

   Reduce the following:

   $$\frac{5}{100} \qquad \frac{3}{21} \qquad \frac{6}{36} \qquad \frac{12}{244} \qquad \frac{2}{4}$$

2. Finding the lowest common denominator of a series of fractions is not always easy. Here are some points to remember:
   If the numerator and denominator are both even numbers, 2 will work as a common denominator, but may not be the smallest one.
   If the numerator and denominator end with 0 or 5, 5 will work as a common denominator, but may not be the smallest one.
   Check to see if the numerator divides evenly into the denominator; this will be the smallest term.
   When all else fails, use the prime number method to find the lowest common denominator: A prime number is a whole number, greater than 1, that can be divided by itself and 1 only (2,3,5,7,11,19,23, etc.).

   Steps: (1) Write down all the denominators in a row, then proceed to divide each denominator by the lowest prime number, until you can no longer use that number, proceed to the next higher prime number and divide using it until it can no longer be used. Continue this procedure until all 1's are obtained. (2) Multiply all the prime numbers used to divide and you will have the lowest common denominator.

EXAMPLE

Fractions: $\frac{7}{16}$ $\frac{5}{9}$ $\frac{13}{30}$ $\frac{7}{22}$

Write down all denominators:

		16	9	30	22
Prime numbers:	2	8	9	15	11
	2	4	9	15	11
	2	2	9	15	11
	2	1	9	15	11
	3	1	3	5	11
	3	1	1	5	11
	5	1	1	1	11
	11	1	1	1	1

2 is smallest prime number. Keep dividing by this number until it no longer will divide into the denominators evenly. Proceed to next higher prime, reuse if possible. Go to next higher prime that will divide in evenly, continue until all 1's are obtained.

Lowest common denominator is

$$2 \times 2 \times 2 \times 2 \times 3 \times 3 \times 5 \times 11 = 7920$$

3. *Adding common fractions.* When denominators are the same figure, add the numerators.

EXAMPLE: $\frac{1}{4} + \frac{2}{4} + \frac{3}{4} = \frac{6}{4}$ $1\frac{1}{2}$

Add the following:

$$\frac{2}{6} + \frac{3}{6} + \frac{4}{6} = \frac{9}{6} = 1\frac{1}{2}$$

$$\frac{1}{100} + \frac{3}{100} + \frac{5}{100} = \frac{9}{100}$$

When the denominators are unlike, change the fractions to equivalent fractions by finding the lowest common denominator.

EXAMPLE: $\frac{2}{5} + \frac{3}{10} + \frac{1}{2} = 1\frac{1}{5}$

(use 10 as common denominator)

Divide 5 into 10 and multiply by 2 $= \dfrac{4}{10}$

Divide 10 into 10 and multiply by 3 $= \dfrac{3}{10}$

Divide 2 into 10 and multiply by 1 $= \dfrac{5}{10}$

Add $\dfrac{4}{10} + \dfrac{3}{10} + \dfrac{5}{10} = \dfrac{12}{10} = 1\frac{1}{5}$

Add the following:

$$\frac{2}{8} + \frac{4}{64} + \frac{5}{16} \qquad \frac{3}{7} + \frac{9}{14} + \frac{1}{28}$$

4. *Adding mixed numbers.* Add the fractions first; then add the whole numbers.

EXAMPLE: $2\frac{3}{4} + 2\frac{1}{2} + 3\frac{3}{8}$

a. Determine common denominator of fractions:

$$\frac{3}{4} = \frac{6}{8}, \qquad \frac{1}{2} = \frac{4}{8}, \qquad \frac{3}{8} = \frac{3}{8}$$

b. Add the fractions:

$$\frac{6}{8} + \frac{4}{8} + \frac{3}{8} = \frac{13}{8} = 1\frac{5}{8}$$

c. Add whole numbers:

$$2 + 2 + 3 = 7$$

d. Add b and c:

$$1\frac{5}{8} + 7 = 8\frac{5}{8} \text{ answer}$$

Add the following:

$$\frac{1}{4} + \frac{3}{4} \qquad \frac{1}{2} + \frac{1}{3} + \frac{1}{6} \qquad \frac{3}{5} + \frac{4}{50}$$

$$\frac{1}{3} + \frac{4}{9} + \frac{3}{19} \qquad \frac{1}{5} + \frac{14}{25} + \frac{11}{50}$$

$$3\frac{3}{10} + 4\frac{2}{5} + 5\frac{3}{15}$$

5. *Subtracting.* To find the least common denominator, subtract the smaller numerator from the larger. Reduce the remainder to its lowest terms.

EXAMPLE: $\dfrac{1}{4} - \dfrac{3}{16} = \dfrac{4}{16} - \dfrac{3}{16} = \dfrac{1}{16}$

6. *Subtracting mixed numbers.* When the numerator of the fraction in the top number is smaller than the

numerator of the bottom number, it is necessary to borrow from the whole number, in the top number.

EXAMPLE: $4\frac{1}{4} - 1\frac{3}{4}$ (Note: you cannot subtract ¾ from ¼)
$3\frac{5}{4} - 1\frac{3}{4} = 2\frac{2}{4} = 2\frac{1}{2}$ (reduced to lowest terms)

Subtract the following:

$$\frac{7}{8} - \frac{3}{6} \qquad \frac{6}{12} - \frac{2}{24} \qquad \frac{1}{3} - \frac{1}{4}$$

$$6\frac{7}{8} - 3\frac{1}{16} \qquad 12\frac{1}{9} - 5\frac{7}{36}$$

Decimals as Fractions

Now let us think of $1.00. The decimal point is after the "1," so this is read "one dollar." A decimal point in front of a number, in regard to the dollar, would make the amount less than a dollar. For example, 75 cents expressed as a fraction of a dollar would be $^{75}/_{100}$. Seventy-five cents expressed as a decimal part of a dollar would be $.75. Twenty-five cents expressed as a fraction of a dollar would be $^{25}/_{100}$. Expressed as a decimal part of a dollar, it would be $.25. (Decimal points will be discussed later in the chapter.)

The fraction $^{25}/_{100}$ is twenty-five hundredths of one hundred or, in this case, of the whole dollar. The fraction $^{75}/_{100}$ is seventy-five hundredths of the hundred, or dollar. Notice the spelling of hundredths. This indicates less than the whole amount and shows that it is different from hundred, or less than one hundred. Be careful to spell hundredths correctly. The same is true of "tenths," "thousandths," and "ten thousandths." They all indicate less than the whole amount.

Multiplication

Multiplying a Whole Number by a Fraction

1. Multiply the whole number by the numerator (top number).
2. Write the answer (product) over the denominator (bottom number).
3. Change the improper fraction to a mixed number.

EXAMPLE: $3 \times \frac{5}{8} = \frac{15}{8} = 1\frac{7}{8}$

Multiply the following:

$$2 \times \frac{3}{4} \qquad 15 \times \frac{3}{5} \qquad 9 \times \frac{3}{33} \qquad 4 \times \frac{9}{28} \qquad 6 \times \frac{5}{100}$$

Multiplying Two Fractions

1. Multiply the numerators (top numbers) together.
2. Multiple the denominators (bottom numbers) together.
3. Reduce your answer to its lowest terms.

EXAMPLES: $\frac{1}{4} \times \frac{2}{3} = \frac{2}{12}$ or reduced $\frac{1}{6}$

$\frac{5}{6} \times \frac{9}{10} = \frac{45}{60}$ or reduced $\frac{3}{4}$

Using Cancellation to Speed Your Work

1. Divide both the numerator and the denominator by the same number.
2. Then multiply both numerators and both denominators for the final answer.

EXAMPLE: $\frac{5}{6} \times \frac{9}{10}$

$$\frac{\overset{1}{\cancel{5}}}{\underset{2}{\cancel{6}}} \times \frac{\overset{3}{\cancel{9}}}{\underset{2}{\cancel{10}}} = \frac{3}{4}$$

Multiplying Mixed Numbers

To multiply mixed numbers change the mixed numbers to improper fractions.

EXAMPLES

$$\overset{+}{3\frac{1}{2}} \times \overset{+}{2\frac{1}{5}} = \frac{7}{2} \times \frac{11}{5} = \frac{77}{10} = 7\frac{7}{10}$$

$$16 \times \overset{+}{2\frac{1}{4}} = \frac{16}{1} \times \frac{9}{4} = \frac{144}{4} = 36$$

Multiply the following:

$$1\frac{2}{3} \times \frac{3}{6} \qquad 1\frac{7}{8} \times 1\frac{1}{4}$$

Multiplying Whole Numbers and Decimals

1. Count as many places in the answer, starting from

the right, as there are places in the decimal involved in the multiplication.
2. The multiplier is the bottom number with the × or multiplication sign before it.
3. The multiplicand is the top number.

EXAMPLES

$$\begin{array}{r} 500 \\ \times\ \ .02 \\ \hline 10.00(10) \end{array} \qquad \begin{array}{r} 1000 \\ \times\ \ .04 \\ \hline 40.00(40) \end{array} \qquad \begin{array}{r} 1000 \\ \times\ \ .009 \\ \hline 9.000(9) \end{array}$$

$$\begin{array}{r} 7.25 \\ \times\ \ 4 \\ \hline 29.00(29) \end{array} \qquad \begin{array}{r} 500 \\ \times\ \ .009 \\ \hline 4.500 \text{(or 5)} \end{array}$$

Rounding the Answer

Note in the last example that the first number after the decimal point in the answer is 5. Instead of the answer remaining 4.5 it becomes the next whole number, 5. This would be true if the answer were 4.5, 4.6, 4.7, 4.8, or 4.9. In each case the answer would become 5. If the answer were 4.1, 4.2, 4.3, or 4.4 the answer would remain 4.

When the first number after the decimal point is 5 or above, the answer becomes the next whole number. When the first number after the decimal point is less than 5, the answer becomes the whole number in the answer.

Multiply the following:

$$\begin{array}{r} 1,200 \\ \times\ \ .009 \end{array} \qquad \begin{array}{r} 575 \\ \times\ \ .02 \end{array} \qquad \begin{array}{r} 515 \\ \times\ \ .02 \end{array} \qquad \begin{array}{r} 510 \\ \times\ \ .04 \end{array}$$

Multiplying a Decimal by a Decimal

1. Multiply the problem as if the numbers were both whole numbers.
2. Count decimal places in the answer, starting from the right, as many decimal places as there are in both of the numbers that were to be multiplied.

EXAMPLE:
$$\begin{array}{r} 3.75 \\ \times\ \ .5 \\ \hline 1.875 = 2 \end{array}$$

There are two decimal places in 3.75 and one decimal place in .5, making three decimal places. Count three decimal places from the right. Round off the answer to 2.

Multiplying Numbers with Zero

EXAMPLES
1. Multiply 223 by 40.

a. Multiply 223 by 0. Write the answer, 0, in the unit column of the answer.
b. Then multiply 223 by 4. Write this answer in front of the 0 in the product.

$$\begin{array}{r} 223 \\ \times\ \ 40 \\ \hline 8920 \end{array}$$

2. Multiply 124 by 304.
a. First multiply 124 by 4. The answer is 496.
b. Now multiply 124 by 0. Write this answer, 0, under the 9 in 496.
c. Multiply 124 by 3. Write this answer in front of the 0 in the product.

$$\begin{array}{r} 124 \\ \times\ \ 304 \\ \hline 496 \\ 3720\ \ \\ \hline 37696 \end{array}$$

Division

Dividing Fractions

1. Change the division sign to a multiplication sign.
2. Invert the divisor (number by which you divide).
3. Multiply the numerators; multiply the denominators.

EXAMPLES

$$4 \div \frac{1}{2} = \frac{4}{1} \times \frac{2}{1} = \frac{8}{1} \text{ or } 8$$

$$\frac{1}{8} \div \frac{1}{4} = \frac{1}{8} \times \frac{4}{1} = \frac{4}{8} \text{ or } \frac{1}{2}$$

4. Reduce the fraction.

EXAMPLES

$$5\% = \frac{5}{100} = \frac{1}{20} \qquad 75\% = \frac{75}{100} = \frac{3}{4}$$

Change the following:

$$25\% = \frac{25}{100} = \qquad\qquad 2\% = \frac{2}{100} =$$

$$15\% = \frac{15}{100} = \qquad\qquad 12\tfrac{1}{2}\% = \frac{12.5}{100} =$$

$$10\% = \frac{10}{100} = \qquad\qquad \tfrac{1}{4}\% = \frac{\tfrac{1}{4}}{100} =$$

$$20\% = \frac{20}{100} = \qquad\qquad 150\% = \frac{150}{100} =$$

$$50\% = \frac{50}{100} = \qquad 4\% = \frac{4}{100} =$$

Changing Percents to Decimal Fractions

1. Omit the percent signs.
2. Insert a decimal point *two places to the left* of the last number, or express as hundredths, decimally.

EXAMPLES: 5% = .05   15% = .15

Change the following:

$$4\% = \qquad 25\% =$$
$$1\% = \qquad 50\% =$$
$$2\% = \qquad 10\% =$$

Note in these examples that those numbers that were already hundredths, such as 10%, 15%, 25%, 50%, merely need to have the decimal point placed in front of the first number, since they are already expressed in hundredths: where 1%, 2%, 4%, 5% needed to have a zero placed in front of the number to express them as hundredths.

Change these percents to decimal fractions:

$$12\tfrac{1}{2}\% = \qquad \tfrac{1}{4}\% =$$

If the percent is a mixed number, it should have the fraction expressed as a decimal. Then change the percent to a decimal by moving the decimal point two places to the left.

EXAMPLES

$$12\tfrac{1}{2}\% = 12.5\% \text{ or } .125$$
$$\tfrac{1}{4}\% = 0.25\% \text{ or } .0025$$

Changing Common Fractions to Percents

1. Divide the numerator by the denominator.
2. Multiply the quotient by 100 and add the percent sign.

EXAMPLE: $\dfrac{1}{50} = 50\overline{)1.00}^{\,.02} = .02 \times 100 = 2\%$

Divide the following:

$$2 \div \frac{3}{8} \qquad \frac{5}{8} \div \frac{7}{10} \qquad \frac{1}{8} \div \frac{1}{6}$$

If the divisor is a whole number, remember that the denominator of a whole number is always 1. Thus, a divisor of 4 becomes ¼ when inverted.

EXAMPLE: $\dfrac{1}{8} \div 4 = \dfrac{1}{8} \times \dfrac{1}{4} = \dfrac{1}{32}$

Divide the following:

$$3\frac{1}{8} \div 2\frac{1}{16}$$

Dividing with a Mixed Number

1. Change the mixed number to an improper fraction.
2. Change the division sign to a multiplication sign.
3. Invert the divisor.

EXAMPLES

$$4\frac{1}{2} \div \frac{3}{4} = \frac{9}{2} \div \frac{3}{4} = \frac{\overset{3}{\cancel{9}}}{\underset{1}{\cancel{2}}} \times \frac{\overset{2}{\cancel{4}}}{\underset{1}{\cancel{3}}} = \frac{6}{1} \text{ or } 6$$

$$6\frac{1}{4} \div 1\frac{1}{4} = \frac{25}{4} \div \frac{5}{4} = \frac{\overset{5}{\cancel{25}}}{\underset{1}{\cancel{4}}} \times \frac{\overset{1}{\cancel{4}}}{\underset{1}{\cancel{5}}} = \frac{5}{1} \text{ or } 5$$

Dividing Decimals

1. If the divisor (number by which you divide) is a decimal, make it a whole number by moving the decimal point to the right of the last figure.
2. Move the decimal point in the dividend (the number dividend) as many places to the right as you moved the decimal point in the divisor.
3. Place the decimal point for the quotient (answer) directly above the new decimal point of the dividend.

EXAMPLES

$$.25\overline{)\,.10\,} = 25\overline{)10.00}^{\,.40} \qquad .03\overline{)9.93\,} = 3\overline{)993}^{\,331}$$

$$.4\overline{)1.68\,} = 4\overline{)16.8}^{\,4.2}$$

Decimal Fractions

When fractions are written in decimal form, the denominators are not written. The word *decimal* means "10."

When reading decimals, the numbers to the left of the decimal point are whole numbers. It helps to think of them as whole dollars.

EXAMPLES

1.	=	one
11.	=	eleven
111.	=	one hundred eleven
1111.	=	one thousand one hundred eleven

Numbers to the right of the decimal point are read as follows:

EXAMPLES

Decimal(s):	Fraction(s):
.1 = one tenth	1/10
.01 = one hundredth	1/100
.465 = four hundred sixty-five thousandths	465/1000
.0007 = seven ten thousandths	7/10000

Here is another way to view reading decimals:

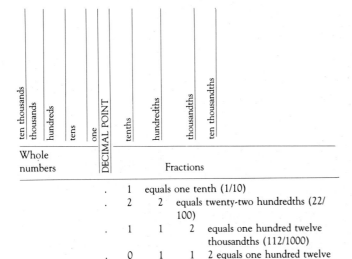

.	1			equals one tenth (1/10)
.	2	2		equals twenty-two hundredths (22/100)
.	1	1	2	equals one hundred twelve thousandths (112/1000)
.	0	1	1	2 equals one hundred twelve ten thousandths (112/10000)

1	.			equals number one
1	0	.		equals number ten
1	0	0	.	equals number one hundred
1	0	0	0	. equals number one thousand

On prescriptions another way of expressing the decimal is by using a slanted line.

EXAMPLES

1	mg	=	0.001 g	=	0/001 g
0.1	mg	=	0.0001 g	=	0/0001 g
30	mg	=	0.030 g	=	0/030 g
100	mg	=	0.100 g	=	0/100 g
1000	mg	=	1.000 g	=	1/0 g
250	mg	=	0.250 g	=	0/250 g

Changing Decimals to Common Fractions

1. Remove the decimal point.
2. Place the appropriate denominator under the number.
3. Reduce to lowest terms.

EXAMPLES

$$.2 = \frac{2}{10} = \frac{1}{5} \qquad .20 = \frac{20}{100} = \frac{1}{5}$$

Change the following:

.3 _____	.25 _____
.4 _____	.50 _____
.5 _____	.75 _____
.05 _____	.002 _____

Changing Common Fractions to Decimal Fractions

Divide the numerator of the fraction by the denominator.

EXAMPLE: $\frac{1}{4}$ means $1 \div 4$ or $4\overline{)1.00}$ with quotient $.25$

Change the following:

$\frac{1}{2}$ means _____	$\frac{3}{4}$ means _____
$\frac{1}{6}$ means _____	$\frac{1}{50}$ means _____
$\frac{2}{3}$ means _____	

Percents

Determining Percent One Number Is of Another

1. Divide the smaller number by the larger number.
2. Multiply the quotient by 100 and add the percent sign.

EXAMPLE: A certain 1000 parts solution is 10 parts drug. What percent of the solution is drug?

$$1000\overline{)10.00} = .01 \qquad .01 \times 100 = 1. \text{ or } 1\%$$

Changing Percents to Fractions

1. Omit the percent sign to form the numerator.

2. Use 100 for the denominator.
3. Reduce the fraction.

EXAMPLES: $5\% = \dfrac{5}{100} = \dfrac{1}{20}$ $75\% = \dfrac{75}{100} = \dfrac{3}{4}$

Change the following:

$25\% = \dfrac{25}{100} =$ $2\% = \dfrac{2}{100} =$

$15\% = \dfrac{15}{100} =$ $12\frac{1}{2}\% = \dfrac{12.5}{100} =$

$10\% = \dfrac{10}{100} =$ $\frac{1}{4}\% = \dfrac{\frac{1}{4}}{100} =$

$20\% = \dfrac{20}{100} =$ $150\% = \dfrac{150}{100} =$

$50\% = \dfrac{50}{100} =$ $4\% = \dfrac{4}{100} =$

Changing Percents to Decimal Fractions

1. Omit the percent signs.
2. Insert a decimal point *two places to the left* of the last number, or express as hundredths, decimally.

EXAMPLES: $5\% = .05$ $15\% = .15$

Change the following:

4% =	25% =
1% =	50% =
2% =	10% =

Note in these examples that those numbers that were already hundredths, such as 10%, 15%, 25%, 50%, merely need to have the decimal point placed in front of the first number, since they are already expressed in hundredths: where 1%, 2%, 4%, 5% needed to have a zero placed in front of the number to express them as hundredths.

Change these percents to decimal fractions:

$12\frac{1}{2}\% =$ $\frac{1}{4}\% =$

If the percent is a mixed number, it should have the fraction expressed as a decimal. Then change the percent to a decimal by moving the decimal point two places to the left.

$12\frac{1}{2}\% = 12.5\%$ or $.125$
$\frac{1}{4}\% = 0.25\%$ or $.0025$

Changing Common Fractions to Percents

1. Divide the numerator by the denominator.
2. Multiply the quotient by 100 and add the percent sign.

EXAMPLE: $\dfrac{1}{50} = 50\overline{)1.00}^{\,.02} = .02 \times 100 = 2\%$

Change the following:

$$\dfrac{1}{400} =$$

$$\dfrac{1}{8} =$$

Changing Decimal Fractions to Percents

1. Move the decimal point two places to the right.
2. Omit the decimal point if a whole number results.
3. Add the percent signs. (This is the same as multiplying the decimal fraction by 100 and adding the percent sign.)

EXAMPLE: $.01 = 1.00 = 1\%$ (or $\dfrac{1}{100}$)

Change the following:

.05	=
.25	=
.15	=
.125	=
.0025	=

Points to Remember in Reading Decimals

1. 1. is the whole number 1. When it is written 1.0 it is still one or 1.
2. The whole number is usually written like this: 1 or 2 or 3 or 4, and so on.
3. The whole number also can be written with the decimal point after the number: 1.0, 2.0, 3.0, 4.0.
4. Can you read this one? 0.1. This is one-tenth. There is one number after the decimal point.
5. Can you read this one? .1. This is also one-tenth. The zero in front of the decimal point does not change its value. One-tenth can be written, then, in two ways: 0.1 and .1.

6. Remember that in writing the number 1. or 1.0, the decimal point is after the number. This makes the number a whole number. It is read the whole number 1.

Ratios

A ratio expresses the relationship that one quantity bears to another.

EXAMPLES

1:5 means 1 part of a drug to 5 parts of a solution.
1:100 means 1 part of a drug to 100 parts of a solution.
1:500 means 1 part of a drug to 500 parts of a solution.

A common fraction can be expressed as a ratio.

EXAMPLE: $\frac{1}{5}$ is the same as 1:5.

The ratio of one amount to an amount expressed in terms of the same unit is the number of units in the first divided by the number of units in the second. The ratio of 2 ounces of a disinfectant to 10 ounces of water is 2 to 10 or 1 to 5 or $\frac{1}{5}$. This ratio may be written $\frac{1}{5}$ or 1:5.

The two numbers compared are called the terms of a ratio. The first term of a true ratio is always one, or 1. This is the simplest form of a ratio.

Changing Ratio to Percent

1. Make the first term of the ratio the numerator of the fraction whose denominator is the second term of the ratio.
2. Divide the numerator by the denominator.
3. Multiply by 100 and add the percent sign.

EXAMPLE: $5:1 = \frac{5}{1} \times 100 = 500\%$

Change the following:

$$1:5 \ =$$

Changing Percent to Ratio

1. Change the percent to a fraction and reduce the fraction to lowest terms.
2. The numerator of the fraction is the first term of the ratio, and the denominator is the second term of the ratio.

EXAMPLE: $\frac{1}{2}\% = \frac{\frac{1}{2}}{100} = \frac{1}{2} \div \frac{100}{1}$

$$= \frac{1}{2} \times \frac{1}{100} = \frac{1}{200} = 1:200$$

Change the following:

$$
\begin{aligned}
2\% &= \\
50\% &= \\
75\% &=
\end{aligned}
$$

Simplifying Ratios

Ratios can be simplified as ratios or as fractions.

EXAMPLE: $25:100 = 1:4$ or $\frac{25}{100} = \frac{1}{4}$

Simplify the following:

$$
\begin{aligned}
4:12 &= \\
5:10 &= \\
10:5 &= \\
75:100 &= \\
\frac{1}{4}:100 &= \\
15:20 &= \\
3:9 &=
\end{aligned}
$$

Proportions

A proportion shows how two *equal* ratios are related. This method is good because it is possible to prove that your answer is correct, and it is especially useful in solutions.

1. Three factors are known. The fourth *unknown* (what you are looking for) is represented by *x*.
2. The first and fourth terms of a proportion are called extremes. The second and third are the means. The product of the means equals the product of the extremes, or multiplying the first and fourth equals the second and third.

EXAMPLE

$$
\begin{array}{cccc}
& \text{multiply} & & \\
\text{extreme} & \text{mean} & \text{mean} & \text{extreme} \\
1 & \times \quad 2 & = \quad 2 & \times \quad 4 \\
& \text{multiply} & & \\
\text{extreme} & & \text{mean} &
\end{array}
$$

Proof: $1 \times 4 = 4$ and $2 \times 2 = 4$

If you did not know one number you could solve for it as follows:

EXAMPLE:
$$
\begin{aligned}
1:2 &= 2:x \\
1x &= 4 \\
x &= 4 \div 1 = 4 \\
x &= 4
\end{aligned}
$$

Proof: $1 \times 4 = 4$ and $2 \times 2 = 4$

Solve the following:

$$6:12 = 24:x$$

Systems of Weights and Measures

Three systems of measurement are used during the calculation, preparation and administration of drugs.

Household Measurements

Household measurements are the least accurate. However, they are often the way pharmacological agents are administered at home. It is this system of measurement the patient has grown up using and therefore understands the best. Household measurements include the use of drops, teaspoons, tablespoons, teacups, cups, glasses, pints, quarts, and gallons. The first three measurements, drops, teaspoons, and tablespoons would be used for medications, depending on the amount prescribed.

Common Household Equivalents

1 quart	=	4 cups
1 pint	=	2 cups
1 cup	=	8 ounces
1 teacup	=	6 ounces
1 tablespoon	=	3 teaspoons
1 teaspoon	=	approximately 60 drops

Apothecary Measurements

The apothecary system of measurement is an ancient system; the word *apothecary* means "pharmacist" or "druggist." Some physicians still order the drugs they want given using the apothecary system. However, the metric system is the preferred system of measurement.

Apothecary Weight. For weighing solids the units are, in increasing order of magnitude (smallest to largest), as follows:

grain (smallest)
scruple
dram
ounce
pound (largest)

The grain was originally derived from the average weight of a grain of wheat. The symbol for grain is "gr." The dram (originally, drachma or drachm) was a Greek silver coin. The symbol for dram is ʒ. The ounce, whose symbol is ℥, is ¹⁄₁₂ of a troy pound. The pound is of Roman origin and signifies a balance.

The symbol "lb" is the abbreviation for the Latin word *libra*, which means pound.

In apothecary weight, 12 ounces equal 1 pound (same weight as those of troy weight). In avoirdupois weight, 16 ounces equal 1 pound. Avoirdupois weight is used in weighing all articles *except* drugs, gold, silver, and precious stones.

20 grains (gr)	=	1 scruple
3 scruples or 60 grains	=	1 dram (ʒ)
		(1 dram = 4 ml or 4 cc)
8 drams or 480 grains	=	1 ounce (℥)
12 ounces	=	1 pound (lb)

Apothecary Volume. For measuring fluids the units are, from smallest to largest, as follows:

minim (smallest)
fluidram
fluidounce
pint
quart
gallon (largest)

The unit of fluid measure is a minim (see Fig. 3.1). This is approximately the quantity of water that would weigh a grain. The symbol for minim is ♏. The symbol "O" is the abbreviation for the Latin word *octarius*. It means an eighth of a gallon and is the same as a pint. The symbol "C" is taken from the latin word *congius*. It means a vessel or container that holds a gallon.

60 minims (♏)	=	1 fluidram (fʒ)
8 fluidrams or 480 minims	=	1 fluidounce (f℥)
16 fluidounces	=	1 pint (pt or O)
2 pints	=	1 quart (qt)
4 quarts	=	1 gallon (C)

It might be of aid to visualize a dram as approximately equal to one teaspoonful in household measure.

The minim (♏) is the approximate equivalent of the drop, but it is not identical to the drop. To help you realize that it is an approximate equivalent to the drop, note the following:

1. A minim of water is approximately equal to 1 drop.
2. A minim of an alcoholic solution, such as tincture of belladonna, equals 2 drops.
3. A minim of ether is about 3 drops.
4. A minim of a gummy substance is less than 1 drop.

Minims should always be measured when the doctor orders a drug in minims. A minim glass should be used for accuracy (see Fig. 3.1). When the doctor orders drops, they may be measured with a medicine dropper.

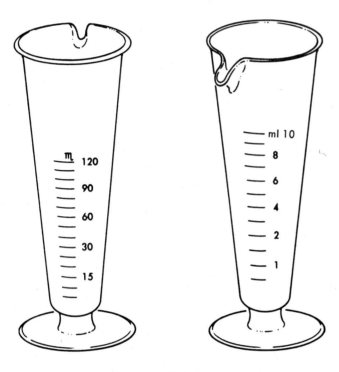

Fig. 3.1. *Fluid measures.*

The abbreviation for drops is "gtt," from the Latin *gutta*, meaning drops.

Symbols and Abbreviations

grains = gr
drams = ℨ
ounces = ℥
minims = ℳ
fluidram = fl ℨ
fluidounces = fl ℥
quart = qt

Dosages in the apothecary system are written in lower case Roman numerals after the unit of measurement.

EXAMPLE: gr ii means 2 grains, ℥ iii means 3 ounces.

On the other hand Arabic numbers are used to write quantities of less than one or mixed fractions.

EXAMPLES: 1/150 gr, 3½ gr

The symbol "ss" may be used for one-half: 1½ grains is written gr iss. The symbol "ss" comes from the Latin *seml, semisis,* meaning half.

EXAMPLE: gr viiss means grains 7½

Metric System

The metric system was invented by the French in the late eighteenth century. A committee of the Acad-emy of Sciences, working under government authority, recommended a standard unit of linear measure. For a basis of measurement they chose a fourth of the earth's circumference measured across the poles. One ten-millionth of this distance was accepted as the standard unit of linear measure.

The committee calculated the distance from the equator to the North Pole from surveys that had been made along the meridian that passes through Paris. The distance divided by 10,000,000 was chosen as the unit of length, or the meter.

Metric standards were adopted in France in 1799. The International Metric Convention met in Paris in 1875, and as a result of this meeting the International Bureau of Weights and Measures was formed. The first task of the International Bureau of Weights and Measures was the preparation of an international standard meter bar and an international standard kilogram weight. Duplicates of these were made for all countries participating in the convention.

A measurement line was selected on the international standard meter bar. The distance between the two lines of measurement on the bar is the official unit of the metric system. The standards given to the United States are preserved in the U.S. Bureau of Standards, Washington, D.C. There are 25 millimeters in 1 inch (2.5 centimeters).

The metric system uses the meter as the unit of length, the liter as the unit of volume, and the gram as the measurement of weight.

Units of Length (Meter)
1 millimeter = 0.001 meaning 1/1000
1 centimeter = 0.01 meaning 1/100
1 decimeter = 0.1 meaning 1/10
1 meter = 1 meter

Units of Volume (Liter)
1 milliliter = 0.001 meaning 1/1000
1 centiliter = 0.01 meaning 1/100
1 deciliter = 0.1 meaning 1/10
1 liter = 1 liter

Units of Weight (Gram)
1 microgram = 0.000001 meaning 1/1000000
1 milligram = 0.001 meaning 1/1000
1 centigram = 0.01 meaning 1/100
1 decigram = 0.1 meaning 1/10
1 gram = 1 gram

Other Prefixes. *Deca* means ten or 10 times as much. *Hecto* means one hundred or 100 times as much. *Kilo* means one thousand or 1000 times as much. These three prefixes can be combined with the words meter, gram, or liter.

EXAMPLES

$$1 \text{ decaliter} = 10 \text{ liters}$$
$$1 \text{ hectometer} = 100 \text{ meters}$$
$$1 \text{ kilogram} = 1000 \text{ grams}$$

Arabic numbers are used to write metric doses.

EXAMPLES: 500 milligrams, 5 grams, 15 milliliters.

Prefixes added to the units (meter, liter, or gram) indicate smaller or larger units. All units are derived by dividing or multiplying by 10, 100, or 1000.

Common Metric Equivalents
1 milliliter (ml)	=	1 cubic centimeter (cc)
1000 milliliters (ml)	=	1 liter (L) = 1000 cubic centimeters (cc)
1000 milligrams (mg)	=	1 gram (g)
1000 micrograms (mcg)	=	1 milligram (mg)
1,000,000 micrograms (mcg)	=	1 gram (g)
1000 grams (g)	=	1 kilogram (Kg)

Conversion of Metric and Apothecary Units (Table 3.1)

Converting Grams to Grains (Milliliters to Minims)
(1 g = 15 grains; 1 ml = 15 ♏)

Multiply the number of grains (or milliliters) by 15:

EXAMPLES

1. Change 30 grams to grains.
$$30 \times 15 = 450 \text{ gr}$$

2. Change 1 gram to grains.
$$1g \times 15gr/g = 15gr$$

Use ratio and proportion.

$$\frac{g}{1} : \frac{gr}{1} :: \frac{g}{15} : \frac{gr}{x}$$

$$x = 15$$
$$1 \text{ g} = \text{gr } 15$$

Converting Grains to Grams

Divide the number of grains by 15 (or multiply by 0.060). (1 gr = 0.060 g)

EXAMPLES

1. Change 30 grains to grams.
$$30 \div 15 = 2 \text{ g}$$

2. Change 5 grains to grams.

$$0.060 \text{ g/gr} \times 5 \text{ gr} = 0.3 \text{ g}$$

Converting Grams to Milligrams (1 g = 1000 mg)

Multiply by 1000 and move the decimal point of the grams three places to the right.

EXAMPLE: The physician orders the patient to have 0.250 g of a drug. The label on the bottle of medicine says 250 mg, meaning that each capsule contains 250 mg of the drug.
To change the gram dose into milligrams multiply 0.250 by 1000 and move the decimal point three places to the right (a milligram is one thousandth of a gram), 0.250 g = 250 mg, so you would give one tablet of this drug.

TRY THIS ONE: The physician orders the patient to have 0.1 g of a drug. The label on the bottle states the strength of the drug is 100 mg.
To change the gram dose into milligrams, move the decimal point three places to the right: 0.1 g = 100 mg, exactly what the bottle label strength states.

Convert the following grams (g) to milligrams (mg):

$$0.2 \text{ g} = \text{_____ mg}$$
$$.250 \text{ g} = \text{_____ mg}$$
$$.125 \text{ g} = \text{_____ mg}$$
$$.0006 \text{ g} = \text{_____ mg}$$
$$0.004 \text{ g} = \text{_____ mg}$$

Converting Milligrams to Grams (1000 mg = 1 g)

Divide by 1000 and move the decimal point of the milligrams three places to the left.

EXAMPLES: 200 mg = 0.2 g
0.6 mg = .0006 g

Convert the following milligrams to grams:

$$0.4 \text{ mg} = \text{_____ g}$$
$$0.12 \text{ mg} = \text{_____ g}$$
$$0.2 \text{ mg} = \text{_____ g}$$
$$0.1 \text{ mg} = \text{_____ g}$$
$$500 \text{ mg} = \text{_____ g}$$
$$125 \text{ mg} = \text{_____ g}$$
$$100 \text{ mg} = \text{_____ g}$$
$$200 \text{ mg} = \text{_____ g}$$
$$50 \text{ mg} = \text{_____ g}$$
$$400 \text{ mg} = \text{_____ g}$$

Can you take the gram dosages in these answers and convert them to milligrams?

Table 3.1
Metric Doses and Apothecary Equivalents

LIQUID MEASURE		WEIGHT	
METRIC	APPROXIMATE APOTHECARY EQUIVALENTS	METRIC	APPROXIMATE APOTHECARY EQUIVALENTS
1000 ml[b]	**1 quart**	**30 g**	**1 ounce**
750 ml	1½ pints	15 g	4 drams
500 ml	**1 pint**	100 g	2½ drams
250 ml	8 fluidounces	7.5 g	2 drams
200 ml	7 fluidounces	6 g	90 grains
100 ml	3½ fluidounces	5 g	75 grains
50 ml	1⅓ fluidounces	3 g	45 grains
30 ml	**1 fluidounce**	2 g	30 grains (½ dram)
15 ml	4 fluidrams	1.5 g	22 grains
10 ml	2½ fluidrams	**1 g**	**15 grains**
8 ml	2 fluidrams	0.75 g	12 grains
5 ml	1¼ fluidrams	0.6 g	10 grains
4 ml	1 fluidram	**0.5 g**	**7½ grains**
3 ml	45 minims	0.4 g	6 grains
2 ml	30 minims	0.3 g	5 grains
1 ml	**15 or 16 minims**	0.25 g	4 grains
0.75 ml	12 minims	0.2 g	3 grains
0.6 ml	10 minims	0.15 g	2½ grains
0.5 ml	8 minims	0.12 g	2 grains
0.3 ml	5 minims	0.1 g	1½ grains
0.25 ml	4 minims	75 mg	1¼ grains
0.2 ml	3 minims	**60 mg**	**1 grain**
0.1 ml	1½ minims	50 mg	¾ grain
0.06 ml	**1 minim**	40 mg	⅔ grain
0.05 ml	¾ minim	**30 mg**	**½ grain**
0.03 ml	½ minim	25 mg	⅜ grain
		20 mg	⅓ grain
		15 mg	**¼ grain**
		12 mg	⅕ grain
		10 mg	⅙ grain
		8 mg	⅛ grain
		6 mg	1/10 grain
		5 mg	1/12 grain
		4 mg	1/15 grain
		3 mg	1/20 grain
		2 mg	1/30 grain
		1.5 mg	1/40 grain
		1.2 mg	1/50 grain
		1 mg	**1/60 grain**
		0.8 mg	1/80 grain
		0.6 mg	**1/100 grain**
		0.5 mg	1/120 grain
		0.4 mg	**1/150 grain**
		0.3 mg	**1/200 grain**
		0.25 mg	1/250 grain
		0.2 mg	1/300 grain
		0.15 mg	1/400 grain
		0.12 mg	1/500 grain
		0.1 mg	1/600 grain

[a] From United States Pharmacopeia XX.
[b] A milliliter (ml) is approximately equivalent to a cubic centimeter (cc). Equivalents in bold type should be memorized.

Converting Ounces to Pints (16 oz = 1 pint)

Divide the number of ounces by 16

EXAMPLE: Convert 320 ounces to pints.

$$320 \div 16 = 20 \text{ pt}$$

Converting Pints to Quarts (2 pt = 1 quart)

Divide the number of pints by 2.

EXAMPLE: Convert 10 pints to quarts.

$$10 \div 2 = 5 \text{ qt}$$

Converting Quarts to Gallons (4 qt = 1 gallon)

Divide the number of quarts by 4.

EXAMPLE: Convert 4 quarts into gallons.

$$4 \div 4 = 1 \text{ G}$$

Solid Dosage for Oral Administration

If the dosage *on hand* and the dosage ordered are both in the same system, the problem is to give the patient the *correct* dosage ordered from what you have.

EXAMPLE: Physician orders patient to have 1.0 g of Gantrisin. The Gantrisin bottle states that each capsule in the bottle contains 0.5 g.
PROBLEM: You do not have the 1.0 g as ordered. How many capsules will you give?
SOLUTION: You may use two methods:

1. $\dfrac{\text{Dosage desired}}{\text{Dosage on hand}} = \dfrac{1.0 \text{ g}}{0.5 \text{ g}} = 2$ You will give two 0.5 g capsules to give the 1.0 g ordered.

2. $\dfrac{\text{g}}{0.5} : \dfrac{\text{Capsule}}{1} :: \dfrac{\text{g}}{1.0} : \dfrac{\text{Capsule}}{x}$ $\begin{aligned} 0.5x &= 1.0 \\ x &= 2 \end{aligned}$

Proof: $0.5 \times 2 = 1.0$
$1.0 \times 1 = 1.0$

EXAMPLE: Physician orders patient to have 1000 mg of ampicillin. You have on hand a bottle of tablets labeled 0.25 g per tablet (0.25 g = 250 mg).
SOLUTION:

1. $\dfrac{\text{Dosage desired}}{\text{Dosage on hand}} = \dfrac{1000 \text{ mg}}{250 \text{ mg}} = 4$ Give four 0.25 g tablets.

2. $\dfrac{\text{mg}}{250} : \dfrac{\text{tablet}}{1} :: \dfrac{\text{mg}}{1000} : \dfrac{\text{tablet}}{x}$ $\begin{aligned} 250x &= 1000 \\ x &= \dfrac{1000}{250} = \end{aligned}$

4 tablets

Proof: $250 \times 4 = 1000$
$1000 \times 1 = 1000$

Solve the following yourself using both rules (desired:on hand) and proportion:

1. Physician orders aspirin 600 mg. You have aspirin gr v per tablet.
2. Physician orders Gantrisin 0.25 g. You have Gantrisin 500 mg per tablet.
3. Physician orders pentobarbital 200 mg. You have pentobarbital 1½ gr capsules.

EXAMPLE: Physician orders 3 g. You have grains.
PROBLEM: How can you give 3 g from grains? To convert grams to grains, multiply the number of grams by 15.
SOLUTION: 3 g × 15 = 45 grains
or 15 : 1 :: x : 3 = gr 45

Prepare 45 grains to give the 3.0 g ordered. Solve the following:

$$
\begin{aligned}
6.0 \text{ g} &= \underline{\hspace{2cm}} \text{ gr} \\
500 \text{ mg} &= \underline{\hspace{2cm}} \text{ gr} \\
60 \text{ mg} &= \underline{\hspace{2cm}} \text{ gr} \\
.1 \text{ g} &= \underline{\hspace{2cm}} \text{ gr}
\end{aligned}
$$

EXAMPLE: Physician orders aspirin gr 45. You have aspirin in grams.
PROBLEM: How can you give aspirin gr 45 from the grams you have on hand? To convert grains to grams, divide the number of grains by 15.
SOLUTION: 45 ÷ 15 = 3 g in gr 45
or 0.06 : 1 :: x : 45 = 3 g

Prepare 3 g to give the gr 45. Solve the following:

$$
\begin{aligned}
\text{gr x} &= \underline{\hspace{2cm}} \text{ g} \\
\text{gr 3} &= \underline{\hspace{2cm}} \text{ mg} \\
\text{gr xv} &= \underline{\hspace{2cm}} \text{ g}
\end{aligned}
$$

Conversion Problems

Some students understand problems in tablet dosage for oral administration if presented with their fractional equivalents as follows:

1. Physician orders patient to receive 2 g of a drug in oral tablet form. The medicine bottle label states the strength on hand is 0.5 g. This means each tablet in the bottle is the strength 0.5 g.

How many tablets would be given to the patient?
1, 2, 3, 4, or 5? Answer: 4
What strength is ordered? 2 g
What strength is on the bottle label? 0.5 g
What is the fractional equivalent of 0.5 g? ½ g
How many ½ (0.5 g) tablets would equal 2 g?

$$2 \div \tfrac{1}{2} = \tfrac{2}{1} \times \tfrac{2}{1} = 4 \text{ tablets}$$

2. Physician orders patient to receive 0.2 mg of a drug in oral tablet form. The medicine bottle label states the strength on hand is 0.1 mg. This means each tablet in the bottle is the strength 0.1 mg.
How many tablets would be given to the patient?
1, 2, 3, or 4? Answer: 2
What strength is ordered? 0.2 mg
What is the fractional equivalent of 0.2 mg? ²⁄₁₀
What strength is on the bottle label (on hand)? 0.1 mg
What is the fractional equivalent of 0.1 mg? ¹⁄₁₀
How many ¹⁄₁₀ mg (0.1 mg) tablets would equal ²⁄₁₀ mg (0.2 mg)? 2

$$\begin{aligned} 0.1 \text{ mg} &= 1 \text{ tablet} \\ +\,0.1 \text{ mg} &= 1 \text{ tablet} \\ \hline 0.2 \text{ mg} &= 2 \text{ tablets} \end{aligned}$$

Dosage desired ÷ Dosage on hand =

or $\tfrac{2}{10} \div \tfrac{1}{10} = \tfrac{2}{10} \times \tfrac{10}{1} = 2 \text{ tablets}$

3. Physician orders patient to receive 0.5 mg of a drug in oral tablet form. The medicine bottle label states the strength on hand is 0.25 mg. This means each tablet in the bottle is the strength 0.25 mg.
How many tablets would be given to the patient?
1, 2, 3, 4, or 5? Answer: 2
What strength is ordered? 0.5 mg
What fractional equivalent equals 0.5 mg? ½ mg
What strength is on the bottle label? 0.25 mg
What fractional equivalent equals the strength on hand? ¼ mg
How many ¼ mg (0.25 mg) tablets would equal ½ mg (0.5 mg)? 2

$$\begin{aligned} 0.25 \text{ mg} &= \tfrac{1}{4} \text{ mg or } 1 \text{ tablet} \\ +\,0.25 \text{ mg} &= \tfrac{1}{4} \text{ mg or } 1 \text{ tablet} \\ \hline 0.50 \text{ mg} &= \tfrac{1}{2} \text{ mg or } 2 \text{ tablets} \end{aligned}$$

Dosage desired ÷ Dosage on hand =

or $\tfrac{1}{2} \div \tfrac{1}{4} = \tfrac{1}{2} \times \tfrac{4}{1} = 2 \text{ tablets}$

4. Physician orders patient to receive 0.25 mg of a drug in oral tablet form. The medicine bottle label states the strength on hand is 0.5 mg. This means that every tablet in the bottle is the strength 0.5 mg.
How many tablets would be given? ½, 1, 1½, 2, 2½, 3, 4, or 5? Answer: ½
What strength did the physician order? 0.25 mg
What is the fractional equivalent of the strength the physician ordered? ¼ mg
What strength is on the bottle label? 0.5 mg
What is the fractional equivalent of the strength on the bottle label (on hand)? ½ mg
Which is less: 0.5 mg (½ mg) or 0.25 mg (¼ mg)? 0.25 mg (¼ mg)
Was the amount ordered less than the strength on hand or more? Less

$$0.5 \text{ mg} = \tfrac{1}{2} \text{ mg or } 1 \text{ tablet}$$
$$0.25 \text{ mg} = \tfrac{1}{4} \text{ mg or half as much or } \tfrac{1}{2} \text{ tablet}$$

or $\tfrac{1}{4} \div \tfrac{1}{2} = \tfrac{1}{4} \times \tfrac{2}{1} - \tfrac{1}{2} \text{ tablet}$

If the medication is also available in 0.25 mg tablets, request that size from the pharmacy. A tablet should be divided only when scored; even then the practice should be avoided.

Liquid Dosage for Oral Administration

1. Physician orders 60 ml of a liquid medication. How many ounces will be given?

   To convert milliliters to ounces, divide milliliters by 30:

$$60 \text{ ml} \div 30 \ (30 \text{ ml} = 1 \text{ oz}) = 2 \text{ oz}$$

2. Physician orders 45 ml. How many ounces will be given?

$$45 \div 30 = 1\tfrac{1}{2} \text{ oz}$$

3. Physician orders 6 drams. How many milliliters (cubic centimeters) will you give?

   To convert drams to milliliters, multiply drams by 4:

$$4(4 \text{ ml} = 1 \text{ dram}) \times 6 = 24 \text{ ml (cc)}$$

Converting Weight to Kilograms (1 lb = 2.2 kg)

Many physicians request that the metric measure be used to record the body weight of the patient.

Since the scales used in many hospitals are still calibrated in pounds, the conversion from pounds to kilograms is required.

1. To convert weight in kilograms to pounds, multiply the kilogram weight by 2.2.

EXAMPLE: 25 kg × 2.2 lb = 55 lb

Convert the following:

$$35 \text{ kg} = \text{_____} \text{ lb}$$
$$16 \text{ kg} = \text{_____} \text{ lb}$$
$$65 \text{ kg} = \text{_____} \text{ lb}$$

2. To convert weight in pounds to kilograms, divide the weight in pounds by 2.2.

EXAMPLE: 140 lb ÷ 2.2 kg = 63.5 kg

Convert the following:

$$125 \text{ lb} = \text{_____} \text{ lb}$$
$$9 \text{ lb} = \text{_____} \text{ lb}$$
$$180 \text{ lb} = \text{_____} \text{ lb}$$

The weight of a liter of water at 40°C is 1 pound.

Fahrenheit and Centigrade (Celsius) Temperatures

It is necessary for the nurse to be familiar with both the centigrade and the Fahrenheit scale. Here are some of the main points about centigrade and Fahrenheit thermometers (Fig. 3.2).

1. Centigrade and Fahrenheit thermometers look alike.
2. Both are made of the same-sized tube containing mercury.
3. The column of mercury in each thermometer rises to the same height when placed in a beaker of freezing water and to the same height in boiling water.
4. The centigrade and Fahrenheit thermometers differ from each other in the way they are graduated.
5. On the centigrade thermometer the point at which water freezes is marked "0."
6. On the Fahrenheit thermometer the point at which water freezes is marked "32."
7. The boiling point in centigrade is 100°.
8. The boiling point in Fahrenheit is 212°.
9. The space between the 0° point and the 100° point on the centigrade scale is divided into equal spaces or degrees.

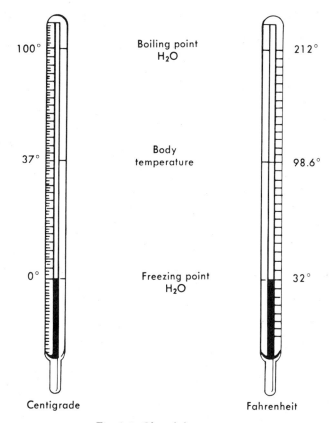

Fig. 3.2. *Clinical thermometers.*

10. The value of graduations (degrees) on the centigrade thermometer differs from the value of degrees on the Fahrenheit thermometer.
11. There are 180 spaces between the freezing and boiling points on the Fahrenheit thermometer.
12. In order to change readings on the centigrade thermometer to the Fahrenheit scale, the centigrade reading is multiplied by 180/100 or 9/5 and then added to 32.
13. To change Fahrenheit reading to centigrade scale, subtract 32 from the Fahrenheit reading and multiply by 5/9.

To understand why thermometer readings are interpreted in the way explained in point 12 and to understand your conversion formula better, read points 4 to 12 again several times.

Formula for Converting Fahrenheit Temperature to Centigrade Temperature

$$(\text{Fahrenheit} - 32) \times \frac{5}{9} = \text{centigrade}$$

$$(F - 32) \times \frac{5}{9} = C$$

EXAMPLE: Change 212°F to C.

$$(F - 32) \times \frac{5}{9} = C$$

$$212 - 32 = 180$$

$$180 \times \frac{5}{9} = \frac{900}{9} = 100°C$$

Convert the following Fahrenheit temperatures to centigrade:

$$98.6°F = \rule{2cm}{0.4pt} C$$
$$102.4°F = \rule{2cm}{0.4pt} C$$
$$95.2°F = \rule{2cm}{0.4pt} C$$

Formula for Converting Centigrade Temperature to Fahrenheit Temperature

$$(Centigrade \times \frac{9}{5}) + 32 = Fahrenheit$$

$$(C \times \frac{9}{5}) + 32 = F$$

EXAMPLE: Change 100°C to F.

$$(C \times \frac{9}{5}) + 32 = F$$

$$100 \times \frac{9}{5} = \frac{900}{5} = 180$$

$$180 + 32 = 212°F$$

Convert the following centigrade temperatures to Fahrenheit:

$$37°C = \rule{2cm}{0.4pt} F$$
$$35°C = \rule{2cm}{0.4pt} F$$
$$41°C = \rule{2cm}{0.4pt} F$$

Try these problems in converting centigrade to Fahrenheit and Fahrenheit to centigrade.

1. The nurse takes the following temperatures with Fahrenheit clinical thermometers: patient A, 104°F; patient B, 99°F; patient C, 101°F. The physician asks what the centigrade temperature is for each patient. Work your problems to convert Fahrenheit temperatures to centigrade. Check your answers. (Answers: patient A, 40°C; patient B, 37.2°C; and patient C, 38.3°C.)
2. The nurse takes the following temperatures with centigrade clinical thermometers: patient D, 37°C; patient E, 37.8°C; patient F, 38°C. The physician asks what the Fahrenheit temperature is for each patient. Work your problems to convert centigrade to Fahrenheit. Check your answers. (Answers: patient D, 98.6°F; patient E, 100°F; and patient F, 100.4°F.)

Many hospitals today have conversion tables available on the wards. This saves time and possibility of error in doing problems. The nurse simply refers to the particular temperature on one scale and finds the conversion listed in a column beside it. However, try to remember the formula for each conversion.

Most larger hospitals currently use electronic thermometers which give centigrade readings or Fahrenheit readings.

Chapter 4

Principles of Medication Administration

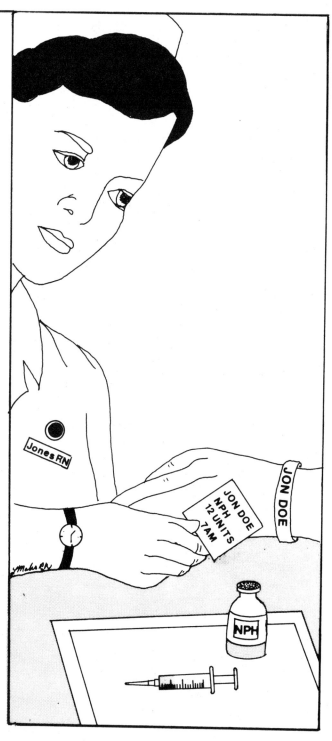

Objectives

After completing this chapter, the student should be able to do the following:

1. Cite legal and ethical considerations inherent in the administration of medications.
2. List the components of the patient's chart and give specific examples of the information found in each section.
3. Describe the advantages and disadvantages of various types of drug distribution systems.
4. Compare the types of commonly used drug orders to existing policies within the practice setting where functioning.
5. Identify the person who is ultimately responsible for the proper transcription of drug orders.
6. Use the nursing process to gather and analyze data in order to detect potential problems that may be encountered during the course of the patient's treatment.
7. Describe the nursing responsibilities associated with drug administration.
8. Apply the RIGHTS of drug administration within the practice setting.
9. Develop a teaching plan; implement and document actual teaching performed relative to drug therapy and monitoring of the therapeutic regimen.

Prior to the administration of medications, it is important that the nurse understands the professional responsibilities associated with medication administration, drug orders, medication delivery systems, and the nursing process as it relates to drug therapy. Lack of knowledge of the nurse's overall responsibilities in the system will, at a minimum, result in delays in receiving and administering medications, but may also result in serious administration errors. Either way, the patient loses, and may unnecessarily suffer.

Legal and Ethical Considerations

The practice of nursing under a professional license is a privilege, not a right. In accepting the privilege, the nurse must understand that this responsibility includes being held accountable for one's actions and judgments during the performance of professional duties. Understanding the Nurse Practice Act and the rules and regulations established by the state boards of nursing for the various levels of entry (i.e., practical nurse, registered nurse, and nurse practitioner) will provide a solid foundation for beginning practice.

In addition to a knowledge of state rules and regulations, nurses must be familiar with the established policies and procedures of the employing health care agency. These policies must adhere to the minimum standards of the state board of nursing, but agency policies may be more stringent than those recognized by the state. Employment within the agency implies the willingness of the professional to adhere to established standards and to work within established guidelines to make necessary changes in the standards. Examples of policy statements relating to medication administration include the following: (1) educational requirements of professionals authorized to administer medications (many health care facilities require that a written test be passed to attest to the necessary knowledge and skills of medication preparation, calculation, and administration prior to being granted approval to administer any medications); (2) approved lists of intravenous solutions and medications that the nurse can start or add to an existing infusion; (3) lists of restricted medications (e.g., antineoplastic agents, magnesium sulfate, allergy extracts, lidocaine,

RhoGAM, Imferon and heparin) that may be administered only by certain personnel.

Prior to the administration of any medication, the nurse must have (1) a current license to practice nursing, (2) a clear policy statement that authorizes the act, and (3) a medication order signed by a licensed physician or dentist. The nurse must understand the individual patient's diagnosis and presenting symptoms that correlate with the rationale for drug use. The nurse should also know why a medication is ordered, the expected actions, usual dosage, route of administration, minor side effects to expect, adverse effects to report, and contraindications of the use of a particular drug. If drugs are to be administered using the same syringe or at the same IV site, drug compatibility should be confirmed prior to administration. If unsure of any of these key medication points the nurse must consult an authoritative resource or the hospital pharmacist *prior* to the administration of a medication. The nurse must be accurate in the calculation, preparation and administration of medications. The nurse must assess the patient to be certain that both therapeutic and adverse effects associated with the medication regimen are reported. Nurses must be able to collect patient data at regularly scheduled intervals and record observations in the patient's chart for evaluation of the effectiveness of the treatment. Claiming unfamiliarity with any of these nursing responsibilities, when an avoidable complication arises, is unacceptable, and is considered negligence of nursing responsibility.

Nurses must take an active role in the education of the patient and family in preparation for discharge from the health care environment. (A person's health will improve only to the extent that the patient understands how to take care of himself or herself.) Specific teaching goals should be developed and implemented. Nursing observations and progress toward mastery of skills should be charted to verify the degree of understanding attained (see Health Teaching later in this chapter).

Patient Charts

The patient's chart is a major source of information that is necessary in patient assessment so that the nurse may make and implement plans for patient care. It is also the place for the nurse to provide a written record documenting nursing assessments performed, observations reported to the physician for further verification, basic nursing measures implemented (e.g., daily bath and treatments), patient teaching performed, and observed responses to therapy.

This document serves as the communications link among all members of the health care team regarding the patient's status, care provided, and progress. It is a legal document that describes the patient's health, lists diagnostic and therapeutic procedures initiated, and the patient's response to these measures. It must be kept current as long as the patient is in the hospital. After the patient's discharge, it is stored in the medical records department until needed again. While in medical records, the chart may be used for research to compare responses to selected therapy in a sampling of patients with similar diagnoses.

Contents of Patient Charts

Although each hospital uses a somewhat different format, the basic patient chart consists of the following:

1. *Summary Sheet*—This sheet identifies the patient by name, address, date of birth, name of attending physician, sex, marital status, allergies, nearest relative, occupation and employer, insurance carrier and other payment arrangements, religious preference, date and time of admission to the hospital, previous hospital admissions, and admitting problem or diagnosis. The date and time of discharge will be added when appropriate.
2. *Physician's Order Form*—The physician orders all procedures and treatments on this form (Fig. 4.1). These orders include general care (activity, diet, frequency of vital signs), laboratory tests to be completed, other diagnostic procedures (e.g., X-rays, ECG, CAT scans, etc.), and all medications and treatments (e.g., physical therapy, occupational therapy, etc.).
3. *Graphic Record*—This is a list of the vital signs, fluid intake and output, activity level, and other information used regularly for assessment of the patient's status (Fig. 4.2a,b).
4. *History and Physical Examination Form*—Upon admission to the hospital, the patient is interviewed by the physician and given a physical examination. The physician records the findings here and lists the problems to be corrected (the diagnoses).
5. *Progress Notes*—The physician uses this sheet to record frequent observations of the patient's health status. In some hospitals, other health professionals,

such as pharmacists, dieticians, and physical therapists, may record observations and suggestions.
6. *Nurses' Notes* (Fig. 4.3)—Here nurses record ongoing assessments of the patient's condition, responses to nursing interventions ordered by the physician (e.g., treatments or medications) or those initiated by the nurse (skin care or patient education); evaluations of the effectiveness of nursing interventions; procedures completed by other health professionals (e.g., wound cleaning by a physician or fitting for a prosthesis by a fitter); other pertinent information such as physician or family visits and the patient's responses after these visits. Entries may be made on the nurses' notes throughout a shift, but general guidelines include the following: (1) completing records immediately after making contacts with, and assessments of, the patient (i.e., when first admitted or returning from a diagnostic procedure or therapy); (2) recording all p.r.n. medications immediately after administration, and the effectiveness of the medication; (3) recording immediately before leaving the patient for extended periods of times, such as lunch or coffee breaks. The nurse should report significant changes in a patient's status or assessments to the charge nurse, in addition to accurately charting the observations in a clear, concise form. The charge nurse will then make a nursing judgment regarding notification of the attending physician.
7. *Laboratory Tests Record*—All laboratory test results are kept together in one section of the chart. Hospitals using computerized reports may list consecutive values of the same test once that test has been repeated several times (such as the electrolytes). Other hospitals may attach small report forms to a full sized backing sheet as each report returns from the laboratory.
8. *Consultation Reports*—When other physicians (or other health professionals) are asked to consult on a patient, the specialist's summary of findings, diagnoses, and recommendations for treatment are recorded in this section.
9. *Other Diagnostic Reports*—Reports of surgery, EEG, ECG, pulmonary function tests, radioactive scans, and X-ray reports are usually recorded in this section.

Additional forms included in a patient's chart depend upon the therapy prescribed. These may include separate medication administration reports; health teaching records; operative and anesthesiology records; recovery room records; physical, occupational, or speech therapy records; inhalation therapy reports; or a diabetic's daily record of insulin dosage, urine, and blood sugar tests. Each page placed in the patient's chart will be imprinted

508-52-1917
Joseph Lorenzo
18 Bush Ave.
Glen Cove, NY
Dr. M. Wells
Unit-6W

DOCTOR'S ORDER SHEET

DATE	TIME	PROB. NO.	ORDERS	DOCTOR	NOTED BY	TIME	CODE NO.
3/18/82	3 PM	6	ERYTHROMYCIN 250 mg p.o. q.6hr.	M. Wells	So		

5 25345-0

Fig. 4.1. *The physician's order form. (From Hahn, A. B., et al.: Pharmacology in Nursing, ed. 15, St. Louis, 1982, The C. V. Mosby Co.)*

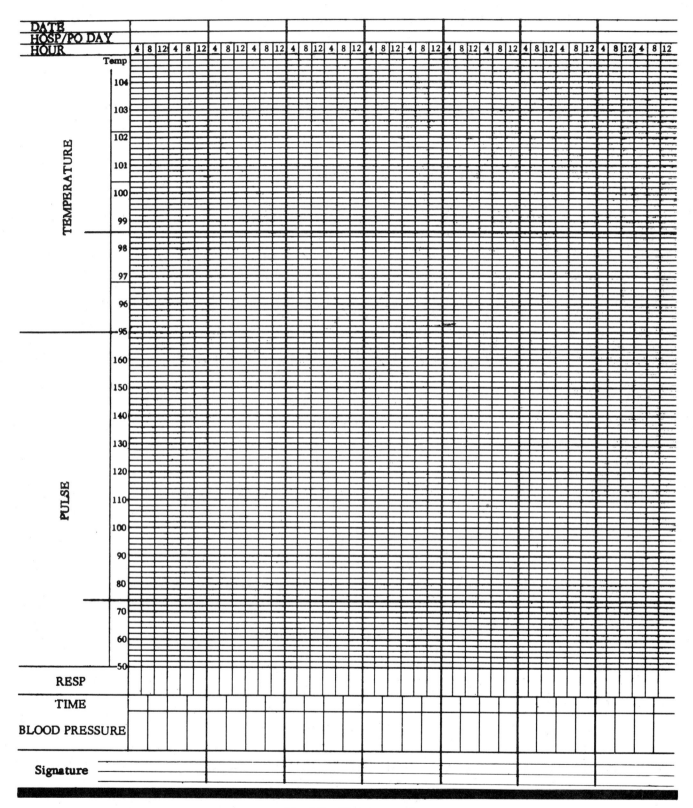

Fig. 4.2a. *Vital sign record.*

DATE							
HT-WT							
HYGIENE:							
Bedbath							
Partial							
Self							
Shower/tub							
Oral							
H.S.							
ACTIVITY:							
Bedrest							
BRP							
BRcBRP							
Dangle							
Chair/W.C.							
Amb							
Other							
Rails	7-3-11	7-3-11	7-3-11	7-3-11	7-3-11	7-3-11	7-3-11
DIET:	8-12-5	8-12-5	8-12-5	8-12-5	8-12-5	8-12-5	8-12-5
NPO							
Liquid							
Soft							
Regular							
Spec.							
HOLD							
OTHER:							

Intake	11-7	7-3	3-11	11-7	7-3	3-11	11-7	7-3	3-11	11-7	7-3	3-11	11-7	7-3	3-11	11-7	7-3	3-11	11-7	7-3	3-11
Oral																					
I.V. or Subq.																					
Blood																					
Other																					
Total 24 Hr. (cc.)																					
Output Urine																					
Total 24 Hr. (cc.) Urine																					
Emesis																					
Other																					
Total 24 Hr. (cc.)																					
Stool																					
Signature																					

Fig. 4.2b. *Patient care record.*

with the patient's name, registration number, and unit or room number. Nurses often use data from all of these sections to formulate a plan of nursing care.

Kardex Records

The Kardex (Fig. 4.4) is a large index-type card usually kept in a flip-file that contains pertinent information such as the patient's name, diagnosis, allergies, schedules of current medications with stop dates, treatments, and the nursing care plan. Since all ordered medications are listed in the Kardex, the nurse can assemble the medication cards (Fig. 4.5) for all assigned patients and verify each medication card against the Kardex. When the unit dose system is used, all medications are still listed on the Kardex or the medication profile, but individual medication cards are not necessary. Although used primarily by nurses, the intent of the Kardex is to make patient data quickly accessible to all members of the health team. The Kardex is often completed in pencil and updated by erasures. Since it is not a legal document, it is destroyed when the patient is discharged from the institution.

Drug Distribution Systems

Prior to the administration of medications, it is important that the nurse understand the overall medication delivery system used at the employing health care agency. Although no two drug distribution systems function exactly alike, three general types are currently being used:

1. The Floor or Ward Stock System—In this system, all but the most dangerous or rarely used medications are stocked at the nursing station in stock containers. This system has been used most often in very small hospitals, and in those where there are no charges directly to the patient for medications, such as in some government hospitals. Some advantages which may exist with the complete floor stock system are (1) ready availability of most drugs, (2) fewer inpatient prescription orders, (3) minimal return of medications. The disadvantages of this type of system are (1) the increased potential for medication errors because of the large array of stock medications to choose from and the lack of review by the pharmacist of each individual patient's medication order; (2) the increased danger of unnoticed drug deterioration, jeopardizing patient safety; (3) economic loss caused by misplaced or forgotten charges and misappropriation of medication by hospital personnel; (4) increased amounts of expired drugs to be discarded; (5) the need for larger stocks and frequent total drug inventories; and (6) storage problems on the nursing units in many hospitals.

2. The Individual Prescription Order System—In this system, medications are dispensed from the pharmacy upon receipt of a prescription or a drug order for an individual patient. The pharmacist usually sends a 3- to 5-day supply of medication in a bottle labeled for a specific patient. Medications, once received at the nurses' station, are placed in the medication cabinet in accordance with institutional practices. Generally, the medication containers are arranged alphabetically by the patient's name; or they may be arranged numerically by the patient's room or bed number.

Time	Output	MEDS/TX/VS	

Fig. 4.3. *Format of nurses' notes.*

JENNIE EDMUNDSON HOSPITAL

PATIENT ASSESSMENT/CARE PLAN

ALLERGIES *Penicillin*

REACTION *Hives on Trunk*   ALLERGY BAND APPLIED ☑

IN EMERGENCY CALL *Mary Doe (wife)* (Home) *323-6421*
     (Name)   (Relationship)   (Phone)
John Jr. (son) (Home) *323-0644*
     (Name)   (Relationship)   (Phone)
     (work) *536-1282*

IV THERAPY *6/1 Heparin lock*
Rotate site 6/4 6/7 6/10 M.D.

CONSULTS/REFERRALS *Dr Krammer — cardiology*

O₂ THERAPY/IPPB *6/1 O₂ 2L N.C. Continuously*
6/5 O₂ PRN Chest pain 2L/N.C.

PHYSICAL THERAPY _____

SUPPORT SERVICES _____

TREATMENTS-OTHER _____

_____

_____

CURRENT MEDS BEING TAKEN *Lanoxin 0.125 mgm qd. Tenormin 50 mgm qd. Procardia 20 mgm qid, Transderm Nitro 5 - patch qid Persantine 25 mgm tid, N+G 1/150 gr PRN chest pain Tylenol gr X PRN headache, minor discomforts*

OPERATIVE PROCEDURE *6/5/84 Cardiac catheterization*
Outcome: 2 Grafts blocked - severe coronary artery disease

DIAGNOSIS *Angina CHF*
Hist MI 7/76 hypertension

05-8/83

Physical Care: Bath *6/1 N.O.*
at bedside c̄ Assistance if pain free

Diet: *6/1 2 gm Na; low cholesterol diet*

Fluid: *As desires. Not to exceed 3000 cc/24 hr*

Help Needed: *N/A*

Miscellaneous: *M.P. basic Rhythm 6/1 S. tachy 120-130*

Daily Lab/Specimens:

Activity/Limitations/Safety
6/1 Bedrest c̄ BRP c̄ pain
Up as desires when pain free. Begin 6/2/84

Elimination: *N.O. Note bowel activity daily. Allow to stand to void.*

Not to SMOKE IN HOSP. D.O.
Smoker *✓ 1/2 pk/day* Dentures *upper only*

Non Smoker _____ Eye Glasses *✓*

Hearing Aid _____ Other *② #4 Telemetry*

I & O *✓*

B.P. *T 40*

T-P-R *q 4°*
(N.O. Apical & Radial pulse q 4 hr)

Weight: *D.O. Daily at brkfst.*

PATIENT CLASSIFICATION
KEY — 0-13 = I   14-18 = II   19 + = III

AMBUL	MEALS	BATH	Pr/Po OP	TRTMTS	TOT
1②3	①23	1②3	2	3·1	PTS = **14**
BTH RM	MEDS	T&ES	UNCONS	AGE	PT
②34	①②2	1 or②	5	2 1	CAT = **2**
					use pencil ONLY

PSYCHIATRIC PATIENT CLASSIFICATION
KEY — 0-15 = I   16-20 = II   21 = III CONSTANT CARE

AMBUL	BATHR'M	TRTMNTS	BEHAVR	TOT PTS
1 2 3	1 2 3 4	· 1		
MEALS	MEDS	PR/PO-OP	5 3 1	
1 2 3	1 or 2	2	PHYS ACT	PAT CAT
BATHE	AGE	MENT ATT	5 3 1	5 3 1
1 2 3	· 1	5 3 1		

ADM DATE *6/1/84*

CHURCH/PARISH *St. Lukes*
RELIGION *Catholic*

90-540

NAME *Doe, Johns*   HOSP.# *43641*   AGE *58*   PHYSICIAN *Fitzgerald*   ROOM NO. *425*

Fig. 4.4. *An example of a Kardex (above and facing).*

This system provides (1) greater patient safety due to the review of prescription orders by both the pharmacist and the nurse prior to administration, (2) less danger of drug deterioration and easier inventory control, (3) smaller total inventories, (4) reduced revenue loss due to improved charging systems and less pilferage. While the dispensing of medication to individual patients is better than the floor stock system, the major disadvantages of this system are the very unwieldy procedures used to schedule, prepare, administer, control, and record the drug distribution and administration process that consume nursing personnel's time.

3. The Unit Dose System—Unit dose drug distribution systems use single unit packages of drugs, dispensed to fill each dosage requirement as it is ordered. Each package is labeled with generic and brand name, manufacturer, lot number, and expiration date. When dispensed by the pharmacy, the individual packages are placed in drawers assigned to individual patients. The drawers are kept in a large "unit dose cabinet" (Fig. 4.6) that is kept at the nurses' station. Under most unit dose systems, the drawers are refilled by the pharmacist every 24 hours. The system was developed in the 1960s to overcome problems with inefficient use of nursing personnel, underutilization of pharmacists, excessively high rates of medication errors, poor drug control, waste of medications, and large inventories. The unit dose system is the safest and most economical method of drug distribution in hospitals today. Advantages of the system include the following: (1) The time normally spent by nursing personnel in preparation of drugs for administration is drastically reduced. (2) The pharmacist has a profile of all medications of each patient, and is therefore able to analyze the prescribed medications for drug interactions or contraindications. This method increases the pharmacist's involvement and better utilizes his or her extensive drug knowledge. (3) No dosage calculations are necessary due to unit-of-use packaging, thus reducing errors. (4) The patient may double check drugs and dosages since each dose is individually packaged and labeled. (5) There is less waste and misappropriation since single units are dispensed. (6) Credit is given to the patient for unused medications, since each dose is individually packaged.

JENNIE EDMUNDSON HOSPITAL — PATIENT ASSESSMENT

	SHORT TERM GOALS	TEACHING/DISCHARGE PLAN LONG TERM GOALS
6/1	1. Achieve normal respiratory status	6/1 1. Include spouse č patient with
6/1	2. Alleviate chest discomforts	cardiac instructions related to
6/3	3. Verbalizations of fears	review of risk factors, CAD process,
		diet restrictions, medication action, dose,
		major side effects, home activity levels
		2. Achieve Maximal activity level allowed

COMPLETED BY **Nancy Smith, R.N.** R.N.
DATE 6/1/84
Time 10:10
(Use pen to complete)

A. Reason for Admission
States "Chest pressure in middle of chest that goes into my jaw č weakness. Chest pain since 11:30 last N.O.C. č little relief č N.T.G.

B. Other Pertinent Conditions
Anterior wall MI 7/76
Hypertension treated since 7/72

C. Hospitalized previously - reason
Appendectomy Age 18
MI 7/76 JEMH
CABG x3 7/76 Bishop Clarkson-Omaha
Angina 2/80 1/84 č present JEMH

D. Mental Status (Level of Consciousness) Fully alert
Orientated x3. Appropriate. Seems preoccupied. States "worried about being able to return to work."
Behavior Anxious about health status

E. Head/neck (ears, nose, eyes, speech)
No recent colds or infections. States "hay fever every spring." Takes no medication for hay fever. Speech clear. Wears glasses during working day.

F. Respiratory (rate, effort, lung sounds, cough, general color)
Rate 26 seems S.O.B. O₂ 2L N.C.
Bilateral basilar rales → fine. States "started coughing late last p.m." Bring up little clear sputum.
Color: Pale
Smoker: ½ pkg/day States "I know I need to stop smoking"

G. Cardiac (Apical rate, rhythm, peripheral pulses, chest pain, presence of edema)
Apical/Radial 128/128. Reg Rhythm. Clear to S₁ & S₂ č soft S₃. Tele: sinus tachy č rare PVC (128-130). Radials strong symmetrically. Pedals faint but symmetrical. Feet cool. Otherwise, skin warm & dry. No peripheral edema. Continues č moderate amount of sternal heaviness radiating into jaw.

H. Gastrointestinal (diet, appetite, bowel activity, tone of abdomen, bowel sounds) Low salt č good appetite. abd. flat. Soft and active bowel sounds. Bowels normal. Move daily.

I. Genitourinary (LMP-female patients, urinary problems) Denies burning or urgency. At times, has difficulty starting stream, yet empties adequately.

J. Extremities (limitations, contractures, skin condition, turgor) Activity limited č chest pain. Well healed surgical scar of sternum č inner aspects of both thighs. No rashes, bruises or abrasions. Turgor Normal.

K. Personal Habits, preferences (bathing, oral hygiene, sleep) Prefers showers. Leaves upper dentures in at Noc. Sleeps 5-7 hr @ Noc Occasionally naps 1-1½ hr @ supper.

L. Psychosocial history (occupation, attitude, behavior, home environment, hobbies, religion) Career Change č CABG-1976 from police work to high school teacher. Enjoys yard & garden work č wife. No children at home. 3 Grandchildren living in Omaha C.B. area. Active church member.
Lives with wife on 4 acres near C. Blfs. Iowa.

Date	Nursing Diagnosis	Nursing Orders	Ini.
6/1 6/3 Renewed	1. Alterations in Comfort Chest pain related to temporary ischemia to myocardial tissue	Bedrest for duration of chest pain č at least 30 min thereafter. O₂ as ordered. Administer N&G as ordered. Provide quiet, restful environment. Note precipitating factors prior to anginal episodes. Note characteristics of chest pain, Location, type, radiation, duration V.S. q 15 min until chest pain resolved. Note skin temperature, color	NS RN
6/1 6/3 Renewed	2. Impaired Respiratory Status related to lung congestion	Head of bed elevated if dyspneic. Administer O₂ as ordered. Note color. Auscultate lungs q 8°. Note presence of rales, cough, frequency and type of sputum. Discourage smoking.	NS RN
6/1 6/3 Renewed	3. Potential for impairment of tissue perfusion related to decreased cardiac output due to heart rate	Apical/radial pulses as ordered. Provide quiet, restful environment. Eliminate cardiac stimulants in diet. ie. caffeine, ice, alcohol, etc. č instruct in same. I&O every 8 hr. Daily at brkfst weight. Attentiveness to fluid restrictions	NS RN
6/7 6/10 6/12	4. Fear of loss of employment related to unfavorable medical diagnosis for self	Approach unhurriedly. Provide atmosphere of encouragement and acceptance. Encourage expression of feelings. Listen attentively & offer feedback to patient's expressed feelings. Explore č patient his strengths & resources. Include spouse if appropriate. Investigate other resources - priest, social worker etc.	NS RN
6/8 6/9	5. Unknowledgeable about hypertension as it relates to medical diagnosis of self (CAD)	Discourage smoking. State reasons. Encourage activity level prescribed be maintained on daily basis & increased as ordered. Encourage adequate rest. Discourage strenuous activity. Dietician to see regarding dietary restrictions. Encourage pt. to ask questions. Teach spouse to take B/P. Teach medications - how & when to use. Explain causes of health problems	NS RN
6/11 6/12	6. Unknowledgeable as to types of activities regarded as safe as relates to medical diagnosis of self (CAD)	Provide list of guidelines for home recovery to include when resumption of activities may occur. e.g., driving, stairs, sexual activity, return to work. Explain aerobic conditioning activity versus isotonic - straining activity - the latter to be avoided. Teach how to take pulse and set normal limits to achieve during exercise. Clearly define exercises. Demonstrate č return demonstration by patient. Demonstrate relaxation/breathing techniques č encourage compliance daily. Reinforce No smoking, giving causes as related to health problems. Encourage post discharge follow-up č physician.	NS RN
6/13	Alterations in health maintenance as relates to medical diagnosis Discharged to home	Home instructions reviewed.	NS RN

Initials and Signature: Nancy Smith RN

NAME **Doe, John**   HOSP.# **43641**   AGE **58**   PHYSICIAN **Fitzgerald**   ROOM NO. **425**

(Under the individual prescription order system, returned bottles of unused medications were destroyed due to fear of contamination.)

An argument occasionally used by nurses against the unit or "single dose" system is that medications are prepared by someone else for the nurse to administer. Nurses have been taught: "Never administer anything you haven't prepared yourself." In principle, this is certainly true. A nurse should not administer any drug mixed and left unlabeled by another individual. However, for years nurses have administered medications that have been prepared and labeled by the pharmacist. The unit dose medication is prepared under rigid controls, and is dispensed only after quality control procedures have been completed by pharmacists. Nurses should always continue to check medications prior to administration. If there is a discrepancy between the Kardex and the medication in the cart, the pharmacist and the original physician's order should be consulted.

At the time of administration, the nurse should check all aspects of the medication order as stated on the medication profile against the medication container removed from the patient's drawer for administration. The number of doses remaining in the drawer for the shift should also be checked. If the number of remaining doses is incorrect, check the medication order prior to continuing with the drug administration. Always consider the possibility that the drug has been discontinued, that someone else has given the dose, or that someone has omitted or given the wrong patient the wrong medication. In the event that an error has been made, report it in accordance with hospital policies.

Narcotic Control Systems

As described in Chapter 1, laws regulating the use of controlled substances have been enacted and are rigidly enforced. Within hospitals, it is a standard policy that controlled substances are issued in single unit packages and are kept in a separate, locked cabinet on each nursing unit. The key to the cabinet is controlled by the head nurse or a designee. When controlled substances are issued to a nursing unit, they are accompanied by an inventory sheet (Fig. 4.7) listing each type of controlled substance being supplied. This record is used to account for the disposition of each type of medication issued. At the time the controlled substance supply is dispensed to the nursing unit by the pharmacist, the nurse receiving the drug supply is responsible for counting and verifying the number and types of controlled substances received. The nurse then signs a record attesting to the accuracy and receipt

of the controlled substances, and locks them in the controlled substances (narcotic) cabinet.

When a controlled substance is ordered for a particular patient, the nurse caring for the patient requests the key to the cabinet to obtain and prepare the medication for administration. At the time of removal from the cabinet, the inventory control record (Fig. 4.7) must be completed indicating time, patient's name, drug, dose, and the signature of the nurse responsible for checking out the controlled substance. If a portion of the medication is to be discarded due to a smaller prescribed dosage, two nurses must check the dosage, preparation, and the portion discarded. Both nurses must then co-sign the inventory control record to verify the transaction. The key is returned to the charge nurse after the dose is obtained and the paperwork is completed.

Prior to the administration of any controlled substance, the patient's chart should be checked to verify that the time interval since the last use of the drug has elapsed, as specified in the physician's orders. (See Chapter 8 for details of monitoring pain and the use of analgesics.) Immediately after the administration of a controlled substance, the chart should be completed by the nurse administering the medication. At appropriate intervals following the administration of a controlled substance, the degree and duration of effectiveness should be recorded in the nurse's notes.

At the end of each shift, the contents of the controlled substances cabinet are counted (inventoried) by two nurses, one from the shift that is about to end and the other from the oncoming shift. Each individual container is counted and the remaining number of tablets, ampules and prefilled syringes is added to the amount used, according to the inventory control record. The amount of each drug remaining, plus the amount recorded as administered to individual patients, should equal the total number issued. During the counting procedure, packages of prefilled syringes that have not been opened are visually inspected to verify that the seal and the cellophane covering are intact. Once the package seal is broken, closer scrutiny of the package is required. These observations should include tilting the package of prefilled syringes to observe the rate of air bubble movement inside the barrel, uniformity of color of the solutions in each of the barrels, and the similarity in fluid level in each of the barrels. The same medication in the same type of syringe should be the same color, travel within the barrel at the same rate, and all fluid levels should be similar. Discrepancies in the number of remaining doses are checked with nursing personnel on the unit to see if all narcotics used have been charted. If this does not reveal the source of the inaccuracy, each patient's chart is checked to be certain that all controlled substances recorded on the individual patient's charts for the shift coincide with the controlled substances inventory record. If the error is still not found, the pharmacy and the nursing service office should be contacted in accordance with the policy of the institution. In the event that the count appears to be accurate but tampering with the contents of the containers is suspected, it should be reported to the pharmacy and the nursing service office. When the controlled substances inventory is complete, the two nurses doing the counting sign the inventory control shift record to verify that the records and inventory are accurate at that point in time.

The Drug Order

Medications for patient use must be ordered by licensed physicians or dentists (or in some states by nurse practitioners) acting within their areas of professional training. Placing an order for a medication or treatment is known as issuing a *prescription*. Initially it may be issued verbally or in written form. Prescriptions issued for nonhospitalized patients use a form similar to that shown in Fig. 4.8, while prescriptions for hospitalized patients are written on the Physician's Order Form (Fig. 4.1). All prescriptions must contain the following elements: the patient's full name, date, drug name, route of administration, dosage, duration of the order, and signature of the prescriber. Additional information may be required for certain types of medications (e.g., for intravenous administration, the concentration, dilution, and rate of flow should be specified, in addition to the method—"IV push" or "continuous infusion").

Types of Medication Orders

Medication orders fall into four categories: the "stat" order, the single order, the standing order, and the p.r.n. order.

1. The *stat* order is generally used on an emergency basis. It means that the drug is to be administered as soon as possible, but only once. For example, if a patient is having a seizure, the physician may order "diazepam 10 mg IV stat," which is meant to be given immediately, and one time only.
2. The *single* order means administration at a certain time, but only one time. For example, a preoperative analgesic may be ordered "Demerol 100 mg I.M. to be given at the time the patient leaves the floor for surgery." Demerol would then be administered at that time, but once only.

3. The *standing* order indicates that a medication is to be given for a specified number of doses. For example, "TACE 72 mg q 12 h ×4 doses." A standing order may also indicate that a drug is to be administered until discontinued at a later date: For example, "Ampicillin 500 mg PO q 6 h."

   In the interest of patient safety, however, all accredited health agencies have policies that automatically cancel an order after a certain number of doses are administered or a certain number of days of therapy have passed (e.g., discontinuation prior to surgery; 72 hours for narcotics; one dose only for anticoagulants; 7 days for antibiotics). A *renewal order* must be written and signed by the physician before the nurse can continue to administer the medication.
4. A *p.r.n.* order means "administer if needed." This order allows a nurse to judge when a medication should be administered based on the patient's need and when it can be safely administered.

Verbal Orders. Health care agencies have policies established with regard to who may accept verbal or telephone orders, and under what circumstances they should be accepted. The practice should be avoided whenever possible, but when a verbal order is accepted, the person who took the order is responsible for accurately entering the order on the order sheet and signing it. The physician must co-sign and date the order, usually within 24 hours.

Nurses' Responsibilities Associated with the Drug Order

Verification of the Drug Order. Once a prescription has been written for a hospitalized patient, the nurse interprets it and makes a professional judgment on its acceptability. Judgments must be made regarding the type of drug, the therapeutic intent, the usual dose, and the mathematical and physical preparation of the dose. The nurse must also evaluate the method of administration in relation to the patient's physical condition, as well as any allergies and the patient's ability to tolerate the dosage form. If any part of an order is vague, the physician who wrote the order should be consulted for further clarification. Patient safety is of primary importance and the nurse assumes responsibility for verification and safety of the medication order. If, after gathering all possible information, it is concluded that it is inappropriate to administer the medication as ordered, the prescribing physician should be notified immediately. An explanation should be given for why the order should not be executed. If the physician cannot be contacted or if the physician does not change the order, the nurse should notify the

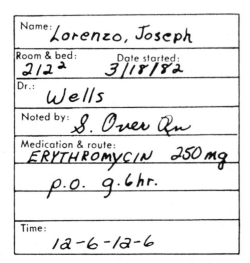

| Name: Lorenzo, Joseph |
| Room & bed: 212² | Date started: 3/18/82 |
| Dr.: Wells |
| Noted by: S. Over Rn |
| Medication & route: ERYTHROMYCIN 250 mg p.o. q. 6 hr. |
| Time: 12 - 6 - 12 - 6 |

Fig. 4.5. *Transcription of a medication order onto the Kardex or a medication card or ticket. (From Hahn, A. B., et al.:* Pharmacology in Nursing, *ed. 15, St. Louis, 1982, The C. V. Mosby Co.)*

director of nurses and/or the nursing supervisor on duty. The reasons for refusal to administer the drug should be recorded in accordance with the policies of the employing institution.

Transcription of the Order. Transcription of the prescriber's order is necessary to put it into action. After verification of an order, a nurse, or another designated person, transcribes the order from the order sheet onto the Kardex or onto a medication card (Fig. 4.5). This data may also be entered into a computer that produces a Kardex. When this process is delegated to a ward clerk or unit secretary, the nurse is still responsible for the verification of all aspects of the medication order. The nurse must sign the original medication order indicating that she received, interpreted, and verified the order. The nurse then sends a carbon copy of the original order to the pharmacy. A small supply is issued either in unit dose, or in a container containing a multi-day supply. The container is labeled with the date, patient's name, room number, and the drug name and strength/dose. When the supply arrives from the pharmacy it is stored in the medication room or in the patient's medication drawer of a medication cart. The nurse administers a drug by following the order on the medication card or drug profile according to the RIGHTS of drug administration.

The Six Rights of Drug Administration

Right Drug

Many drugs have similar spellings and variable concentrations. *Prior* to the administration of the medi-

cation, it is imperative to compare the exact spelling and concentration of the prescribed drug with the medication card or drug profile and the medication container. Regardless of the drug distribution system used, the drug label should be read at least 3 times:

1. Before removing the drug from the shelf or unit dose cart;
2. Before preparing or measuring the actual prescribed dose;
3. Before replacing the drug on the shelf or before opening a unit dose container (just prior to administering the drug to the patient).

Right Time

When scheduling the administration time of a medication, factors such as timing abbreviations, standardized times, consistency of blood levels, absorption, diagnostic testing, and the use of p.r.n. medications must be considered.

1. Standard Abbreviations—The drug order specifies the frequency of drug administration. Standard abbreviations used as part of the drug order specify the times of administration (see Appendixes A and B). The nurse should also check institutional policy concerning administration of medications. Hospitals often have standardized interpretations for abbreviations (e.g., "q 6 h" may mean 0600, 1200, 1800, and 2400; "q.i.d." may mean 0800, 1200, 1600, and 2000). The nurse must memorize and utilize standard abbreviations in interpreting, transcribing, and administering medications accurately.

2. Standardized Administration Times—For patient safety, certain medications are administered at specific times. This allows laboratory work or ECGs to be completed first, in order to determine the size of the next dose to be administered. For example, warfarin or digoxin would be administered at 1300, if ordered by the physician.

3. Maintenance of Consistent Blood Levels—The schedule for the administration of a drug should be planned to maintain consistent blood levels of the drug in order to maximize the therapeutic effectiveness.

4. Maximum Drug Absorption—The schedule for oral administration of drugs must be planned to prevent incompatibilities and maximize absorption. Certain drugs require administration on an empty stomach. Thus, they are given one hour before or two hours after meals. Other medications should be given with foods to enhance absorption or reduce irritation. Still other drugs are not given with dairy products or antacids. It is important to maintain the recommended schedule

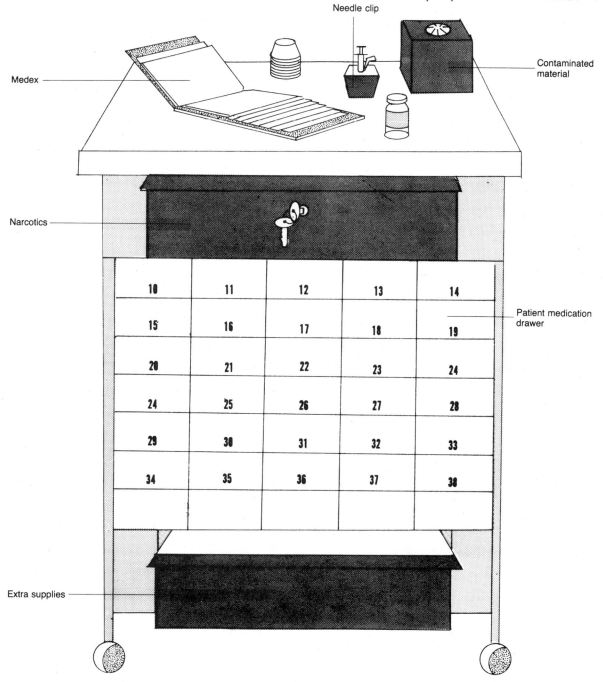

Needle clip

Medex

Contaminated material

Narcotics

10	11	12	13	14
15	16	17	18	19
20	21	22	23	24
24	25	26	27	28
29	30	31	32	33
34	35	36	37	38

Patient medication drawer

Extra supplies

Fig. 4.6. *A unit dose cabinet.*

of administration for maximum therapeutic effectiveness.

5. Diagnostic Testing—Determine whether any diagnostic tests have been ordered for completion prior to initiating or continuing therapy. Before beginning antimicrobial therapy, assure that all culture specimens (e.g., blood, urine, or wound) have been collected. If a physician has ordered serum levels of the drug, coordinate the administration time of the medication with the time the phlebotomist is going to draw the blood sample. Timing is important; if not done at the same time intervals in the same patient, the data gained is of little value.

6. P.R.N. Medications—Prior to the administration of any p.r.n. medication, the patient's chart should be checked to assure that the drug has not been administered by someone else, or that the specified time interval has passed since the medication was last ad-

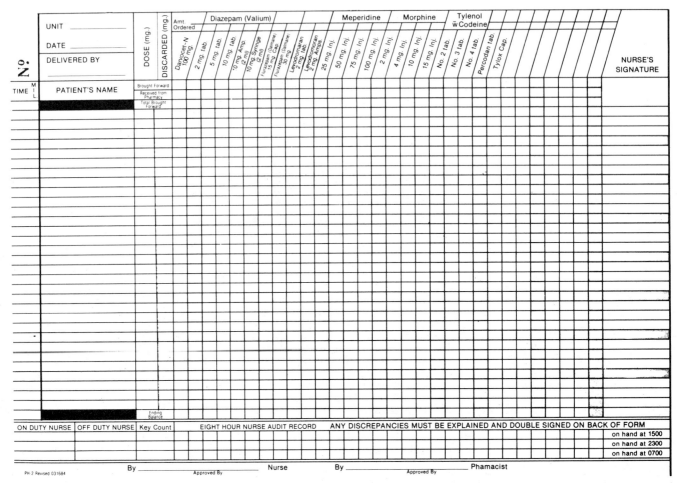

Fig. 4.7. *Controlled-substances inventory form. (Courtesy of University Hospital, The University of Nebraska Medical Center; Copyright, Board of Regents of the University of Nebraska, Lincoln, Nebraska.)*

ministered. When a p.r.n. medication is given, it should be charted immediately. Record the response to the medication.

Right Dose

Check the drug dosage ordered against the range specified in reference books available at the nurses' station.

1. Abnormal Hepatic or Renal Function—Always consider the hepatic and renal function of the specific patient who will receive the drug. Depending on the rate of drug metabolism and route of excretion from the body, certain drugs require a reduction in dosage to prevent toxicity. Conversely, patients being dialyzed may require higher than normal doses. Whenever a dosage is outside the normal range for that drug, it should be verified *prior* to administration. Once verification has been obtained, a brief explanation should

be recorded in the nurse's notes and on the Kardex (or drug profile) so that others administering the medication will have the information and the physician will not be repeatedly contacted with the same questions.

2. Pediatric and Geriatric Patients—Specific doses for some drugs are not yet firmly established for the elderly and for the pediatric patient. The nurse should question any order outside the normal range *prior* to administration. For pediatric patients, the most reliable method is by proportional amount of body surface area or body weight. (See Appendixes E and H.)

3. Nausea and Vomiting—If a patient is vomiting, oral medications should be withheld and the physician contacted for alternate medication orders, since the parenteral or rectal route may be preferred. Investigate the onset of the nausea and vomiting. If it began after the start of the medication regimen, consideration should be given to rescheduling the oral medication. Administration with food usually decreases gastric irritation. Consult with a physician for changes in orders.

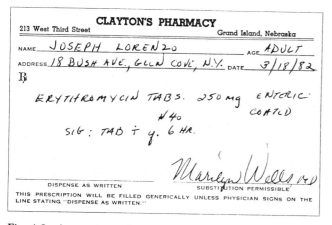

CLAYTON'S PHARMACY

213 West Third Street   Grand Island, Nebraska

NAME *JOSEPH LORENZO* AGE *ADULT*

ADDRESS *18 BUSH AVE., GLEN COVE, N.Y.* DATE *3/18/82*

℞

ERYTHROMYCIN TABS. 250 mg ENTERIC COATED

#40

SIG: TAB ī q. 6 HR.

Marilyn Wells M.D.

—————————————   ———————————————
DISPENSE AS WRITTEN   SUBSTITUTION PERMISSIBLE

THIS PRESCRIPTION WILL BE FILLED GENERICALLY UNLESS PHYSICIAN SIGNS ON THE LINE STATING "DISPENSE AS WRITTEN."

Fig. 4.8. *A prescription, listing patient name, patient address, date, drug and strength, number of tablets, directions for use, and the physician's signature.*

4. Accurate Dose Forms—Do not break a tablet unless it is scored. Consult with the pharmacy about other available dosage forms.

5. Accurate Calculations—Safety should always be maintained when calculating a drug dose. Whenever a dosage is questionable, or when fractional doses are calculated, check the dosage with another qualified individual. Most hospital policies require that certain medications (e.g., insulin, heparin, IV digitalis preparations) be checked by two qualified nurses prior to administration.

6. Correct Measuring Devices—Accurate measurement of the volume of medication prescribed is essential. **Fractional Doses Require the Use of a Tuberculin Syringe, While Insulin Is Always Measured in an Insulin Syringe That Corresponds to the Number of Units in 1 ml** (U-100 insulin is measured in a U-100 syringe).

Right Patient

When using the medication card system, compare the name of the patient on the medication card with the patient's identification bracelet. With the unit dose system, compare the name on the drug profile with the individual's identification bracelet. When checking the bracelet under either system, always check for allergies, as well. Some institutional policies require that the individual be called by name as a means of identification. This practice must take into consideration the patient's mental alertness and orientation. It is much safer to ALWAYS check the identification bracelet.

1. Pediatric Patients—Never ask children their names as a means of positive identification. Children may change beds, try to avoid you, or seek attention by identifying themselves as someone else. Check identification bracelets EVERY TIME.

2. Geriatric Patients—It is a wise policy to check identification bracelets, in addition to verbally confirming names. In a long term care setting, residents usually do not wear identification bracelets. In these instances, only a person who is familiar with the residents should administer medications.

Many errors may be avoided by carefully following the practices just presented. Make it a habit to check the identification bracelet EVERY TIME a medication is administered. The adverse effects of administration of the wrong medication to the wrong patient and the potential for a lawsuit can thus be avoided.

Right Route

The drug order should specify the route to be used for the administration of the medication. Never substitute one dosage form of medication for another unless the physician is specifically consulted, and an order for the change is obtained. There can be a great variation in the absorption rate of the medication through various routes of administration. The intravenous route delivers the drug directly into the bloodstream. This route provides the fastest onset, but also the greatest danger of potential adverse effects such as tachycardia and hypotension. The intramuscular route provides the next fastest absorption rate, based upon availability of blood supply. This route can be quite painful, as is the case with many antibiotics. The subcutaneous route is next fastest, based on blood supply. In some instances the oral route may be as fast as the intramuscular route, depending on the medication being given, the dosage form (liquids are absorbed faster than tablets), and whether there is food in the stomach. The oral route is usually safe if the patient is conscious and able to swallow. The rectal route should be avoided, if possible, due to irritation of mucosal tissues and erratic absorption rates. In case of error, the oral and rectal routes have the advantage of recoverability for a short time after administration.

Right Drug Preparation and Administration. Maintain the highest standards of drug preparation and administration. Focus your entire attention on the calculation, preparation and administration of the ordered medication. A drug reconstituted by a nurse should be clearly labeled with the patient's name, the dose or strength per unit of volume, the date and time the drug was reconstituted, the amount and type of diluent used, the expiration date and/or time, and the initials or name of the nurse who prepared it. Once reconstituted, the drug should be stored according to the manufacturer's recommendation.

- CHECK the label of the container for the drug name, concentration and route of appropriate administration.
- CHECK the patient's chart, Kardex, or identification bracelet for allergies. If no information is found, ask the patient, prior to the administration of the medication, if he or she has any allergies.
- CHECK the patient's chart or Kardex for rotation schedules of injectible medications.
- CHECK medications to be mixed in one syringe with a list approved by the hospital or the pharmacy for compatibility. Normally, all drugs mixed in a single syringe should be administered within 15 minutes after mixing. Immediately prior to administration, ALWAYS CHECK the contents of the syringe for clarity and the absence of any precipitate; if either is present, do not administer the contents of the syringe.
- CHECK the patient's identity EVERY TIME a medication is administered.
- DO approach the patient in a firm but kind manner that conveys the feeling that cooperation is expected.
- DO adjust the patient to the most appropriate position for the route of administration (e.g., for oral medications, sit the patient upright to facilitate swallowing). Have appropriate fluids ready before administration.
- DO remain with the patient to be certain that all medications have been swallowed.
- DO use every opportunity to teach the patient and family about the drug being administered.
- Do give simple and honest answers or explanations to the patient regarding the medication and treatment plan.
- DO use a plastic container, medicine cup, medicine dropper, oral syringe, or nipple to administer oral medications to an infant or small child.
- DO reward the child who has been cooperative by giving praise; comfort and hold the uncooperative child after completing the medication administration.
- DO NOT prepare or administer a drug from a container that is not properly labeled, or from a container where the label is not fully legible.
- DO NOT give any medication prepared by another individual other than the pharmacist. ALWAYS check the drug name, dosage, and route of administration against the order. Student nurses must know the practice limitations instituted by the hospital or school and which medications can be administered under what level of supervision.

- DO NOT return an unused portion or dose of medication to a stock supply bottle.
- DO NOT attempt to administer any drug orally to a comatose patient.
- DO NOT leave a medication at the patient's bedside to be taken "later"; remain with the individual until the drug is taken and swallowed.
- DO NOT dilute a liquid medication form unless there are specific written orders to do so.
- BEFORE DISCHARGE: (1) Explain the proper method of taking prescribed medications to the patient (e.g., do not crush or chew enteric-coated tablets, or any capsules; sublingual medication is placed under the tongue, and is not taken with water). (2) Stress the need for punctuality in the administration of medications, and what to do if a dosage is missed. (3) Teach the patient to store medications separately from other containers and personal hygiene items. (4) Provide the patient with written instructions reiterating the medication names, schedules, and how to obtain refills. Write the instructions in a language understood by the patient, and use LARGE, BOLD LETTERS when necessary.

Right Documentation

Documentation of nursing actions and patient observations has always been an important ethical responsibility, but now it is becoming a major medicolegal consideration, as well. Indeed, it is becoming known as the SIXTH RIGHT. Always chart the following information: date and time of administration, name of medication, dosage, route, and site of administration. Documentation of drug action should be made in the regularly scheduled assessments for changes in the disease symptoms the patient is exhibiting. Promptly record and report adverse symptoms observed. Document health teaching performed and evaluate and record the degree of understanding exhibited by the patient.

- DO record when a drug is *not* administered and why.
- DO NOT record a medication until after it has been given.

The Nursing Process

The nursing process is the foundation for clinical practice. It provides the framework for consistent nursing actions, using a problem solving process rather than an intuitional approach. All patient care activities initiated by the nurse should follow the nursing process. It provides a systematic method of identifying patient problems, particularly those related to drug therapy, and helps determine what measures must be taken to correct the problems. The process incorporates four phases: (1) assessment, (2) planning of goals, (3) implementation of plans, and (4) evaluation.

Assessment is an ongoing process that starts with the admission of the patient and is completed at discharge. In relating the nursing process to the nursing functions associated with medications, assessment includes evaluating the patient's need for medication, as well as any problems the patient has that are related to drug therapy. The nurse must have a knowledge of the patient's diagnosis and of the drugs being administered. The nurse must be able to use pharmacological references to answer questions that arise.

Assessment information is gathered from a variety of sources. The patient's chart usually serves as the basis for starting to research the patient. Additional sources of information include the family and friends, other members of the health care team, and performance of ongoing nursing assessments and observations. Examples of ongoing assessment activities include visiting with the patient, monitoring vital signs, and observing therapeutic effects, adverse effects, and potential drug interactions.

One goal of the initial nursing interview should be to evaluate the individual's view of the existing problems and readiness to accept health care. Many beginning practitioners fail to take the time to set an empathetic tone and establish a conducive atmosphere prior to initiation of the interview process. The nurse should provide an initial orientation to the hospital surroundings, then start the interview in a quiet, private place. A calm manner and attention to the patient's expressed and implied needs can serve to reduce stress and establish a feeling of sincerity, warmth, and understanding. As the interview progresses, the nurse should strive to clarify the patient's perspective of the symptoms present.

Another important aspect of the initial nursing interview is the establishment of a *medication history* for the patient. Keeping in mind the patient's mental alertness and ability to provide accurate answers (which may have to be verified by the physician or family members) the nurse should carefully review the following: (1) any medications currently being taken by the patient, both prescription and over-the-counter; (2) whether the patient has brought any medications from home (the nurse should consult the hospital policy regarding the use and storage of these medications to prevent inadvertent dual administration by both the nurse and the patient); (3) previous medications taken by the patient for extended periods of time (including analgesics or laxatives); (4) known allergies to any type of medication.

The nurse should be careful to allow the patient, or a responsible family member, to answer completely and fully. The nurse should not use statements such as "You aren't taking any other medications, are you?," but rather, should allow the patient to respond fully to the question, "What other medications are you taking?" All responses should be charted.

After gathering clinical and psychosocial information, the nurse must establish *nursing diagnoses* that clearly identify the individual's problems and needs. The nursing diagnoses should reflect only the problems that nurses are qualified and licensed to treat within the scope of nursing practice. These diagnoses serve as a basis for formulating the *care plan* and implementing nursing interventions. Consideration should be given to allowing the patient to maintain control of appropriate events within the overall delivery of care. Goal statements should be formulated in brief, measurable, behavioral terms. They should direct the care toward the attainment of broader, long-term goals, such as the return of the patient to a normal pattern of living. When setting priorities, consider the disease process exhibited by the presenting symptoms, the diagnostic data, the patient's preferences, and the degree of urgency reflected by the individual's current status. When completed, the care plan should be entered in the Kardex or on the chart.

During the *implementation* phase, the actual care planned is delivered. Although the phases in the nursing process are descriptively pictured as separate entities, they are, in fact, performed on a continuum. While providing patient care, assessments should be performed continually, and additional information gathered to *evaluate* the effectiveness of the care being provided. Modifications in the care plan are made as frequently as necessary, in order to promote optimal care based on sound nursing judgments and scientific rationale. Regular nursing notes are recorded to identify changing needs as well as completed goals. The formal plan should be revised and communicated clearly to all who provide care for the individual patient.

Table 4.1 describes the principles of the nursing process. Table 4.2 provides an overview of the application of the nursing process to the nursing responsibilities associated with drug therapy.

Health Teaching

In the past, health teaching was considered an abstract form of intervention that occurred only if a specific need existed at discharge (and the physician approved of providing the information to the patient). Health teaching has evolved to the current state of development of formal learning objectives to direct the patient toward attainment of goals based on in-

Table 4.1
*Principles of the Nursing Process**

ASSESSMENT	PLANNING	INTERVENTION	EVALUATION
Collect all relevant data associated with the individual patient's diagnosis to detect potential problems needing intervention.	Prioritize the problems identified from the assessment data, with the most severe or life-threatening first. Other problems are arranged in ascending order of importance. (Maslow's hierarchy is frequently used as a basis for prioritizing; other approaches may be equally valid.)	Perform the nursing intervention planned to achieve the individualized short- and long-term goals.	Evaluation is an ongoing process that occurs at every phase of the nursing process. Review and analyze the data regarding the patient and modify the care plan so that goals of care (usually, returning the patient to the highest level of functioning) are attained.
Based on the data collected, formulate a statement of the behaviors or problems of concern and the cause. This is referred to as a *nursing diagnosis*. (Check hospital policies for the level of nursing required for this function.)	Develop short- and long-term patient goals in measurable statements to describe the behavior to be observed.		Unrealistic goals may require revision or discontinuation.
	Plan nursing approaches to correlate with each identified long-term goal. More than one short-term goal may be required to actually lead to the broader, more encompassing long-term goals.		Follow a systematic approach to recording progress, depending on the setting and charting methods used.

* For additional information on the theory and application of the nursing process, see textbooks on nursing practice.

dividual needs. Today, health teaching is an important nursing responsibility that carries with it legal implications for failure to provide education or to document health teaching provided for the patient.

The content to be taught to the patient should be thoroughly planned in advance and should be provided in increments that the patient is capable of mastering. The goals must include the entire therapeutic regimen: an understanding of the meaning of the diagnosis; diet; exercise and activity; medication; monitoring tests; treatments; scheduled follow-up care; and special equipment or supply needs. During the development of the goals, the nurse must consider the patient's intellectual level and potential for mastery of skills requiring visual acuity, fine motor movement, and coordination. The complete teaching plan should be in the Kardex or on the patient's chart. Each segment should be expressed in measurable, behavioral terms (see Table 4.3). Once the goals have been formulated, they should not be considered to be "etched in stone," but should be re-evaluated throughout the course of treatment and modified, if necessary. All teaching should be documented in the nurse's notes or on the health teaching record (Fig. 4.9a,b,c), along with observations that verify the degree of understanding or proficiency of skill mastered. As mastery of an item is

attained, it should be checked off on the Kardex or health teaching record in the patient's chart.

Assessing the patient's readiness for learning is crucial to success. When the patient's anxiety is high, the ability to focus on details is reduced. The nurse should anticipate time periods during the hospitalization when teaching can be more effectively implemented. Some teaching is most successful when done spontaneously, such as when the patient asks direct questions regarding progress toward discharge. Conversely, the nurse must learn to anticipate inopportune times to initiate teaching, such as during times of withdrawal after first learning of a poor diagnosis.

The approach to the patient is important. Many times nurses and physicians do not take the time to discuss the benefits of the total treatment plan with the individual patient and/or family. Adult learners must usually see a need to learn before they personally invest their time in the learning process. If patients understand the benefits to be gained, they will frequently adhere more closely to the plan. We often forget that patients can leave the hospital and choose to abandon the treatment plan. The faith patients have in the physicians prescribing the plan and the nurses who teach the plan can significantly influence the outcome of therapy.

Table 4.2
The Nursing Process Applied to the Patient's Pharmacologic Needs

ASSESSMENT	PLANNING	INTERVENTION	EVALUATION
Data collection			
Collect data on patient symptoms; disease process as based on the history and physical, patient, and/or family information; nursing assessments and interview.	Identify and prioritize: • Potential patient problems • Baseline assessment data to be monitored to evaluate the patient's symptoms • Anticipated drug side effects and those to report	Perform the identified baseline patient assessments on a regularly scheduled basis (i.e., blood pressure, pulse, respirations, pain level [frequency, duration, activity associated with onset], leg pain).	Analyze data collected on a continuum; chart and report *changes* of significance in the baseline data and/or patient's status. Report escalating of symptoms or ineffective response to drug therapy.
Drug history: Ask questions in a simple, direct manner to elicit information regarding drugs currently being taken, or those taken during the preceding year. Ask about over-the-counter drugs used on a regular or casual basis.	Plan to monitor patients total drug needs. Develop goals to deal with any drug interactions, incompatibilities, or diagnostic tests potentially affected by drugs being administered.	Perform drug preparation, scheduling, and administration to coincide with specific patient needs or problems.	Analyze data collected on a continuum.
Ask about any prior drug "allergies" and specifics of the "reaction" and treatment used.	Plan to monitor patient's at risk for the development of an allergic reaction.	Implement monitoring parameters.	Analyze observed symptoms for potential drug reaction or interactions.
Age and disease process present.	Plan modifications in dosage, administration technique, and observations based on the individual's age and physiologic status that may indicate a problem with drug absorption, distribution, metabolism, or excretion. Confirm drug dosages BEFORE administering any drug in question.	Implement the proper administration of confirmed drug dosages.	As therapy continues, analyze the patient's weight, mental status, and disease processes that may be indicative of a problem with drug absorption, distribution, metabolism, or excretion. Report abnormal laboratory values or *changes* in the patient's baseline assessment data.
Body weight	Plan to weigh the patient daily or as needed.	Perform the procedure of weighing the patient at the same time, in the same weight clothing, on the same scale at the intervals ordered.	Report weight gains or losses. This is of particular importance with some types of drugs such as digitalis glycosides, corticosteroids, thyroid medications, and chemotherapy.
Metabolic rate	Plan nursing intervention to correlate with diseases that alter metabolic rate (i.e., hyperthyroidism, hypothyroidism, congestive heart failure).	Institute nursing measures directed at nutritional status, activity/exercise needs, environmental alterations needed.	Analyze effectiveness of approaches utilized. Observe closely for an increase or decrease in therapeutic effect.
Monitoring parameters			
Laboratory data (See Appendix for normal values): Review data to determine potential problems in the absorption, distribution, metabolism and elimination of the prescribed drug.	Following hospital policies for ordering and assisting with laboratory/diagnostic tests. Always check for drugs that may interact with scheduled laboratory tests.		

(*Table 4.2 continues on p. 56.*)

Table 4.2 (*continued*)

ASSESSMENT	PLANNING	INTERVENTION	EVALUATION
Monitoring parameters (*cont.*)			
Hepatic function	SGOT, SGPT, alkaline phosphatase, LDH	Complete appropriate forms to order the tests; assist in drawing of blood samples and in providing patient support during procedure.	As soon as results are received on the unit, report any diagnostic value outside the normal range to the physician.
Renal function	Serum creatinine BUN (Blood Urea Nitrogen) Urinalysis (UA)	Same as above. Same as above. Collect urine sample by clean catch or, if ordered, by catheterization. Check for drugs being given and and record on urinalysis slip.	Elevated serum creatinine levels generally indicate renal disease. Elevated levels occur in renal disease, dehydration, a high protein diet, or a catabolic state. Depressed levels are found in severe hepatic damage, overhydration, and malnutrition. Always report RBCs, casts, crystals, proteinurea, glycosuria, high or low pH, or specific gravity outside the normal range (1.001–1.017).
In addition to the above tests, the following tests may be used to monitor disease and drug therapy.			
Infectious disease Assessment for site/source of the infection.	Culture and sensitivity (C&S)	Collect specimen properly to maintain sterility of the culture tip so that the source examined is the only surface touched by the sterile swab. Label appropriately; take to lab immediately.	Report results of a culture and sensitivity promptly; of particular importance are results that indicate that the drug being administered is not effective against the organism cultured.
Complete blood count	Plan intervention based on the organism, the site of the infection, fever, hematuria, and drainage.	Implement nursing measures to deal effectively with the patient's needs—fever, pain, drainage, and degree of precautions appropriate to the organism.	Elevated WBCs, bands, segs, lymphocytes need to be reported to the physician. Analyze subsequent CBC reports for significant changes. Continue performing baseline assessments to detect degree of responsiveness to therapy.
Monitoring of drug levels			
Routinely monitored: digitalis glycosides, theophyllines, aminoglycosides, lithium, lidocaine, phenytoin, procainamide, quinidine.	Plan to requisition the laboratory tests ordered by the physician to monitor serum blood levels at the scheduled times. Assure that the patient will be available at the required times.	Record drug name, dosage, and times and route of administration on requisition.	Therapeutic doses of certain drugs can be established through a combination of monitoring of serum levels and patient assessments of essential data. Example: Aminophylline—The patient's age and disease factors modify the dosage needs. Therefore patients with cardiac, pulmonary, or renal dysfunction may require serum concentration as a guide to dosage. **The current clinical status of the patient is always important; therefore, regular assessments specifically planned to detect**

Table 4.2 (*continued*)

ASSESSMENT	PLANNING	INTERVENTION	EVALUATION
Monitoring of drug levels (*cont.*)			
			therapeutic and toxic activity is imperative to effective patient management.
			Check specific drug monographs for other drugs that may alter laboratory results. Report results promptly for the physician's evaluation.
Other laboratory tests	Prothrombin time (PT) (for warfarin) Partial thromboplastin time (PTT) (for heparin)	Requisition the prescribed laboratory test so that the drug dosage can be ordered by the physician. Perform nursing assessments associated with anticoagulant therapy and the disease process specifically being treated.	Be certain the correct date and patient data are relayed to the physician when seeking or confirming the anticoagulant drug order. Always double check the date, time, and specific dosage of the anticoagulant drug order. Anticoagulants should be checked with a second qualified nurse at the time of preparation and administration.
	Blood glucose and urine glucose	Withhold daily insulin until blood sugar sample is drawn. Test urine for glucose as ordered or ac and HS.	Correlate the results of the laboratory reports to the patient's status and degree of response to drug therapy. Carefully evaluate patient symptoms for hyper- and hypoglycemia. Report laboratory data and patient status changes to the physician.
Nursing research of prescribed drugs			
Drug action			
Consult "General Nursing Considerations" in specific drug monographs to correlate drug action and monitoring parameters to the patient's presenting symptoms and disease process.	Develop goal statements for monitoring presence or absence of response. Plan the administration schedule to correlate with known information about time of administration in relation to food, tests, and planned sleep.	Assess the patient for baseline data before administering the drug; perform subsequent assessments at regular intervals to collect data to evaluate therapeutic response to the drug. Administer the prescribed drug: 　RIGHT patient 　RIGHT drug 　RIGHT dose 　RIGHT route 　RIGHT time 　RIGHT documentation	Document all assessments by carefully recording all pertinent observations in the patient's chart. Analyze the collected data and compare to the baseline data gathered before initiation of drug therapy. Report significant changes in the patient's status.
Side effects to expect	Consult specific drug monographs for side effects to expect. Plan assessments to detect and intervention to manage these as they occur.	Monitor the patient for development of expected side effects; implement measures designed to effectively manage or minimize effects. Assist patient to understand and cope with specific symptoms as developed.	Once expected side effects develop, it is important to evaluate the nursing measures designed to minimize or reduce the effects. Report lack of responsiveness. Modify intervention appropriately. Analyze the patient's level of tolerance of the side effects.

(*Table 4.2 continues on p. 58.*)

Table 4.2 (*continued*)

ASSESSMENT	PLANNING	INTERVENTION	EVALUATION
Side effects to expect (*cont.*)	Plan specific teaching that incorporates side effects to expect.	Teach which side effects to expect and how to alleviate discomfort. Encourage the patient to discuss relevant symptoms with the physician and to adhere to the medication prescribed. Suggest discussion of symptoms and encourage cooperative planning for modifications in the medications taken. Discourage discontinuance or self-adjusted dosages.	Document specific teaching performed and the degree of understanding observed through direct questioning and return demonstrations. Analyze verbal and nonverbal behaviors observed to detect patient response to suggestion of cooperative goal-setting between the physician and patient.
Side effects to report	Plan nursing assessments and intervention for side effects that are serious and require reporting. Develop a specific teaching plan that incorporates teaching of side effects to report. Plan teaching of necessary monitoring parameters (i.e., blood pressure, pulse, respirations, daily weights, other).	Perform regularly scheduled nursing assessments to detect any side effects from drug therapy that should be reported. Perform health teaching of the observations the patient should make and the findings that require reporting. Teach and repeat at appropriate intervals to achieve patient/family mastery.	Analyze data collected on a continuum. Report deviations appropriately. Carefully evaluate the patient's attitude toward compliance with drug therapy and intent to report problems for discussion and needed modifications. Evaluate the degree of accuracy attained by the patient or family members. Refer to social services or community agencies if assistance is needed at time of discharge.
Patient understanding of drug therapy	Plan teaching of drug name, dosage, route of administration, and exact time schedule. Record overall teaching plan on the Kardex or chart. Plan teaching of medications taken on a p.r.n. basis (e.g., nitroglycerin) and establish goals to evaluate understanding of frequency and dose, repeating of dose, lack of response. Plan teaching of any self-administration techniques (i.e., oral, inhalation, injection, rectal, other).	Throughout the hospitalization, discuss medication information and how it will benefit the course of treatment. Seek cooperation and understanding of the following points so that medication compliance may be enhanced: 1. Name 2. Dosage 3. Route and administration times 4. Anticipated therapeutic response 5. Side effects to expect 6. Side effects to report 7. What to do if a dosage is missed 8. When, how, or if to refill the medication prescription Teach name of drug being taken, symptoms that can be relieved by the p.r.n. drug, when to take it, amount to take, what to do if not effective.	Document teaching and understanding achieved. Try role playing a situation, or when appropriate during hospitalization, have the patient describe what needs to be done. Document the individual's understanding of the directions given. Try role playing a situation, or when appropriate during hospitalization, have the patient describe what needs to be done. Validate the patient/significant other's understanding by return demonstration. Document teaching of administration techniques and degree of understanding in nurse's notes.

Table 4.2 (*continued*)

ASSESSMENT	PLANNING	INTERVENTION	EVALUATION
Patient understanding of drug therapy (*cont.*)		Teach administration techniques to be used at home. Give simple written instructions to follow at home.	
Patient understanding of entire treatment plan	Develop goal statements for teaching the individual's care that will assist the patient in gaining knowledge of *all* aspects of self-care for the disease process present (i.e., nutritional status, activity or exercise modifications, psychological, medication, physical therapy, other). Incorporate assessments to determine the individual's readiness and capability to learn, degree of understanding, and tolerance for needed alterations.	Implement planned nursing measures appropriate to the specific disease process affecting the individual. Incorporate teaching techniques (i.e., visual aids, demonstrations and return demonstrations, role playing, other).	Analyze the patient's response to *each* component of the entire treatment plan. Throughout the course of teaching, evaluate the degree of understanding exhibited by having the patient perform appropriate activities (e.g., choose the therapeutic diet from the hospital menu, etc.). Evaluate the tolerance exhibited to restrictions and modifications implemented, or to drug side effects expected and present. Document all facets of health teaching performed, degree of understanding attained, or intolerances observed or experienced.

Table 4.3
Sample Teaching Plan for a Patient with Diabetes Mellitus Taking One Type of Insulin[*]

Understanding of Health Condition
- Assess the patient's and family's understanding of diabetes mellitus.
- Clarify the meaning of the disease in terms the patient is able to understand.
- Establish learning goals through mutual discussion. Arrange to teach most important data first. Set dates for teaching of content after discussion with patient.

Food and Fluids
- Arrange for the patient, family members, and significant others to attend nutrition lectures and demonstrations on food preparation.
- Reinforce knowledge of exchange lists by tactful questioning and by giving the patient a chance to practice food selections for daily meals from menus provided.
- Explain management of the diabetic diet during illness (i.e., nausea and vomiting, need for increase in fluid) and when to contact the physician.
- Stress interrelationship of food and onset, peak, and duration of the prescribed insulin.

Monitoring Tests
- Demonstrate the collection and testing of urine and blood samples as appropriate.
- Validate understanding by having the patient collect, test, and record results of the testing for the remainder of the hospitalization.
- Stress performing urine or blood testing before meals and at bedtime.
- Explain the importance of regular follow-up laboratory studies (i.e., fasting blood sugar) to monitor the patient's degree of control.

Medications and Treatments
- Teach the name, dose, route of administration, desired action, storage, and refilling of the type of insulin prescribed.
- Explain the principles of insulin action, onset, peak, and duration (see Index).
- Demonstrate preparation and administration of the prescribed dose of insulin.
- Teach site location and rotation schedule for self-administration of insulin.
- Give specific instructions on reading the syringe to be used at home (glass or disposable plastic).
- Teach sterilization of glass syringe and needle, and storage and assembly, if necessary.

Table 4.3 (*continued*)

- Cite usual times for "reactions," signs and symptoms of hypoglycemia or hyperglycemia, and management of each complication.
- Validate the patient's understanding of the side effects to expect and those that require reporting.
- Teach and validate family members' and significant others' understanding of the signs and symptoms of hypoglycemia and hyperglycemia, and management of each complication.

Personal Hygiene
Discuss the management of personal hygiene measures of great importance to the patient with diabetes mellitus:
- Regular foot care
- Meticulous oral hygiene and dental care
- Care of cuts, scratches, minor and major injuries
- Stress management and needed alterations in insulin dosage, and reporting to physician for guidance and discussion.

Activities
- Assist the patient to develop a detailed time schedule for usual activities of daily living. Incorporate diabetic care needs into the schedule.
- Encourage maintenance of all usual activities of daily living; discuss anticipated problems and possible interventions.
- Correlate personal care needs not only in the home environment, but also in the work setting as appropriate. (Consider involvement of the industrial nurse if available in the work setting.)
- Discuss effects of an increase or decrease in activity level on the management of the diabetes mellitus.

Home or Follow-Up Care
- Arrange for outpatient or physician follow-up appointments and for scheduling ordered laboratory tests.
- Tell the individual to seek assistance from the physician or from the nearest emergency room service for problems that may develop.
- Arrange appropriate referral to community health agencies if needed.
- Complete a Diabetic Alert card or other means of alerting people to the individual's needs (i.e., identification necklace or bracelet).

Special Equipment and Instructional Materials
- Develop a list of equipment and supplies to be purchased; have a family member purchase and bring to the hospital for use during teaching sessions (urine or blood glucose monitoring supplies, syringes, needles and sterilizing equipment, alcohol, cotton balls, etc.).
- Show audiovisual materials available on insulin preparation, storage, administration, urine testing, etc.
- Develop a written record (see Chapter 15) and assist the patient to maintain pertinent data during hospitalization.

Other
- Teach measures to make travel easier.
- Tell the patient of the American Diabetes Association and material available through this resource.

---

* Each item listed needs to be assessed for the individual's current knowledge base and level of understanding throughout the course of teaching. The process is reassessed and the teaching continued until the patient masters all facets of self-care needs. With the advent of shorter hospitalizations, inpatient and outpatient teaching may be necessary. Referral to community-based health care agencies may be necessary. Discharge charting and referral should carefully document those facets of the teaching plan mastered and those to be taught. The physician should be notified of deficits in learning ability and/or mastery of needed elements in the teaching plan.

Mutual goal setting that starts with the needs the patient views as important, may act as a motivator for the learning process. Start, whenever possible, with simple, attainable goals in order to build the patient's confidence.

Develop a data collection form for the patient to record responses to treatments (see the template in Appendix L). The data collection form is an excellent tool for providing encouragement while teaching the patient a systematic method for recording responses to the therapy as treatment progresses. Use of the data collection form should be continued after discharge and it should be taken to the physician's office as a part of the follow-up visits. If, in the patient's mind, obstacles are encountered, they should be discussed with the physician and nursing staff for modification.

As the patient progresses in the mastery of the medication regimen, more complex information should be taught. Using the example in Table 4.3, once the patient is able to name the drug and dosage, as well as the onset, peak, and duration of the action, the nurse should progress to teaching the actual administration technique, control of the expected side effects, and which adverse effects to report. Management of adverse reactions, such as an insulin overdose, would be taught toward the end of the plan, after the patient is familiar with routine responses. Constant feedback, praise, and reinforcement of the tasks being taught is important to mastery achievement and a continued commitment to learning by the patient.

JENNIE EDMUNDSON MEMORIAL HOSPITAL

PREOPERATIVE TEACHING GUIDE

DATE	TOPIC DISCUSSED/METHODS USED	PATIENT'S RESPONSE	INSTRUCTOR

CONTENT

1. Understanding of consent form.

2. Anesthesiologist's visit.

3. Food and fluid restrictions (NPO p̄ 2400).

4. Bowel preparation.

5. H.S. sedation.

6. Physical care AM before surgery— bathing, removing nail polish, dentures, etc.

7. Surgical skin prep if applicable.

8. Preoperative medications—effects and safety implications.

9. Postop safety and prevention of complications
   a) Activity limitations and expectations (only up with assistance)
   b) Taking of frequent vital signs
   c) Leg exercises

10. Postop respiratory care and turning—explain and have patient demonstrate
    a) Turning side to side
    b) Coughing/deep breathe
    c) Splinting wound

11. Postop expectations and measures/ medications that will be used to relieve pain.

12. Postop plan for food and fluid restrictions/rationale. How long patient will be NPO. Progressive dietary plan— liquid to solid. I & O record kept 24 hours.

13. Nasogastric and other tubes, catheters, drains, IV therapy, and other special equipment.

14. Description of O.R. holding area (e.g., how transported, taken via cart), stay in R.R., and the surgical waiting room for family members.

* List the date, number of topic discussed, and what method used (e.g., booklet title, discussion) in the appropriate column. Patient's response and signature of instructor must be entered for each topic discussed.

Fig. 4.9. (a–c) *Patient teaching forms (a above and b and c next two pages).*

PATIENT & FAMILY TEACHING

Specify: Date, instructional content, and/or instructional material	Taught to Patient	Taught to Family	Patient Comments and/or Return Demonstration/Instructor Signature
1. Understanding of health condition:			
2. Food & fluid.			
3. X-rays — tests — treatments			
4. Medications & precautions			
5. Activities			
6. Home or follow-up care			
7. Special equipment & instructional materials given to patient			
8. Other			
• ☑ means teaching complete			

90-570

DISMISSAL INSTRUCTIONS

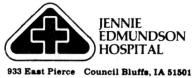

JENNIE EDMUNDSON HOSPITAL

933 East Pierce   Council Bluffs, IA 51501

I. Diet: _____

    Instructions given _____

    Business Office Notified   ☐ Yes   ☐ No

    Stop   ☐ Yes   ☐ No

II. Medications: Dose/Times to Take

    Medications _____

_____

_____

_____

_____

_____

_____

    Family or significant others instructed ☐ *

    Medications which should *NOT* be taken:

_____

_____

III. Activity: ·

_____

_____

_____

    Family or significant others instructed ☐ *

IV. Follow-up care (appointment): _____

_____

V. Special Instructions (wound care, special treatments, etc.):

_____

_____

_____

    Family or significant others instructed ☐ *

    Date: _____ Signature _____

                                     Instructor

I understand the above discharge instructions and feel they have been explained to my satisfaction.

Date: _____ Signature _____

* Check ☑ when family or significant others taught.

63

Chapter 5

Preparation and Administration of Medications by the Enteral Route

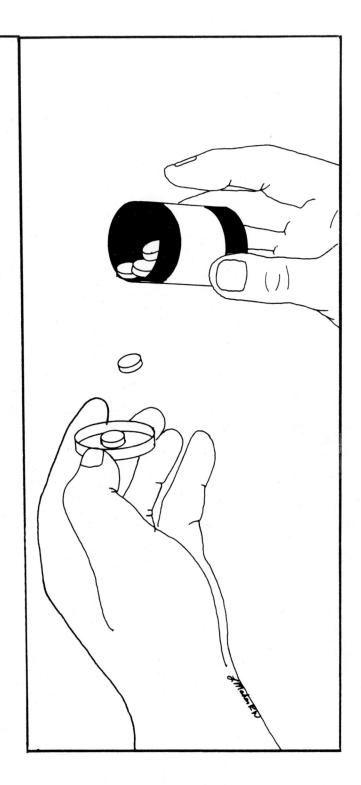

Objectives

After completing this chapter, the student should be able to do the following:

1. Cite the advantages and disadvantages of using the enteral route for drug administration.
2. Differentiate between various oral dosage forms and techniques involved in the use of each.
3. Explain usual equipment used to administer medications accurately via the enteral route.
4. Describe the principles of measurement of medications using a unit dose package, medicine cup, dropper, teaspoon, and oral syringe.
5. Contrast medication administration principles and techniques using the unit dose and medication card systems of delivery.
6. Describe the 6 RIGHTS of medication administration.
7. Use the procedures and principles cited to practice and perfect the preparation and administration of medications in solid and liquid forms via the enteral route.

The routes of drug administration can be classified into three categories: the enteral, the parenteral, and the percutaneous routes. The enteral route refers to those drugs administered directly into the gastrointestinal tract by oral, rectal, or nasogastric routes. The oral route is safe, most convenient, and relatively economical, and dosage forms are readily available for most medications. In the event of a medication error or intentional drug overdose, much of the drug can be retrieved for a reasonable time after administration. Disadvantages of the oral route are that it has the slowest and least dependable rate of absorption (and thus onset of action) of the commonly used routes of administration because of the frequent changes in the gastrointestinal environment produced by food, emotion, and physical activity. Another limitation on this route is that a few drugs, such as insulin and gentamicin, are destroyed by digestive fluids and must be administered parenterally for therapeutic activity. This route should not be used if the drug may harm or discolor the teeth or if the patient is vomiting, has gastric or intestinal suction, is likely to aspirate, or is unconscious and unable to swallow.

An alternative for those patients who cannot swallow or who have had oral surgery is the nasogastric route. The primary purpose of the nasogastric route is to bypass the mouth and pharynx. Advantages and disadvantages are quite similar to those of the oral route. The irritation caused by the tube in the nasal passage and throat must be weighed against the relative immobility associated with continuous intravenous infusions, expense, and the pain and irritation of multiple injections.

Administration via the rectal route has the advantages of bypassing the digestive enzymes and avoiding irritation of the mouth, esophagus, and stomach. It may also be a good alternative when nausea or vomiting is present. Absorption via this route varies depending on the drug product, the ability of the patient to retain the suppository or enema, and fecal material that is present.

Administration of Oral Medications

Dosage Forms

Capsules. Capsules are small, cylindrical gelatin containers (Fig. 5.1) that hold dry powder or liquid

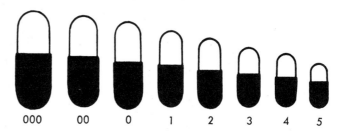

Fig. 5.1. *Various sizes and numbers of gelatin capsules, actual size. (From Bergersen, B. S.: Pharmacology in Nursing, ed. 14, St. Louis, 1979, The C. V. Mosby Co.)*

medicinal agents. They are available in a variety of sizes and are a convenient way of administering drugs with an unpleasant odor or taste. They do not require coatings or additives to improve the taste. The color and shapes of capsules, as well as the manufacturer's symbols that are on the capsule surface, are means of identifying the product.

Timed-release Capsules. Timed-release or sustained-release capsules (Fig. 5.2) provide a gradual but continuous release of drug because the granules within the capsule dissolve at different rates. The advantage of this delivery system is that it reduces the number of doses administered per day. Trade names indicating

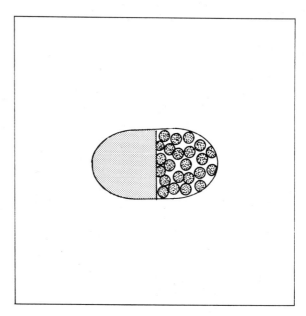

Fig. 5.2. *Timed-release capsule.*

that the drug is a timed-release product are Spansules, Gyrocaps, and Plateau Caps. The timed-release capsules should NOT be crushed or chewed or the contents emptied into food or liquids, since this may alter the absorption rate and could result in either drug overdose or subtherapeutic activity.

Lozenges. Lozenges are flat disks containing a medicinal agent in a suitably flavored base. The base may be a hard sugar candy or the combination of sugar with sufficient mucilage to give it form. Lozenges are held in the mouth to dissolve slowly, which releases the therapeutic ingredients.

Pills. Pills are an obsolete dosage form that are no longer manufactured due to the development of capsules and compressed tablets. Laypersons still use the term to refer to tablets and capsules.

Tablets. Tablets are dried, powdered drugs that have been compressed into small disks. In addition to the drug, tablets also contain one or more of the following ingredients: binders (adhesive substances that allow the tablet to stick together); disintegrators (substances that encourage dissolution in body fluids); lubricants (required for efficient manufacturing); and fillers (inert ingredients to make the tablet size convenient). Tablets are sometimes scored or grooved (Fig. 5.3); the indentation may be used to divide the dosage. Whenever possibile it is best to request the exact dosage prescribed rather than attempt to divide a tablet.

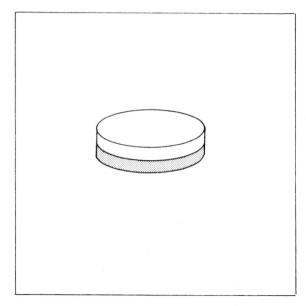

Fig. 5.4. *Layered tablet.*

Tablets can be formed in layers (Fig. 5.4). This method allows otherwise incompatible medications to be administered at the same time.

An enteric-coated tablet (Fig. 5.5) has a special coating that resists dissolution in the acidic pH of the stomach but is dissolved in the alkaline pH of the intestines. Enteric-coated tablets are often used for administering medications that are destroyed in an acid pH. Enteric-coated tablets must NOT be crushed or chewed. The active ingredients will be released prematurely and be destroyed in the stomach.

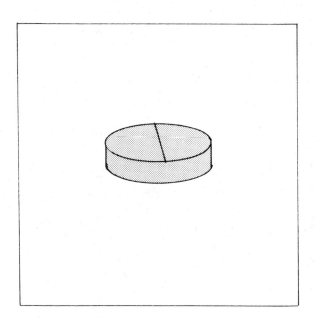

Fig. 5.3. *Scored tablet.*

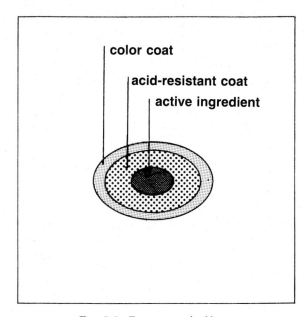

Fig. 5.5. *Enteric coated tablet.*

Elixirs. Elixirs are clear liquids made up of drugs dissolved in alcohol and water. Elixirs are used primarily when the drug will not dissolve in water alone. After the drug is dissolved in the elixir, flavoring agents are frequently added to improve taste. The alcohol content of elixirs is highly variable, depending on the solubility of the drug.

Emulsions. Emulsions are dispersions of small droplets of water in oil or oil in water. The dispersion is maintained by emulsifying agents such as sodium lauryl sulfate, gelatin, or acacia. Emulsions are used to mask bitter tastes or provide better solubility to certain drugs.

Suspensions. Suspensions are liquid dosage forms that contain solid, insoluble drug particles dispersed in a liquid base. All suspensions should be shaken well before administration to assure thorough mixing of the particles.

Syrups. Syrups contain medicinal agents dissolved in a concentrated solution of sugar, usually sucrose. Syrups are particularly effective for masking the bitter taste of a drug. Many preparations for pediatric patients are syrups, since children tend to like the flavored base.

Equipment

Unit Dose or Single Dose. "Unit dose or single dose" packaging (Fig. 5.6) provides a single dose of medication in one package, ready for dispensing. The package is labeled with generic and brand names, man-

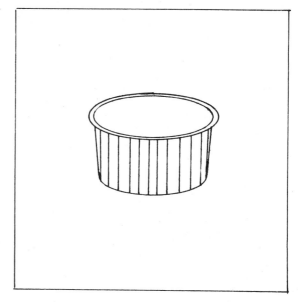

Fig. 5.7. *Soufflé cup.*

ufacturer, lot number, and date of expiration. Depending on the distribution system, the patient's name may be added to the package by the pharmacy.

Soufflé Cup. A small paper or plastic cup (Fig. 5.7) may be used to transport solid medication forms, such as a capsule or tablet, to the patient to prevent contamination by handling. A tablet that must be crushed can be placed between two soufflé cups and then crushed with a pestle. This powdered form of the tablet can then be administered in a solution if soluble, or it may be mixed with a small amount of food, such as applesauce.

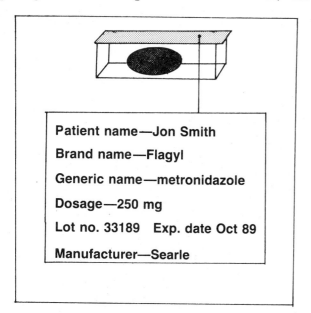

Patient name—Jon Smith

Brand name—Flagyl

Generic name—metronidazole

Dosage—250 mg

Lot no. 33189   Exp. date Oct 89

Manufacturer—Searle

Fig. 5.6. *Unit dose package.*

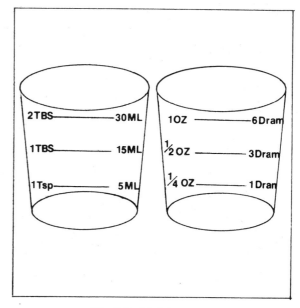

2 TBS — 30 ML 1 OZ — 6 Dram

1 TBS — 15 ML $\frac{1}{2}$ OZ — 3 Dram

1 Tsp — 5 ML $\frac{1}{4}$ OZ — 1 Dram

Fig. 5.8. *Medicine cup.*

Table 5.1
Commonly Used Measurement Equivalents

HOUSEHOLD MEASUREMENT	APOTHECARY MEASUREMENT	METRIC MEASUREMENT
2 Tbsp	1 oz (6–8 drams)*	30 ml
1 Tbsp	½ oz (3–4 drams)*	15 ml
2 tsp	⅓ oz	10 ml
1 tsp	⅙ oz (1 dram)	5 ml

* Some sources list 1 teaspoonful as equivalent to 1 dram; others refer to it as 1⅓ drams or 1¼ drams. For practical purposes, 1 teaspoonful equals 5 ml, therefore, 1 oz would have 6 drams. (If using 1⅓ dram = 1 teaspoonful, an ounce would equal 8 drams.)

Medicine Cup. The medicine cup (Fig. 5.8) is a glass or plastic container that has three scales (apothecary, metric, and household) for the measurement of liquid medications. The medicine cup should be carefully examined before pouring any medication to assure that the proper scale is being used for measurement (see Table 5.1). The medicine cup is inaccurate for the measurement of doses smaller than 1 teaspoonful, although it is reasonably accurate for larger volumes. A syringe comparable to the volume to be measured should be be used for smaller volumes. For volumes less than 1 cc, a tuberculin syringe should be used.

Medicine Dropper. The medicine dropper (Fig. 5.9) may be used to administer eye drops, ear drops, and, occasionally, pediatric medications. There is great variation in the size of the drop formed, so it is quite important to use only the dropper supplied by the manufacturer for a specific liquid medication. Before

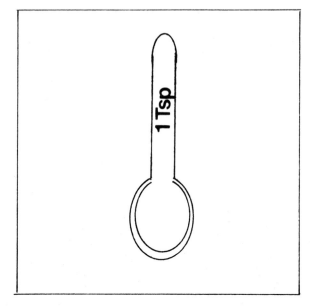

Fig. 5.10. *Measuring teaspoon.*

drawing medication into a dropper, become familiar with the calibrations on the barrel. Once the medication is drawn into the barrel, the dropper should not be tipped upside down. The medication will run into the bulb, causing some loss of the medication. Medications should not be drawn into the dropper and then transferred to another container for administration since part of the medication will adhere to the second container, which will diminish the dose delivered.

Teaspoons. Doses of most liquid medications are prescribed in terms using the teaspoon (Fig. 5.10) as

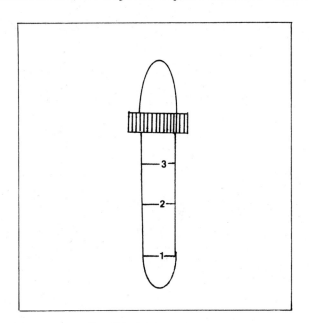

Fig. 5.9. *Medicine dropper.*

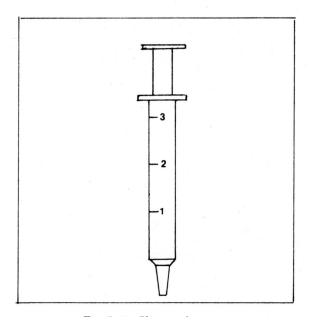

Fig. 5.11. *Plastic oral syringe.*

the unit of measure. However, there is great variation between the volumes measured by various teaspoons within the household. Within the hospital, 1 teaspoonful is converted to 5 ml (see Table 5.1) and is read on the metric scale of the medicine cup. For home use, an oral syringe is recommended. If not available, a teaspoon used specifically for baking may be used as an accurate measuring device.

Oral Syringes. Plastic oral syringes (Fig. 5.11) may be used to measure liquid medications accurately. Various sizes are available to measure volumes from 0.1 ml to 15 ml.

Nipples. An infant feeding nipple (Fig. 5.12) with additional holes may be used for administering oral medications to infants. (See Techniques of Administration.)

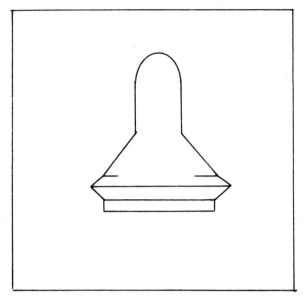

Fig. 5.12. *Nipple.*

Administration of Solid-Form Oral Medications

Technique

MEDICATION CARD SYSTEM
Equipment:
 Medication tray
 Soufflé cup or medicine cup
 Medication cards
1. Wash hands.
2. Gather medication cards and and verify against Kardex and/or physician's order for accuracy.
3. Gather remainder of equipment.
4. Read the entire medication card.
5. Obtain the medication prescribed from the cabinet.
6. COMPARE the label on the container against the medication card:
  RIGHT PATIENT
  RIGHT DRUG
  RIGHT ROUTE OF ADMINISTRATION
  RIGHT DOSAGE
  RIGHT TIME OF ADMINISTRATION
7. Open lid of the bottle; pour correct number of capsules or tablets into the lid; return any extras to the container using the lid. (DO NOT touch the medication with your hands!)
8. Transfer correct number of tablets or capsules from the lid to a soufflé cup or medicine cup.
9. COMPARE the information on the medication card against the label on the stock bottle and the quantity of drug placed in the cup.
10. Replace lid of container.

11. RECHECK the 5 RIGHTS of of the medication order.
12. Return the medication container to the shelf in the cabinet.
13. Place the patient's medication cup on the medication tray with the medication card directly behind the medication (Fig. 5.13).
14. Proceed to the patient's bedside when all medications are assembled for administration.
  —Check the patient's identification bracelet and verify against the medication card.
  —Explain what you are doing.
  —Check pertinent patient monitoring parameters (i.e., apical pulse, respiratory rate, etc.).
  —Hand medication to patient for placement in the mouth.

UNIT DOSE SYSTEM
Equipment:
 Medication cart
 Medication profile
1. Wash hands.
2. Read the patient medication profile for drugs and times of administration.
3. Obtain the medication prescribed from the drawer assigned to the patient in the medication cart.
4. Check the label on the unit dose package against the patient medication profile.
  RIGHT PATIENT
  RIGHT DRUG
  RIGHT ROUTE OF ADMINISTRATION

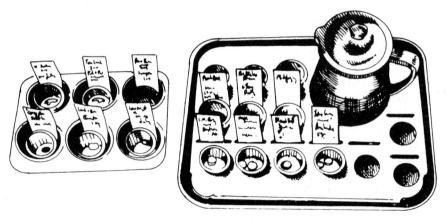

Fig. 5.13. *Tray for medication card system.*

RIGHT DOSAGE
RIGHT TIME OF ADMINISTRATION

5. Check the number of doses remaining in the drawer. (If the number of doses remaining is not consistent, investigate!)
6. Check the 5 RIGHTS of the medication order on the patient medication profile and unit dose package as removed from drawer.
7. Proceed to the bedside:
   —Check patient's identification bracelet and verify against the profile.
   —Explain what you are doing.
   —Check pertinent patient monitoring parameters (i.e., apical pulse, respiratory rate, etc.).
8. Hand the medication to the patient and allow him/ her to read the package label.
9. Retrieve the unit dose package and open it, placing the contents in the patient's hand for placement in the mouth.

General Principles of Solid-Form Medication Administration

1. Give the most important medication first.
2. Allow the patient to drink a small amount of water to moisten the mouth to make swallowing the medication easier.
3. Have the patient place the medication well back on the tongue. Offer appropriate assistance.
4. Give the patient liquid to swallow the medication. Encourage keeping the head forward while swallowing.
5. A full glass of fluid should be encouraged to ensure that the medication reaches the stomach and to dilute the drug to decrease the potential for irritation.
6. Always remain with the patient while the medication is taken. DO NOT leave the medication at the bed-

side unless an order exists to do so (medication such as nitroglycerin may be ordered for the bedside).
7. Discard the medication container (i.e., soufflé cup or unit dose package).

Documentation

Provide the RIGHT DOCUMENTATION of medication administration and responses to drug therapy:

1. Chart: Date, time, drug name, dosage, and route of administration.
2. Perform and record regular patient assessments for the evaluation of the therapeutic effectiveness (i.e., blood pressure, pulse, output, improvement or quality of cough and productivity, degree and duration of pain relief, etc.).
3. Chart and report any signs and symptoms of adverse drug effects.
4. Perform and validate essential patient education about the drug therapy and other essential aspects of intervention for the disease process affecting the individual.

Administration of Liquid-Form Oral Medications

Technique

MEDICATION CARD SYSTEM
Equipment:
   Medication tray
   Plastic syringe or medicine cup
   Medication cards
   1. Wash hands.
   2. Gather medication cards and and verify against Kardex and/or physician's order for accuracy.

3. Gather remainder of equipment.
4. Read the entire medication card.
5. Obtain the medication prescribed from the cabinet.
6. COMPARE the label on the container against the medication card:
   RIGHT PATIENT
   RIGHT DRUG
   RIGHT ROUTE OF ADMINISTRATION
   RIGHT DOSAGE
   RIGHT TIME OF ADMINISTRATION
7. Shake medication, if required.
8. Remove lid and place upside down on a flat surface to prevent contamination.
9. Proceed with one of the measuring techniques below:
   Measuring with a medicine cup:
   —Hold the bottle of liquid so that the label is in the palm of the hand. This prevents the contents from smearing the label during pouring.
   —Examine the medicine cup and locate the exact place to where the measured volume should be measured; place your fingernail at this level.
   —While holding the medicine cup straight at eye level, pour the prescribed volume.
   —Read the volume accurately at the level of the meniscus (Fig. 5.14).
   —COMPARE the information on the medication card against the label on the stock bottle and the quantity of drug placed in the cup.
   —Replace lid of container.
   —RECHECK the 5 RIGHTS of of the medication order.
   —Return the medication container to the shelf in the cabinet.

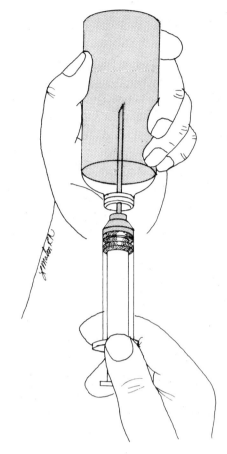

Fig. 5.15. *Removing medication directly from a bottle.*

—Place the patient's medication cup on the medication tray with the medication card directly behind the medication (Fig. 5.13).
—Proceed to the patient's bedside when all medications are assembled for administration.
Measuring in an oral syringe (see Chapter 6 for reading calibrations of a syringe):
—Select a syringe in a size comparable to the volume to be measured.
—*Method 1:* With a large bore needle attached to the syringe, draw up the prescribed volume of medication. The needle is not necessary if the bottle opening is large enough to receive the syringe (Fig. 5.15).
—*Method 2:* Using the cup and the method described above, pour the amount of medication needed into a medicine cup, then use a syringe to measure the prescribed volume (Fig. 5.16).
—COMPARE the information on the medication card against the label on the stock bottle and the volume of drug drawn into the syringe.

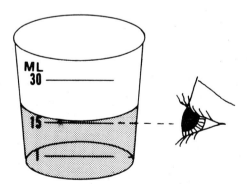

Fig. 5.14. *Reading meniscus. The meniscus is caused by the surface tension of the solution against the walls of the container. The surface tension causes the formation of a concave or hollowed curvature on the surface of the solution. Read the level at the lowest point of the concaved curve.*

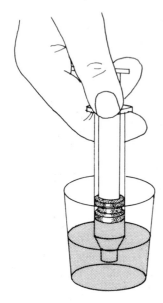

Fig. 5.16. *Filling a syringe directly from a medicine cup.*

—Replace the container lid.
—RECHECK the 5 RIGHTS of of the medication order.
—Return the medication container to the shelf of the cabinet.
—Place the patient's medication on the medication tray with the medication card directly under the syringe.
—Proceed to the patient's bedside when all medications are assembled for administration.
10. Check the patient's identification bracelet and verify against the medication card.
11. Explain what you are doing.
12. Check pertinent patient monitoring parameters (i.e., apical pulse, respiratory rate, etc.).
13. Hand medication cup to patient for placement of the contents in the mouth.

Unit Dose System
Equipment
    Medication cart
    Medication profile
1. Wash hands.
2. Read the patient medication profile for drugs and times of administration.
3. Obtain the medication prescribed from the drawer assigned to the patient in the medication cart.
4. Check the label on the unit dose package against the patient medication profile:
    RIGHT PATIENT
    RIGHT DRUG
    RIGHT ROUTE OF ADMINISTRATION
    RIGHT DOSAGE
    RIGHT TIME OF ADMINISTRATION

5. Check the number of doses remaining in the drawer. (If the number of doses remaining is not consistent, investigate!)
6. Check the 5 RIGHTS of the medication order on the patient medication profile and unit dose package as removed from drawer.
7. Proceed to the bedside:
    —Check patient's identification bracelet and verify against the profile.
    —Explain what you are doing.
    —Check pertinent patient monitoring parameters (i.e., apical pulse, respiratory rate, etc.).
8. Hand the medication to the patient and allow him/her to read the package label.
9. Retrieve the unit dose package and open it, placing the container in the patient's hand for placement of the contents in the patient's mouth.

General Principles of Liquid-Form Oral Medication Administration

For an adult or child:

1. Give the most important medication first.
2. Never dilute a liquid medication unless specifically ordered to do so.
3. Always remain with the patient while the medication is taken. DO NOT leave the medication at the bedside unless an order exists to do so.

For an infant:

1. Check the infant's identification bracelet and verify against the medication card or profile.
2. Be certain that the infant is alert.
3. Position the infant so that the head is slightly elevated (Fig. 5.17).
4. Administration:

Oral Syringe or Dropper

—Place the syringe or dropper between the cheek and gums, halfway back into the mouth. This placement will lessen the chance that the infant will spit out the medication with tongue movements.
—Slowly inject, allowing the infant to swallow medication. (Rapid administration may cause choking and aspiration!)

Nipple

—When the infant is awake (and preferably hungry), place the nipple in the infant's mouth. When the baby starts to suck, place the medication in the back of the nipple with a syringe or dropper

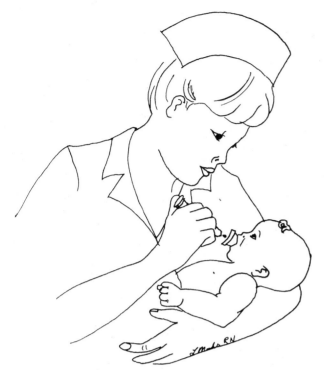

Fig. 5.17. *Position the infant in a "football hold" with the head slightly elevated. Place the nipple in the infant's mouth. When the baby starts to suck, place the medication in the back of the nipple and allow the baby to suck.*

and allow the baby to suck it in (Fig. 5.17). (The size of the nipple holes may need to be enlarged for suspensions and syrups.) Follow with milk or formula, if necessary.

Documentation

Provide the RIGHT DOCUMENTATION of the medication administration and responses to drug therapy:

1. Chart: Date, time, drug name, dosage, and route of administration.
2. Perform and record regular patient assessments for the evaluation of therapeutic effectiveness (i.e., blood pressure, pulse, output, improvement or quality of cough and productivity, degree and duration of pain relief, etc.).
3. Chart and report any signs and symptoms of adverse drug effects.
4. Perform and validate essential patient education about the drug therapy and other essential aspects of intervention for the disease process affecting the individual.

Administration of Medications by the Nasogastric Tube

Medications are administered via a nasogastric (NG) tube to patients who have impaired swallowing, are comatose, or have a disorder of the esophagus. Whenever possible, a liquid form of a drug should be used for NG administration. If it is necessary to use a tablet or capsule, the tablet should be crushed and the capsule pulled apart and the powder sprinkled in approximately 30 ml of water. (DO NOT crush enteric-coated tablets or timed-release capsules.)

Equipment

Glass of water
5 to 10 ml syringe (adult patient)
1 ml syringe (young child)
Stethoscope
Medication
Bulb syringe with catheter tip

Technique

Refer to the sections on the administration of solid-form or liquid-form oral medications for preparation of dosages.

1. Proceed to the patient's bedside when all medications are assembled for administration.
2. Check the patient's identification bracelet and verify against the medication card or drug profile.
3. Explain what you are going to do.
4. Sit the patient upright and check the location of the nasogastric tube before administering any liquid (Fig. 5.18).
   —*Method 1:* Aspirate part of the stomach contents using the bulb syringe (Fig. 5.18a). Return of stomach contents confirms correct tube placement. If contents are not returned, use methods 2, 3, and/or 4 to assess the location of the tube tip.
   —*Method 2:* Place a stethoscope over the stomach area; listen as 5 to 10 ml (adult) (0.5 up to 5 ml for child) of air are inserted (Fig. 5.18b). A gurgling sound should be heard if the nasogastric tube is properly placed. Withdraw the amount of air inserted. (Although a bulb syringe is frequently used to insert the air, a syringe with an adapter may also be used for more accurate measurement.)
   —*Method 3:* Place the unclamped NG tube next to the ear and listen for any crackling noise (Fig.

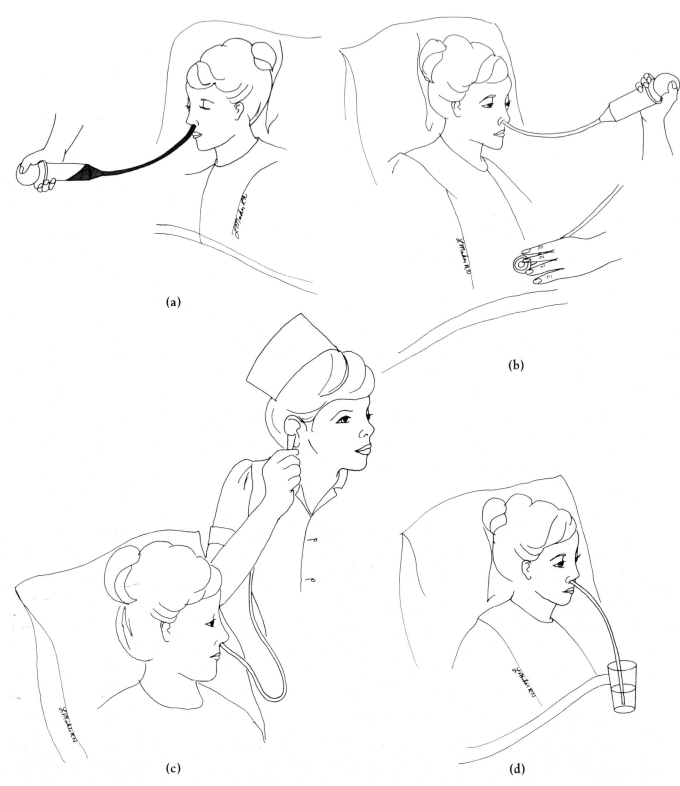

Fig. 5.18. *Checking the location of the nasogastric tube. (a) Aspiration of stomach contents. (b) Place a stethoscope over the stomach area; listen for a "gurgling" sound as air is inserted. (c) Listen for "crackling" sounds indicating placement of nasogastric tube in the lung. (d) Place the end of the nasogastric tube in a glass of water. Watch for bubbling with respirations, indicating placement of the tube in the lung.*

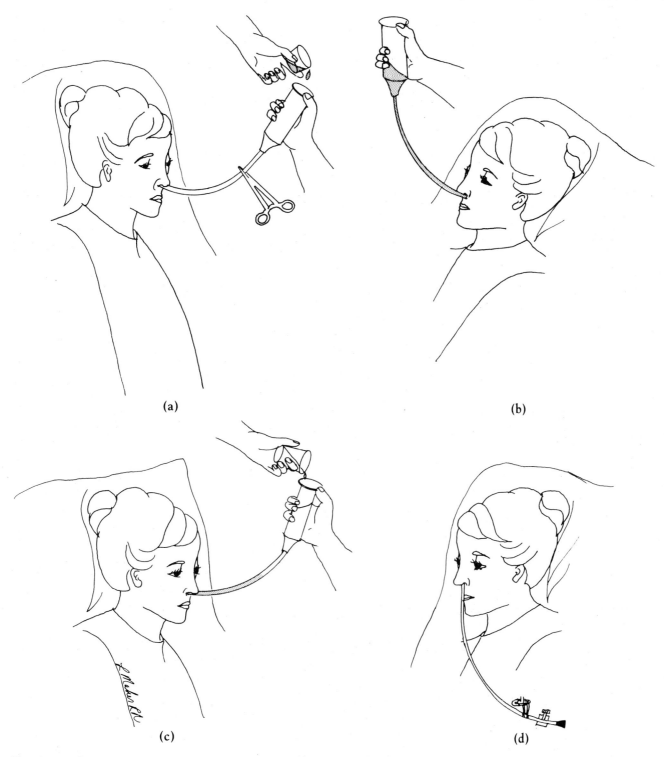

(a)

(b)

(c)

(d)

Fig. 5.19. *Administering medication via nasogastric tube. (a) Clamp nasogastric tube; attach a bulb syringe; and pour prescribed medication into syringe portion. (b) Unclamp tubing and allow the medication to flow in by gravity. (c) When medication is low in the syringe portion, pour in water to allow for thorough flushing of the medication from the tubing. (d) Clamp tubing and secure end in place. Do not reattach to suction (if being used) for at least 30 minutes.*

5.18c); if the crackling sounds are heard, the tube may be in the lung. Check method 4.

—*Method 4:* Place the end of the NG tube in a glass of water (Fig. 5.18d). Watch for bubbling with respirations which would indicate the nasogastric tube is in the lung, not in the stomach. If bubbling does occur, get assistance and/or replace the nasogastric tube correctly.

5. Once the placement of the NG tube in the stomach is confirmed
   —Clamp the tubing and attach the bulb syringe; pour the medication into the syringe while the tubing is still clamped (Fig. 5.19a).
   —Unclamp the tubing and allow the medication to run in by gravity (Fig. 5.19b); add the specified amount of water (at least 50 ml) (Fig. 5.19c) to flush the medication through the tube and into the stomach; clamp the tubing as soon as the water has flowed through the bulb syringe (Fig. 5.19d).
   —Clamp the tubing at the end of the medication administration. DO NOT attach to the suction source for at least 30 minutes, since the medication will be suctioned out.
   —Give oral hygiene, if needed.

Documentation

Provide the RIGHT DOCUMENTATION of medication administration and responses to drug therapy:

1. Chart: Date, time, drug name, dosage, and route of administration. Include all fluids administered on intake record.
2. Perform and record regular patient assessments for the evaluation of the therapeutic effectiveness (i.e., blood pressure, pulse, output, improvement or quality of cough and productivity, degree and duration of pain relief, etc.).
3. Chart and report any signs and symptoms of adverse drug effects.
4. Perform and validate essential patient education about the drug therapy and other essential aspects of intervention for the disease process affecting the individual.

Administration of Rectal Suppositories

Dosage Form

Suppositories (Fig. 5.20) are a solid form of medication designed for introduction into a body orifice. At body temperature, the substance dissolves and is absorbed by the mucous membranes. Suppositories should be stored in a cool place to prevent softening. If a suppository becomes soft and the package has not yet been opened, hold the foil-wrapped suppository under cold running water, or place in ice water for a short time until it hardens.

Equipment

Finger cot or disposable glove
Water-soluble lubricant

Technique

1. Wash hands and assemble the necessary equipment and the prescribed rectal suppository.
2. COMPARE the label on the container against the medication card or drug profile:
   RIGHT PATIENT
   RIGHT DRUG
   RIGHT ROUTE OF ADMINISTRATION
   RIGHT DOSAGE
   RIGHT TIME OF ADMINISTRATION
3. Proceed to the patient's bedside.
4. Check the patient's identification bracelet and verify against the medication card or drug profile.
5. Explain what you are going to do.
6. Check pertinent patient monitoring parameters (i.e., time of last defecation, severity of nausea or vomiting, respiratory rate, etc.) as appropriate to the medication to be administered.
7. Whenever possible, have the patient defecate.
8. Provide for patient privacy; position and drape to avoid unnecessary exposure (Fig. 5.21a).
9. Put on a disposable glove or finger cot (index finger for an adult; fourth finger for infants).
10. Ask the patient to bend the uppermost leg toward the waist.
11. Unwrap the suppository and apply a small amount of water-soluble lubricant to the tip of it. (If lubricant is not available, use plain water to moisten;

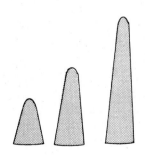

Fig. 5.20. *Rectal suppositories.*

DO NOT use Vaseline or mineral oil.) (Fig. 5.21b and c.)

12. Place the tip of the suppository at the rectal entrance and ask the patient to take a deep breath and exhale through the mouth (many patients will have an involuntary rectal gripping when the suppository is pressed against the rectum). Gently insert the suppository (Fig. 5.21d) about an inch beyond the orifice past the internal sphincter.

13. Ask the patient to remain lying on the side for 15 to 20 minutes to allow melting and absorption of the medication.

14. In children, it is necessary to gently but firmly compress the buttocks and hold in place for the same time period to prevent expulsion.

15. Discard used materials and wash hands thoroughly.

Documentation

Provide the RIGHT DOCUMENTATION of medication administration and responses to drug therapy:

1. Chart: Date, time, drug name, dosage, and route of administration.

2. Perform and record regular patient assessments for the evaluation of the therapeutic effectiveness (i.e., when given as a laxative, chart color, amount, and consistency of stool; if given for pain relief, chart the degree and duration of pain relief; if given as an antiemetic, the degree and duration of relief of nausea and/or vomiting).

3. Chart and report any signs and symptoms of adverse drug effects.

4. Perform and validate essential patient education about the drug therapy and other essential aspects of intervention for the disease process affecting the individual.

Administration of a Disposable Enema

Dosage Form

A prepackaged, disposable-type enema solution of the type prescribed by the physician.

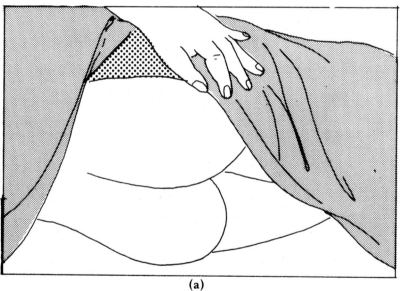

(a)

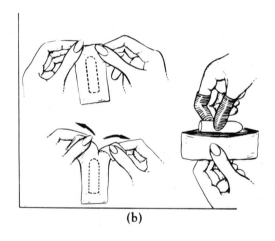

(b)

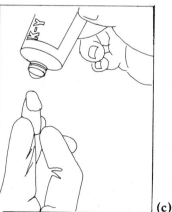

(c)

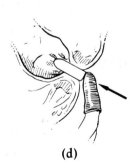

(d)

Fig. 5.21. *Administering a rectal suppository. (a) Position patient on side and drape. (b) Unwrap suppository and remove from package. (c) Apply water-soluble lubricant. (d) Gently insert suppository about an inch past the internal sphincter.*

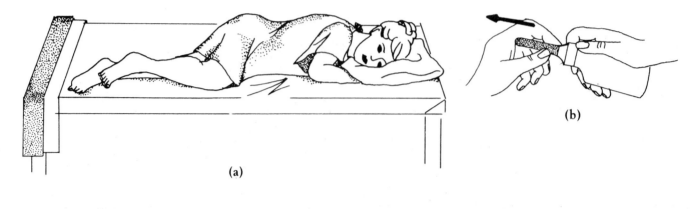

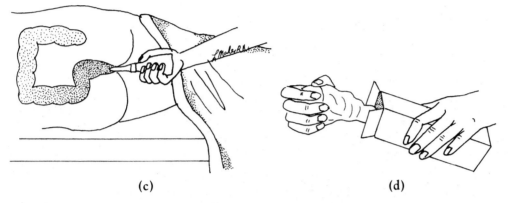

Fig. 5.22. *Administering a disposable enema (Fleet enema). (a) Place patient in a left lateral position, unless knee-chest position has been specified. (b) Remove protective covering from rectal tube and lubricate tube. (c) Insert lubricated rectal tube into rectum and dispense solution by compressing plastic container. (d) replace used container in original wrapping for disposal.*

Equipment

Toilet tissue
Bedpan, if patient is not ambulatory
Water-soluble lubricant
Prescribed disposable enema kit

Technique

1. Wash hands and assemble the necessary equipment and the prescribed rectal enema.
2. COMPARE the label on the container against the medication card or drug profile:
   RIGHT PATIENT
   RIGHT DRUG
   RIGHT ROUTE OF ADMINISTRATION
   RIGHT DOSAGE
   RIGHT TIME OF ADMINISTRATION
3. Proceed to the patient's bedside.
4. Check the patient's identification bracelet and verify against the medication card or drug profile.
5. Explain what you are going to do.
6. Check pertinent patient monitoring parameters (i.e., time of last defecation).

7. Provide for patient privacy; position patient on left side; drape to avoid unnecessary exposure (Fig. 5.22a).
8. Remove protective covering from the rectal tube and lubricate (Fig. 5.22b).
9. Insert lubricated rectal tube into the rectum and insert solution by compressing plastic container (Fig. 5.22c).
10. Replace used container in its original container for disposal (Fig. 5.22d).
11. Encourage the patient to hold the solution for a short period of time (30 minutes) before defecating.
12. Assist the patient to a sitting position on the bedpan or to the bathroom, as orders permit.
13. Tell the patient NOT to flush the toilet until you return and can see the results of the enema. Instruct the patient regarding the location of the call light in case assistance is needed.
14. Wash hands thoroughly.

Documentation

Provide the RIGHT DOCUMENTATION of medication administration and responses to drug therapy:

1. Chart: Date, time, drug name, dosage, and route of administration.
2. Perform and record regular patient assessments for the evaluation of the therapeutic effectiveness (i.e., color, amount, and consistency of stool).
3. Chart and report any signs and symptoms of adverse drug effects.
4. Perform and validate essential patient education about the drug therapy and other essential aspects of intervention for the disease process affecting the individual.

Chapter 6

Preparation and Administration of Medications by the Parenteral Routes

Objectives

After completing this chapter, the student should be able to do the following:

1. Cite advantages and disadvantages of using the intradermal, subcutaneous, intramuscular, and intravenous drug administration routes.
2. Read the calibrations of the minim, cubic centimeter, or milliliter scales on different types of syringes.
3. Explain the calibration and use of an insulin syringe.
4. Differentiate between the points where the volume of medication is read on a glass or plastic syringe.
5. Give examples of volumes of medication that can best be measured in a tuberculin syringe, rather than a larger volume syringe.
6. State the advantages and disadvantages of using prefilled syringes.
7. Explain the system of measurement used to define the inside diameter of a syringe.
8. Compare the usual volume of medication that can be administered at one site when giving a drug by the intradermal, subcutaneous, or intramuscular routes.
9. State the criteria used for the selection of the correct needle gauge and length.
10. Differentiate between the techniques for preparing drugs using ampules, vials, and Mix-O-Vials.
11. Practice and perfect the preparation of medications using the various dosage forms for parenteral administration.
12. Practice and perfect the technique of preparing two different drugs in one syringe, such as insulins or preoperative medications.
13. Use the procedures and principles cited for the preparation and administration of intradermal, subcutaneous, intramuscular, or intravenous medications.

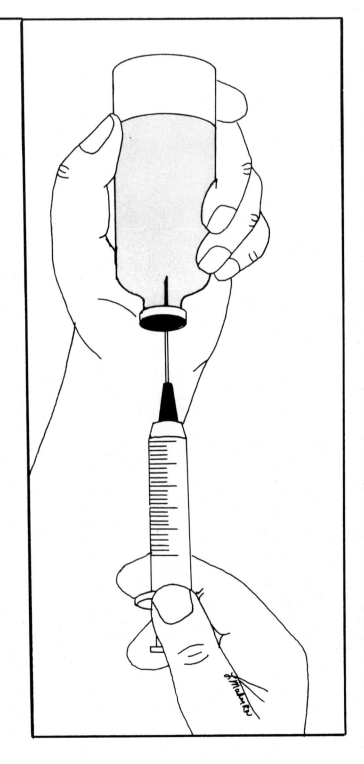

The routes of drug administration may be classified into three categories: the enteral, the parenteral, and the percutaneous routes. The term *parenteral* means administration by any route other than the enteral, or gastrointestinal, tract. Technically, this definition could include topical or inhalation administration. However, as ordinarily used, *parenteral route* refers to intradermal, subcutaneous, intramuscular, or intravenous injections.

When drugs are given parenterally rather than orally, (1) the onset of drug action is generally more rapid but of shorter duration, (2) the dosage is often smaller, since drug potency tends not to be immediately altered by the stomach or liver, and (3) the cost of drug therapy is often greater. Drugs are administered by injection when it is important that all of the drug be absorbed as rapidly and completely as possible or at a steady, controlled rate, or when a patient is unable to take a medication orally because of nausea and vomiting.

Injection of drugs requires skill and special care because of the trauma at the site of needle puncture, the possibility of infection, the chance of allergic reaction, and because once it is injected, the drug is irretrievable. Therefore, it is important that medications are prepared and administered carefully and accurately. Precautions must be taken to assure that (1) aseptic technique is used to avoid infection and (2) accurate drug dosage, proper rate of injection and proper site of injection is used to avoid harm such as abscesses, necrosis, skin sloughing, nerve injuries, prolonged pain, or periosteitis. Thus, parenteral administration of drugs requires specialized knowledge and manual skill to ensure safety and therapeutic effectiveness.

Equipment Used in Parenteral Administration

Syringes

The syringe (Fig. 6.1) has three parts:
—The *barrel* is the outer portion on which the calibrations for the measurement of the drug volume are located (Fig. 6.2).
—The *plunger* is the inner, cylindrical portion that fits snugly into the barrel. This portion is used to draw up and eject the solution from the syringe.

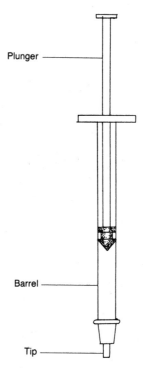

Fig. 6.1. *Parts of a syringe.*

—The *tip* is the portion that holds the needle. There are two types of tips, the plain tip and the Luer-Lok.

Syringes are made of glass or a hard plastic material. Each type has advantage and disadvantages to use.

Glass Syringes. Advantages of the glass syringe include economy, easy-to-read calibrations, and availability in a wide range of sizes. In addition, they can be cleaned, packaged, sterilized, and reused. Disadvantages of the glass syringe are that it is easily breakable, time-consuming to clean and resterilize, and that the plunger may become loose with extended use, which causes medication to "creep" between the plunger and the barrel. This results in an inaccurate dose being administered to the patient.

Plastic Syringes. Advantages of the plastic syringe include availability in a wide range of sizes, prepackaging with and without needles in a wide variety of gauges and needle lengths, disposability, and convenience. Disadvantages of the plastic syringe include expense,

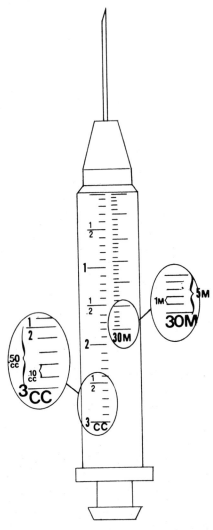

Fig. 6.2. *Reading the calibrations of a 3 cc syringe.*

one-time use, and, in some instances, the unclear calibrations.

Syringe Calibration

The syringe is calibrated in *minims* (ɱ) and *milliliters* (ml) or *cubic centimeters* (cc) (Fig. 6.2). The most commonly used syringes are 1, 3, and 5 cc syringes, but 10, 20, and 50 cc syringes are also available. (*Note:* Technically, millimeter is a measure of volume, while cubic centimeter is a three-dimensional measure of space. Even though it is technically inappropriate, many syringes are labeled in "cc" rather than "ml.")

Reading the Calibration of the Syringe

Minim Scale (ɱ). Using Figure 6.2 as a guide, note that 1 minim is indicated by *each* smaller line on the calibrated scale marked (ɱ). Each of the longer lines

on the scale equals 5 minims. Remember that 16 minims equals 1 ml or 1 cc.

Milliliter Scale (ml). Milliliters (or cubic centimeters) are read on the scale marked ml or cc (Figs. 6.2 and 6.4). The shorter lines represent 0.1 cc. The longer lines on this scale each represent 0.5 cc (1 ml = 1 cc).

Insulin Syringe. The insulin syringe has a scale specifically calibrated for the measurement of insulin. The most commonly used size is U-100 since most insulin is now manufactured in this concentration. However, some patients may still be using insulin in the 40 unit per ml (U-40) concentration and these individuals need to use the syringe that corresponds to this concentration.

The U-100 syringe (Fig. 6.3a) holds 100 units of insulin per cc. On the scale, the shorter lines represent 2 units measured, while the longer lines measure 10 units of insulin. Low-dose insulin syringes (Fig. 6.3b) may be used for patients receiving 50 units or less of U-100 insulin. The shorter lines on the scale of the low-dose insulin syringe measure 1 unit, while the longer lines each represent 5 units.

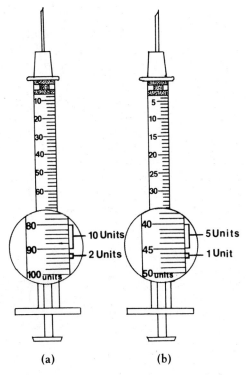

Fig. 6.3. *Calibration of (a) U-100 insulin syringe and (b) low-dose insulin syringe.*

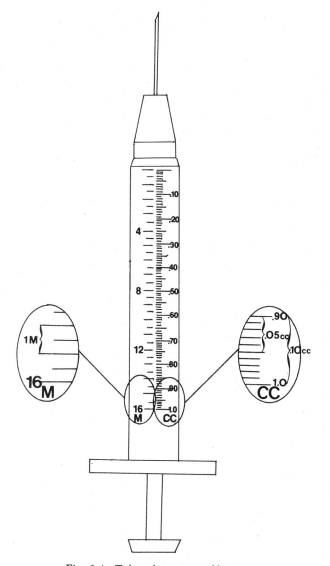

Fig. 6.4. *Tuberculin syringe calibration.*

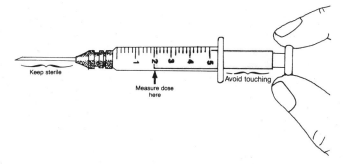

Fig. 6.5. *Reading measured amount of medication in a glass syringe.*

disposable plastic syringes are read at the point where the rubber flange of the syringe plunger is parallel to the calibration scale of the barrel (Fig. 6.6). Also note the area of the needle to keep sterile and the area on the syringe plunger to avoid touching.

Prefilled Syringes

There are several manufacturers that supply a premeasured amount of medication in a disposable cartridge-needle unit. These units are called by brand names such as Tubex and Carpuject. The cartridge contains the amount of drug for one standard dose of medication. The drug name, concentration, and volume are clearly printed on the cartridge. Certain brands of prefilled cartridges require a holder that corresponds to the type of cartridge being used (Fig. 6.7a,b). Advantages of the prefilled syringe include the time saved in preparation of a standard amount of medication for one injection and the diminished chance of contamination between patient and hospital personnel, since the cartridge is in a sealed unit, used once, and discarded. Disadvantages include additional expense, the need for different holders for different cartridges, and the limitation of the volume of a second medication that may be added to the cartridge.

Tuberculin Syringe. The tuberculin syringe (Fig. 6-4) was originally designed to administer tuberculin. Today it is used to accurately measure small volumes of medication. The volume may be measured on either the cubic centimeter or minim scale, depending on how the medication was ordered. The syringe holds a total of 1 cc or 16 minims. On the minim scale, the longer lines represent 1 minim, while the shorter lines measure 0.5 (5/10 or 1/2) minim. On the cubic centimeter scale, each of the longest lines represents 0.1 (1/10) cc, the intermediate lines equal 0.05 (5/100) cc, and the shortest lines are 0.01 (1/100) cc.

The volumes within glass syringes are read at the point where the plunger is directly parallel with the calibration on the syringe (Fig. 6.5). Volumes within

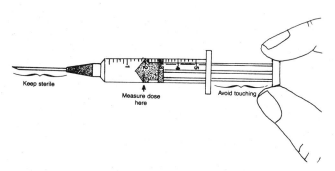

Fig. 6.6. *Reading measured amount of medication in a plastic syringe.*

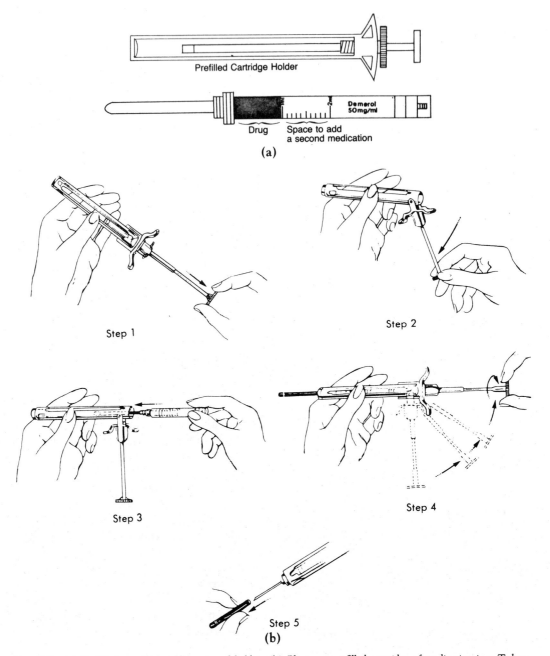

Fig. 6.7. (a) *Prefilled cartridge-needle unit and holder.* (b) *Placing a prefilled cartridge of medication in a Tubex.*

The Needle

Parts of the Needle. The needle parts (Fig. 6.8) are the hub, shaft, and beveled tip. The angle of the bevel can vary; the longer the bevel, the easier the needle penetration.

Needle Gauge. The needle gauge is the diameter of the hole through the needle. The larger the number (which indicates the gauge), the smaller the hole. The gauge number is marked on the hub of the needle as well as on the outside of the disposable package. The proper needle gauge is usually selected based upon the viscosity (thickness) of the solution to be injected. A thicker solution requires a larger diameter; thus, a smaller gauge number is chosen (Fig. 6.9).

Needles for Intravenous Administration. All needles, if long enough, may be used to administer medications or fluids intravenously, but special equipment has been designed for this purpose.

The *butterfly, scalp,* and *wing-tipped* needles (Fig. 6.10) are short, sharp-tipped needles designed to minimize tissue injury during insertion. The "winged" area can be pinched together to form a handle while the needle is being inserted, then laid flat against the skin to form a base for anchoring with tape. These needles

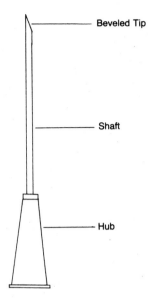

Fig. 6.8. *Parts of a needle.*

come in gauges 17–27. A short plastic tubing with a plastic adapter at the end is attached to the needle. Butterfly needles are commonly used for venipuncture in infants and as "heparin locks" to allow patient mobility.

Plastic needles or *over-the-catheter* needles (Fig. 6.11a) are actually stainless steel needles coated with a teflonlike plastic. After penetrating the vein, the metal needle is removed, leaving the plastic catheter in place. This unit is used when intravenous therapy is expected to continue for several days or more. The rationale for use of the plastic catheter is that it does not have a sharp tip that may cause venous irritation and extravasation.

Intracatheters (Fig. 6.11b) use a large-bore needle for venipuncture. Then a 4–6-inch sterile, smaller-gauge plastic catheter is advanced through the needle into the vein. The needle is withdrawn and the skin

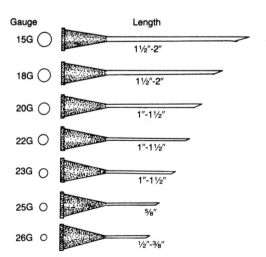

Fig. 6.9. *Needle length and gauge.*

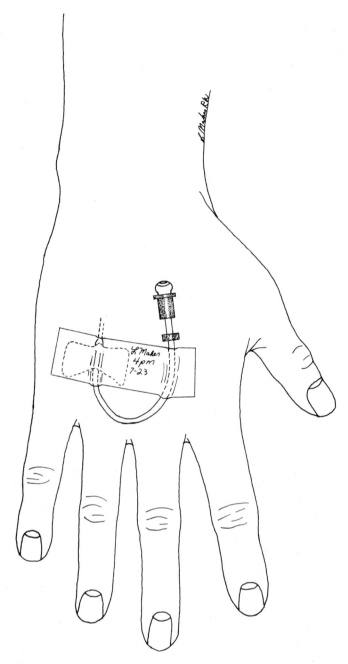

Fig. 6.10. *Butterfly, scalp, or wing-tipped needle in place as a heparin lock.*

forms a seal around the plastic catheter. The intravenous administration set is attached directly to the plastic catheter. This type of catheter is often used for hyperalimentation solutions and for IVs that will be running for a week or more.

Selection of the Syringe and Needle

The size of the syringe used is determined by the volume of medication to be administered, the degree of accuracy needed in measurement of the dose, and the type of medication to be administered.

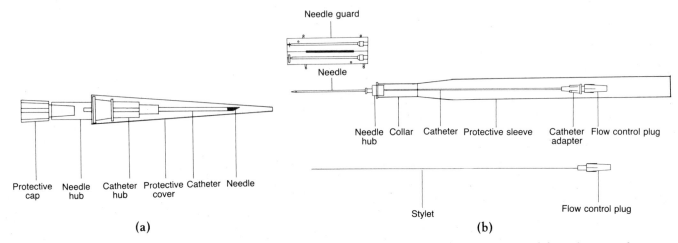

Fig. 6.11. (a) *Over-the-needle catheter. This unit is used when intravenous therapy is expected to continue several days.* (b) *Intracatheters use a large-bore needle for venipuncture, then a 4–6-inch sterile, small gauge plastic catheter is advanced through the needle into the vein. The needle is withdrawn and the skin forms a seal around the plastic catheter.*

Needle selection should be based upon the correct gauge for the viscosity of the solution, and the correct needle length for delivery of the medication to the correct site (i.e., subcutaneous, intramuscular, or intravenous). Table 6.1 may be used as a guideline to select the proper volume of syringe and length and gauge of needle for adult patients.

In small children and older infants, the usual maximum volume for intramuscular injection at one site is 1 ml. In small infants the muscle mass may only be able to tolerate 0.5 (5/10 or 1/2) ml. For older children, the amount should be individualized; generally, the larger the muscle mass, the greater the similarity to the adult volume for one injection site. Pediatric intramuscular injections routinely use a 25–27 gauge needle 1–1½ inches long, depending on assessment of the depth of the muscle mass in the child.

Clinical Example: Selection of Needle Length. Assess the depth of the patient's tissue for administration (muscle tissue for intramuscular administration, subcutaneous tissue for subcutaneous injection) and then choose a needle length to correspond with the findings.

EXAMPLE: Compare the muscle depth of a 250-lb obese, sedentary female to the muscle depth of a 105-lb debilitated adult patient. The obese individual may require a 3–5-inch needle, the frail person a 1–1½ inch needle. A child may need a 1 inch needle (Fig. 6.12).

Packaging of Syringes and Needles

Always inspect and verify the sterility of the syringe and needle to be used to prepare and administer a parenteral medication. Check cloth wrappers for holes,

Table 6.1
Selection of Syringe and Needles

ROUTE	VOLUME	GAUGE	LENGTH
Intradermal	0.01–0.1 ml	25–27 g	⅜–½ inch
Subcutaneous	0.5–2 ml	25–27 g	Individualize based on depth of appropriate tissue at site of injection.†
Intramuscular	0.5–2 ml*	20–22 g	
Intravenous	1–2000 ml	20–22 g (solutions) 15–19 g (blood)	½–1¼ inch (butterfly) ½–2 inch (regular needles)

* Divided doses are generally recommended for volumes that exceed 2–3 ml, particularly for medications that are irritating to the tissues.

† When judging the needle length, allow an extra ¼–½-inch length to remain above the skin surface when the injection is administered. In the rare event of a needle breaking, this allows a length of needle to protrude above the skin to grasp for removal.

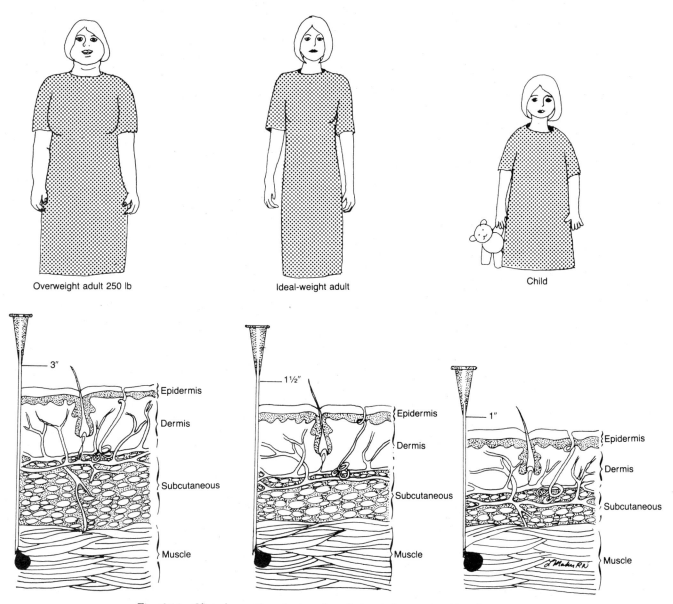

Fig. 6.12. *Clinical example: selection of needle length for intramuscular administration.*

signs of moisture penetrating the wrapper, and the date of expiration. With prepackaged disposable items, check for continuity of the wrapper, loose lids or needle guards, and for any penetration of the paper or plastic container by the needle.

Intravenous Administration Sets. Intravenous administration sets (Fig. 6.13a,b,c) are available with a variety of attachments (i.e., volume and size of drip chamber, "piggyback" portals, filters, drug administration chamber, clamps or rollers), but all sets have an insertion spike, a drip chamber, plastic tubing with a control clamp, a rubber injection portal, a needle

adapter, and a protective cap over the needle adapter. The type of system used by a particular hospital is usually determined by the manufacturer of the physiologic solutions used by the institution. Each manufacturer makes adaptations to fit a specific type of glass or plastic large-volume solution container. A crucial point to remember about administration sets is that the drops delivered by drip chambers vary between different manufacturers. Macrodrip chambers (Fig. 6.13a,c) provide 10, 15 or 20 drop/ml, while microdrip chambers (Fig. 6.13b) deliver 60 drops/ml of solution. It is essential to read the label of the box before opening it.

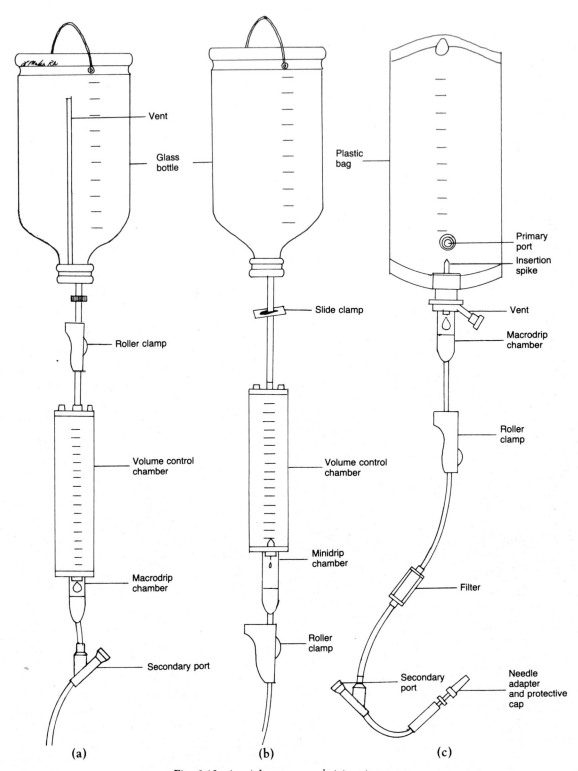

Fig. 6.13. (a–c) *Intravenous administration sets.*

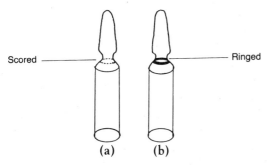

Fig. 6.14. *(a) scored and (b) ringed ampules.*

Parenteral Dosage Forms

All parenteral drug dosage forms are packaged so that the drug is sterile and ready for reconstitution (if needed) and administration.

Ampules

Ampules are glass containers that usually contain a single dose of a medication. The container may be scored (Fig. 6.14a) or have a darkened ring around the neck (Fig. 6.14b). This marking is the location at which the ampule is broken open for withdrawing the medication.

Vials

Vials are glass containers that contain one or more doses of a sterile medication. The mouth of the vial is covered with a thick rubber diaphragm (Fig. 6.15b) through which a needle must be passed to remove the medication. Prior to use, the rubber diaphragm is sealed by a metal lid (Fig. 6.15a) to insure sterility. The medication in the vial may be in solution, or may be a sterile powder to be reconstituted just prior to the time of administration.

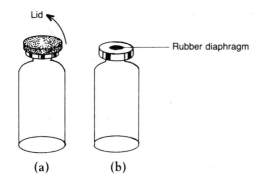

Fig. 6.15. *(a) metal lid and (b) rubber diaphragm vials.*

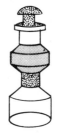

Fig. 6.16. *Mix-O-Vial.*

Mix-O-Vials

Mix-O-Vials are glass containers with two compartments (Fig. 6.16). The lower chamber contains the drug (solute) and the upper chamber contains a sterile diluent (solvent). Between the two areas is a rubber stopper. A single dose of medication is normally contained in the Mix-O-Vial. At the time of use, pressure is applied on the top rubber diaphragm plunger. This forces the solvent and the rubber stopper to fall into the bottom chamber, dissolving the drug. A needle is then placed through the top plunger-diaphragm to withdraw the solution. (Change the needle after drug withdrawal since puncturing the plunger-diaphragm may dull the needle bevel.)

Large Volume Solution Containers

Intravenous solutions are available in both glass and plastic containers in a variety of types and concentrations (Table 6.2) and volumes ranging from 100 to 2000 ml. Both the glass and plastic containers are vacuum sealed. The glass bottles are sealed with a hard rubber stopper, then a metal disk, followed by a metal cap. Just before use, the metal cap and disk are removed, exposing the hard rubber stopper. The insertion spike of the IV administration set is pushed into a specifically marked area on the rubber stopper. Some brands also have another opening in the rubber stopper that serves as an air vent. Other brands locate the air vent on the administration set (Fig. 6.13c). As the solution runs out of the container, it is replaced with air.

Plastic bags are somewhat different in that the entire bag and solution is sealed inside another plastic bag for removal just before administration. When the insertion spike is forced into the specifically marked portal, an internal seal is broken, allowing the solution to flow into the tubing.

Some drugs, such as antibiotics, are administered by intermittent infusion through an apparatus known as a *tandem setup, piggyback* (IVPB), or *IV rider* (Fig. 6.17). They are given by a setup that is secondary to the primary IV infusion and that is hung in tandem

Table 6.2
*Types of Intravenous Solutions**

SOLUTION	INGREDIENTS	ABBREVIATION
Electrolyte solutions	5% Dextrose in water	D5W
	10% Dextrose in water	D10W
	0.9% Sodium chloride (Normal Saline)	N.S.
	Ringer's lactate	R.L.
	5% Dextrose in 0.2% sodium chloride	D5/.2
	5% Dextrose in 0.45% sodium chloride	D5/.45
	5% Dextrose in Ringer's Lactate	D5/LR
Nutrient solutions		
Carbohydrate	Dextrose 5–25%	D5–25
Amino acids	Novamine	
	Travasol	
	Nephramine	
Lipids	Intralipid	
	Liposyn	
Blood volume	Hetastarch	
expanders	Dextran	
	Albumin	
	Plasma	
Alkalinizing solutions	Sodium bicarbonate	
	Tromethamine (THAM)	
	Lactate solutions	
Acidifying solutions	Ammonium chloride	

* A representative listing, not intended to be inclusive.

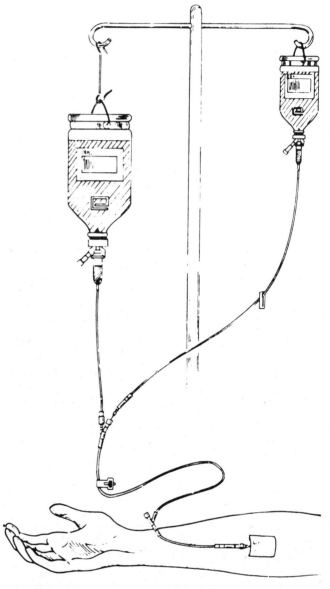

Fig. 6.17. *Tandem, secondary, or "piggyback" intermittent administration setup. This illustrated a "piggyback" setup. Note that the smaller bottle is hung higher than the primary bottle.*

and connected to the primary setup. The secondary setup may consist of a drug infusion from a small volume of fluid in either a small bag or bottle (up to 250 ml) (Fig. 6.17) or from a volume-control set (also known as a Volutrol, Pediatrol, or Buretrol) (Fig. 6.13a,b). A volume-control set is made up of a calibrated chamber hung under the primary IV solution container that can provide the necessary 50–250 ml of diluent per dose of drug. Most intermittent diluted drug infusions are infused over 20–60 minutes.

Preparation of Parenteral Medication

Equipment

Drug in sterile, sealed container
Syringe of the correct volume
Needles of the correct gauge and length
Antiseptic swab
Special equipment based on the route of administration (i.e., heparin lock for insertion, IV administration set for starting intravenous infusion)

Technique

These are standard procedures for preparing all parenteral medications:

1. Wash hands *before* proceeding to prepare any medication or handling of sterile supplies. During the actual preparation of a parenteral medication, the primary rule is "sterile-to-sterile and unsterile-to-unsterile" when handling the syringe and needle.
2. Use the 5 RIGHTS of medication preparation and administration throughout the procedure:

RIGHT PATIENT
RIGHT DRUG
RIGHT ROUTE OF ADMINISTRATION
RIGHT DOSAGE (AMOUNT AND CON-
CENTRATION)
RIGHT TIME OF ADMINISTRATION

3. Check the drug dosage form ordered against the source you are holding to prepare.
4. Check compatibility charts or contact the pharmacist before mixing two medications or adding medication to an intravenous solution.
5. Check medication calculations. When in doubt about a dose, check it with another qualified nurse. (Most hospital policies require that fractional doses of medications and doses of heparin and insulin be checked by two qualified personnel prior to administration.)
6. Be knowledgeable of the hospital policy regarding limitations on the types of medications to be administered by nursing personnel.
7. Prepare the drug in a clean, well-lighted area, using aseptic technique throughout the entire procedure.
8. Concentrate on this procedure; assure accuracy in preparation.

Guidelines for Preparing Medications

To prepare a medication from an *ampule*:

1. Move all of the solution to the bottom of the ampule, flicking the side of the glass container with the fingers to displace the medication from the top portion of the ampule (Fig. 6.18a).
2. Cover the ampule neck area with a sterile gauze pledget or antiseptic swab while breaking the top off (Fig. 6.18b). Discard the swab and top.
3. Using an aspiration (filter) needle (Fig. 6.18c), withdraw the medication from the ampule (Fig. 6.18d,e).
4. Remove the aspiration needle from the ampule and point the needle vertically (Fig. 6.18f). Pull back on the plunger (this allows air to enter the syringe) (Fig. 6.18g) and replace the filter needle with a new sterile needle (Fig. 6.18h,i) of the appropriate gauge and length for administration.
5. Push the plunger slowly until the medication appears at the tip of the needle (Fig. 6.18j); or measure the amount of air to be included to allow total clearance of the medication from the needle when injected. (Never add air to a syringe that is to be used to administer an intravenous medication.)

Drugs in a *vial* may be in solution ready for administration (Fig. 6.19) or may be in a powdered form for reconstitution prior to administration. To prepare medication from a vial:

A. *Reconstitution of a sterile powder*
   1. Read the accompanying literature from the manufacturer and follow specific instructions for reconstituting the drug ordered. Add only the diluent specified by the manufacturer.
   2. Cleanse the rubber diaphragm of the vial of diluent with an antiseptic swab (Fig. 6.19a).
   3. Pull back on the plunger of the syringe to fill with an amount of air equal to the volume of solution to be withdrawn (Fig. 6.19b).
   4. Insert the needle through the rubber diaphragm; inject air (Fig. 6.19c).
   5. Withdraw the measured volume of diluent required to reconstitute the powdered drug (Fig. 6.19d,e). Remove the needle from the diaphragm of the diluent container.
   6. Recheck the type and volume of diluent to be injected against the type and amount required.
   7. Remove the needle and replace with a new, sterile needle (use principles illustrated in Fig. 6.18 h,i,j). Tap the vial containing the powdered drug to break up the caked powder (Fig. 6.19f). Wipe the rubber diaphragm of the vial of powdered drug with a new antiseptic swab (Fig. 6.19g).
   8. Insert the needle in the diaphragm and inject the diluent into the powder (Fig. 6.19h).
   9. Remove the syringe and needle from the rubber diaphragm.
   10. MIX THOROUGHLY to ensure that the powder is entirely dissolved BEFORE withdrawing the dose (Fig. 6.19i).
   11. Label the reconstituted medication:
       • Date, time of reconstitution
       • Volume and type of diluent added
       • Name of reconstituted drug
       • Concentration of reconstituted drug
       • Expiration date and time
       • Name of person reconstituting drug
       Store according to manufacturer's instructions.
   12. Change the needle as described before. Attach a needle of the correct gauge and length to administer the medication to the patient.

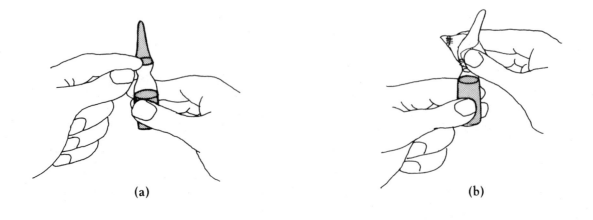

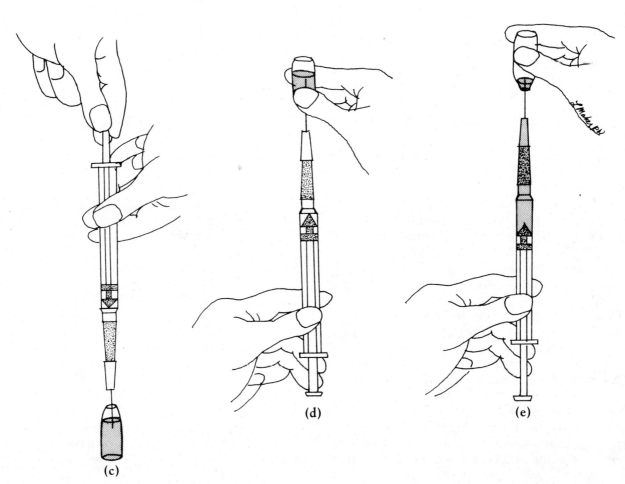

Fig. 6.18. *Withdrawing from an ampule and changing needle. (a) Displace medication from top portion of ampule. (b) Cover ampule neck area with gauze sponge while breaking top off. (c) Filter needle. (d) Withdraw medication from ampule. (e) Note that needle must be lowered to withdraw all solution from ampule.*

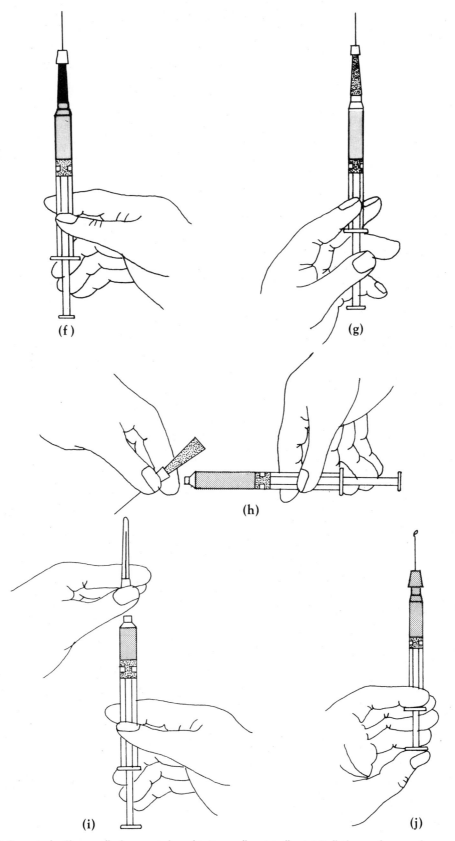

Fig. 6.18. (cont.). *(f) Remove the filter needle from ampule and point needle vertically. (g) Pull plunger downward to remove drug from needle. (h) Remove filter needle. (i) Replace filter needle with correct size needle for administering medication. (j) Slowly push plunger until a drop of medication appears at needle tip. Recheck medication prepared against drug order.*

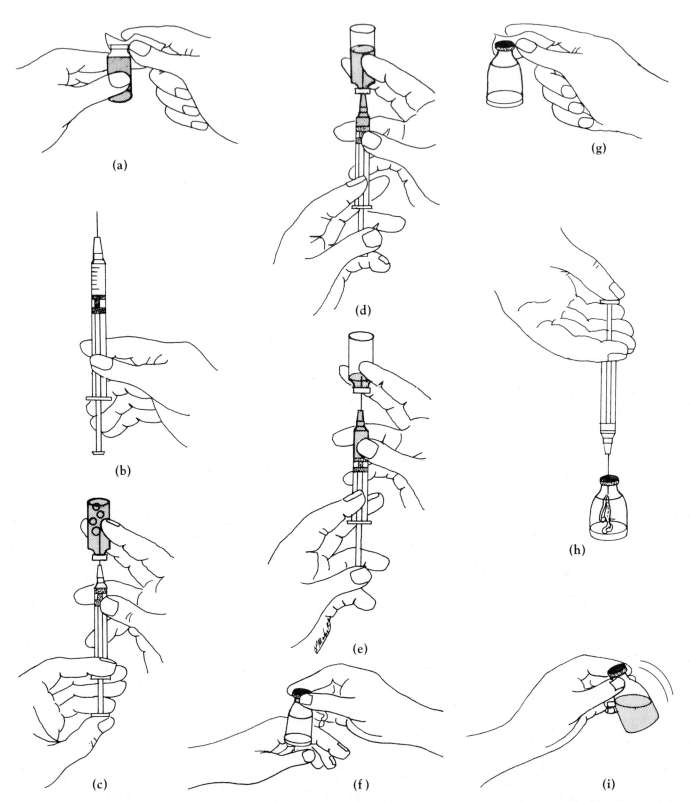

Fig. 6.19. *Removal of a volume of liquid from a vial. (a) Cleanse rubber diaphragm of the vial. (b) Pull back on plunger of syringe to fill with an amount of air equal to the volume of solution to be withdrawn. (c) Insert the needle through the rubber diaphragm; inject air. (d) withdraw the volume of diluent required to reconstitute the drug. (e) Move needle downward to facilitate removal of diluent. Change the needle as illustrated in Fig. 6.18h, i, j. (f) Tap the container with the powdered drug to break up the "caked" powder. (g) Wipe the rubber diaphragm of the vial of powdered drug with a new antiseptic swab. (h) Insert the needle in the rubber diaphragm and inject the diluent into the powdered drug. (i) Mix thoroughly to ensure the powdered drug is dissolved prior to withdrawing the prescribed dose.*

94

*B. Removal of a volume of liquid from
   a vial (Fig. 6.19a–e):*

1. Calculate the volume of medication required
   for the prescribed dose of medication to be
   administered.
2. Cleanse the rubber diaphragm of the vial
   of diluent with an antiseptic pledget.
3. Pull back on the plunger of the syringe to
   fill with an amount of air equal to the volume
   of solution to be withdrawn.
4. Insert the needle through the rubber diaphragm; inject air.
5. Withdraw the volume of drug required to
   administer the prescribed dosage.
6. Recheck all aspects of the drug order.
7. Change the needle as described before. Attach a needle of the correct gauge and length
   to administer the medication to the patient.

To prepare a drug from a *Mix-O-Vial:*

1. Check the drug order against the medication you
   have for administration.
2. To mix:
   —Tap the container in the hand a few times to
   break up the caked powder.
   —Remove the plastic lid protector (Fig. 6.20a).

—Push firmly on the diaphragm-plunger. The
   downward pressure dislodges the divider between
   the two chambers (Fig. 6.20b,c).
—Mix thoroughly to ensure that the powder is
   COMPLETELY DISSOLVED before drawing up
   the medication for administration.
—Cleanse the rubber diaphragm and remove the
   drug in the same manner as described for removal
   of a volume of liquid from a vial (see Fig. 6.19a–
   e).

Preparing Two Medications in One Syringe.
Occasionally two medications may be drawn into the
same syringe for a single injection. This is most commonly done when preparing a preoperative medication
or when two types of insulin are ordered to be administered at the same time. Since mixing insulins is
a routine procedure, it will be used to illustrate the
technique (Fig. 6.21).

1. Check the compatibility of the two drugs to be
   mixed before starting to prepare the medications.
2. Check the labels of the medications against the
   medications order.
3. Check
   Type: NPH, Regular, Lente, other
   Concentration: U-100 is most common
   Expiration Date: DO NOT use if outdated

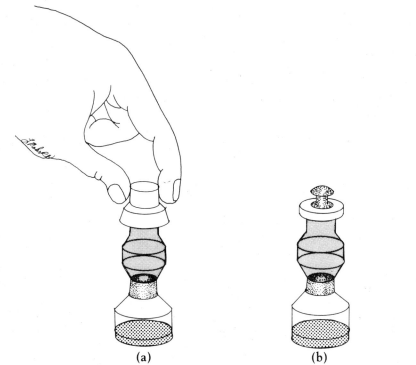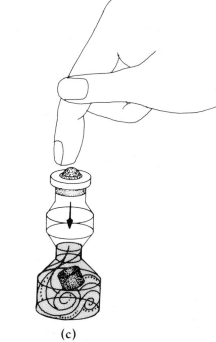

(a)   (b)   (c)

Fig. 6.20. *Mix-O-Vial. (a) Remove plastic lid protector. (b) Powdered drug is in lower half; diluent is in upper half. (c) Push firmly on the diaphragm-plunger. Downward pressure dislodges the divider between the two chambers.*

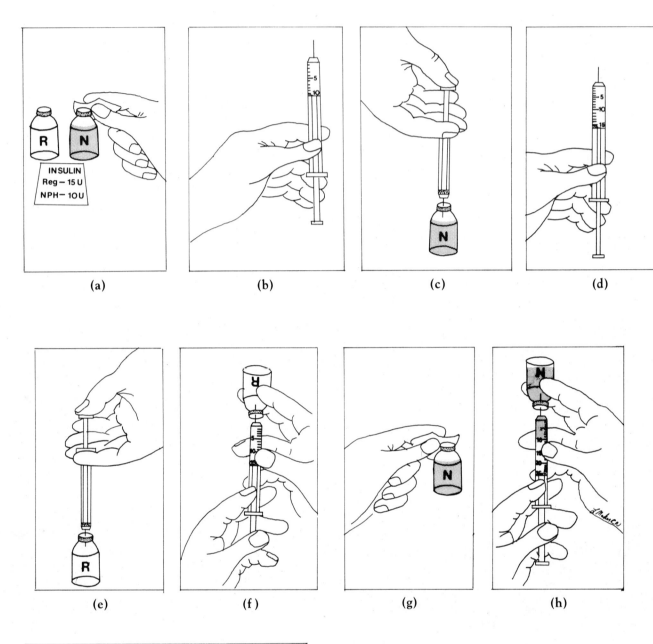

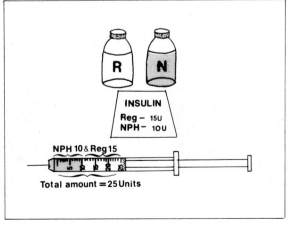

(a)   **(b)**   **(c)**   **(d)**

(e)   **(f)**   **(g)**   **(h)**

(i)

Fig. 6.21. *Preparing two drugs in one syringe. (a) Check insulin order; cleanse top of both vials with an antiseptic swab. (b) Pull back on plunger to an amount equal to the volume of longer-acting insulin. (c) Insert needle through the rubber diaphragm of the longer-acting insulin; inject air. Remove needle and syringe; do not remove insulin. (d) Pull back the plunger on the syringe to a point equal to the volume of the shorter-acting insulin ordered. (e) Insert needle through the rubber diaphragm; inject air. (f) Invert the bottle and withdraw the volume of shorter-acting insulin ordered. Check amount withdrawn against amount ordered. (g) Rewipe the lid of the longer-acting insulin. (h) Insert needle; withdraw the specified amount of longer-acting insulin. (i) Remove the needle and syringe; recheck the drug order against the labels on the insulin containers and the amount in the syringe. Pull plunger back slightly and proceed to mix two insulins (tilt syringe back and forth gently); change needle.*

Appearance: Clear, cloudy, precipitate present?
Temperature: Should be at room temperature
4. Philosophies: There are two philosophies concerning which way insulins should be mixed. In one procedure, the volume of the shorter-acting insulin is drawn into the syringe first, followed by the longer-acting insulin. The rationale for this approach is that if a small amount of short-acting insulin is accidently displaced into the second (longer-acting insulin) bottle, the onset, peak, and duration of the longer-acting insulin will not be appreciably affected. If done in reverse order, the shorter-acting insulin would have its onset, peak, and duration affected due to the contamination by the longer-acting preparation.

In the second procedure, the opposite is advocated. The rationale for this approach is that since the longer-acting insulin is cloudy, a change in clarity would be immediately visible if the longer-acting insulin contaminated the normally clear second (shorter-acting) insulin during preparation.

We strongly recommend the use of the first procedure, but encourge you to check your institution's procedure manual for details.
5. Procedure:
- Roll the bottle between the palms of the hands to thoroughly mix the contents. DO NOT SHAKE.
- Check the insulin order and calculations of the preparation with another qualified nurse, in accordance with hospital policy.
- Cleanse the top of BOTH vials with separate antiseptic swabs (Fig. 6.21a).
- Pull back the plunger on the syringe to an amount equal to the volume of the longer-acting insulin ordered (Fig. 6.21b).
- Insert the needle through the rubber seal of the longer-acting insulin bottle; inject air (Fig. 6.21c). (Do not inject air into the insulin solution because it may break up insulin particles.)
- Remove the needle and syringe. (Do not withdraw insulin at this time.)
- Pull back the plunger on the syringe to an amount equal to the volume of the shorter-acting insulin ordered (Fig. 6.21d).
- Insert the needle through the rubber seal of the second bottle; inject air (Fig. 6.21e). Invert the bottle and withdraw the volume of shorter-acting insulin ordered (Fig. 6.21f). *Note:* Check for bubbles in the insulin, flick the side of the syringe with the fingers to displace the bubbles, then recheck the amount in the syringe.
- Check the medication order against the label of the container and the amount in the syringe.
- Rewipe the lid of the longer-acting insulin container

(Fig. 6.21g); recheck the drug order against this container; insert the needle of the syringe containing the shorter-acting insulin and withdraw the specified amount of longer-acting insulin (Fig. 6.21h). Be careful NOT to inject any of the first type of insulin already in the syringe into the vial.
- Remove the needle and syringe; recheck the drug order against the label on the insulin container and the amount in the syringe (Fig. 6.21i).
- Withdraw a small amount of air into the syringe and mix the two medications. Remove air carefully so that part of the medication is not displaced.
- Change needles and proceed to administer subcutaneously.

Preparation of Medications for Use in the Sterile Field during an Operative Procedure. The following principles apply to the operating room:

1. All medications used during an operative procedure must remain sterile.
2. All medication containers (ampules, vials, "piggyback," and blood bags) used during the operative procedure should remain in the operating room until the entire procedure is completed. (In case a question arises, the container is available.)
3. Do not save an unused portion of medication for use in another operative procedure. Discard at the end of the operative procedure or send the patient's medication to the patient care unit with the patient, if appropriate (i.e., antibiotic ointment for a patient having ophthalmic surgery).
4. Adhere to hospital policies concerning handling and storage of medications in the operating room.
5. ALWAYS tell the surgeon the name and dosage or concentration of the medication or solution being handed to him or her.
6. ALWAYS repeat the entire medication order back to the surgeon at the time the request is made to verify all aspects of the order. If in doubt, repeat again until accuracy is certain.

The following technique is used to prepare medications for use in the sterile operative field.

1. Prepare the drug prescribed according to the directions.
2. Always check the accuracy of the drug order against the medication being prepared at least three times during the preparation phase: (1) when first removed from the drug storage area; (2) immediately before removing the solution for use on the sterile field;

(3) immediately after completing the transfer of the medication/solution to the sterile field. ALWAYS tell the surgeon the name and dose or concentration of the medication/solution when passing it to him or her for use.

3. The circulating (nonsterile) nurse retrieves the medication from storage, reconstitutes as needed, and turns the medication container so the scrubbed (sterile) nurse can read the label. It is best to read the label aloud to assure that both individuals are verifying the contents against the verbal order from the surgeon.

The following two methods may be used:

Method 1:

1. The circulating (nonsterile) nurse cleanses the top of the vial or breaks off the top of the ampule, as described above.
2. The scrubbed (sterile) person chooses a syringe of the correct volume for the medication to be withdrawn and attaches a large-bore needle to facilitate removal of the solution from the container.
3. The circulating (nonsterile) nurse holds the ampule or vial in such a way that the scrubbed (sterile) person can easily insert the sterile needle tip into the medication container (Fig. 6.22a).
4. The scrubbed person pulls back the plunger on the syringe until all the medication prescribed has been withdrawn from the container and from the needle used to withdraw the medication.
5. The needle is disconnected from the syringe and left in the vial or ampule (Fig. 6.22b).

6. The medication container is again shown to the scrubbed person and read aloud to verify all components of the drug prepared against the medication/solution requested.

Method 2:

1. The circulating (nonsterile) nurse removes the entire lid of the vial with a bottle opener, cleanses the rim of the vial, and pours the medication directly into a sterile medicine cup held by the scrubbed nurse.
2. The scrubbed person continues drug preparation on the sterile field in accordance with the intended use (i.e., irrigation, injection).

Regardless of the method used to transfer the medication to the sterile field, both the sterile scrubbed person and the nonsterile circulating nurse should know the location and exact disposition of each medication on the sterile field.

Administration of Medication by the Intradermal Route

Intradermal injections are made into the dermal layer of skin just below the epidermis (Fig. 6.23). Small volumes, usually 0.1 ml, are injected to produce a wheal. The absorption from intradermal sites is slow, making it the route of choice for allergy sensitivity tests, desensitization injections, local anesthetics, and vaccinations.

Equipment

Medication to be injected
Tuberculin syringe with 26 gauge, ¼, ⅜, or ½ inch needle, OR a special needle and syringe for allergens
Metric ruler, if skin-testing procedure

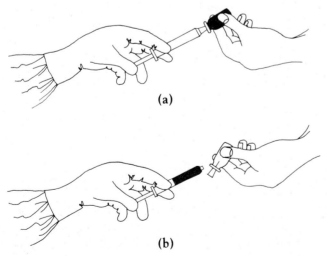

Fig. 6.22. *Preparing a medication in the operating room. (a) Circulating (unsterile) nurse holds vial to facilitate the "scrubbed" (sterile) person to insert the sterile needle tip into the medication container. (b) The needle is disconnected from the syringe and left in the vial.*

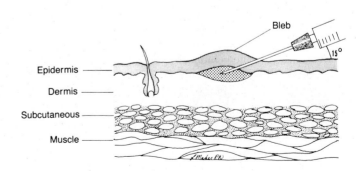

Fig. 6.23. *Intradermal injection technique.*

Sites

Intradermal injections may be made on any skin surface, but the site should be hairless and receive little friction from clothing. The upper chest, scapular areas of the back, and the inner aspect of the forearms are most commonly used (Fig. 6.24a,b).

Technique

The example of technique uses allergy sensitivity testing. CAUTION: Do not start any type of allergy testing unless emergency equipment is available in the immediate area in case of an anaphylactic response. Personnel should be familiar with the procedure to follow if an emergency does arise.

1. Check with the patient before starting the testing to be sure that he or she has not taken any antihistamines or anti-inflammatory agents (i.e., aspirin, ibuprofen, corticosteroids) for 24 to 48 hours preceding the tests. If the patient has taken antihistamines or anti-inflammatory agents, check with the physician before proceeding with the testing.
2. Cleanse the selected area thoroughly with an antiseptic pledget. Use circular motions starting at the planned site of injection, continuing outward in ever-widening circular motions to the periphery. Allow the area to air-dry.
3. Prepare the designated solutions for injection using aseptic technique. Usual volumes to be injected range between 0.01 and 0.05 ml. A control injection of normal saline or diluent is also administered.
4. Insert the needle at a 15° angle with the needle bevel upward. The solution being injected is deposited in the space immediately below the skin; remove the needle quickly. A small *bleb* will appear on the surface of the skin as the solution enters the intradermal area (Fig. 6.23). Be careful not to inject into the subcutaneous space.
5. Chart the times, agents, concentrations, and amounts injected (Fig. 6.24c). Make a diagram in the patient's chart numbering each location. Record what agent and concentration was injected at each site. (Subsequent "readings" of each area are then performed and charted on this record.)
6. Follow directions for the time of the "reading" of the skin testing being performed. Inspection of the injection sites should be performed in good light. Generally, a positive reaction (development of a wheal) to a dilute strength of suspected allergen is considered clinically significant. Measure the diameter in millimeters of erythema, and palpate and measure the size of any induration. Record this

information in the patient's chart. No reaction should be noted at the control site.

The technique described above can easily be modified for desensitization injections and vaccinations.

Patient Teaching

Tell the patient the time, date, and place to return to have the test sites read. Tell the patient not to wash or scrub the area until the injections have been read.

If the patient develops an area of severe burning or itching, he or she should try not to scratch. Tell the patient to report immediately the development of any breathing difficulty, severe hives, or rashes. He or she should go to the nearest emergency room if unable to reach the physician who prescribed the skin tests.

Documentation

Provide the RIGHT DOCUMENTATION of the medication administration and responses to drug therapy.

1. Chart: Date, time, drug name, dosage, and site of administration (Fig. 6.24c).
2. Perform a reading of each site after the application, as directed by the physician or the policy of the health care agency.
3. Chart and report any signs and symptoms of adverse drug effects.
4. Perform and validate essential patient education about the drug therapy and other essential aspects of intervention for the disease process affecting the individual.

Commonly used readings of reactions and appropriate symbols are listed below.

+	(1 +)	Redness of skin present (erythema)
+ +	(2 +)	Redness and solid elevated lesions up to 5 mm in diameter (erythema and papules)
+ + +	(3 +)	Erythema, papules, and vesicles (blisterlike areas 5 mm or less in diameter)
+ + + +	(4 +)	Generalized fusing of blistered areas

Medication Administration Via the Subcutaneous Route

Subcutaneous injections are made into the loose connective tissue between the dermis and muscle layer

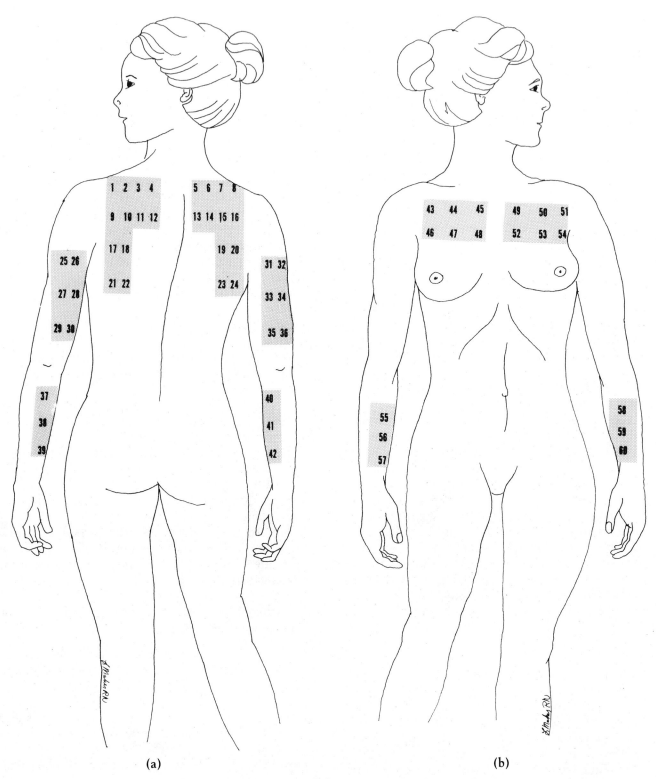

Fig. 6.24. (*Legend on opposite page.*)

Reading Chart for Intradermal Testing

Patient Name: _____
Identification Number: _____
Physician Name: _____

DATE:	TIME:	AGENT	CONCENTRATION	AMOUNT INJECTED	SITE NUMBER:*	Reading Time in Hours or minutes, i.e., 30 min. or 24, 48, or 72 hours		

* Refer to diagram of sites, Figure 6.24a,b.
  —Follow directions for the "reading" of the skin testing performed.
  —Inspect sites in a good light
  —Record reaction in upper half of box using the following guidelines, i.e., [2+]
  +   (1+)   Redness of skin present (erythema)
  + +   (2+)   Redness and solid elevated lesion up to 5 mm in diameter (erythema and papules).
  + + +   (3+)   Erythema, papules and vesicles (blister-like areas 5 mm or less in diameter).
  + + + +   (4+)   Generalized fusing of blisters.
  —Record measurement of induration (process of hardening) in mm. in lower half of box, i.e., [5mm]

(c)

Fig. 6.24. *Intradermal sites. (a) Posterior view. (b) Anterior view. (c) Reading chart for intradermal testing.*

(Fig. 6.25). Absorption is slower and drug action is generally longer with subcutaneous injections than with intramuscular or intravenous injections. If the circulation is adequate, the drug is completely absorbed from the tissue.

Many drugs cannot be administered by this route since no more than 2 ml can ordinarily be deposited at a subcutaneous site. The drugs must be quite soluble and potent enough to be effective in small volume, without causing significant tissue irritation. Drugs commonly injected into the subcutaneous tissue are heparin and insulin.

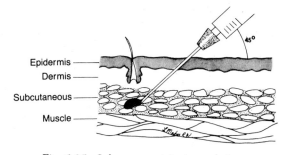

Fig. 6.25. *Subcutaneous injection technique.*

Equipment

Syringe Size. Choose a syringe that corresponds to the volume of drug to be injected at one site. The usual amount injected subcutaneously at one site is 0.5–2 ml. Correlate syringe size with the size of the patient and the tissue mass.

Needle Length. Assess each patient so that the needle length selected will deposit the medication into the subcutaneous tissue, not muscle tissue. Needle lengths of ⅜, ½, and ⅝ inch are routinely used. It is prudent to leave an extra ¼ inch of needle extending above the skin surface in case the needle breaks.

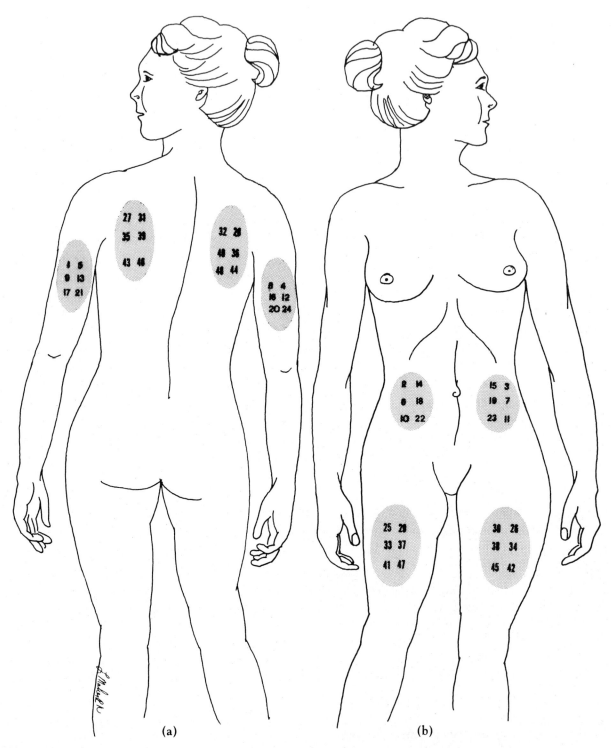

Fig. 6.26. *Subcutaneous injection sites and rotation plan.* (a) *Posterior view.* (b) *Anterior view.*

Needle Gauge. Commonly used gauges for subcutaneous injections are 25–27 gauge.

Sites

Common sites used for the subcutaneous administration of medications include upper arms, anterior thighs, and abdomen (Fig. 6.26a,b). Less common areas are the buttocks and upper back or scapular region.

A plan for rotating injection sites should be developed for all patients who require repeated injections (Fig. 6.26a,b). The anterior view (Fig. 6.26b) illustrates areas easily used for self-administration. The posterior view (Fig. 6.26a) illustrates less commonly used areas that may be used by other persons injecting the medication.

Technique

1. Prepare the medication as described before:
2. Check the accuracy of the drug order against the medication being prepared at least three times during the preparation phase: (1) when first removing the drug from the storage area; (2) immediately after preparation; and (3) immediately before administration.
3. Check your hospital policy regarding whether 1–2 minims of air are added to the syringe AFTER accurately measuring the prescribed volume of drug for administration. (*Philosophy:* The rationale for adding the air is that it will result in the needle being completely cleared of all medication at the time of injection. Conversely, if the volume of medication is completely drawn into the syringe before changing the needle, the drug volume ordered will still be administered as long as the same size needle is used for drawing up and injection. Thus, the needle should not need to be completely cleared of medication by air during administration. This issue can be critical when small volumes of potent drugs are administered to infants.)
4. Consult the master rotation schedule for the patient so that the drug is administered at the correct site.
5. Identify the patient prior to administration of the medication by checking the bracelet.
6. Explain what you are going to do.
7. Position the patient appropriately.
8. Expose the selected site and locate the landmarks.
9. Cleanse the skin surface with an antiseptic pledget starting at the injection site and working outward in a circular motion toward the periphery.
10. Let the area air-dry.
11. Consult the institution's policy regarding which of the following methods to use.
    Method 1:
    Grasp the skin area of the site selected, spread, hold firmly, and insert the needle quickly at a 45 degree angle; aspirate (DO NOT ASPIRATE FOR HEPARIN) and slowly inject the medication. If the aspiration draws blood, withdraw the needle and prepare an entirely new medication for administration (new syringe, needle, and drug).
    Method 2:
    Grasp the skin area of the site selected and create a small roll or "bunch." Insert the needle quickly at a 90° angle, aspirate (DO NOT AS-

PIRATE FOR HEPARIN), and slowly inject the medication. If the aspiration draws blood, withdraw the needle and prepare an entirely new medication for administration (new syringe, needle, and drug).
12. As the needle is withdrawn, apply gentle pressure to the site with an antiseptic pledget.
13. Provide emotional support for the patient.

Documentation

Provide the RIGHT DOCUMENTATION of the medication administration and response to drug therapy:

1. Chart: Date, time, drug name, dosage, and route of administration.
2. Perform and record regular patient assessments for the evaluation of the therapeutic effectiveness (i.e., blood pressure, pulse, output, improvement or quality of cough and productivity, degree and duration of pain relief, etc.).
3. Chart and report any signs and symptoms of adverse drug effects.
4. Perform and validate essential patient education about the drug therapy and other essential aspects of intervention for the disease process affecting the individual.

Administration of Medication by the Intramuscular Route

Intramuscular (IM) injections are made by penetrating a needle through the dermis and subcutaneous tissue into the muscle layer. The injection deposits the medication deep within the muscle mass (Fig. 6.27). Absorption is more rapid than from subcutaneous injections because muscle tissue has a greater blood

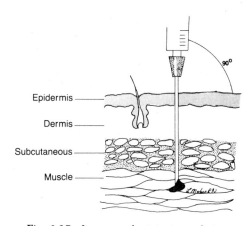

Fig. 6.27. *Intramuscular injection technique.*

supply. Site selection is especially important with intramuscular injections because incorrect placement of the needle may cause damage to nerves or blood vessels. A large, healthy muscle free of infection or wounds should be used.

Equipment

Syringe Size. Choose a syringe that corresponds to the volume of drug to be injected at one site. The usual amount injected intramuscularly at one site is 0.5–2 ml. In infants and children, the amount should not exceed 0.5–1 ml. Correlate syringe size with the size of the patient and the tissue mass. In adults, divided doses are generally recommended for amounts in excess of 3 ml; 1 ml may be injected in the deltoid area. Other factors that influence syringe size include the type of medication and site of administration, thickness of subcutaneous fatty tissue, and the age of the individual.

Needle Length. Assess each patient so that the needle length selected will deposit the medication into the muscular tissue (Fig. 6.12). There is a significant difference among needle lengths appropriate for an obese patient, an infant, or an emaciated or debilitated patient. Needle lengths commonly used are 1–1½ inches long, although longer lengths may be required for an obese person. When estimating needle length, it is prudent to leave an extra ¼ inch of needle extending above the skin surface in case the needle breaks.

Needle Gauge. Commonly used gauges for intramuscular injections are 20–22 gauge.

Sites

Common sites used for the intramuscular administration of medication include the following:

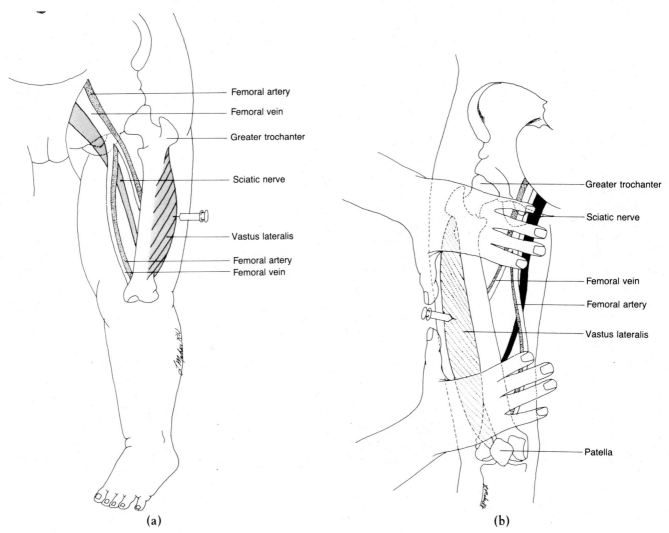

Fig. 6.28. *Vastus lateralis muscle.* (a) *Child/infant.* (b) *Adult.*

Vastus Lateralis Muscle. This muscle is located on the anterior lateral thigh away from nerves and blood vessels. The midportion is one handbreadth below the greater trochanter and one handbreadth above the knee (Fig. 6.28a,b). It is generally the preferred site for IM injections in infants since it has the largest muscle mass for that age group. The vastus lateralis muscle is also a good choice for an injection site in healthy, ambulatory adults (Fig. 6.28b). It will accomodate a large volume of medication and permits good drug absorption. In the elderly, debilitated, or nonambulatory adult, the muscle should be carefully assessed before injection since significantly less muscle mass may be present. If muscle mass is insufficient, an alternative site should be selected.

Rectus Femoris Muscle. The rectus femoris muscle lies just medial (Fig. 6.29a,b) to the vastus lateralis muscle, but does not cross the midline of the anterior thigh. The injection site is located in the same manner as the vastus lateralis muscle. It may be used in both children and adults when other sites are unavailable. A primary advantage to its use is that it may be used more easily by patients for self-administration. A disadvantage is that the medial border is quite close to the sciatic nerve and major blood vessels (Fig. 6.29a,b). If the muscle is not well developed, injections in this site may also cause considerable discomfort.

Gluteal Area. The gluteal area is a commonly used site of injection because it is free of major nerves and blood vessels. It must not be used in children under 3 years of age because the muscle is not yet well-developed from walking. The area may be divided into two distinct injection sites: (1) the ventrogluteal area and (2) the dorsogluteal area.

Ventrogluteal area: This site is easily accessible when the patient is in a prone, supine, or side-lying position.

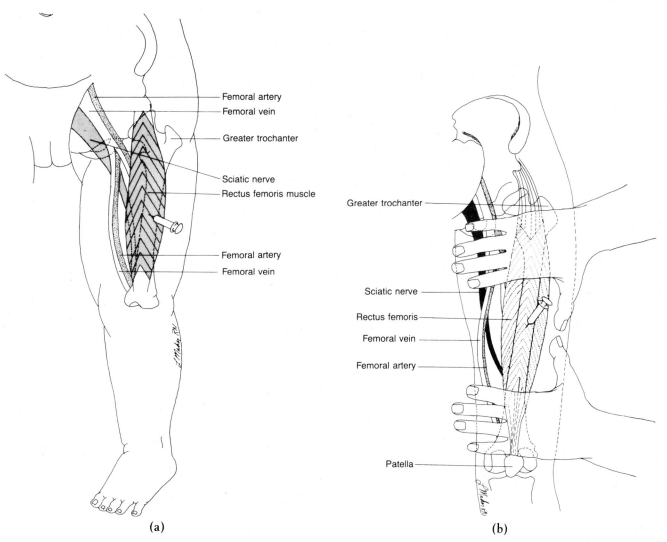

Fig. 6.29. *Rectus femoris muscle.* (a) *Child/infant.* (b) *Adult.*

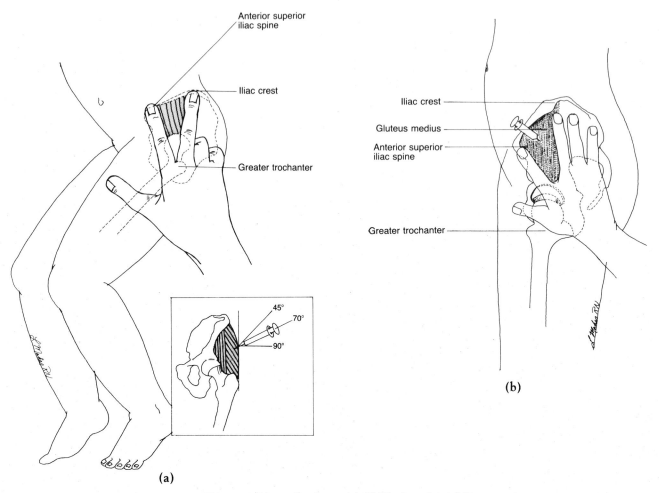

Fig. 6.30. *Ventrogluteal site.* (a) *Child/infant.* (b) *Adult.*

It is located by placing the palm of the hand on the lateral portion of the greater trochanter, the index finger on the anterior superior iliac spine, and the middle finger extended to the iliac crest. The injection is made into the center of the "V" formed between the index and middle fingers with the needle directed slightly upward toward the crest of the ilium (Fig. 6.30a,b). Pain on injection can be minimized if the muscle is relaxed. The patient can aid in relaxation by pointing the toes inward while lying in a prone position (Fig. 6.31) or by flexing the upper leg if lying on the side (Fig. 6.32).

Dorsogluteal area: To use this injection site (Fig. 6.33a,b), the patient must be placed in a prone position on a flat table surface. The site is identified by drawing an imaginary line from the the posterior superior iliac spine to the greater trochanter of the femur. The injection should be given at any point between the imaginary straight line and below the curve of the iliac crest (hipbone). The syringe should be held perpendicular to the flat table surface with the needle directed on a straight back-to-front course. Pain on injection can be minimized if the muscle is relaxed. The patient can aid in relaxation by pointing the toes inward while lying in a prone position (Fig. 6.31).

Deltoid Muscle. The deltoid muscle is frequently used because of ease of access in the standing, sitting, or prone positions. However, it should be used in infants only when the volume to be injected is quite small, the drug is nonirritating, and the dose will be quickly absorbed. In adults, the volume should be limited to 2 cc or less and the substance must not cause irritation. Caution must also be exercised to avoid the clavicle, humerus, acromion, the brachial vein and artery, and the radial nerve. The injection site (Fig. 6.34a,b) of the deltoid muscle is located by drawing an imaginary line across the armpit at the level of the axilla and the lower edge of the acromion. The lateral borders of the rectangle are vertical lines parallel to the area one-third and two-thirds of the way around the outer lateral aspect of the arm.

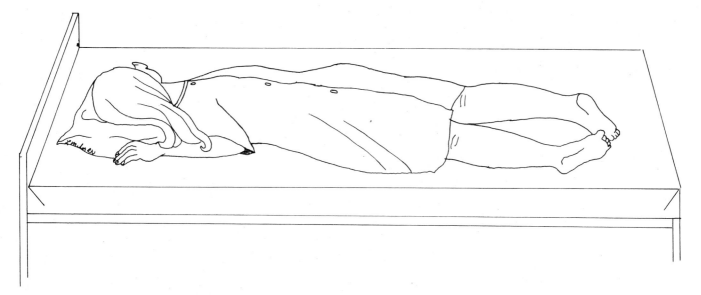

Fig. 6.31. *Prone position. Toes pointed to promote muscle relaxation.*

Site Rotation

A master plan for site rotation should be developed and used for all patients requiring repeated injections (Fig. 6.35a,b).

Technique

1. Prepare the medication as described before.
2. Check the accuracy of the drug order against the medication being prepared at least three times during the preparation phase: (1) when first re-moving the drug from the storage area; (2) im-mediately after preparation; and (3) immediately before administration.
3. Check your hospital policy regarding whether 1–2 minims of air should be added to the syringe AFTER accurately measuring the prescribed volume of drug for administration. (The rationale for adding the air is that it will result in the needle being completely cleared of all medication at the time of injection. Conversely, if the volume is com-pletely drawn into the syringe before changing the needle, the drug volume ordered will still be

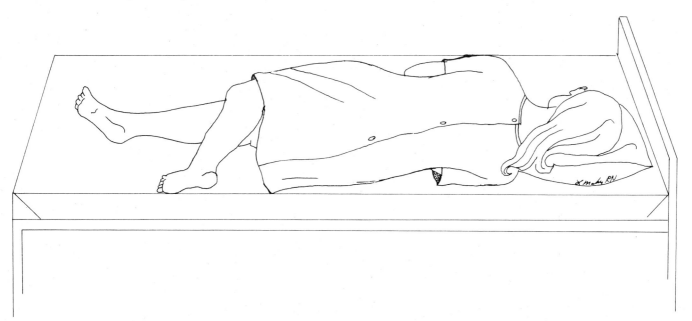

Fig. 6.32. *Patient lying on side. Flexing upper leg promotes muscle relaxation.*

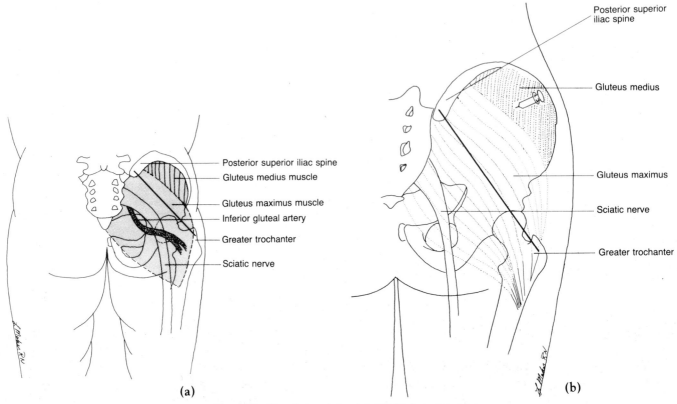

Fig. 6.33. *Dorsal gluteal site.* (a) *Child/infant.* (b) *Adult.*

administered as long as the same size needle is used for drawing up and injection. Thus, the needle should not need to be completely cleared of medication by air during administration. This issue can be critical when small volumes of potent drugs are administered repeatedly to infants.)

4. Consult the master rotation schedule for the patient so that the drug is administered at the correct site (Fig. 6.35).
5. Identify the patient prior to administration of the medication by checking the bracelet.
6. Explain what you are going to do.
7. Position the patient appropriately (see Figs. 6.31 and 6.32 for relaxation techniques).
8. Expose the selected site and locate the landmarks.
9. Cleanse the skin surface with an antiseptic pledget starting at the injection site and working outward in a circular motion toward the periphery.
10. Let the area air-dry.
11. Insert the needle at the correct angle and depth for the site being used.
12. Aspirate. If no blood returns, slowly inject the medication using gentle, steady pressure on the plunger. OR,
13. Aspirate. If blood does return, place an antiseptic pledget over the injection site as the needle is withdrawn. Start the procedure over with a new syringe, needle, and medication.

14. After removing the needle, apply gentle pressure to the site. Massage can increase the pain if the muscle mass is stressed by the amount of medication given.
15. Apply a small bandage to the site.
16. Provide emotional support of the patient. Children should be given comfort during and after the injection. Sometimes letting a child hold your hand or say "ouch" helps. Praise the patient for assistance and cooperation.

The Z-Track Method. The use of a Z-track technique (Fig. 6.36a,d) may be appropriate for medications that are particularly irritating or that stain the tissue. Check the hospital policy concerning which personnel may administer by this method.

1. Expose the dorsogluteal site (Fig. 6.36a). Calculate and prepare the medication, and add 0.5 cc of air to ensure that the drug will clear the needle. Position the patient and cleanse the area for injection as previously described. Never inject into the arm or other exposed site.
2. Stretch the skin approximately 1 inch to one side (Fig. 6.36b).
3. Insert the needle. Choose a needle of sufficient length to insure *deep* muscle penetration.

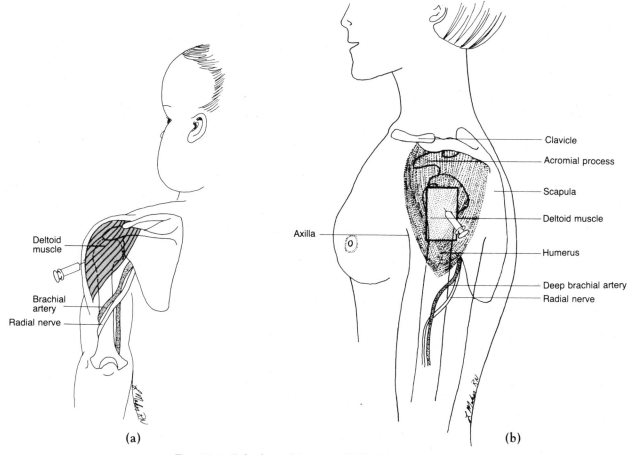

Fig. 6.34. *Deltoid muscle site.* (a) *Child/infant.* (b) *Adult.*

4. Aspirate and follow previous guidelines for use of the dorsogluteal site.
5. Gently inject the medication and wait approximately 10 seconds (Fig. 6.36c).
6. Remove the needle and allow the skin to return to the normal position (Fig. 6.36d).
7. DO NOT massage the injection site.
8. If further injections are to be made, alternate between dorsogluteal sites.
9. Walking will help absorption. Vigorous exercise or pressure on the injection site (e.g., tight girdle) should be temporarily avoided.

Administration of Medications by the Intravenous Route

Intravenous (IV) administration of medication places the drug directly into the bloodstream, bypassing all barriers to drug absorption. Large volumes of medications can be administered into the vein, there is usually less irritation, and the onset of action is the most rapid of all parenteral routes. Drugs may be given by direct injection with a needle and syringe, but more commonly drugs are given intermittently or by continuous infusion through an established IV line.

Intravenous drug administration is usually more comfortable for the patient, especially when several doses of medication must be administered daily. However, use of the intravenous route requires time and skill to establish and maintain an IV site, the patient tends to be less mobile, and there is a greater possibility of infection and severe adverse reactions from the drug.

Dosage Forms

Medications for intravenous administration are available in ampules, vials, and prefilled syringes. Be certain that the label specifically states "for IV use."

Intravenous physiologic solutions come in a variety of volumes and concentrations in glass or plastic containers (Table 6.2).

Equipment

Tourniquet
Administration set with appropriate needle, drip chamber, and filter
Medication
Physiologic solution ordered

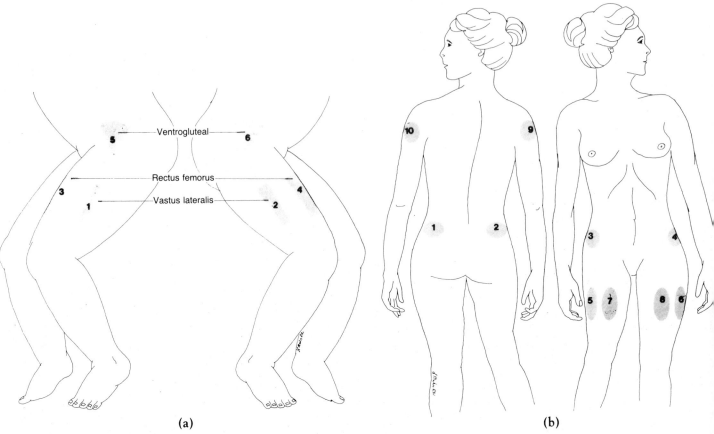

Fig. 6.35. *Intramuscular master rotation plan. (a) Infant/child. Note that the deltoid site may also be used in an infant or child, however, the volume of medication must be quite small and the drug nonirritating. (b) Adult. In an adult, avoid the use of the rectus femoris (numbers 7 and 8) unless other sites are not available, due to the pain produced when this site is used and the location of the sciatic nerve, femoral artery and vein. If used, be certain to insert the needle lateral to the midline.*

Sterile dressing materials
Antiseptic solution
Syringe and needle (if by bolus)
Armboard
Tape
Standard IV pole or rod
Heparin lock, "piggyback," and additional solutions, as appropriate

Sites

When selecting a site, consider the length of time intravenous therapy will be required. If a prolonged course of treatment is anticipated, start the first IV in the hand (Fig. 6.37). The metacarpal veins, dorsal vein network, cephalic, and basilic vein are commonly used. To avoid irritation and leakage from a previous puncture site, the subsequent venipuncture sites should be made above the earlier site. Refer to Fig. 6.38 for the veins of the forearm area which could be used for additional venipuncture sites.

- Avoid the use of vessels over bony prominences or joints unless absolutely necessary.
- In the elderly, the use of the veins in the hand area may be a poor choice due to the fragility of the skin and veins in this area.
- Veins commonly used in infants and children for intravenous administration are on the back of the hand, dorsum of the foot, or the temporal region of the scalp (Fig. 6.39).
- If possible, do not use the veins of the lower extremities because of the danger of developing thrombi and emboli.
- Do not use veins with varicosities or an extremity with impaired blood flow (e.g., the affected side following a mastectomy and lymph node dissection).
- *Never start an IV in an artery!*

General Principles of Intravenous Medication Administration

- Be certain medications to be administered intravenously are thoroughly dissolved in the correct volume and type of solution. *Always* follow the manufacturer's recommendations.

- Use in-line filters as recommended.
- DO NOT administer any drug or IV solution that is hazy or cloudy, or has foreign particles or a precipitate in it.
- DO NOT mix any other drugs with blood or blood products (e.g., albumin).
- DO NOT administer a drug in an IV solution if the compatibility is not known.
- Drugs must be entirely infused through the IV line before adding a second medication to the IV line.
- Once mixed, know the length of time an agent remains stable; all unused IV solutions should be returned to the pharmacy if not used within 24 hours.
- Check the hospital policy for the definition of "TKO" (to keep open). It is usually interpreted as "an infusion rate of 10 ml/hr" and should infuse less than 500 ml/24 hours.

- Shade IV solutions that contain drugs that should be protected from light (e.g., hyperalimentation solutions, nitrofurantoin, amphotericin B, nitroprusside).
- Administration sets should be changed every 24–48 hours (check hospital policy). The sets must be labeled with the date and time initiated, the date to change the set, and the nurse's initials.
- Whenever a patient is receiving IV fluids, monitor intake and output accurately. Report declining hourly outputs and those of less than 30–40 ml/hour.
- Never "speed up" an IV flow rate to "catch up" when the volume to be infused has fallen behind. In certain cases, this could be dangerous. The physician should be consulted, particularly with patients who have cardiac, renal, or circulatory impairment.

Technique

1. Prepare the medication as described before.

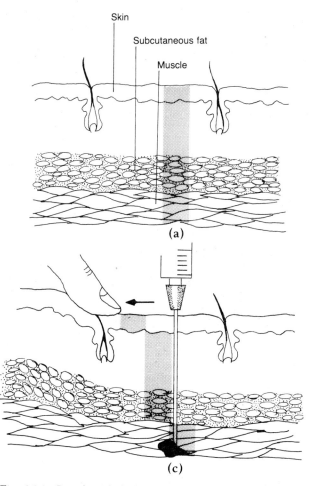
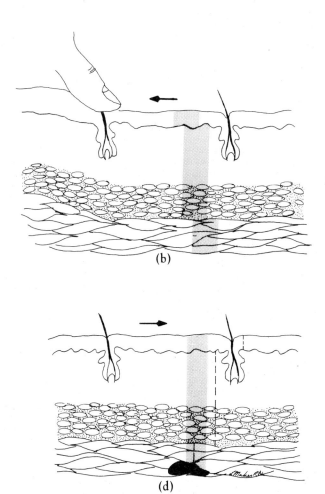

Fig. 6.36. *Z-track method of intramuscular injection. (a) Tissue prior to starting Z tracking. (b) Stretch skin slightly to one side, approximately one inch. (c) Gently inject the medication; wait approximately 10 seconds. (d) Remove needle and allow skin to return to normal position. Do not massage injection site.*

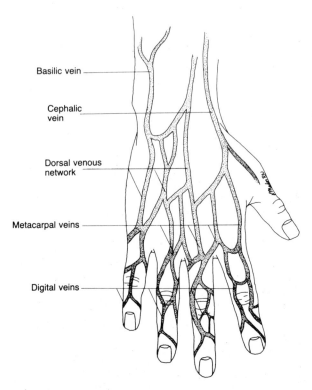

Fig. 6.37. Intravenous sites on the hand.

Basilic vein

Cephalic vein

Dorsal venous network

Metacarpal veins

Digital veins

Venipuncture. Follow these steps in performing venipuncture.

1. Wash hands thoroughly.
2. Position the patient appropriately. Immobilize an infant or child for patient safety, if necessary.
3. Apply the tourniquet using a slip knot 2–6 inches above the site chosen (shaded area in Fig. 6.40a). Inspect the area to identify a vein of sufficient size

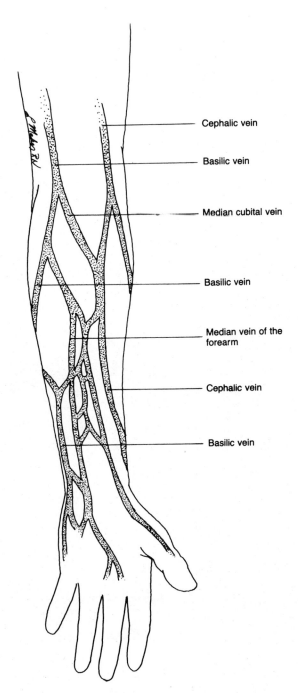

Cephalic vein

Basilic vein

Median cubital vein

Basilic vein

Median vein of the forearm

Cephalic vein

Basilic vein

Fig. 6.38. Veins in the forearm used as intravenous sites.

2. Check the accuracy of the drug order against the medication and/or solution being prepared at least three times during the preparation phase: (1) when first removing the drug/solution from the storage area; (2) immediately after preparation; and (3) immediately before administration. Check the expiration date on the solution.
3. Determine that the drug being added to an existing IV line is compatible with the physiologic solution in the line by reviewing hospital policies or by consulting the pharmacist.
4. Using aseptic technique, prepare the IV solution, check for particulate matter, and label the container with the patient's name, medications added, start time, stop time, hourly intervals between, and number of container (i.e., #1, #2, #3). Insert the administration set, clearing the line of air; reclamp the tubing. (Have the sterile cover for the adapter tip of the line available to cover the tip as soon as the line is completely flushed.)
5. *Identify the patient by checking the bracelet prior to initiating any intravenous procedure.*
6. Explain what you are going to do.
7. Before initiating intravenous therapy or administering IV medications, perform baseline assessments of the patient's current vital signs and state of hydration.

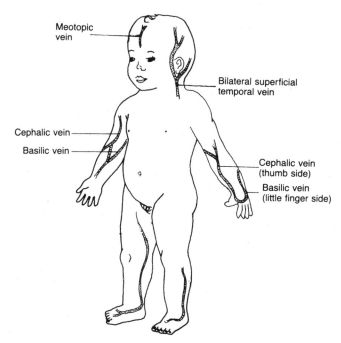

Fig. 6.39. *Veins in infants and children used as intravenous sites.*

Labels on figure:
- Meotopic vein
- Bilateral superficial temporal vein
- Cephalic vein
- Basilic vein
- Cephalic vein (thumb side)
- Basilic vein (little finger side)

to accommodate the needle and provide adequate anchorage. Palpate the vein to feel the depth and direction (Fig. 6.40b,c). To dilate the vein, it may be necessary to (1) place the extremity in a dependent position, (2) massage the vein against the direction of blood flow, (3) have the patient open and close the hand repeatedly, (4) lightly thump the vein with your fingertips, or (5) remove the tourniquet and apply a heating pad or warm, wet towels to the extremity for 15–20 minutes and then start the process all over.

4. Cleanse the skin surface with the antiseptic starting at the site of entry and working outward in a circular motion toward the periphery (Fig. 6.40d).
5. Let the area air-dry.
6. Provide tension on the skin surface to stretch the skin and stabilize the vein.

When using an *administration set* or a *needle and syringe*: (1) Hold the needle (bevel up) at an angle slightly less than 45° (Fig. 6.40e) and penetrate the skin surface approximately ½ inch below the intended entry site into the vein; decrease the angle to 15° (Fig. 6.40f) and slowly advance the needle along the course of the vein. (2) When blood flow is established, connect the tubing to the needle, release the tourniquet, and anchor the needle and tubing to the arm or hand with tape (Fig. 6.41) and dressing as prescribed by hospital policy. (3) Adjust the rate of flow of the solution

$$\frac{\text{ml of solution} \times \text{number of drops/ml}}{\text{hours of administration} \times 60 \text{ minutes}} = \text{drops/minute}$$

(4) Regulate the flow by counting the drops for 15 seconds, multiply by 4, and adjust clamp on tubing for the appropriate rate.

When using a *plastic needle* (Fig. 6.42): (1) Proceed as above until blood flow is established (Fig. 6.41a) (2) Remove the inner needle (Fig. 6.42b), connect the tubing to the plastic needle (Fig. 6.42c), release the tourniquet, and anchor the needle (Fig. 6.41) and tubing to the arm or hand with tape and dressing, according to hospital policy. (3) Adjust the rate of flow solution:

$$\frac{\text{ml of solution} \times \text{number of drops/ml}}{\text{hours of administration} \times 60 \text{ minutes}} = \text{drops/minute}$$

(4) Regulate the flow by counting the drops for 15 seconds, multiply by 4, and adjust clamp on tubing for the appropriate rate.

Regardless of the apparatus used, mark the tape with the date and time of insertion and the initials of the nurse who started it (Fig. 6.41c).

Many types of infusion pumps are available and the nurse should become familiar with the type used in his or her practice setting. Remember that the use of any type of equipment does not remove responsibility for visible monitoring of the rate of infusion and the infusion site at regularly scheduled intervals. Whenever an infusion pump is used, the danger of infiltration is increased.

Administration of Medications into an Established IV Line

1. Prepare the medication as described before.
2. Identify the patient using the bracelet and explain what you are going to do.
3. Swab the self-sealing portal of the injection site with an antiseptic sponge.
4. Using a short needle on the syringe, puncture the portal site. (The short needle reduces the possibility of penetrating the opposite wall of the portal.)
5. Draw back the plunger of the syringe until blood flow is seen in the tubing at the venipuncture site to establish that the line is open into the vein.
6. While pinching the IV tubing *above* the portal to stop flow, inject the prescribed medication into the IV line at a rate recommended by the manufacturer.
7. When all the medication is administered, withdraw the needle from the portal and reestablish the flow rate as ordered. (Flushing the IV line is not recommended because the medication still in the line would be administered as a bolus. This is contrary to the manufacturer's safety recommendation. Sudden boluses of certain medications may also cause severe hypotension or other signs of toxicity.)

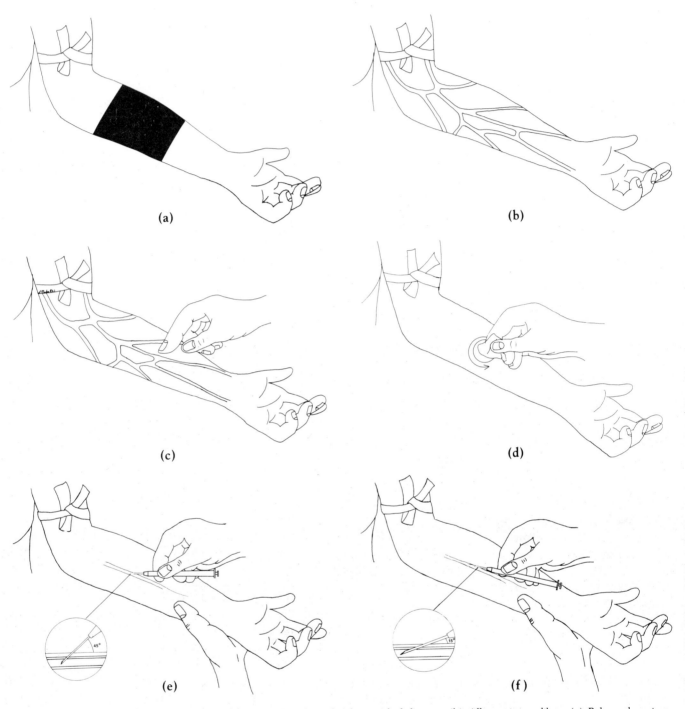

Fig. 6.40. (a) *Apply tourniquet using a slip knot 2–6 inches above the chosen (shaded) area.* (b) *Allow veins to dilate.* (c) *Palpate the vein to feel the depth and direction.* (d) *Cleanse the skin surface with an antiseptic, starting at the anticipated site of entry, working outward in a circular motion to the periphery.* (e) *Hold the needle (bevel up) at an angle slightly less than 45° to penetrate the skin surface.* (f) *Decrease the angle to 15° and slowly advance the needle along the course of the vein.*

Administration of Medication by a Heparin Lock
(Fig. 6.10)

1. Select a syringe several cc larger than that required by the volume of the drug. This allows room for aspiration of blood to assure placement of the needle and to allow blood to mix with the drug solution.
2. Prepare the medication as described before.
3. Identify the patient using the armband and explain what you are going to do.
4. Swab the self-sealing rubber diaphragm with an

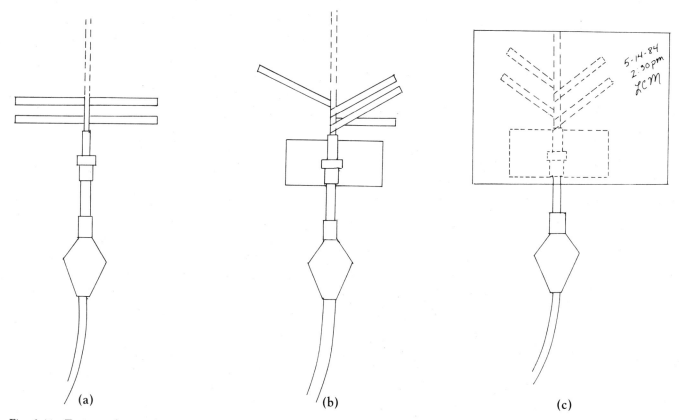

(a)   **(b)**   **(c)**

Fig. 6.41. *Taping a plastic catheter or needle. (a) Place two small adhesive strips under the needle or plastic catheter with the adhesive side up. (b) Cross adhesive tapes one at a time to secure the plastic catheter or needle. The larger piece of tape is placed under the hub with adhesive side up. (It will adhere to larger tape to be applied later.) (c) A larger piece of tape completes the stabilization of the plastic needle or catheter. Mark the date and time of insertion and the nurse's initials or signature.*

antiseptic sponge and hold the sides of the injection port with your free hand.

5. Using a short, small-gauge needle, puncture the rubber diaphragm and gently pull back on the plunger for blood return.
6. If blood return is established, inject the medication at the rate specified by the manufacturer.
7. Periodically pull back on the plunger to mix blood with the drug solution and to assure that the needle is in the vein.
8. After administration, withdraw the needle from the diaphragm.
9. Remove the syringe and insert another syringe containing (usually) 1–2 ml of normal saline to flush the remaining drug from the butterfly line.
10. Flush the lock with 1 ml of heparin (10 unit/ml to 100 unit/ml as directed by hospital policy). *Always* verify heparin dosage with another qualified nurse.

The heparin in the lock should be replaced (1) when initially placed, (2) after administering medications, (3) after withdrawing blood samples, or (4)

every 8 hours if medications are not administered more frequently.

Check the hospital policy to determine how long a heparin lock may remain in place before changing it. Monitor the lock venipuncture site as you would any other venipuncture site.

Adding a Medication to an Intravenous Bag, Bottle, or Volume Control

1. Prepare the medication as described before.
2. Identify the patient using the bracelet and explain what you are going to do.
3. Identify the injection port on the specific type of IV container or volume control set to be used; cleanse the portal with an antiseptic swab.
4. Insert the sterile needle into the correct injection port and slowly add the prescribed medication to the intravenous solution. Always check to be certain the medication is being added to a compatible solution of sufficient amount to insure proper dilution of the medication as specified by the manufacturer.
5. For a volume control apparatus, fill the volume chamber with the specified amount of intravenous

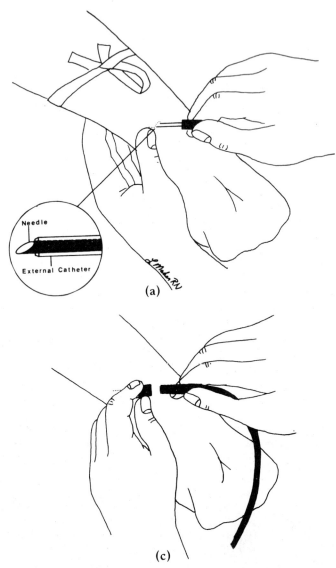

(a)

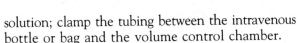

(c)

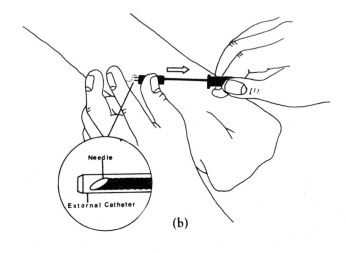

(b)

Fig. 6.42. *(a) "Over-the-catheter" type needle (see also Fig. 6.11a). When using a plastic needle, proceed as described in Fig. 6.40a-e, until blood flow is established. (b) After the catheter has been advanced into the vein, remove the inner needle by withdrawing from the plastic needle. (c) Connect the tubing to the plastic needle hub; release tourniquet.*

solution; clamp the tubing between the intravenous bottle or bag and the volume control chamber.

6. Add the medication, as described before, via the cleansed injection port.
   —Adjust the rate of flow solution:

$$\frac{\text{ml of solution} \times \text{number of drops/ml}}{\text{hours of administration} \times 60 \text{ minutes}} = \text{drops/minute}$$

7. Regulate the flow by counting the drops for 15 seconds, multiply by 4, and adjust clamp on tubing for the appropriate rate. *Note:* When IV medications are administered by a volume control apparatus, calculation of the rate of infusion to administer the drug over the proper time must include an allowance for the volume of the fluid in the IV tubing *and* the volume of medication.

8. Affix a label to the container. Indicate the medication name, dosage, date and time prepared, rate of infusion, length of infusion time, and the nurse's signature.

Adding a Medication with a Piggyback or Secondary Set

1. Prepare the medication as described before and add to an IV bag or bottle.
2. Identify the patient using the bracelet and explain what you are going to do.
3. Insert the administration set into the container, attach a short sterile needle, clear the line of air, and clamp the tubing.
4. Connect to the primary IV tubing in one of the following ways:
   Piggyback—Arrange the piggyback container so that it is elevated higher than the primary container (Fig. 6.17). Cleanse the secondary portal

with an antiseptic swab and insert the needle, thereby connecting the piggyback tubing to the port of the tubing of the primary solution. Secure in place.

Secondary set—Arrange both the primary and secondary containers at the same height and connect the secondary tubing to the port of the tubing of the primary solution in the same manner as described for piggybacks.

5. Always check specific orders for the infusion rate and sequence of solution or medication administration. Clamp the tubing of the primary solution if ordered to do so.
6. Affix a label to the container. Indicate the medication name, dosage, date and time prepared, rate of infusion, length of infusion time, and the nurse's signature.

Changing to the Next Container of IV Solution

1. Monitor the rate of infusion at least once per hour. When the container nears completion, notify the nurse responsible for adding the next container.
2. Slow the rate to keep the vein open if the level of solution in the container is low.
3. Using aseptic technique, clamp the tubing and quickly exchange the new container for the empty one. Fill the chamber at least half full; then unclamp.
4. Adjust the flow rate as previously described, and inspect the injection site.

Discontinuing an Intravenous Infusion

You will need the following equipment to discontinue an IV infusion
Tourniquet
Sterile sponges
Dressing materials
Tape
Perform the following technique:

1. Check the physician's orders. Verify that all intravenous solutions and medications have been completed.
2. Check the patient's identity using the bracelet before discontinuing the intravenous solutions.
3. Explain what you are going to do.
4. Adequately expose the intravenous site.
5. Clamp the intravenous tubing.
6. Loosen the tape at the venipuncture site while simultaneously stabilizing the needle to prevent venous damage.
7. Review hospital policy regarding the placement of a tourniquet. (Some health care agencies state that a tourniquet should be applied prior to removal of the needle or intravenous catheter in case the tip breaks during removal. Other agencies state that the tourniquet should be loosely attached to the limb, but not tightened unless necessary.)
8. Using a gauze pad, gently apply pressure with the nondominant hand to the venipuncture site. Withdraw the needle, pulling out parallel to the skin surface. Inspect the tip of the needle or catheter to be sure it is intact. Release the tourniquet, if in place.
9. Continue to hold the IV site firmly until all bleeding ceases. If the venipuncture site was in the antecubital fossa, have the patient flex the elbow to hold the gauze in place.
10. Apply a small dressing as stated by policy.
11. Provide patient comfort. Remove and discard intravenous apparatus.

Provide the RIGHT DOCUMENTATION of termination of intravenous therapy.

1. Chart: date and time of termination.
2. Perform and record regular patient assessments (i.e. site data, size of site and color of skin at injection site).
3. Chart and report any signs of adverse effects (i.e. redness, warmth, swelling, and/or pain at the intravenous site).

Monitoring Intravenous Therapy

Prior to initiating therapy, perform baseline patient assessments to evaluate the patient's current status. Report at appropriate intervals throughout the course of treatment.

The patient and the intravenous site should be checked at least every hour for flow rate, infiltration (tenderness, redness, puffiness), and adverse effects. If the flow rate is falling behind schedule:

1. Check for mechanical obstruction of the tubing (closed clamp, kinking) or filter and either irrigate or change the tubing.
2. Check the drip chamber. If less than half full, squeeze it to fill more completely. (Do not overfill.)
3. Check to make sure that the IV container is not empty. Also check to make sure the container is higher than 3 feet above the venipuncture site. The incorrect height may inadvertently occur if the patient is repositioned or the bed height is readjusted.

4. Check for tubing that has fallen below the venipuncture site. If a significant amount has fallen, elevate and carefully coil the tubing near the site of venipuncture.
5. Check to determine whether the bevel of the needle is pushing against the wall of the vein. Do this by CAUTIOUSLY raising or lowering the angle of the needle slightly to see if flow is restored. If so, reposition slightly using a gauze pad in the most appropriate location.
6. Check the temperature of the solution being infused. Cold solutions can cause spasms in the vein.
7. Check to assure that a restraint or blood pressure cuff applied to the arm has not interfered with the flow.
8. If it appears that the syringe is clotted, DO NOT attempt to clear the needle by flushing with fluid. This will dislodge the clot and may cause a thromboembolus. *Aspirate* the needle with a syringe to dislodge the clot.

Phlebitis or Infection

If signs of redness, warmth, swelling, and burning pain along the course of the vein are present, infection or phlebitis may be developing. Confirm the presence of these signs with the supervising nurse; then discontinue the IV. Insert a new IV using all new equipment at a different site. Many hospitals also require that the infection control nurse be notified, and that the site of phlebitis or infection be treated with hot or cold compresses.

Extravasation

Inspect the IV site at regular intervals for extravasation. Whenever a change in the limb's color, size, or skin integrity is observed, compare with the opposite limb. Apply a tourniquet *proximal* to the infusion site to constrict the flow. Continued flow with the tourniquet in place confirms infiltration. DO NOT rely on blood backflow into the tubing when the container is lowered. The venipuncture site could still be patent, but a laceration in the vessel may allow extravasation. Know the policies of your institution concerning the treatment of extravasation. Here are some general guidelines:

1. Stop the infusion.
2. Elevate the affected limb.
3. Remove the needle, as described above.
4. Apply heat to the site of extravasation to produce vasodilation and drug absorption.

5. Contact the physician for the possible use of antidotes to minimize tissue damage.

Air in Tubing

If an air bubble is found in IV tubing, clamp the tubing immediately. Swab either the injection site in the rubber hub near the needle or the "piggyback" portal (whichever is closest to the air bubble) with an antiseptic sponge. Using sterile technique, insert a needle and syringe into the entry site below the air bubble and withdraw the air pocket.

If air has actually entered the patient via the IV tubing, turn the patient on the left side with the head in a dependent position. Administer oxygen and notify the physician immediately.

Circulatory Overload and Pulmonary Edema

Signs of circulatory overload due to excessive volumes of fluid are engorged neck veins, dyspnea, reduced urine output, edema, weak and rapid pulse, and shallow, rapid respirations. The signs of pulmonary edema are dyspnea, cough, anxiety, rales, rhonchi, and frothy sputum. When these symptoms develop, slow the IV immediately to a "keep open" rate. Place the patient in a sitting position, start oxygen, collect vital signs, and summon the physician immediately. Gather equipment for application of rotating tourniquets, but do not apply until an order is received.

Pyrogenic Reaction

A pyrogenic reaction should be suspected if the patient develops sudden onset of chills, fever, headache, nausea, and vomiting. Check the patient's vital signs, stop the IV, and notify the physician of the findings immediately.

Save the unused portion of solution. Return it to the pharmacy or laboratory for testing as specified by hospital policy.

Pulmonary Embolism

A pulmonary embolus may occur from foreign materials injected into the vein or from a blood clot that breaks loose. Emboli can be prevented by (1) using an in-line filter, (2) completely dissolving any medications added to a solution, (3) using proper diluents for reconstitution, (4) using IV solutions that are clear and have no visible signs of foreign matter or precipitate, and (5) avoiding the use of veins in the lower extremities.

Documentation

Provide the RIGHT DOCUMENTATION of the medication administration and responses to drug therapy:

1. Chart: Date, time, drug name, dosage, and route of administration.
2. Perform and record regular patient assessments for the evaluation of the therapeutic effectiveness (i.e., blood pressure, pulse, intake and output, lung-field sounds, respiratory rate, pain at infusion site, etc.).
3. Chart and report any signs and symptoms of adverse drug effects.
4. Perform and validate essential patient education about the drug therapy and other essential aspects of intervention for the disease process affecting the individual.

Chapter 7

Preparation and Administration of Medications By Percutaneous Routes

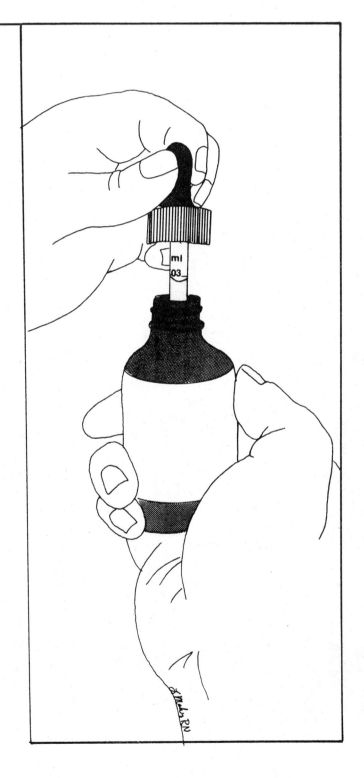

Objectives

After completing this chapter, the student should be able to do following:

1. Identify medication forms used for each type of percutaneous medication administration.
2. Explain the equipment, sites, and technique used to administer medications percutaneously.
3. Develop a written record for the documentation of significant patient symptoms and course of progress during treatment.
4. Incorporate patient teaching as a part of the medication administration procedure.
5. Chart the medication administration and health teaching performed.

Percutaneous administration refers to application of medications to the skin or mucous membranes for absorption. Methods of percutaneous administration include topical application of ointments, creams, powders, or lotions to the skin, instillation of solutions onto the mucous membranes of the mouth, eye, ear, nose, or vagina, and inhalation of aerosolized liquids or gases for absoprtion through the lungs. The primary advantage of the percutaneous route is that the action of the drug, in general, is localized to the site of application, which reduces the incidence of systemic side effects. Unfortunately, the medications are sometimes messy and difficult to apply. In addition they usually have a short duration of action and thus require more frequent reapplication.

Administration of Topical Medications to the Skin

Absorption of topical medications can be influenced by the drug concentration, the length of time the medication is in contact with the skin, the size of the affected area, the thickness of the skin, the hydration of tissues, and the degree of skin disruption.

Administration of Creams, Lotions, and Ointments

Dosage Forms

Creams. Creams are semisolid emulsions containing medicinal agents for external application. The cream base is generally nongreasy and can be removed with water. Many available over-the-counter creams are used as moisturizing agents.

Lotions. Lotions are usually aqueous preparations that contain suspended materials. They are commonly used as soothing agents to protect the skin and relieve rashes and itching. Some lotions have a cleansing action, whereas others have an astringent or drawing effect. To prevent increased circulation and itching, lotions should be gently but firmly patted on the skin, rather than rubbed in. Shake all lotions thoroughly immediately before application and use sparingly to avoid waste.

Ointments. Ointments are semisolid preparations of medicinal substances in an oily base such as lanolin or petrolatum. This type of preparation can be applied directly to the skin or mucous membrane and generally cannot be removed by water. The base helps keep the medicinal substance in prolonged contact with the skin.

Wet Dressings. Solutions frequently used for wet dressings include potassium permanganate, silver nitrate, or Burow's solution. When used, these substances are added to plain water or physiologic saline at room temperature. If making the potassium permanganate from tablets, always strain the solution PRIOR to use. Potassium permanganate and silver nitrate *stain everything*. Use measures to prevent unnecessary staining.

Equipment

Prescribed cream, lotion, or ointment
2 × 2 gauze sponges
Cotton-tipped applicators
Tongue blade
Gloves

Sites

Skin surfaces affected by the disorder being treated.

Techniques

1. Wash hands and assemble the equipment.
2. Use the 5 RIGHTS of medication preparation and administration throughout the procedure.
   RIGHT PATIENT
   RIGHT DRUG
   RIGHT ROUTE OF ADMINISTRATION
   RIGHT DOSAGE
   RIGHT TIME OF ADMINISTRATION
3. Provide privacy for the patient and give a thorough explanation of what you are going to do.
4. Place the patient in a position so the surface where the topical materials are to be applied is exposed.

Assess current status of symptoms. Provide for patient comfort before starting therapy.

5. Cleansing: Follow the specific orders of the physician for cleansing of the site of application. *Oil-based* products may be removed with cottonseed oil and gauze. *Coal tar* products may be removed with corn oil and gauze. *Water-* or *alcohol-based* products may be removed with soap and water or water alone.

6. Application: Use gloves during the application process. Many of the agents used may be absorbed through the skin of both the patient and the person applying the medication. *Lotions:* Shake well until a uniform appearance of the solution is obtained. *Ointments or creams:* Use a tongue blade to remove the desired amount from a wide-mouth container; sqeeze the amount needed onto a tongue blade or cotton-tipped applicator from a tube-type container. Apply lotions firmly, but gently, by dabbing the surface. Apply ointments and creams with a gloved hand using firm but gentle strokes. Creams are gently rubbed into the area.

7. Dressings: Check specific orders regarding the type of dressing to be used. If a dressing is to be applied, spread the prescribed amount of ointment directly on the dressing material with a tongue blade; the impregnated dressing material can then be applied to the affected skin surface. Secure the dressing in place.

8. Wet Dressings: Wring out wet dressings to prevent dripping. Always completely remove and reapply potassium permanganate or silver nitrate dressings prevent excessive chemical irritation from build-up of residue at the site of application. Secure the dressing in place. A binder or Montgomery tapes may be needed for dressings requiring frequent changes.

9. Clean up the area and equipment used and make sure the patient is comfortable after the application procedure.

10. Wash hands.

Patient Teaching

1. If appropriate, teach the patient to apply the medication and dressings.
2. Teach personal hygiene measures appropriate to the underlying cause of the skin condition (e.g., acne, contact dermatitis, infection).
3. When dressings are ordered, discuss materials readily available at home, such as clean, old muslin sheets or cloth diapers with no cotton filling. Or suggest the purchase of gauze and other necessary supplies.

4. Stress gentleness and moderation in the amount of medication to be applied.
5. Emphasize that the patient must avoid touching or scratching the affected area.
6. Tell the patient to wash hands before and after touching the affected area or applying the medication. Stress the prevention of spread of infection, when present.

Documentation

Provide the RIGHT DOCUMENTATION of the medication administration and responses to drug therapy.

1. Chart: Date, time, drug name, dosage, and route of administration.
2. Perform and record regular patient assessments for the evaluation of the therapeutic effectiveness (i.e., change in size of affected area, reduced drainage, decreased itching, lowered temperature with an infection, etc.).
3. Chart and report any signs and symptoms of adverse drug effects as well as a narrative description of the area being treated.
4. Develop a written record for the patient to use in charting progress for evaluation of the effectiveness of the treatments being used. List the patient symptoms (e.g., rash on lower leg with redness and vesicles present; decubitus ulcer on the sacrum). List the data to be collected regarding the medication prescribed and the effectiveness (e.g., vesicles now crusted, weeping, or appear to be drying; redness in lower leg is lessening; area of decubitus is extending, remaining the same, or shrinking).
5. Perform and validate essential patient education about the drug therapy and other essential aspects of intervention for the disease process affecting the individual.

Patch Testing for Allergens

Patch testing is a method used to identify patient's sensitivity to contact materials (i.e., soaps, pollens, dyes, etc.). The suspected allergens (antigens) are placed in direct contact with the skin surface and covered with nonsensitizing, nonabsorbent tape. Unless marked irritation appears, the patch is usually left in place for 48 hours, then removed. The site is left open to air for 15 minutes, and then "read." A positive reaction is noted by the presence of redness and swelling, and indicates allergy to the specific antigen.

Intradermal tests may also be used to determine allergenicity to specific antigens. See Chapter 6 for further information on intradermal administration of allergens.

Equipment

Alcohol for cleansing the area
Solutions of suspected antigens
2 × 2 inch pieces of typewriter paper
1 × 1 inch gauze pads
Droppers
Mineral or olive oil
Water
Hypoallergenic tape
Record for charting data on substances applied and responses

Sites

The back, arms, or thighs are commonly used. (DO NOT use the face or areas receiving friction from clothing.) Selected areas are spaced every 2 to 3 inches apart. The type of allergen applied and the site of application are documented on the patient's chart (Fig. 7.1).

Technique

CAUTION: DO NOT start any type of allergy testing unless emergency equipment is available in the immediate area in case of an anaphylactic response. Personnel should be familiar with the procedure to follow if an emergency does arise.

1. Check with the patient before starting the testing to be sure that he or she has not taken any antihistamines or anti-inflammatory agents (i.e., aspirin, ibuprofen, corticosteroids) for 24 to 48 hours preceding the tests. If the patient has taken an antihistamine or anti-inflammatory agent, check with the physician before proceeding with the testing.
2. Wash hands and assemble the equipment.
3. Use the 5 RIGHTS of medication preparation and administration throughout the procedure.
   RIGHT PATIENT
   RIGHT DRUG
   RIGHT ROUTE OF ADMINISTRATION
   RIGHT DOSAGE
   RIGHT TIME OF ADMINISTRATION
4. Provide privacy for the patient and give a thorough explanation of what you are going to do.
5. Place the patient in a position so the surface where the test materials are to be applied is horizontal. Provide patient comfort before starting testing.

6. Cleanse the selected area thoroughly using an alcohol pledget. Use circular motions starting at the planned site of injection and continuing outward in ever-widening circular motions to the periphery. Allow the area to air-dry.
7. Prepare the designated solutions using aseptic technique.
8. Follow specific directions of the employing health care agency for the application of liquid and solid forms of suspected allergens. Generally, a dropper is used to apply suspected liquid contact-type materials; solid materials are applied directly to the skin surface and then moistened with mineral or olive oil.
9. After application, each area used should be covered first with a 1 × 1 gauze followed by a 2 × 2 piece of typewriter paper; secure with hypoallergenic tape. (If the patient is known to be allergic to all types of tape, consider the use of a binder.)
10. Chart the times, agents, concentrations, and amounts applied. Make a diagram in the patient's chart numbering each location. Record what agent and concentration was placed at each site. Subsequent readings of each area are then performed and charted on this record.
11. Follow directions for the time of the reading of the skin testing being performed. Inspection of the testing sites should be performed in good light. Generally, a positive reaction (development of a wheal) to a dilute strength of suspected allergen is considered clinically significant. Measure the diameter of erythema in millimeters and palpate and measure the size of any induration. Record this information in the patient's chart. No reaction should be noted at the control site.

Patient Teaching

1. Tell the patient the time, date, and place of the return visit to have the test sites read.
2. Tell the patient not to take a bath or shower until the patches are read and removed.
3. If the patient develops an area of severe burning or itching, lift the patch and gently wash the area. Tell the patient to report immediately the development of any breathing difficulty, severe hives, or rashes. The patient should be told to go to the nearest emergency room if unable to reach the physician who prescribed the skin tests.

Documentation

Provide the RIGHT DOCUMENTATION of the medication administration and responses to drug therapy.

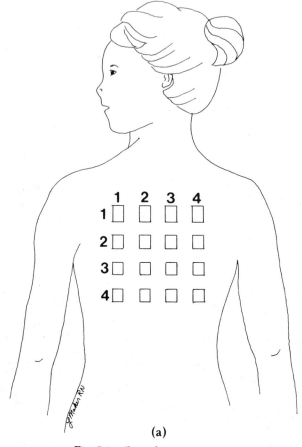

(a)

Fig. 7.1. *(Legend on opposite page.)*

1. Chart: Date, time, drug name, dosage, and site of administration (Fig. 7.1).
2. Read each site 24–28 hours after the application, as directed by the physician or policy of the health care agency.
3. Chart and report any signs and symptoms of adverse drug effects.
4. Perform and validate essential patient education about the testing and other essential aspects of intervention for the disease process affecting the individual.

Commonly used readings of reactions and appropriate symbols are listed below.

+	(1+)	Redness of skin present (erythema)
+ +	(2+)	Redness and solid elevated lesions up to 5 mm in diameter (erythema and papules)
+ + +	(3+)	Erythema, papules, and vesicles (blisterlike areas 5 mm or less in diameter)
+ + + +	(4+)	Generalized fusing of blistered areas

Administration of Nitroglycerin Ointment

Dosage Form

Nitroglycerin ointment (Nitro-Bid; Nitrol) provides relief of anginal pain for several hours longer than sublingual preparations. When properly applied, nitroglycerin ointment is particularly effective against nocturnal attacks of anginal pain. Specific instructions for nitroglycerin ointment are reviewed in this text because it is the only ointment currently available for which dosage is critical to the success of use. (See Chapter 10, Drugs Affecting the Cardiovascular System.)

Equipment

Nitroglycerin ointment
Applicator paper
Clear plastic wrap
Nonallergenic adhesive tape

Sites

Any area without hair may be used. Most people prefer the chest, flank, or upper arm areas (Fig. 7.2).

Patient Name: _____
Identification Number: _____
Physician Name: _____

DATE:	TIME:	AGENT	CONCENTRATION	AMOUNT INJECTED	SITE NUMBER:*	Reading Time in Hours or minutes i.e. 30 min. or 24, 48, 72 hours		

* Refer to diagram of sites, Figure 6.24a,b.
—Follow directions for the "reading" of the skin testing performed.
—Inspect sites in a good light
—Record reaction in upper half of box using the following guidelines, i.e.,
   +   (1⁺) Redness of skin present (erythema)
   + +   (2⁺) Redness and solid elevated lesion up to 5 mm in diameter (erythema and papules).
   + + + (3⁺) Erythema, papules and vesicles (blister-like areas 5 mm or less in diameter).
   + + + + (4⁺) Generalized fusing of blisters.
—Record measurement of induration (process of hardening) in mm. in lower half of box, i.e.,

(b)

Fig. 7.1. *Patch test for contact dermatitis.* (a) *(opposite) Patch testing sites.* (b) *Reading chart, patch testing.*

(Do NOT shave an area to apply the ointment; shaving may cause skin irritation.)

Techniques

1. Wash hands and assemble the equipment.
2. Use the 5 RIGHTS of medication preparation and administration throughout the procedure.
   RIGHT PATIENT
   RIGHT DRUG
   RIGHT ROUTE OF ADMINISTRATION
   RIGHT DOSAGE
   RIGHT TIME OF ADMINISTRATION
3. Provide privacy for the patient and give a thorough explanation of what you are going to do.
4. Place the patient in a position so the surface where the topical materials are to be applied is exposed. Provide patient comfort before starting therapy.
5. Lay the dose-measuring applicator paper with the print side DOWN on the site (Fig. 7.3a). (The ointment will smear the print.)

6. Squeeze a ribbon of ointment of the proper length onto the applicator paper.
7. Place the measuring applicator on the skin surface at the site chosen on the rotation schedule, ointment side DOWN. Spread in a thin, uniform layer under the applicator. DO NOT RUB IN. Leave the paper in place. *Note:* Use of the applicator paper allows you to measure the prescribed dose and prevents absorption through the fingertips as you apply the medication (Fig. 7.3b).
8. Cover the area where the paper is placed with plastic wrap and tape it in place.
9. Wash hands after applying the ointment.

Patient Teaching

1. Guide the patient in learning how to apply the ointment.
2. Tell the patient that the medication may discolor clothing. Use of clear plastic wrap protects clothing.
3. When the dose is regulated properly, the ointment may be used every 3 to 4 hours and at bedtime.

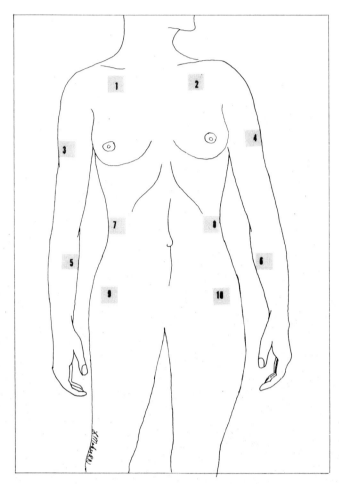

Fig. 7.2. *Sites for nitroglycerin application.*

4. Tell the patient to wash hands after application to remove any nitroglycerin that came in contact with the fingers.

5. When terminating the use of this topical ointment, the dose and frequency of application should be gradually reduced over a 4- to 6-week period. Tell the patient to contact the physician if he or she feels that the dosage needs to be adjusted. Encourage the patient not to discontinue the medication abruptly. (See Chapter 10, Drugs Affecting the Cardiovascular System, for further information.)

Documentation

Provide the RIGHT DOCUMENTATION of the medication administration and responses to drug therapy.

1. Chart: Date, time, drug name, dosage, site, and route of administration.

2. Perform and record regular patient assessments for the evaluation of therapeutic effectiveness (i.e., blood pressure, pulse, output, degree and duration of pain relief, etc.).

3. Chart and report any signs and symptoms of adverse drug effects.

4. Perform and validate essential patient education about the drug therapy and other essential aspects of intervention for the disease process affecting the individual.

Administration of Nitroglycerin Topical Disks

Dosage Form

The nitroglycerin transdermal patch provides controlled release of nitroglycerin through a semipermeable

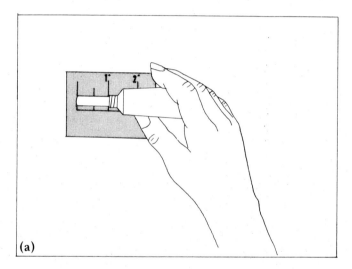

(a)

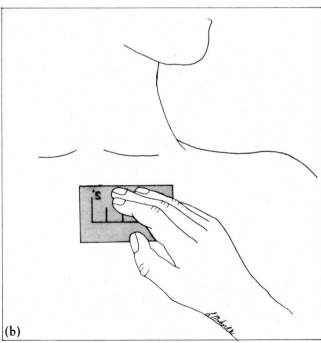

(b)

Fig. 7.3. *Administering nitroglycerine topical ointment.* (a) *Lay applicator paper print side down, and measure ribbon of ointment.* (b) *Apply applicator to skin site, ointment side down. Spread in a uniform layer under applicator; leave paper in place.*

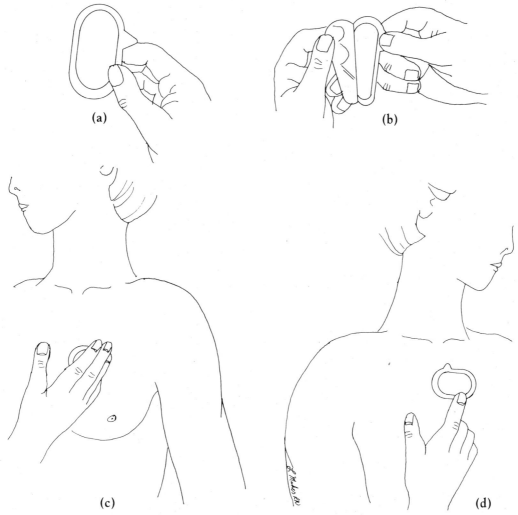

Fig. 7.4. *Administering nitroglycerin topical disks (Trans-Derm Nitro®). (a) Carefully pick up the system lengthwise, with the tab up. (b) Remove clear plastic backing from system at the tab. Do not touch inside of exposed system. (c) Place the exposed adhesive side of the system on the chosen skin site; press firmly with the palm of the hand. (d) Circle the outside edge of the system with one or two fingers. (Courtesy of CIBA Pharmaceutical Co., Summit, New Jersey.)*

membrane for 24 hours when applied to intact skin. The dosage released depends upon the surface area of the disk in contact with the skin surface. Therapeutic effects can be observed in about 30 minutes after attachment and for about 30 minutes after removal. (See Chapter 10, Drugs Affecting the Cardiovascular System.)

Equipment

Nitroglycerin transdermal disk
Shaving equipment as appropriate for the site and skin condition

Sites

Any area without hair may be used. Most people prefer the chest, flank, or upper arm areas. Develop a rotation schedule for use (Fig. 7.2).

Techniques

1. Wash hands and assemble the equipment.
2. Use the 5 RIGHTS of medication preparation and administration throughout the procedure.
   RIGHT PATIENT
   RIGHT DRUG
   RIGHT ROUTE OF ADMINISTRATION
   RIGHT DOSAGE
   RIGHT TIME OF ADMINISTRATION
3. Provide for patient privacy and give a thorough explanation of what is to be done.
4. Place the patient in a position so the surface where the topical materials are to be applied is exposed. Provide for patient comfort.
5. Apply the small adhesive topical disk (Fig. 7.4a–d) once daily to one of the sites recommended by the rotation schedule.

6. Wash hands after application.

Patient Teaching

1. Guide the patient in learning how and when to apply the disks.
2. Trans-Derm Nitro and Nitro-Dur may be worn while showering; Nitrodisc should be replaced after bathing or showering.
3. If a disk becomes partially dislodged, the patient should discard it and apply a new one. The patient should apply the disk to the next rotation site.
4. Sublingual nitroglycerin may be necessary for anginal attacks, especially while the dosage is being adjusted.

Documentation

Provide the RIGHT DOCUMENTATION of the medication administration and responses to drug therapy.

1. Chart: Date, time, drug name, dosage, and route of administration.
2. Perform and record regular patient assessments for the evaluation of therapeutic effectiveness (i.e., blood pressure, pulse, degree and duration of pain relief, etc.).
3. Chart and report any signs and symptoms of adverse drug effects.
4. Perform and validate essential patient education about the drug therapy and other essential aspects of intervention for the disease process affecting the individual.

Administration of Topical Powders

Dosage Form

Powders are finely ground particles of medication contained in a talc base. They generally produce a cooling, drying, or protective effect where applied.

Equipment

Prescribed powder

Site

To the skin surface of the body, as prescribed.

Technique

1. Wash hands.
2. Use the 5 RIGHTS of medication preparation and administration throughout the procedure:

RIGHT PATIENT
RIGHT DRUG
RIGHT ROUTE OF ADMINISTRATION
RIGHT DOSAGE
RIGHT TIME OF ADMINISTRATION

3. Provide privacy for the patient and give a thorough explanation of what you are going to do.
4. Place the patient in a position so the surface where the topical materials are to be applied is exposed. Provide patient comfort before starting therapy.
5. Wash and thoroughly dry the affected area before applying the powder.
6. Apply powder by gently shaking the container. This distributes the powder evenly over the area. Gently smooth over the area for even coverage.

Patient Teaching

Tell the patient to clean and reapply powder to external surface as directed by the physician. The patient should avoid inhaling the powder during application.

Documentation

Provide the RIGHT DOCUMENTATION of the medication administration and responses to drug therapy.

1. Chart: Date, time, drug name, dosage, site, and route of administration.
2. Perform and record regular patient assessments for the evaluation of therapeutic effectiveness.
3. Chart and report any signs and symptoms of adverse drug effects.
4. Perform and validate essential patient education about the drug therapy and other essential aspects of intervention for the disease process affecting the individual.

Administration of Medications to Mucous Membranes

Drugs are well absorbed across mucosal surfaces, and it is easy to obtain therapeutic effects. However, mucous membranes are highly selective in absorptive activity and differ in sensitivity. In general, aqueous solutions are quickly absorbed from mucous membranes, whereas oily liquids are not. Drugs in suppository form can be used for local effects on the mucous membranes of the vagina, urethra, or rectum. A drug may be inhaled and absorbed through the mucous membranes of the nose and lungs. It may be dissolved and absorbed by the mucous membranes of the mouth, or applied to the eyes or ears for local action. Or it may be painted, swabbed, or irrigated on a mucosal surface.

Administration of Sublingual and Buccal Tablets

Dosage Forms

Sublingual tablets are designed to be placed under the tongue for dissolution and absorption through the vast network of blood vessels in this area. Buccal tablets are designed to be held in the buccal cavity (between the cheek and molar teeth) for absorption from the blood vessels of the cheek. The primary advantage of these routes of administration is the rapid absorption and onset of action since the drug passes directly into systemic circulation with no immediate pass through the liver, where extensive metabolism usually takes place. Contrary to most other forms of administration to mucous membranes, the action from these dosage forms is usually systemic, rather than localized to the mouth.

Equipment

Prescribed medication. Note: The medications available to be administered by this route are forms of nitroglycerin. Once the self-administration technique is taught, the patient should carry the medication or keep it readily available at bedside for use as needed.

Site

Sublingual area (under tongue) (Fig. 7.5a) or buccal pouch (between molar teeth and cheek) (Fig. 7.5b).

Technique

For Administration by the Nurse. Refer to Chapter 5, Administration of Solid-Form Oral Medications, for correct technique with either the medication card system or the unit dose system.

1. Wash hands and assemble the equipment.
2. Use the 5 RIGHTS of medication preparation and administration throughout the procedure:
   RIGHT PATIENT
   RIGHT DRUG
   RIGHT ROUTE OF ADMINISTRATION
   RIGHT DOSAGE
   RIGHT TIME OF ADMINISTRATION
3. Provide privacy for the patient and give a thorough explanation of what you are going to do.

4. Place the medication under the tongue (sublingual) (Fig. 7.5a) or between the upper molar teeth and the cheek (buccal) (Fig. 7.5b). The tablet is meant to dissolve in these locations. Do not administer with water. Encourage the patient to allow the drug to dissolve where placed.
5. Wash your hands.

Teaching Self-Administration. Explain the exact placement of the medication and the dosage and frequency of taking the medication. The patient should be told what side effects to expect, what adverse effects to report, where to carry the medication, how to store the medication, and how to refill the prescription when needed. (See Chapter 10, Drugs Affecting the Cardiovascular System, Nitroglycerin.)

Documentation

Provide the RIGHT DOCUMENTATION of the medication administration and responses to drug therapy.

1. Chart: Date, time, drug name, dosage, site, and route of administration.
2. Perform and record regular patient assessments for the evaluation of therapeutic effectiveness (i.e., blood pressure, pulse, degree and duration of pain relief, number of doses taken, etc.).
3. Chart and report any signs and symptoms of adverse drug effects.
4. Perform and validate essential patient education about the drug therapy and other essential aspects of intervention for the disease process affecting the individual.

Note: When the patient is self-administering a medication, the nurse is still responsible for all aspects of the charting and monitoring parameters to document the drug therapy and response achieved.

Administration of Eye Drops and Ointment

Dosage Form

Medications for use in the eye should be labeled OPHTHALMIC. If not labeled as such, do not administer to the eye. Ocular solutions are sterile, easily administered, and usually do not interfere with vision when instilled. Allow eye medication to warm to room temperature before administration.

Ocular ointments do cause alterations in visual acuity. However, they have a longer duration of action than solutions.

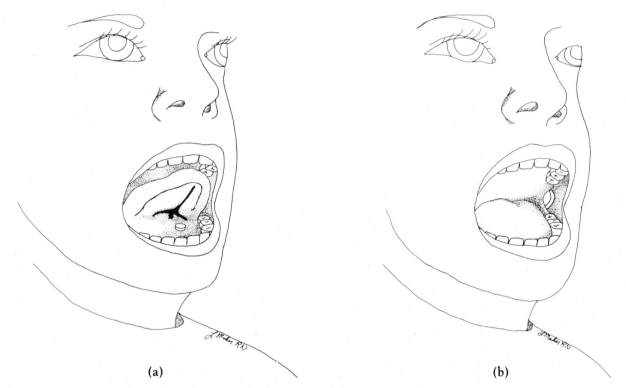

Fig. 7.5. *Placing medication in the mouth.* (a) *Under the tongue (sublingual).* (b) *In the buccal pouch.*

Always use a separate bottle or tube of eye medication for each patient. (See Chapter 18, Drugs Affecting the Eye.)

Equipment

Eye drops or ointment prescribed (check strength carefully)
Dropper (use only the dropper supplied by the manufacturer)
Paper tissues and/or sterile cotton balls
Sterile eye dressing (pad), as appropriate
Normal saline solution, if needed for cleaning off exudate

Site

Eye(s). O.D. = right eye, O.S. = left eye, O.U. = both eyes.

Techniques

1. Wash hands and assemble the *ophthalmic* medication.
2. Use the 5 RIGHTS of medication preparation and administration throughout the procedure.
   RIGHT PATIENT
   RIGHT DRUG
   RIGHT ROUTE OF ADMINISTRATION
   RIGHT DOSAGE
   RIGHT TIME OF ADMINISTRATION
3. Provide privacy for the patient and give a thorough explanation of what you are going to do.
4. Position the patient so that the back of the head is firmly supported on a pillow and the face is directed toward the ceiling. With children, restraints may be necessary if the child is too young to voluntarily cooperate. Always ensure patient safety.
5. Check to be certain that you have the correct medication according to the 5 RIGHTS. Inspect the affected eye to determine the current status. As appropriate, remove exudate from the eyelid and eyelashes using sterile saline solution. Always use a seperate cotton ball for each wiping motion. Start at the inner canthus and wipe outward.
6. Expose the lower conjunctival sac by applying gentle traction to the lower lid at the bony rim of the orbit.
7. Approach the eye from below with the medication dropper or tube of ointment. (Never touch the eye dropper or ointment tip against the eye or face.)
   Drops (Fig. 7.6):
   ● Have the patient look upward over your head.
   ● Drop the specified number of drops into the conjunctival sac. Never drop directly onto the eyeball.
   ● After instilling the drops, apply gentle pressure, using a cotton ball, to the inner corner of the

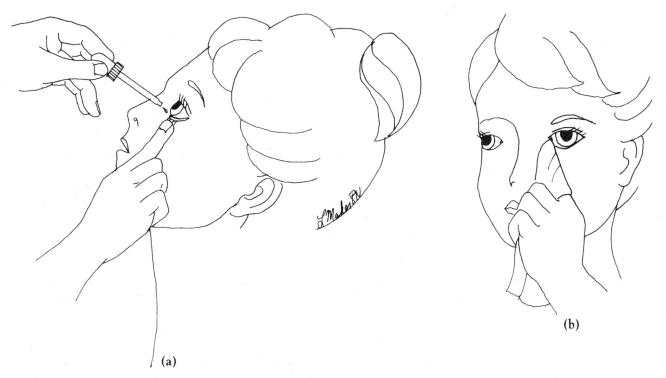

Fig. 7.6. *Administering ophthalmic drops. (a) Have the patient look upward; apply gentle traction to lower lid to expose conjunctival sac. Instill drops into sac. (b) Using a tissue, apply gentle pressure to the inner corner of eyelid on bone for one to two minutes.*

eyelid on the bone for approximately 1 to 2 minutes. This prevents the medication from entering the canal where it would be absorbed in the vascular mucosa of the nose and produce systemic effects. It also ensures an adequate concentration of medication in the eye.

- When more than one type of eye drop is ordered for the same eye, wait 1 to 5 minutes between instillation of the different medications. Use only the dropper provided by the manufacturer. Apply a sterile dressing as ordered.

Ointment:

- Gently squeeze the ointment in a strip fashion into the conjunctival sac (Fig. 7.7). Do not allow the tip to touch the patient.
- Tell the patient to close the eye(s) gently and move the eyes with the lid shut, as if looking around the room, to spread the medication. Apply a sterile dressing as ordered.

8. Wash hands after the application.

Patient Teaching

1. Guide the patient in learning how to apply his or her own ophthalmic medication.
2. Tell the patient to wipe the eye(s) gently from the nose outward to prevent contamination between the eyes and possible spread of infection, and to use a separate tissue to wipe each eye.
3. Have the patient wash hands frequently and avoid touching the eye or immediate areas surrounding it, especially when an infection is present. Dispose of tissues in a manner that prevents spread of an infection.
4. Stress punctuality in administration of eye medications, especially when used for treating infections or increased intraocular pressure.

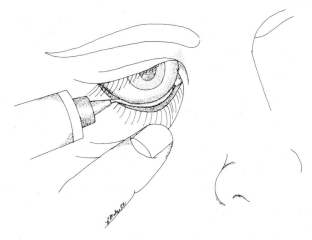

Fig. 7.7. *Administering ophthalmic ointment. To instill the ointment, gently pull the lower lid down as patient looks upward. Squeeze ophthalmic ointment into lower sac. Avoid touching tube to eyelid.*

5. Tell the patient to discard eye medications that have changed color, become cloudy, or contain particles. (If the patient's visual acuity is reduced, someone else should check clarity.)
6. The patient must not use over-the-counter eye washes without first consulting the physician managing the eye disorder.
7. Emphasize the need for careful follow-up of any eye disorder until the physician releases the patient from further care.

Documentation

Provide the RIGHT DOCUMENTATION of the medication administration and responses to drug therapy:

1. Chart: Date, time, drug name, dosage, site, and route of administration.
2. Perform and record regular patient assessments for the evaluation of therapeutic effectiveness (i.e., redness, discomfort, visual activity, changes in infection or inflammatory reaction, degree and duration of pain relief, etc.).
3. Chart and report any signs and symptoms of adverse drug effects.
4. Perform and validate essential patient education about the drug therapy and other essential aspects of intervention for the disease process affecting the individual.

Administration of Ear Drops

Dosage Form

Ear drops are a solution containing a medication which is used for the treatment of localized infection or inflammation of the ear. Medications for use in the ear should be labeled OTIC. If not labeled as such, do not administer to the ear. Ear drops should be warmed to room temperature before use, and separate bottles of ear drops should be used for each patient.

Equipment

Otic solution prescribed
Dropper provided by the manufacturer

Site

Ear(s)

Techniques

1. Wash hands and assemble the equipment.

2. Use the 5 RIGHTS of medication preparation and administration throughout the procedure:
   RIGHT PATIENT
   RIGHT DRUG
   RIGHT ROUTE OF ADMINISTRATION
   RIGHT DOSAGE
   RIGHT TIME OF ADMINISTRATION
3. Provide privacy for the patient and give a thorough explanation of what you are going to do.
4. Place the patient in a position so the affected ear is directed upward.
5. Assess the ear canal for wax accumulation. If wax is present, get an order to irrigate the canal before instilling the ear drops.
6. Allow the medication to warm to room temperature, shake well, and draw up into the dropper.
7. Administration: *Children under 3 years of age:* Restrain the child, turn the head to the appropriate side, and gently pull the earlobe *downward* and *back* (Fig. 7.8a). Instill the prescribed number of drops into the canal. Do not allow the dropper tip to touch any part of the ear. *Children over 3 years of age and adults:* Enlist cooperation, or restrain as necessary, turn the head to the appropriate side, and gently pull the earlobe *upward* and *back* (Fig. 7.8b) to straighten the external auditory canal. Instill the prescribed number of drops into the canal. Do not allow the dropper tip to touch any part of the ear.
8. Have the patient remain on the side for a few minutes following instillation; insert a cotton plug *loosely* if ordered.
9. Repeat the procedure if ear drops are ordered for both ears.

Patient Teaching

1. Explain the importance of administering the medication as prescribed.
2. Teach self-administration or administration to another person as appropriate.

Documentation

Provide the RIGHT DOCUMENTATION of the medication administration and responses to drug therapy:

1. Chart: Date, time, drug name, dosage, site, and route of administration.
2. Perform and record regular patient assessments for the evaluation of therapeutic effectiveness (i.e., redness, pressure, degree, and duration of pain relief, color and amount of drainage, etc.).
3. Chart and report any signs and symptoms of adverse drug effects.

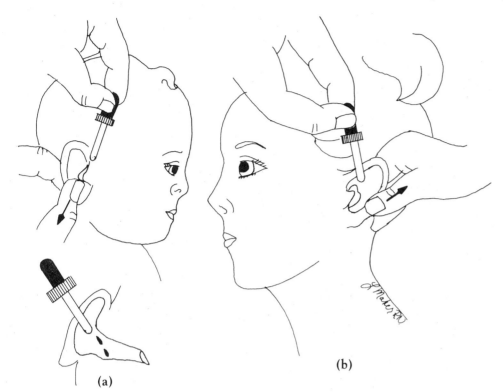

(a)

(b)

Fig. 7.8. *Administering ear drops. (a) Pull earlobe downward and back in children under three years of age. (b) Pull earlobe upward and back in patients over three years of age.*

4. Perform and validate essential patient education about the drug therapy and other essential aspects of intervention for the disease process affecting the individual.

Administration of Nose Drops

Nasal solutions are used to treat temporary disorders affecting the nasal mucous membrane. Always use the dropper provided by the manufacturer and provide each patient with a separate bottle of nose drops.

Equipment

Nose drops prescribed
Dropper supplied by the manufacturer
Tissue to blow the nose

Site

Nostril(s)

Techniques

1. Wash hands and assemble the equipment.
2. Use the 5 RIGHTS of medication preparation and administration throughout the procedure:
    RIGHT PATIENT
    RIGHT DRUG

RIGHT ROUTE OF ADMINISTRATION
RIGHT DOSAGE
RIGHT TIME OF ADMINISTRATION

3. Provide privacy for the patient and give a thorough explanation of what you are going to do.
4. Administration (Fig. 7.9):
    Adults and older children
    - Instruct the patient to gently blow the nose.
    - Have the patient lie down and hang the head backward over the edge of the bed.
    - Draw the medication into the dropper. Hold the dropper just above the nostril and instill the medication.
    - After a brief time, have the patient turn the head to the other side and repeat the administration process in the second nostril, if needed.
    - Have the patient remain in this position for 2 to 3 minutes to allow the drops to remain in contact with the nasal mucosa.
    Infants and young children
    - Position the infant or small child with the head over the edge of the bed or pillow. Or, use the "football" hold to immobilize the infant.
    - Administer nose drops in the same manner as for the adult.
    - For the child who is cooperative, offer praise. Provide appropriate comforting and personal contact for all children or infants.
5. Have paper tissues available for use if absolutely necessary to blow the nose.

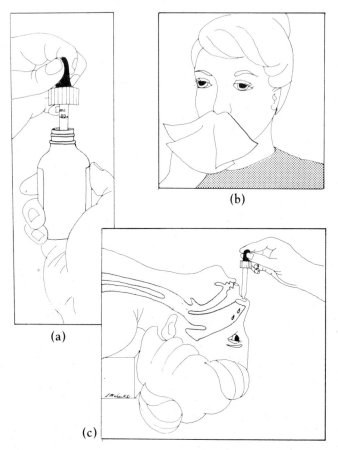

Fig. 7.9. *Administering nose drops. (a) Gently blow nose. (b) Open medication and draw up to calibration on dropper. (c) Instill medication. Have patient remain in position for two to three minutes. Repeat on other side if necessary.*

Patient Teaching

Guide the patient in learning self-administration of nose drops of necessary. Tell the patient that overuse of the nose drops can cause a "rebound effect," which causes the symptoms to become worse. If symptoms have not resolved after a week of nasal drop therapy, the physician should be consulted again.

Documentation

Provide the RIGHT DOCUMENTATION of the medication administration and responses to drug therapy:

1. Chart: Date, time, drug name, dosage, site, and route of administration.
2. Perform and record regular patient assessments for the evaluation of the therapeutic effectiveness (i.e., nasal congestion, degree and duration of relief achieved, improvement in overall status, etc.)
3. Chart and report any signs and symptoms of adverse drug effects.

4. Perform and validate essential patient education about the drug therapy and other essential aspects of intervention for the disease process affecting the individual.

Administration of Nasal Spray

The mucous membranes of the nose absorb aqueous solutions very well. When applied as a spray, the small droplets of solution containing medication coat the membrane and are rapidly absorbed. The advantage of spray over drops is less waste of medication, since some of the drops often run down the back of the throat before absorption can take place. As with drops, each patient should have a personal container of spray.

Equipment

Nasal spray prescribed
Paper tissues to blow the nose

Site

Nostril(s)

Techniques

1. Wash hands and assemble the equipment.
2. Use the 5 RIGHTS of medication preparation and administration throughout the procedure:
   RIGHT PATIENT
   RIGHT DRUG
   RIGHT ROUTE OF ADMINISTRATION
   RIGHT DOSAGE
   RIGHT TIME OF ADMINISTRATION
3. Provide privacy for the patient and give a thorough explanation of what you are going to do.
4. Instruct the patient to gently blow the nose (Fig. 7.10a–c).
5. Sit the patient upright.
6. Block one nostril.
7. Holding the spray bottle upright, shake the bottle.
8. Immediately after shaking, insert the tip into the nostril. Ask the patient to inhale through the open nostril and squeeze a puff of spray into the nostril at the same time.
9. Have paper tissues available for use if absolutely necessary to blow the nose.

Patient Teaching

Guide the patient in learning self-administration of nose drops if necessary. Tell the patient that overuse

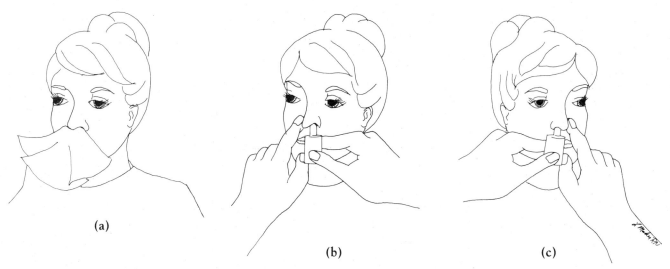

(a) **(b)** **(c)**

Fig. 7.10. *Administering nasal spray. (a) Gently blow nose. (b) Block one nostril; shake bottle, insert tip into nostril and squeeze a puff of spray while inhaling through the open nostril.*

of nasal spray can cause a "rebound effect," which causes the symptoms to become worse. If symptoms have not resolved after a week of nasal spray therapy, the physician should be consulted again.

Documentation

Provide the RIGHT DOCUMENTATION of the medication administration and responses to drug therapy:

1. Chart: Date, time, drug name, dosage, site, and route of administration.
2. Perform and record regular patient assessments for the evaluation of therapeutic effectiveness (i.e., nasal congestion, degree and duration of relief achieved, improvement in overall status, etc.).
3. Chart and report any signs and symptoms of adverse drug effects.
4. Perform and validate essential patient education about the drug therapy and other essential aspects of intervention for the disease process affecting the individual.

Administration of Medications by Inhalation

The respiratory mucosa may be medicated by means of inhalation of sprays (nebulae) or aerosols. Nebulae are sprayed into the throat by a nebulizer. Aerosols use a flow of air or oxygen under pressure to disperse the drug throughout the respiratory tract. Oily preparations should not be applied to the respiratory mucosa since the oil droplets may be carried to the lung and cause lipid pneumonia (see also Chapter 11, Drugs Affecting the Respiratory System.)

Equipment

Liquid aerosol or spray forms of medications for inhalation

Site

Respiratory tract

Techniques

1. Wash hands and assemble the equipment.
2. Use the 5 RIGHTS of medication preparation and administration throughout the procedure:
   RIGHT PATIENT
   RIGHT DRUG
   RIGHT ROUTE OF ADMINISTRATION
   RIGHT DOSAGE
   RIGHT TIME OF ADMINISTRATION
3. Provide privacy for the patient and give a thorough explanation of what you are going to do.
4. Place the patient in a sitting position. This allows maximum lung expansion.
5. Prepare the medication according to the prescribed directions and fill the nebulizer with diluent. (This may be done before sitting the patient up if time is a factor to the patient's well-being.)
6. Direct the patient to exhale through pursed lips.
7. Put the nebulizer mouthpiece in the mouth: DO NOT seal the lips completely.
8. Activate the inhalation equipment while simultaneously having the patient inhale and breathe to full capacity.
9. Direct the patient to exhale *slowly* through pursed lips.

10. WAIT approximately 1 minute and repeat the sequence according to the physician's directions, or until all of the medication in the nebulizer is used.
11. Clean the equipment according to the manufacturer's directions.
12. Assist the patient to a comfortable postion.
13. Wash hands.

Patient Teaching

1. As appropriate to the circumstances, teach the patient or significant others to operate the nebulizer to be used at home.
2. Explain the operation and cleansing of the equipment.
3. Have the patient or significant others administer the treatment using the equipment and medications prescribed for at-home use before discharge.
4. Stress the need to perform the procedure exactly as prescribed and to report any difficulties experienced after discharge for physician evaluation.

Documentation

Provide the RIGHT DOCUMENTATION of the medication administration and responses to drug therapy:

1. Chart: Date, time, drug name, dosage, and route of administration.
2. Perform and record regular patient assessments for the evaluation of therapeutic effectiveness (i.e., blood pressure, pulse, improvement or quality of breathing, cough and productivity, degree and duration of pain relief, ability to operate the nebulizer, activity and exercise restrictions, etc.).
3. Chart and report any signs and symptoms of adverse drug effects.
4. Perform and validate essential patient education about the drug therapy and other essential aspects of intervention for the disease process affecting the individual.

Administration of Vaginal Medications

Women with gynecologic disorders may require the administration of a medication intravaginally, usually for localized action. Vaginal medications may be creams, jellies, tablets, foams, suppositories, or irrigations (douches). The creams, jellies, tablets, and foams are inserted using special applicators provided by the manufacturer, while suppositories are usually inserted with a gloved index finger. (See below for Administration of Vaginal Douches.)

Equipment

Prescribed medication
Vaginal applicator
Perineal pad
Water-soluble lubricant (for suppository)
Gloves
Paper towel

Site

Vagina

Techniques

1. Wash hands and assemble the equipment.
2. Use the 5 RIGHTS of medication preparation and administration throughout the procedure:
   RIGHT PATIENT
   RIGHT DRUG
   RIGHT ROUTE OF ADMINISTRATION
   RIGHT DOSAGE
   RIGHT TIME OF ADMINISTRATION
3. Provide privacy for the patient and give a thorough explanation of what you are going to do. Have the patient void to ensure that the bladder is empty.
4. Fill the applicator with the prescribed tablet, jelly, cream, or foam.
5. Place the patient in the lithotomy position and elevate the hips with a pillow. Drape the patient to prevent unnecessary exposure.
6. Administration. *For creams, foams, and jellies:* With the gloved, nondominant hand, spread the labia to expose the vagina. Assess the status of presenting symptoms (i.e., color of discharge, volume, odor, level of discomfort). Gently insert the vaginal applicator as far as possible into the vagina and push the plunger to deposit the medication (Fig. 7.11). Remove the applicator and wrap it in a paper towel for cleaning later. *For suppositories:* Unwrap a vaginal suppository that has warmed to room temperature and lubricate with a water-soluble lubricant. Lubricate the gloved, dominant index finger. With the gloved, nondominant hand, spread the labia to expose the vagina. Insert the suppository (rounded end first) as far into the vagina as possible with the dominant index finger.
7. Remove glove by turning inside out; place on paper towel for later disposal.
8. Apply a perineal pad to prevent drainage onto the patient's clothing or bed.

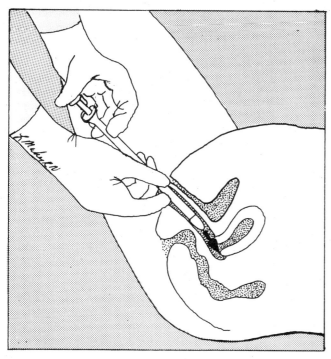

Fig. 7.11. *Applying vaginal medication. Gently insert the vaginal applicator as far as possible into the vagina and push plunger to deposit the medication.*

9. Instruct the patient to remain in a supine position with hips elevated for 5 to 10 minutes to allow melting and spreading of the medication.
10. Dispose of all waste and wash your hands.

Patient Teaching

1. Guide the patient in learning how to correctly administer the medication.
2. The applicator should be washed in warm soapy water after *each* use.
3. Review personal hygiene measures such as wiping from the front to the back after voiding or defecating.
4. Tell the patient not to douche and to abstain from sexual intercourse after inserting the medication.
5. With most types of infection, both the male and female partners require treatment. Partners should abstain from sexual intercourse until both partners are cured to prevent reinfections.

Documentation

Provide the RIGHT DOCUMENTATION of the medication administration and responses to drug therapy:

1. Chart: Date, time, drug name, dosage, and route of administration.

2. Perform and record regular patient assessments for the evaluation of the therapeutic effectiveness (i.e., type of discharge present, irritation of labia, discomfort, degree and duration of pain relief, etc.).
3. Chart and report any signs and symptoms of adverse drug effects.
4. Perform and validate essential patient education about the drug therapy and other essential aspects of intervention for the disease process affecting the individual.

Administration of a Vaginal Douche

Douches (irrigants) are used for washing the vagina. It is a procedure that is not necessary for normal female hygiene, but may be required if a vaginal infection and discharge are present. It should also be noted that douches are not effective methods of birth control.

Equipment

Douche bag with tubing and nozzle
Douche solution

Site

Vagina

Techniques

1. Wash hands and assemble the equipment.
2. Use the 5 RIGHTS of medication preparation and administration throughout the procedure:
   RIGHT PATIENT
   RIGHT DRUG
   RIGHT ROUTE OF ADMINISTRATION
   RIGHT DOSAGE
   RIGHT TIME OF ADMINISTRATION
3. Provide privacy for the patient and give a thorough explanation of what you are going to do.
4. Ask the patient to void prior to the procedure.
5. If teaching this procedure to a patient for home use, the patient would customarily recline in a bathtub. Depending on the patient's condition in the hospital, this too could occur. However, it may be necessary to place the patient on a bedpan and drape for privacy.
6. Hang the douche bag on an IV pole, about 12 inches above the vagina.
7. Cleanse the vulva by allowing a small amount of solution to blow over the vulva and between the labia.

8. Gently insert the nozzle, directing the tip backward and downward 2 to 3 inches.
9. Hold the labia together to facilitate filling the vagina with solution. Rotate nozzle periodically to help irrigate all parts of the vagina.
10. Intermittently release the labia allowing the solution to flow out.
11. When all the solution has been used, remove the nozzle. Have the patient sit up and lean forward to thoroughly empty the vagina.
12. Pat the external area dry.
13. Clean all equipment with warm soapy water after *every* use; rinse with clear water and allow to dry.
14. Thoroughly clean and disinfect the bathtub, if used.
15. Wash hands.

Patient Teaching

1. Guide the patient in learning how to correctly administer the douche.
2. Explain that the bag and tubing should be washed in warm soapy water after each use so as not to become a source of reinfection.
3. Review personal hygiene measures such as wiping from the front to the back after voiding or defecating.

4. Explain that douching is not recommended during pregnancy.
5. With most types of infection, both the male and female partners require treatment. Partners should abstain from sexual intercourse until both partners are cured to prevent reinfections.

Documentation

Provide the RIGHT DOCUMENTATION of the medication administration and responses to drug therapy:

1. Chart: Date, time, drug name, dosage, and route of administration.
2. Peform and record regular patient assessments for the evaluation of therapeutic effectiveness (i.e., type of discharge present, irritation of labia, discomfort, degree and duration of pain relief, etc.).
3. Chart and report any signs and symptoms of adverse drug effects.
4. Perform and validate essential patient education about the drug therapy and other essential aspects of intervention for the disease process affecting the individual.

Unit III

Drugs
Affecting
Body
Systems

Chapter 8

Drugs Affecting the Central Nervous System

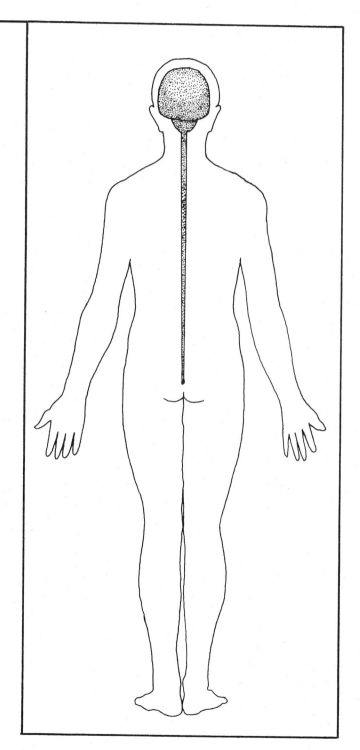

Objectives

After completing this chapter, the student should be able to do the following:

1. Explain the major action (effects) of drugs used to treat disorders of the central nervous system.
2. Identify baseline data the nurse should collect on a continuous basis for comparison and evaluation of drug effectiveness.
3. Identify important nursing assessments and interventions associated with the drug therapy and treatment of diseases associated with the central nervous system.
4. Identify health teaching essential for a successful treatment regimen.

The Central Nervous System

All human functions, from the most complex (abstract reasoning and creative thought) to the most basic (heart rate and respiration), require coordination to perform as a whole. The main coordinator of these functions is the central nervous system.

The central nervous system consists of the brain, the spinal cord, and many nerve cells called neurons. External-world information, such as sound, sight, smell, touch, and taste, and internal-world information, such as oxygen or carbon dioxide blood levels, body temperature, and muscle tension, are integrated. Instructions are relayed to the appropriate cells or tissues to produce the necessary actions and environmental adjustments. Information concerning these actions and adjustments is again relayed to the central nervous system. This feedback permits continuous adjustment in the instructions sent to various tissues for efficient control of body function.

Drugs act to decrease or increase the activity of nerve centers and conducting pathways. Many stimulants and depressants for the brain, the spinal cord, or specific centers of each have been developed, and the effects of such drugs can be predicted accurately. Drugs contained in this chapter are subdivided into sections based on their primary use.

Sedative-Hypnotic Agents

Sleep

Sleep is a state of unconsciousness from which a patient can be aroused by appropriate stimulus. It is a naturally occurring phenomenon that occupies about one third of an adult's life. It is a different state of unconsciousness from that produced by deep anesthesia or coma.

What constitutes optimal or sound sleep is a characteristic of each individual patient, but adequate sleep is important. Natural sleep is a rhythmic progression through four stages that provide physical and mental rest. Stages I and II are light sleep periods that allow easy arousal. Stage III is a transition from the lighter

to the deeper state of sleep, stage IV. Each stage is characterized by a specific set of brainwave activities. Stage IV sleep is called deep sleep and is dreamless, very restful, and associated with a 10% to 30% decrease in blood pressure, respiratory rate, and basal metabolic rate.

In a normal night of sleep, a person will rhythmically cycle through the four stages of sleep. About every 90 minutes or so, a patient will develop a sleep pattern called paradoxical sleep, or REM sleep. It is superimposed on stages I and II of sleep. This type of sleep represents up to 20% of sleep time and is characterized by rapid eye movements (REM), dreaming, increased heart rate, irregular breathing, secretion of stomach acids, and some muscular activity. REM sleep appears to be an important time for our subconscious minds to release anxiety and tension and reestablish a psychic equilibrium.

Insomnia is the most common sleep disorder known. It is defined as the inability to sleep. Insomnia is not a disease but a symptom of physical or mental stress. It is usually mild and lasts for only a few nights. Common causes are changes in lifestyle or environment (such as hospitalization), pain, illness, excess consumption of products containing caffeine, eating large or "rich" meals shortly before bedtime, or anxiety. *Initial* insomnia is the inability to fall asleep when desired, *intermittent* insomnia is the inability to stay asleep, and *terminal* sleep is characterized by early awakening with the inability to fall asleep again.

Measures that may be taken to alleviate or avoid insomnia include eliminating environmental and human noises and providing the patient with such comforts as back rubs, better ventilation, clean linens, a bedpan or urinal if needed, a change of position, extra pillows, an extra blanket, light nourishment (such as warm milk, hot chocolate, one or two crackers), and reassurance (listening to the patient's concerns).

If these measures are not successful, a sedative-hypnotic may be prescribed. A hypnotic is a drug that produces sleep. A sedative quiets the patient and gives a feeling of relaxation and rest, not necessarily accompanied by sleep. Hypnotics and sedatives are not always different drugs; their effects may depend on the dose and the condition of the patient. A small dose of a drug may act as a sedative, whereas a larger dose of the same drug may act as a hypnotic and produce sleep.

A good hypnotic should provide the following action within a short period: a restful natural sleep, a duration of action that will allow the patient to awaken at the usual time, a natural awakening with no "hangover" effects, and no danger of habit formation. Unfortunately, the ideal hypnotic is not available. The most frequently used sedative-hypnotics do increase total sleeping time, especially in stages II and IV; however, they also decrease the number of REM periods and the total time in REM sleep. When REM sleep is decreased, there is a strong tendency to "make it up." Compensatory, or "rebound," REM sleep seems to occur even when hypnotics are used for only 3 or 4 days. After chronic administration of sedative-hypnotic agents, REM rebound may be severe, accompanied by restlessness and vivid nightmares. Depending on the frequency of hypnotic administration, normal sleep patterns may not be restored for weeks. It is suspected that the effects of REM rebound may enhance chronic use of—and dependence on—these agents to avoid the unpleasant consequences of rebound.

The sedative-hypnotics may be classified into three groups: the barbiturates, the benzodiazepines, and the miscellaneous agents (see Tables 8.1, 8.2, and 8.3).

General Nursing Considerations for Patients Receiving Sedative-Hypnotics

Nurses can control many of the factors that cause sleep disturbances in the hospital setting. Therefore all efforts should be made to facilitate sleep within this new and strange environment prior to the administration of a hypnotic agent. This is a nursing challenge to be met by implementing nursing measures that will alleviate anxiety and provide for basic comfort needs.

Sedative-hypnotics may also be prescribed as a preanesthetic medication. If so, the primary purpose is to produce a restful sleep and thereby reduce anxiety in preparation for the planned surgical intervention.

PATIENT CONCERNS: NURSING INTERVENTION/RATIONALE

Insomnia

Assess the patient's usual pattern of sleep and obtain information on the pattern of sleep disruption (e.g., difficulty in falling asleep, unable to sleep the entire night, or awakening in the early morning hours unable to return to a restful sleep).

Ask the patient about the amount of sleep (hours) he or she considers normal and how insomnia is managed at home. If the patient is taking medications, determine the drug, dose, and frequency of administration.

Anxiety Level

Assess the patient's exhibited degree of anxiety. Is it really a sedative-hypnotic the patient needs, or is it someone to *listen* and intervene therapeutically?

Patients with persistent insomnia should be carefully monitored for the number of "naps" taken during the daytime. Investigate the type of activities performed immediately prior to retiring for sleep. A quiet "unwinding" time may be helpful. For children, try a bedtime story that is pleasant and soothing, not one that will cause anxiety or fear.

Environmental Control

Provide for adequate ventilation, subdued lighting, correct room temperature, and control of traffic in and out of the patient's room.

Organize nursing activities so that the patient is disturbed as infrequently as possible while maintaining safe nursing care.

Provide for the patient's well-being and personal safety. Leave a night light on, place the call light within reach, and if appropriate, put the bed in the *low* position with the side rails up. Do *not* allow a patient who has been medicated to smoke in bed.

Nutritional Needs

Help the patient avoid products containing caffeine, such as coffee, tea, soft drinks, and chocolate. Limit the total daily intake of these items and give warm milk and crackers as a bedtime snack.

Routine Orders

Many physicians order a sedative-hypnotic on a p.r.n. basis. Do not offer it unless the patient is having difficulty sleeping and other measures to meet his or

Table 8.1

Example of a Written Record for Patients Receiving Sleeping Pills

Medications	Color	To be taken

Name _____

Physician _____

Physician's phone _____

Next appt.* _____

	Parameters	Day of discharge							Comments
Time:	Arising								
	Bedtime								
	Last cup of coffee								
Sleep pattern	Took ____ hr. or min. to get to sleep.								
	Awaken during night; takes ____ hr. or min. to get back to sleep.								
	Slept all night								
	Couldn't sleep								
	Went right to sleep								
Dreams	Dreamed all night								
	No. of dreams								
	Did not dream								
Feelings the next morning?	Very tired when I woke up.								
	Awoke refreshed.								
Exercise	No desire to exercise								
	Usual routine, including work.								
	Unable to work								
Stress level No time to relax Time to relax 10 5 1									
Medication	Took (#) sleeping pills								

*Please bring this record with you to your next appointment.
Use the back of this sheet for additional information.

her comfort and psychological needs have failed to produce the desired effect. Never leave a medication at the bedside "in case" it is needed later.

p.r.n.

If giving p.r.n. medications, assess the record for the effectiveness of the therapy. It is sometimes necessary to repeat a medication if an order exists to do so. This is up to the nurse's discretion based on the evaluation of a particular patient's needs.

A paradoxical response may occur if the patient is showing increasing signs of excitement, restlessness, euphoria, or confusion. In such cases, it would be harmful to repeat the medication.

Reassess the underlying cause of sleeplessness. Is it really pain control that is needed? If so, repeating the order for a hypnotic will not meet the patient's needs.

When a medication is administered, carefully assess the patient at regular intervals for therapeutic and adverse effects.

Personal Comfort

Position the patient for maximum comfort, provide a back rub, encourage the patient to empty his or her bladder, and be certain that bedding is clean and dry. Take time to meet patients' individual needs and calm their fears. Foster a trusting relationship.

Patient Teaching Associated with Sedative-Hypnotic Therapy

PATIENT CONCERNS: NURSING INTERVENTION/RATIONALE

Communication and Responsibility

Encourage open communication with the patient concerning frustrations and anger as attempts are made to adjust to the diagnosis and need for treatment. The patient must be guided to gain insight into the disorder to assume the responsibility for the continuation of treatment. Keep emphasizing those things the patient can do to alter the progression of the disease including

maintenance of good general health through adequate rest, activity, and proper nutrition.

Nutrition

Teach appropriate nutrition information concerning the basic four food groups, adequate intake of fluids, and use of vitamins. Place the information at the educational level of the patient.

Caffeine consumption should be reduced or discontinued. Introduce the patient to decaffeinated products that can be substituted for previously used foods containing caffeine.

For insomnia, suggest warm milk about 30 minutes prior to the patient's attempting to sleep.

Environmental Control

Encourage the patient to provide for insomnia relief by attempting to sleep in the proper environment— a quiet, darkened room free from distractions.

Activity and Exercise

Plan daily activities so that sufficient exercise is obtained and the individual is tired enough to sleep. Also plan a quiet "unwinding" time prior to retiring for the night.

Stress Management

Some stressors that create insomnia may be within the work environment; therefore involvement of the industrial nurse along with a thorough exploration of work factors may be appropriate.

Teach the patient relaxation techniques and personal comfort measures, such as a warm bath, to relieve stress.

Referral for mastery of biofeedback or other techniques to reduce stress levels may be necessary.

Stress produced within the dynamics of the family may require professional counseling.

Encourage the patient to express *feelings* openly with regard to stress and insomnia. The adjustment to this situation involves working through great personal fears, frustrations, hostilities, and resentments.

Try to identify the coping mechanisms the person uses in response to stress and identify methods of channeling these toward positive realistic goals and alternatives to the use of medication.

Expectations of Therapy

Discuss the expectations of therapy and the degree of relief from previous symptoms that caused the need for medications.

If a substance-abuse problem exists, denial and manipulation may be major problems. See a mental health text for appropriate nursing intervention.

Changes in Expectations

Assess changes in expectations as therapy progresses and the patient gains understanding and skill in the management of the diagnosis.

Changes in Therapy through Cooperative Goal-Setting

Work mutually with the patient to encourage adherence to the treatment as prescribed. When the patient feels that a change should be made in a treatment plan, encourage discussion with the physician.

Written Record

Enlist the patient's aid in developing and maintaining a written record of monitoring parameters (e.g., extent of insomnia, time frequency, see Table 8.1) and response to prescribed therapies for discussion with the physician. The patient should be encouraged to bring this record on follow-up visits.

Fostering Compliance

Discuss medication information and how it will benefit the course of treatment. Seek cooperation and understanding of the following points so that medication compliance may be enhanced:

1. Name.
2. Dosage: Lowest dose for the shortest time possible.
3. Route and administration times: Do not leave medication at bedside; the patient may forget and repeat the dose too frequently.
4. Anticipated therapeutic response: When sedative-hypnotics are prescribed, the degree of response the patient anticipates should be discussed. All attempts should be made to substitute changes in daily activities, control of the environment, or assistance with underlying problems rather than the use of this medication.
5. Side effects to expect: Sedation, lethargy, and "morning hangover" or grogginess.
6. Side effects to report: Excessive drowsiness, slurred speech, tremors, alteration in mental alertness and the ability to use sound judgment, motor incoordination, mental depression, hives, rash, pruritis, fever.
7. What to do if a dosage is missed: Ignore it and substitute alternative methods of relaxation whenever possible.
8. When, how, or if to refill the medication: Try to avoid refills of sedative-hypnotic agents.

Difficulty in Comprehension

If it is evident that the patient or the patient's family is not understanding all aspects of continuing therapy being prescribed (e.g., administration and monitoring of medications, exercises, diets, follow-up appointments), consider use of social service or visiting nurse agencies.

Associated Teaching

Always inform the physician or dentist of any prescription or over-the-counter medication being taken.

Over-the-counter medications should not be taken without discussion first with the physician or pharmacist.

Always report side effects of rash, itching, or hives immediately. Nausea, vomiting, or diarrhea should also be reported for the physician's evaluation if it is a new symptom.

Keep all medications out of the reach of children.

If pregnancy is suspected, consult an obstetrician as soon as possible about continuation of medication therapy.

At Discharge

Items to be sent home with the patient should include the following:

1. Written instructions for the item's use.
2. Items labeled in a level of language and size of print appropriate for the patient.
3. If needed, include identification cards or bracelets.

4. Include a list of additional supplies to be purchased after discharge.
5. A schedule for follow-up appointments.

Barbiturates

The first barbiturate was placed on the market as a sedative-hypnotic in 1903. It became so successful that chemists identified some 2500 barbiturate compounds, of which more than 50 were distributed commercially. Barbiturates became such a mainstay of therapy that fewer than a dozen other sedative-hypnotic agents were successfully marketed through 1960. The release of the first benzodiazepine (chlordiazepoxide) in 1961 started the decline in the use of barbiturates. There are, however, several barbiturate compounds still prescribed today (see Table 8.2).

Barbiturates can reversibly depress the activity of all excitable tissues. The central nervous system is particularly sensitive, but the degrees of depression (ranging from mild sedation to deep coma and death) depend on the dosage, route of administration, tolerance from previous use, degree of excitability of the central nervous system at the time of administration, and condition of the patient. Usual hypnotic doses produce mild respiratory depression similar to that of natural sleep; with large doses, the rate, depth, and volume of respiration are markedly diminished.

Barbiturates are classified according to their duration of action: ultrashort, short, intermediate, and long acting. Since the duration of action depends on the dose and the rate of metabolism of the barbiturate, it is important to use the duration-of-action information as a guideline only.

Barbiturate-induced sleep varies from normal sleep in that there is decreased REM time. With chronic administration of hypnotic doses, the amount of REM sleep gradually returns to normal as tolerance develops to the REM suppressant effect. When barbiturate therapy is discontinued, a rebound increase in REM sleep occurs in spite of the tolerance. Irregularities in REM sleep cycles may take weeks to dissipate fully.

Barbiturates are used primarily for their sedative and hypnotic effects. Long-acting barbiturates (i.e., phenobarbital, metharbital) are also used for their anticonvulsant activity. The ultrashort-acting agents (methohexital, thiopental) may be administered intravenously as general anesthetics.

Side Effects

The habitual use of barbiturates may result in physical dependence. Rapid discontinuance of barbiturates after long-term use of high dosages may result in symptoms similar to alcohol withdrawal. They may vary from weakness and anxiety to delirium and grand mal seizures. Treatment consists of cautious and gradual withdrawal of barbiturates over a 2- to 4-week period.

General adverse effects of barbiturates include drowsiness, lethargy, headache, muscle or joint pain, and mental depression. Barbiturate "hangover" frequently occurs after administration of hypnotic doses of the long-acting barbiturates. Patients may display a dulled affect, subtle distortion of mood, and impaired coordination.

Elderly patients and those in severe pain may respond paradoxically to barbiturates with excitement, euphoria, restlessness, and confusion.

Hypersensitivity reactions to barbiturates are infrequent but may be serious. Barbiturate therapy should be discontinued immediately if the patient develops symptoms of hypersensitivity.

Rarely, barbiturates may induce blood dyscrasias.

Availability

See Table 8.2.

Dosage and Administration

See Table 8.2.

Nursing Interventions

See also General Nursing Considerations for Patients Receiving Sedative-Hypnotics.

**PATIENT CONCERNS:
NURSING INTERVENTION/RATIONALE**

Side Effects to Expect

"Hangover," Sedation, Lethargy

Patients may complain of "morning hangover," blurred vision, and transient hypotension on arising.

Explain to the patient the need for arising first to a sitting position, equilibrating, and then standing. Assistance with ambulation may be required.

If hangover becomes troublesome, there should be a reduction in the dosage or a change in the medication or both.

People working around machinery, driving a car, pouring and giving medicines, or performing other duties

Table 8.2
Barbiturates

GENERIC NAME	BRAND NAME	AVAILABILITY	ADULT ORAL DOSAGE	COMMENTS
Amobarbital	Amytal	Tablets: 15, 30, 50, 100 mg Capsules: 65, 200 mg Elixir: 44 mg/5 ml	Sedation: 30–50 mg 2–3 times daily Hypnosis: 100–200 mg 30 minutes before bedtime	Intermediate-acting; Schedule II. Used primarily as a daytime sedative, and bedtime hypnotic. May also be used as a sedative prior to anesthesia or during labor. Elixir contains 34% alcohol. Also available for rectal, IM, and IV use.
Aprobarbital	Alurate	Elixir: 40 mg/5 ml	Sedation: 40 mg 3 times daily Hypnosis: 40–160 mg prior to bedtime	Intermediate-acting; Schedule III. Used primarily as a daytime sedative, and bedtime hypnotic. Elixir contains 20% alcohol.
Butabarbital	Butisol, Butatran, Butalan	Tablets: 15, 30, 50, 100 mg Capsules: 15, 30 mg Elixir: 30, 33.3 mg/5 ml	Sedation: 15–30 mg 3–4 times daily Hypnosis: 50–100 mg at bedtime	Intermediate-acting; Schedule III. Used primarily as a daytime sedative, and bedtime hypnotic. Elixir contains 7% alcohol.
Mephobarbital	Mebaral	Tablets: 32, 50, 100, 200 mg	Sedation: 32–100 mg 3–4 times daily Anticonvulsant: 400–600 mg daily	Long-acting: Schedule IV. Used primarily as an anticonvulsant; may also be used as a daytime sedative.
Metharbital	Gemonil	Tablets: 100 mg	Anticonvulsant: up to 600–800 mg daily	Long-acting; Schedule III. Used as an anticonvulsant, usually in combination with other anticonvulsant agents.
Pentobarbital	Nembutal	Capsules: 30, 50, 100 mg Elixir: 18.2 mg/5 ml	Sedation: 30 mg 3–4 times daily Hypnosis: 100 mg at bedtime	Short-acting, Schedule II. Used primarily as a daytime sedative, and bedtime hypnotic. May also be used as a preanesthetic sedative. Elixir contains 18% alcohol. Also available for IM and IV use.
Phenobarbital	Luminal, Solfoton, Barbita	Tables: 8, 15, 16, 30, 32, 65, 100 mg Capsules: 16, 65 mg Drops: 16 mg/ml Liquid: 15 mg/5 ml Elixir: 20 mg/5 ml	Sedation: 8–30 mg 2–3 times daily Hypnosis: 100–320 mg Anticonvulsant: 50–100 mg 2–3 times daily	Long-acting; Schedule IV. Used most commonly now as an anticonvulsant. May also be used as a daytime sedative, preanesthetic, or hypnotic agent. Also available for IM and IV use.
Secobarbital	Seconal	Tablets: 100 mg Capsules: 50 and 100 mg Elixir: 22 mg/5 ml	Sedation: 30–50 mg Hypnosis: 100–200 mg at bedtime	Short-acting; Schedule II. Used primarily as a daytime sedative or bedtime hypnotic. Therapy is not recommended for longer than 14 days. Elixir contains 12% alcohol. Also available for IM and IV use.
Talbutal	Lotusate	Tablets: 120 mg	Hypnosis: 120 mg 15–30 minutes before bedtime	Intermediate-acting Schedule III. Used as a hypnotic for less than 14 days.

in which they must remain mentally alert, should not take these medications while working.

Side Effects to Report

Excessive Use or Abuse

Assist the patient to recognize the abuse problem. Identify underlying needs and plan for more appropriate management of those needs.

Discuss the case with the physician and make plans to cooperatively approach gradual withdrawal of the medications being abused.

Provide for emotional support of the individual; display an accepting attitude—be kind but firm.

Paradoxical Response

Provide supportive physical care and safety during these responses.

Assess the level of excitement and deal calmly with the individual. During periods of excitement, protect people from harm and provide for physical channeling of energy (e.g., walk with them).

Seek change in the medication order.

Hypersensitivity

Report symptoms of hives, pruritus, rash, high fever, or inflammation of mucous membranes for evaluation by the physician. Withhold further barbiturate administration until physician's approval has been granted.

Blood Dyscrasias

Routine laboratory studies (RBC, WBC, and differential counts) should be scheduled. Stress the patient's returning for this laboratory work.

Monitor for the development of sore throat, fever, purpura, jaundice, or excessive and progressive weakness.

Drug Interactions

Drugs That Increase Toxic Effects

Antihistamines, alcohol, analgesics, anesthetics, tranquilizers, valproic acid, chloramphenicol, monoamine oxidase inhibitors, and other sedative-hypnotics: Monitor the patient for excessive sedation and reduce the dosage of the barbiturate if necessary.

Phenytoin

The effects of barbiturates on phenytoin are variable. Serum levels may be ordered, and a change in phenytoin dosage may be required. Observe patients for increased seizure activity and for signs of phenytoin toxicity: nystagmus, sedation, and lethargy.

Barbiturates Decrease the Effects of

Warfarin. Monitor the prothrombin time and increase the dosage of warfarin if necessary.

Digitoxin. Monitor the digitoxin serum levels for signs of increased congestive heart failure: dyspnea, orthopnea, edema. The dosage of digitoxin may need to be increased.

Estrogens. This drug interaction may be critical in patients receiving oral contraceptives containing estrogen. If patients develop spotting and breakthrough bleeding, a change in oral contraceptives and the use of alternative forms of contraception should be considered.

Corticosteroids, Propranolol, Doxycycline, Antidepressants, Quinidine, and Chlorpromazine. The patient should be monitored for signs of increased activity of the illness for which the medication was prescribed. Dosage increases may be necessary or the barbiturate may have to be discontinued.

Benzodiazepines

Benzodiazepines, as a class of compounds, have been extremely successful products from a marketing and safety standpoint. A major advantage over the barbiturate and nonbarbiturate sedative-hypnotics is the wide safety margin between therapeutic and lethal dosages. Intentional and unintentional overdoses of several hundred times the normal therapeutic doses are well tolerated and are not fatal.

Over 2000 benzodiazepine derivatives have been identified, and over 100 have been tested for sedative-hypnotic or other activity. While there are many similarities among the benzodiazepines, they are difficult to characterize as a class. This is so because certain benzodiazepines are effective anticonvulsants, others serve as antianxiety agents, while still others are used as sedative-hypnotics (see Index). It is thought that they are all similar in mechanisms of action as CNS depressants, but individual derivatives act more selectively at specific sites, thus allowing for a variety of uses.

Four benzodiazepine derivatives are used as sedative-hypnotics (see Table 8.3). When benzodiazepine therapy is started, patients feel a sense of deep or refreshing sleep. Benzodiazepine-induced sleep varies, however, from normal sleep in that there is less REM sleep. With chronic administration, the amount of REM sleep gradually increases as tolerance develops to the REM suppressant effects. When benzodiazepines are discontinued, a rebound increase in REM sleep occurs in spite of the tolerance. During the rebound period, the number of dreams stay about the same, but many of the dreams are reported to be bizarre in nature. After chronic use of most benzodiazepines, there is also a rebound in insomnia. Consequently it is important to use these agents only for short courses of therapy.

Side Effects

The more common side effects of benzodiazepines are extensions of their pharmacologic properties. Drowsiness, fatigue, lethargy, and "morning hangover" are relatively common.

Table 8.3
Benzodiazepines Used for Sedation-Hypnosis

GENERIC NAME	BRAND NAME	AVAILABILITY	ADULT ORAL DOSAGE	COMMENTS
Flurazepam	Dalmane	Capsules: 15, 30 mg	Hypnosis: 15–30 mg at bedtime	Long-acting; Schedule IV. Used for short-term treatment of insomnia, up to 4 weeks. Morning hangover may be significant. Rebound insomnia and REM sleep occur less frequently.
Lorazepam	Ativan	Tablets: 0.5, 1, 2 mg	Hypnosis: 2–4 mg at bedtime	Used primarily for insomnia, but may also be used for preoperative anxiety. IM, IV administration also available.
Temazepam	Restoril	Capsules: 30, 50 mg	Hypnosis: 15–30 mg at bedtime	Intermediate-acting; Schedule IV. Used for insomnia. Minimal if any "morning hangover." Rebound insomnia may occur.
Triazolam	Halcion	Tablets: 0.25, 0.5 mg	Hypnosis: 0.25–0.5 mg at bedtime	Short-acting; Schedule IV. Used for insomnia, but tends to lose effectiveness within 2 weeks. Tapering therapy is recommended to reduce rebound insominia. Rapid onset of action. No "morning hangover."

The habitual use of benzodiazepines may result in physical and psychological dependence. Rapid discontinuance of benzodiazepines after long-term use may result in symptoms similar to alcohol withdrawal. They may vary from weakness and anxiety to delirium and grand mal seizures. The symptoms may not appear for several days after discontinuation. Treatment consists of gradual withdrawal of benzodiazepines over a 2- to 4-week period.

Benzodiazepines should be administered with caution to patients with a history of blood dyscrasias or hepatic damage.

Availability

See Table 8.3.

Dosage and Administration

See Table 8.3.

Nursing Interventions

See also General Nursing Considerations for Patients Receiving Sedative-Hypnotics.

**PATIENT CONCERNS:
NURSING INTERVENTION/RATIONALE**

Side Effects to Expect

"Hangover," Sedation, Lethargy

Patients may complain of "morning hangover," blurred vision, and transient hypotension on arising.

Explain to the patient the need for arising first to a sitting position, equilibrating, and then standing. Assistance with ambulation may be required.

If hangover becomes troublesome, there should be a reduction in the dosage or a change in the medication or both.

Persons who are working around machinery, driving a car, pouring and giving medicines, or performing other duties in which they must remain mentally alert should not take these medications while working.

Side Effects to Report

Excessive Use or Abuse

Assist the patient to recognize the abuse problem. Identify underlying needs and plan for more appropriate management of those needs.

Discuss the case with the physician and make plans to cooperatively approach gradual withdrawal of the medications being abused.

Provide for emotional support of the individual; display an accepting attitude—be kind but firm.

Blood Dyscrasias

Routine laboratory studies (RBC, WBC, and differential counts) should be scheduled. Stress the patient's returning for these tests.

Monitor for the development of a sore throat, fever, purpura, jaundice, or excessive and progressive weakness.

Hepatotoxicity

The symptoms of hepatotoxicity are anorexia, nausea, vomiting, jaundice, hepatomegaly, splenomegaly, and abnormal liver function tests (elevated bilirubin, SGOT, SGPT, alkaline phosphatase, prothrombin time).

Drug Interactions

Drugs That Increase Toxic Effects

Antihistamines, alcohol, analgesics, anesthetics, tranquilizers, narcotics, cimetidine, and other sedative-hypnotics.

Smoking

Smoking enhances the metabolism of the benzodiazepines. Larger dosages may be necessary to maintain sedative effects in patients who smoke.

Miscellaneous Sedative-Hypnotic Agents

The nonbarbiturate, nonbenzodiazepine sedative-hypnotics are listed in Table 8.4. All have somewhat variable effects on REM sleep, development of tolerance, and rebound REM sleep and insomnia. Because of the safety factor, the use of these agents is diminishing in favor of the benzodiazepines.

Side Effects

The habitual use of these sedative-hypnotic agents may result in physical dependence. Rapid discontinuance after long-term use may result in symptoms similar to alcohol withdrawal. They may vary from weakness and anxiety to delirium and grand mal seizures. Treat-

ment consists of gradual withdrawal over a 2- to 4-week period.

General adverse effects include drowsiness, lethargy, headache, muscle or joint pain, and mental depression. "Morning hangover" frequently occurs after administration of hypnotic doses. Patients may display dulled affect, subtle distortion of mood, and impaired coordination. Some patients experience transient restlessness and anxiety before falling asleep.

Elderly patients and those in severe pain may respond paradoxically with excitement, euphoria, restlessness, and confusion.

Hypersensitivity reactions are infrequent but may be serious. Therapy should be discontinued immediately if the patient develops symptoms of hypersensitivity.

Availability

See Table 8.4.

Dosage and Administration

See Table 8.4.

Nursing Interventions

See also General Nursing Considerations for Patients Receiving Sedative-Hypnotics.

PATIENT CONCERNS: NURSING INTERVENTION/RATIONALE

Side Effects to Expect

"Hangover," Sedation, Lethargy

Patients may complain of "morning hangover," blurred vision, and transient hypotension on arising.

Explain to the patient the need for arising first to a sitting position, equilibrating, and then standing. Assistance with ambulation may be required.

If hangover becomes troublesome, there should be a reduction in the dosage or a change in medication or both.

Persons who are working around machinery, driving a car, pouring and giving medicines, or performing other duties in which they must remain mentally alert should not take these medications while working.

Table 8.4

Miscellaneous Sedative-Hypnotic Agents

GENERIC NAME	BRAND NAME	AVAILABILITY	ADULT ORAL DOSAGE	COMMENTS
Acetylcarbomal	Paxarel, Sedamyl	Tablets: 250 mg	Sedation: 250–500 mg 2–3 times daily	Short-acting Metabolized to bromide, prolonged use may result in bromide toxicity. Discontinue use if dizziness, impaired thought and memory, incoordination (bromism) develop. Rarely used today because of availability of safer and more effective sedatives.
Chloral Hydrate	Nactec, Oradate, Aquachloral	Capsules: 250–500 mg Syrup: 250, 500 mg/5 ml Elixir: 500 mg/5 ml Suppositories: 325, 500, 650 mg	Sedation: 250 mg 3 times daily after meals Hypnosis: 500 mg to 1 g 15–30 minutes before bedtime	The original "Mickey Finn"; Schedule IV. Used primarily as a bedtime hypnotic, but also is used as a preoperative sedative because it does not depress respirations or cough reflex. May cause nausea; administer with full glass of water. Do not chew capsules. See Drug Interactions.
Ethchlorvynol	Placidyl	Capsules: 100, 200, 500, 750 mg	Hypnosis: —Usual dose 500 mg at bedtime —100–200 mg may be administered if patient wakes up after 500–750 mg	Short-acting; Schedule IV. Used for short-term insomnia. Therapy is not recommended beyond 1 week.
Ethinamate	Valmid	Capsules: 500 mg	Hypnosis: 500 mg to 1 g 20 minutes before bedtime	Short-acting; Schedule IV. Used for short-term insomnia; loses effectiveness after about 7 days.
Glutethimide	Doriden	Tablets: 250, 500 mg Capsules: 500 mg	Hypnosis: 250–500 mg at bedtime	Short-acting; Schedule III. Used for short-term insomnia; not recommended for use beyond 3–7 days. See Drug Interactions.
Methyprylon	Noludar	Tablets: 50, 200 mg Capsules: 300 mg	Hypnosis: 200–400 mg 15–30 minutes before bedtime	Intermediate-acting; Schedule III. Used for short-term insomnia; requires 45 minutes for sleep, but lasts 5–8 hours.
Paraldehyde	Paral	Liquid: 30 ml (for oral or rectal use)	Sedation: 4–8 ml	Bitter-tasting, unpleasant odor; administer in milk or iced fruit juice to mask taste and odor. Dispense only in a glass container. Do not use a plastic spoon or container. Used predominantly as a sedative in treating delirium tremens. This agent imparts a strong, foul odor to the breath for up to 24 hours after administration. The patient is often unaware of the foul smell. Schedule IV.
Triclofos	Triclos	Tablets: 750 mg Liquid: 1.5 g/15 ml	Hypnosis: 1500 mg 15–30 minutes before bedtime	See Chloral Hydrate.

Restlessness, Anxiety

These side effects are usually mild and do not warrant discontinuation of the medication. Encourage the patient to try to relax and let the sedative effect take over.

Safety measures such as maintenance of bed rest, side rails, and observation should be used during this period.

Dosage and Administration

Paraldehyde

Dilute oral form in milk or iced fruit juice to mask taste and odor.

Dispense only in a glass container; do not use a plastic spoon or container.

Drug Interactions

CNS Depressants

CNS depressants, including sleeping aids, analgesics, anesthetics, narcotics, tranquilizers, and alcohol, will increase the sedative effects of the sedative-hypnotics.

Warfarin

Glutethimide and ethchlorvynol may diminish the anticoagulant effects of warfarin. Monitor the prothrombin time and increase the dosage of warfarin if necessary.

Chloral hydrate may enhance the anticoagulant effects of warfarin. Observe for the development of petechiae, ecchymoses, nosebleeds, bleeding gums, dark tarry stools, and bright red or "coffee-ground" emesis. Monitor the prothrombin time and reduce the dosage of warfarin if necessary.

Disulfiram

Disulfiram may prolong the activity of paraldehyde. Monitor the patient for excessive sedation.

Clinitest

Chloral hydrate may produce false-positive Clinitest results. Use Clinistix or Tes-tape to measure urine glucose.

Parkinson's Disease

Parkinson's disease, or paralysis agitans, is a chronic disorder of the central nervous system. An estimated 200,000 to 400,000 patients in the United States are afflicted by this disorder, and an estimated 40,000 new cases are diagnosed annually. Characteristic symptoms are muscle tremors, slowness of movement, muscle weakness with rigidity, and alterations in posture and equlibrium. The cause of Parkinson's disease is unknown, but it is thought to reflect an imbalance in neurotransmitters within the brain. There is a relative excess of acetylcholine and an absolute deficiency of dopamine in the basal ganglia.

Treatment of parkinsonism remains palliative rather than curative. Goals are to provide maximal relief of symptoms and to maintain some independence of movement and activity. Drug therapy includes the use of anticholinergic agents to inhibit the relative excess in cholinergic activity and levodopa, carbidopa, bromocriptine, or amantadine to enhance dopaminergic activity.

General Nursing Considerations for Patients with Parkinson's Disease

Parkinson's disease has an impact on the entire family unit. The disease frequently occurs during middle adult years when the high expenses of educating a family or the years of planning and saving for retirement are at a peak.

The patient and family need assistance to learn the medical regimen aimed at controlling the symptoms and maintaining the patient at an optimal level of participation in the activities of daily living. The drug therapy presents the potential for many side effects that all involved parties must understand.

Nurses can have a major influence in the positive use of coping mechanisms as the patient and family express varying degrees of anxiety, frustration, hostility, conflict, and fear. The primary goal of nursing intervention should be to keep the patient socially interactive and participatory in daily activities. This can be accomplished through the use of physical therapy, adherence to the drug regimen, and management of the course of treatment.

PATIENT CONCERNS: NURSING INTERVENTION/RATIONALE

Characteristics of Parkinsonism

Facial Appearance

The patient typically appears expressionless, as if wearing a mask; eyes are wide open and fixed in position. Some patients have almost total eyelid closure.

Tremors

Tremors are often observed in the hands and may involve the jaw, lips, and tongue. A "pill rolling" motion in the fingers and thumbs is a characteristic movement. Tremors are usually reduced with voluntary movement.

Assess the degree of tremor involvement and specific limitations in activities being affected by the tremors.

Salivation

As a result of excessive cholinergic activity, patients salivate excessively. As the disease progresses, patients may be unable to swallow all secretions and will frequently drool.

Dyskinesia

Dyskinesia is the impairment of the individual's ability to perform voluntary movements. This symptom commonly starts in one arm or hand. It is usually most noticeable because the patient ceases to swing the arm on the affected side while walking.

As the dyskinesia progresses, movement, especially in small muscle groups, becomes slow and jerky. This motion is often referred to as "cogwheel rigidity." Muscle soreness, fatigue, and pain are associated with the prolonged muscle contractibility. The patient develops a shuffling gait, and once-automatic movements such as getting out of a chair or walking require a concentrated effort to be accomplished.

Along with the shuffling gait, the head and spine flex forward and the shoulders become rounded and stooped.

As mobility deteriorates, steps quicken and become shorter. Propulsive, uncontrolled movement forward or backward is evident. Patient safety becomes a primary consideration.

Emotional Lability

The disease does *not* affect the intellectual capacity of the patient. The chronic nature of the disease and physical impairment produce mood swings and serious depression.

Patient Assessment

Assess the patient's degree of alertness and orientation to name, place, and time prior to initiating therapy. Also assess the quality, rate, volume, and flow of speech.

Evaluate the patient's strengths and resources available to assist in working with the disease.

Activity and Exercise

Assess the individual's current level of exercise and compare it to daily life prior to diagnosis.

Stress

Take a detailed history of how the patient has controlled physical and mental stress in the past.

Family Resources

Establish what family resources are available and determine the closeness of the family unit during daily as well as stress-producing events.

Strive to develop a trusting relationship by listening and providing support for patient and family concerns.

Patient Teaching Associated with Antiparkinson Therapy

PATIENT CONCERNS: NURSING INTERVENTION/RATIONALE

Communication and Responsibility

Encourage open communication with the patient concerning frustrations and anger as attempts are made to adjust to the diagnosis and need for treatment. The patient must be guided to gain insight into the disorder to assume the responsibility for the continuation of the treatment. Keep emphasizing those things the patient can do to alter the progression of the disease, including the factors listed below.

Posture

The minimization of deformities is imperative to the long-term well-being of the patient. Erect posture and joint mobility through active and passive exercise must be maintained.

Head and Neck

Perform prescribed exercises to maintain head and neck strength, mobility, and erectness. Encourage the patient to lie on a firm mattress without a pillow.

Gait Training

Prescribed gait training is essential if the patient is to delay the onset of shuffling and propulsion of the gait.

Nutrition

As the disease progresses, dietary modification will be necessary.

Adequate fluid intake to maintain hydration and foods to promote bulk and stool softness should be used to minimize constipation.

Vitamins should not be given unless recommended by the physician. Pyridoxine (B$_6$) will reduce the therapeutic effect of levodopa.

The type and consistency of foods given must be individualized to the current symptoms. In advanced disease, many patients have difficulty swallowing. Because of fatigue and difficulty in eating, assistance appropriate to the degree of impairment should be given. Do not rush the individual when he or she is eating and cut foods in bite-sized pieces. Plan six smaller meals rather than three large meals.

Self-reliance

Encourage patients to perform all activities of daily living they are able to do. Do not "take over"; encourage self-maintenance. Provide for socialization and activities such as hobbies.

Stress Management

The avoidance of stress and the need for relaxation are essential; symptoms such as tremors are enhanced by anxiety.

Depression and mood alterations are secondary to disease progression (e.g., lack of ability to participate in sex, immobility, incontinence) and may be expected.

Expectations of Therapy

Discuss the expectations of therapy. With medications such as levodopa, several weeks of therapy may be required before any degree of improvement in symptoms may be noted.

Generally, patients expect an increase in joint mobility and relief from rigidity and tremor activity. When excessive salivation and drooling are present, relief from these symptoms is desired.

Because of the many side effects from these drugs, individualized teaching of the patient and family is imperative.

Cooperatively, set realistic goals. Family members and the patient need assistance in the establishment and continued refinement of goals as the symptoms of disease improve or worsen.

Changes in Expectations

Assess changes in expectations as therapy progresses and the patient gains understanding and skill in the management of the diagnosis.

Changes in Therapy through Cooperative Goal-Setting

Work mutually with the patient to encourage adherence to the treatment prescribed. When the patient feels that a change should be made in a treatment plan encourage discussion first with the physician.

Written Record

Enlist the patient's aid in developing and maintaining a written record (Table 8.5) of monitoring parameters (e.g., degree of tremor relief, stability, changes in mobility and rigidity, sedation, constipation, drowsiness, mental alertness or deviations) and response to prescribed therapies for discussion with the physician. Patients should be encouraged to bring this record with them on follow-up visits.

Fostering Compliance

Throughout the hospitalization, discuss medication information and how it will benefit the course of treatment. Seek cooperation and understanding of the following points so that medication compliance may be increased:

1. Name.
2. Dosage.
3. Route and administration times: Sudden withdrawal of medication may precipitate a parkinsonian crisis characterized by anxiety, sweating, and tachycardia and an exacerbation of tremors, rigidity, and dyskinesia. Administer medication after meals to prevent gastric irritation.
4. Anticipated therapeutic response: Improved gait, posture, speech, mobility, and ability to perform activities of daily living. Decreased salivation and sweating may be observed with anticholinergic agents.
5. Side effects to expect: Nausea, vomiting, and anorexia can be reduced by administering medications after meals or with food. Orthostatic hypotension may be manifested by dizziness and weakness, particularly during initiation of therapy or therapy changes. Confusion, disorientation, mental depression, insomnia, and hallucinations require careful assessment. With anticholinergic agents, constipation is to be anticipated. Careful dietary management aimed at adequate fluid intake and sufficient bulk are important. Dryness in the mouth

Table 8.5

Example of a Written Record for Patients Receiving Antiparkinson Agents

Medications	Color	To be taken

Name _____

Physician _____

Physician's phone _____

Next appt.* _____

Parameters		Day of discharge							Comments
Weight									
Blood pressure									
Pulse									
Tremor relief or pain relief — Little relief / Moderate relief / Good relief (10 — 5 — 1)									
Mobility and rigidity — gait training, working or not? No improvement / Less rigidity (10 — 5 — 1)									
Control of secretions? Worse / Improved / No problem (10 — 5 — 1)									
Alertness and orientation to time, person, and place (T.P.P.). Poor / Good (10 — 5 — 1)									
Exercise: Note present level of activity: Walking, getting out, performing range of motion (R.O.M.) exercises.									
Bowel and bladder	Constipated = C Normal = N (Check one)	C___ N___	C___ N___	C___ N___	C___ N___	C___ N___	C___ N___	C___ N___	
	Difficulty urinating = D								
	Occasional problem urinating								
Dietary needs	No problem eating or drinking.								
	Drinks (_#_) glasses fluid per day.								
	Needs frequent small meals.								
	Needs a lot of time to eat.								
Socialization Withdrawn / Active, involved (10 — 5 — 1)									

*Please bring this record with you to your next appointment.
Use the back of this sheet for additional information.

156

may be relieved by sucking on hard candy or ice chips, or by chewing gum.

6. Side effects to report: Changes in mental clarity, tachycardia, palpitations, apparent deterioration of clinical status. Dosage adjustments may be required.
7. What to do if a dosage is missed; and when, how, or if to refill the medication: Sudden withdrawal of medications may produce a parkinsonian crisis. Keep an adequate supply of medications available.

Difficulty in Comprehension

If it is evident that the patient or family does not understand all aspects of continuing therapy being prescribed (i.e., administration and monitoring of medications, exercises, diets, follow-up appointments), consider use of social service or visiting nurse agencies.

Associated Teaching

Always inform the physician or dentist of any prescription or over-the-counter medication being taken.

Over-the-counter medications should not be taken without first discussing with the physician or pharmacist; this includes vitamin preparations.

Always report side effects of rash, itching, or hives immediately. Nausea, vomiting, or diarrhea should also be reported for the physician's evaluation if it is a new symptom.

Take all of the medication as prescribed for the full course of treatment. Do not discontinue use when feeling improved; do not save for future use or give medicine to another individual. Sudden discontinuation of certain medications may produce harmful effects.

Keep all medications out of the reach of children.

If pregnancy is suspected, consult an obstetrician as soon as possible about continuation of medication therapy.

At Discharge

Items to be sent home with the patient should include the following:

1. Written instructions for the item's use.
2. Items labeled in a level of language and size of print appropriate for the patient.
3. If needed, include identification cards or bracelets.

4. Include a list of additional supplies to be purchased after discharge (e.g., eating aids, walker).
5. A schedule for follow-up appointments.

Drugs Used to Treat Parkinson's Disease

Amantadine Hydrochloride (ah-man'tah-deen) Symmetrel (sim'eh-trel)

Amantadine is a compound developed originally to treat viral infections. It was administered to a patient with parkinsonism who also had the Asian flu. During the course of therapy for the flu, the patient showed definite improvement in the parkinsonian symptoms. The exact mechanism of action is unknown but appears to be unrelated to the drug's antiviral activity. Amantidine seems to slow the destruction of dopamine, thus making the small amount present more effective. It may also aid in the release of dopamine from its storage sites. Unfortunately, about half the patients who benefit from amantadine therapy will begin to notice a reduction in benefit after 2 or 3 months. An increase in dosage or temporary discontinuation followed by a reinitiation of therapy several weeks later may restore the therapeutic benefits.

Side Effects

Most of the adverse effects of amantadine therapy are dose related and reversible. Common side effects include confusion, disorientation, mental depression, dizziness and light-headedness, nervousness, insomnia, and gastrointestinal complaints manifested by nausea, anorexia, abdominal discomfort, and constipation.

A dermatologic condition known as livido reticularis is frequently observed in conjunction with amantadine therapy. It is characterized by diffuse, rose-colored mottling of the skin, often accompanied by pedal edema, predominantly in the extremities. It is more noticeable when the patient is standing or exposed to cold. It is reversible within 2 to 6 weeks after discontinuation of amantadine but generally does not require discontinuation of therapy.

Amantadine should be used with caution in patients with a history of seizure activity, liver disease, uncontrolled psychosis, or congestive heart failure. Amantadine may cause an exacerbation of these disorders.

Availability

PO—100 mg capsules, 50 mg/5 ml syrup.

Dosage and Administration

Adult
PO—Initially, 100 mg 2 times daily. Maximum daily dose is 400 mg.

Nursing Interventions

See also General Nursing Considerations for Patients with Parkinson's Disease.

PATIENT CONCERNS: NURSING INTERVENTION/RATIONALE

Side Effects to Expect

Confusion, Disorientation, Mental Depression

Perform a baseline assessment of the patient's degree of alertness and orientation to name, place, and time *prior* to initiating therapy. Make regularly scheduled subsequent evaluations of mental status and compare findings. Report development of alterations.

Dizziness, Light-headedness, Anorexia, Nausea, Abdominal Discomfort

These side effects are usually mild and tend to resolve with continued therapy. Encourage the patient not to discontinue therapy without first consulting the physician. Provide for patient safety during periods of dizziness or light-headedness.

Livido Reticularis (skin mottling)

These side effects are usually mild and tend to resolve with continued therapy. Symptoms are enhanced by exposure to the cold or by prolonged standing. Encourage the patient not to discontinue therapy without first consulting the physician.

Side Effects to Report

Liver Disease

The symptoms of liver disease are anorexia, nausea, vomiting, jaundice, hepatomegaly, splenomegaly, and abnormal liver function tests (elevated bilirubin, SGOT, SGPT, alkaline phosphatase, prothrombin time).

Seizure Disorders, Psychosis

Provide for patient safety during episodes of dizziness; report symptoms for further evaluation.

Dyspnea, Edema

If amantadine is used with patients who have a history of congestive heart failure, assess lung sounds, additional edema, and weight gain on a regular basis.

Dosage and Administration

Administration Schedule

Because of the possibility of insomnia, plan the last dose to be administered in the afternoon, not at bedtime.

Drug Interactions

Anticholinergic Agents (trihexyphenidyl benztropine, procylidine, diphenhydramine)

Amantidine may exacerbate the side effects of anticholinergic agents that may also be used to control the symptoms of parkinsonism. Confusion and hallucinations may gradually develop. The dosage of either or both amantidine and the anticholinergic agent should be reduced.

Bromocriptine Mesylate (bro-mo′krip-teen)
Parlodel (par-lo′del)

Bromocriptine stimulates dopamine receptors in the basal ganglia of the brain. Since parkinsonian patients are deficient of dopamine in this neurologic center, there is marked improvement in the symptoms of the disease with bromocriptine therapy. Bromocriptine appears to be nearly as effective as levodopa in treating parkinsonism and is occasionally useful with patients who are no longer benefiting from levodopa therapy.

Side Effects

Side effects with bromocriptine therapy are very common, particularly when the dosage is greater than 15 to 20 mg daily. They can be minimized by starting with low dosages, then increasing dosages gradually to effective levels, and by administering medication in the evening with food. If severe side effects do appear, they can also be minimized by reducing the dosage for a few days, then increasing the dosage more gradually.

Side effects based on organ system are as follows:

Gastrointestinal. Nausea, vomiting, anorexia, abdominal cramps, and constipation on long-term use are very common.

Neurologic. Involuntary movements, headache, migraine, dizziness, light-headedness, and sedation have been reported. Patients taking doses greater than 100 mg daily have a higher incidence of delusions, confusion, hallucinations, and a painful burning of the skin, usually of the feet and hands, accompanied by a mottled redness of the affected areas.

Cardiovascular. Orthostatic hypotension is very common, particularly with higher dosages.

Other side effects. Dryness of the mouth, double vision, nasal congestion, and metallic taste may also occur.

Availability

PO—2.5 tablets and 5 mg capsules.

Dosage and Administration

Adult

PO—Initially, 1.25 mg 2 times daily with meals. Increase the dosage by 2.5 mg/day every 2 to 4 weeks. The dosage must be adjusted according to the patient's response and tolerance. Dosages in the 50 to 100 mg daily range are not uncommon for maximal therapeutic benefit.

Nursing Interventions

See also General Nursing Considerations for Patients with Parkinson's Disease.

PATIENT CONCERNS:
NURSING INTERVENTION/RATIONALE

Side Effects to Expect

Gastrointestinal Effects

Most of these effects may be minimized by temporary reduction in dosage, administration with food, and use of stool softeners for constipation.

Side Effects to Report

Neurologic

As described above, neurologic effects often occur with higher dosages.

Peform a baseline assessment of the patient's degree of alertness and orientation to name, place, and time *prior* to initiating therapy. Make regularly scheduled subsequent evaluations of mental status and compare findings. Report development of alterations.

Provide for patient safety, be emotionally supportive, and assure the patient that these adverse effects dissipate within 2 to 3 weeks of discontinuing therapy.

Orthostatic Hypotension

Monitor the blood pressure daily in both the supine and standing positions.

Anticipate the development of postural hypotension and take measures to prevent an occurrence. Teach the patient to rise slowly from a supine or sitting position; encourage the patient to sit or lie down if feeling "faint."

Dosage and Administration

PO

Dosage must be adjusted according to the patient's response and tolerance.

Side effects can be minimized by starting with small doses, then increasing the dosage gradually, and by administering medication with food in the evening.

Drug Interactions

Levodopa

Bromocriptine and levodopa have additive neurological effects.

This interaction may be advantageous because it often allows a reduction in dosage of the levodopa.

Antihypertensive Agents

Dosage adjustment of the antihypertensive agent is frequently necessary because of excessive orthostatic hypotension.

Carbidopa (kar'be-do-pah), **Levodopa**
Sinemet (sin'eh-met)

Sinemet is a combination of carbidopa and levodopa used for treating the symptoms of Parkinson's disease.

Carbidopa is an enzyme inhibitor that reduces the metabolism of levodopa, allowing a greater portion of the administered levodopa to reach the desired receptor sites in the basal ganglia. Carbidopa reduces the dose of levodopa required by approximately 75%. When administered with levodopa, carbidopa increases both plasma levels and the plasma half-life of levodopa. Patients with irregular, "on and off" responses to levodopa do not show benefit from Sinemet.

Side Effects

Carbidopa has no effect when used alone; it must be used in combination with levodopa. The side effects seen with combined therapy are actually an enhancement of the effects of levodopa because the carbidopa is allowing more levodopa to reach the brain. See Levodopa.

Availability

PO—Sinemet is a combination product containing both carbidopa and levodopa. The combination product is available in ratios of 10/100, 25/100, and 25/250 mg of carbidopa/levodopa respectively.

Dosage and Administration

Adult

PO—Patients not currently receiving levodopa: Initially, Sinemet 10/100 or 25/100 3 times daily, increasing by 1 tablet every other day until a dosage of 6 tablets daily is attained. As therapy progresses and patients show indications of needing more levodopa, substitute Sinemet 25/250, 1 tablet 3 to 4 times daily. Increase by 1 tablet every other day to a maximum of 8 tablets daily.

Drug Interactions

Sinemet may be used to treat parkinsonism in conjunction with amantadine or anticholinergic agents. The dosages of all medications may need to be reduced due to combined therapy. See also Levodopa.

Nursing Interventions

See also General Nursing Considerations for Patients with Parkinson's Disease. See also Levodopa.

Levodopa (le-vo-do′pah) **Larodopa** (lar-oh-do′pah), **Dopar** (do′par)

As stated in the introductory remarks on Parkinson's disease, the symptoms of parkinsonism are thought to result from an absolute deficiency of dopamine and a relative excess of acetylcholine. Dopamine itself, when administered orally, does not enter the brain. Levodopa does cross into the brain, and is metabolized to dopamine where it replaces the dopamine deficiency in the basal ganglia.

About 75% of patients with parkinsonism respond favorably to levodopa therapy, but after a few years the response diminishes, becomes more uneven, and is accompanied by many more side effects. This loss of therapeutic effect reflects the progression of the underlying disease process.

Side Effects

Levodopa causes many side effects but most are dose-related and reversible. Side effects vary greatly, depending on the stage of the disease.

Side effects based on organ system are as follows:

- *Gastrointestinal.* Nausea, vomiting, and anorexia are frequently reported at the initiation of therapy.
- *Cardiovascular.* Orthostatic hypotension and arrhythmias such as sinus tachycardia and premature ventricular contractions occur.
- *Central nervous system.* Abnormal involuntary movements occur in half the patients taking levodopa more than 6 months. These movements are observed as chewing motions, bobbing of the head and neck, facial grimacing, active tongue movements, and rocking movements of the trunk.
- *Psychiatric.* Levodopa may cause nightmares, restlessness, anxiety, insomnia, depression, dementia, loss of memory, and hallucinations. Reduction in dosage may control these symptoms.
- *Ophthalmic.* All patients should be screened for the presence of closed-angle glaucoma. Levodopa may precipitate an acute attack of angle-closure glaucoma. Patients with open-angle glaucoma can safely use levodopa in conjunction with miotic therapy.

Levodopa therapy may cause abnormalities in laboratory tests:

- False-positive tests for urinary ketones are reported with Ketostix and Labstix. Acetest tablets are generally not affected.
- False-negative tests for urine glucose are reported with Tes-tape and Clinistix. A false-positive "trace" reading with Clinitest may also occur.
- The urine may turn red to black on exposure to air or alkaline substances (bowl cleaners). Patients should be told not to be alarmed.

Availability

PO—100, 250, and 500 mg tablets and capsules.

Dosage and Administration

Adult

PO—Initially, 0.5 to 1 g daily in divided doses, administered with food. Do not exceed 8 g per day. Therapy for at least 6 months may be necessary to determine full therapeutic benefits.

Nursing Interventions

See also General Nursing Considerations for Patients with Parkinson's Disease.

**PATIENT CONCERNS:
NURSING INTERVENTION/RATIONALE**

Side Effects to Expect

Nausea, Vomiting, Anorexia

These effects can be reduced by slowly increasing the dose, dividing the total daily dose into 4 to 6 doses, and administering the medication with food or antacids.

Orthostatic Hypotension

Although generally mild, levodopa may cause some degree of orthostatic hypotension manifested by dizziness and weakness, particularly when therapy is being initiated. Tolerance usually develops after a few weeks of therapy.

Monitor the blood pressure daily in both the supine and standing positions.

Anticipate the development of postural hypotension and take measures to prevent an occurrence. Teach patients to rise slowly from a supine or sitting position; encourage them to sit or lie down if feeling "faint."

Side Effects to Report

Chewing Motions, Bobbing, Facial Grimacing, Rocking Movements

These involuntary movements occur in about half the patients taking levodopa more than 6 months. A reduction in dosage may be beneficial.

Nightmares, Depression, Confusion, Hallucinations

Perform a baseline assessment of the patient's degree of alertness and orientation to name, place, and time *prior* to initiating therapy. Make regularly scheduled subsequent evaluations of mental status and compare findings. Report development of alterations.

Provide for patient safety during these episodes.

Reduction in the daily dosage may control these adverse effects.

Tachycardia, Palpitations

Take the pulse at regularly scheduled intervals. Report for further evaluation.

Dosage and Administration

Glaucoma

All patients should be screened for the presence of angle-closure glaucoma *prior* to the initiation of therapy.

Patients with open-angle glaucoma can safely use levodopa.

PO

Administer medication with food or milk to reduce gastric irritation.

Drug Interactions

Phenelzine, Isocarboxazid

These agents unpredictably exaggerate the effects of levodopa. They should be discontinued at least 14 days before the administration of levodopa.

Isoniazid

Use with caution in conjunction with levodopa. Discontinue isoniazid if patients taking levodopa develop hypertension, flushing, palpitations, and tremor.

Pyridoxine

Pyridoxine (vitamin B_6) in oral doses of 5 to 10 mg reverses the toxic and therapeutic effects of levodopa. Normal diets contain less than 1 mg of pyridoxine, so dietary restrictions are not necessary. The ingredients of multiple vitamins should be considered, however.

There is a pyridoxine-free multiple vitamin (Larobec) made specifically for patients taking levodopa.

Diazepam, Chlordiazepoxide, Papaverine, Phenylbutazone, Clonidine, Phenytoin

These agents appear to cause a deterioration in the therapeutic effects of levodopa. Use with caution in patients with parkinsonism and discontinue if there is a deterioration in the patient's clinical status.

Phenothiazines, Reserpine, Haloperidol, Methyldopa

A side effect associated with these agents is a parkinson-like syndrome. Since this will nullify the therapeutic effects of levodopa, do not use concurrently.

Ephedrine, Epinephrine, Isoproterenol, Amphetamines

Levodopa may increase the therapeutic and toxic effects of these agents. Monitor for tachycardia, arrhythmias, and hypertension. Reduce the dose of these agents if necessary.

Antihypertensive Agents

Dosage adjustment of the antihypertensive agent is frequently necessary because of excessive orthostatic hypotension.

Ketostix, Labstix

This drug may produce false-positive urine ketone results with these products. Use Acetest tablets.

Clinitest

This drug may produce a false-positive "trace" of urinary glucose.

Tes-tape, Clinistix

This drug may produce false-negative urine glucose results with these products.

Bowl Cleaners

The metabolites of this drug will react with toilet-bowl cleaners to turn the urine a red to black color. This may also occur if the urine is exposed to air for long periods of time. Inform the patient that there is no cause for alarm.

Anticholinergic Agents

It is hypothesized that parkinsonism is induced by the imbalance of neurotransmitters in the basal ganglia of the brain. The primary imbalance appears to be a deficiency of dopamine, with a relative excess of the cholinergic neurotransmitter acetylcholine. Anticholinergic agents are thus used to reduce hyperstimulation caused by excessive acetylcholine. The anticholinergic agents reduce the severity of the rigidity, sweating, drooling, depression, and tremor that characterize parkinsonism. Anticholinergic agents may be useful for patients with minimal symptoms, for those unable to tolerate the side effects of levodopa, and for those who have not benefited from levodopa therapy. Combination therapy with levodopa and anticholinergic agents is also successful in controlling symptoms of the disease more completely in about half the patients already stabilized on levodopa therapy.

Side Effects

Most side effects observed with anticholinergic agents are direct extensions of their pharmacologic properties. Frequently seen adverse effects that usually dissipate with therapy are dryness and soreness of the mouth and tongue, blurring of vision, dizziness, mild nausea, and nervousness.

Psychiatric disturbances such as mental confusion, delusions, euphoria, paranoia, loss of memory, and hallucinations may be indications of overdosage.

Other side effects include constipation; urinary hesitancy or retention; tachycardia; palpitations; and mild, transient hypotension.

All patients should be screened for the presence of closed-angle glaucoma. Anticholinergic agents may precipitate an acute attack of angle-closure glaucoma. Patients with open-angle glaucoma can safely use anticholinergic agents in conjunction with mitotic therapy.

Availability

See Table 8.4.

Dosage and Administration

Adult
PO—See Table 8.6.

Nursing Interventions

See also General Nursing Considerations for Patients with Parkinson's Disease.

Table 8.6
Agents with Anticholinergic Properties Used to Treat Parkinsonism

GENERIC NAME	BRAND NAME	AVAILABILITY	INITIAL DOSE (PO)	MAXIMUM DAILY DOSE (MG)
Benztropine mesylate	Cogentin	Tablets: 0.5, 1, 2 mg	0.5–1 mg at bedtime	6
Biperiden hydrochloride	Akineton	Tablets: 2 mg	2 mg 1–3 times daily	10
Diphenhydramine hydrochloride	Benadryl	Tablets: 50 mg Capsules: 25, 50 mg Elixir: 12.5 mg/5 ml Syrup: 12.5 mg/5 ml		
Ethopropazine hydrochloride	Parsidol	Tablets: 10, 50 mg	50 mg 1–2 times daily	600
Orphenadrine hydrochloride	Disipal	Tablets: 50 mg	50 mg 3 times daily	150–250
Procyclidine hydrochloride	Kemadrin	Tablets: 5 mg	2 mg 3 times daily	15–20
Trihexyphenidyl hydrochloride	Artane, Tremin	Tablets: 2, 5 mg Sustained release capsules: 5 mg Elixir: 2 mg/5 ml	1 mg daily	12–15

PATIENT CONCERNS: NURSING INTERVENTION/RATIONALE

Side Effects to Expect

Blurred Vision, Constipation, Urinary Retention, Dryness of Mucosa of the Mouth, Throat, and Nose

These symptoms are the anticholinergic effects produced by these agents. Patients taking these medications should be monitored for the development of these side effects.

Dryness of the mucosa may be relieved by sucking hard candy or ice chips, or by chewing gum.

If patients develop urinary hesitancy, assess for distension of the bladder. Report to the physician for further evaluation.

Give stool softeners as prescribed. Encourage adequate fluid intake and foods to provide sufficient bulk.

Caution the patient that blurred vision may occur and make appropriate suggestions for personal safety of the individual.

Side Effects to Report

Nightmares, Depression, Confusion, Hallucinations

Perform a baseline assessment of the patient's degree of alertness and orientation to name, place, and time *prior* to initiating therapy. Make regularly scheduled subsequent evaluations of mental status and compare findings. Report development of alterations.

Provide for patient safety during these episodes.

Reduction in the daily dosage may control these adverse effects.

Orthostatic Hypotension

Although the instance is infrequent and generally mild, all anticholinergic agents may cause some degree of orthostatic hypotension manifested by dizziness and weakness, particularly when therapy is being initiated.

Monitor the blood pressure daily in both the supine and standing positions.

Anticipate the development of postural hypotension and take measures to prevent an occurrence. Teach the patient to rise slowly from a supine or sitting position; encourage the patient to sit or lie down if feeling "faint."

Palpitations, Arrhythmias

Report for further evaluation.

Dosage and Administration

Glaucoma

All patients should be screened for the presence of angle-closure glaucoma *prior* to the initiation of therapy.

Patients with open-angle glaucoma can safely use anticholinergic agents. Monitoring of intraocular pressure should be performed on a regular basis.

PO

Administer medication with food or milk to reduce gastric irritation.

Drug Interactions

Amantadine, Tricyclic Antidepressants, Phenothiazines

These agents may enhance the anticholinergic side effects. Developing confusion and hallucinations are characteristic of excessive anticholinergic activity. Dosage reduction may be required.

Levodopa

Large doses of anticholinergic agents may slow gastric emptying and inhibit absorption of levodopa. An increase in the dosage of levodopa may be required.

Psychotropic Agents

General Nursing Considerations for Patients Receiving Psychotropic Agents

Perform a baseline assessment of the individual's mental status. On succeeding occasions, repeat the evaluation and compare the findings to the original data.

Patients experiencing altered thinking, behavior, or feelings need careful evaluation of both verbal and nonverbal actions. Many times, there is an inconsistency between the thoughts, feelings, and behaviors displayed and so-called normal responses of individuals in a similar set of circumstances.

A complete history of the patient's previous responses to crises can serve as a basis for anticipating response to current events. One should evaluate the degree of reaction of the patient to the perceived threat and decide on the appropriateness of the reaction to the situation.

Try to identify the defense mechanisms currently being employed by the patient to cope with the circumstances. Question in your mind whether the coping mechanism is effective.

During severe levels of anxiety, as well as during periods of depression, the nurse should deal calmly and quietly with the individual and provide for personal well-being and safety.

At a time appropriate to the patient's ability to focus on the problems, alternative methods of handling the anxiety or depression may be explored.

Observe the patient during initial treatment with medications for increased anxiety and changes in levels of depression, or for oversedation, which would require a dosage adjustment.

PATIENT CONCERNS: NURSING INTERVENTION/RATIONALE

General Appearance

Observe the patient on admission and succeeding occasions for the following:

Personal grooming and appropriateness of dress to the occasion.

Posture: stooped, erect, slumped?

Facial expression: tense, worried, sad, angry, expressionless?

General motor activity: check gestures, gait, presence or absence of tremors, ability to perform gross or fine motor movements.

Speech: tone, clarity, pace, appropriateness; does the conversation flow in a logical sequence?

Level of Consciousness

Assess the individual's orientation to time, place, and person.

Evaluate the coherency, relevancy, and organization of thoughts.

Mood (affect)

State whether the mood being displayed is consistent with the circumstances being described (e.g., the person is speaking of death yet is smiling).

Terms usually used to describe affect are euphoric, depressed, aggressive, blunted (lack of normal range of emotions). Note any disturbances in thoughts, such as hallucinations, phobias, or delusions.

Memory

Ask questions to ascertain the individual's memory of recent and past events.

Judgment

Observe the patient during social interactions for the appropriateness of the mannerisms and responses displayed.

Sensory Perception

Ask questions to uncover any impairment of the five senses.

Developmental Pattern

Compare the individual's behavior and responses with the "normals" for the patient's age.

Psychological Assets

Does the individual have the ability to form close relationships? Can the patient function independently? What financial resources are available? Who forms the individual's support group?

Degree of Depression

Assess for signs of depression: loneliness, apathy, withdrawal, or isolation.

Be particularly alert for statements of failure, hopelessness, or self-hatred.

Observe for appetite, symptoms of headache, fatigue, and activity levels. Ask questions to identify any particular sleep pattern being experienced.

If the individual is suspected of being suicidal, ask the patient if he or she has ever thought about suicide. If the response is yes, get more details. Is a specific plan formulated? How often do these thoughts occur?

Take all thoughts of suicide seriously and provide for the patient's personal safety. Record and *report* all findings promptly to the physician.

Patient Teaching Associated with Psychotropic Therapy

PATIENT CONCERNS: NURSING INTERVENTION/RATIONALE

Communication and Responsibility

Encourage open communication with the patient concerning frustrations and anger as attempts are made to adjust to the diagnosis and need for treatment. The patient must be guided to gain insight into the disorder to assume the responsibility for the continuation of the treatment. Keep emphasizing those things the patient can do to alter the progression of disease, including maintenance of general health, nutritional needs, adequate rest and appropriate exercise, and continuation of prescribed medication therapy.

Expectations of Therapy

Discuss the expectations of therapy (e.g., level of interaction and socialization, degree of depression relief, frequency of use of therapy, sexual activity, maintenance of mobility, ability to maintain activities of daily living and/or work).

Changes in Expectations

Assess changes in expectations as therapy progresses and the patient gains understanding and skill in the management of the diagnosis.

Identify underlying stressors and appropriate coping mechanisms to reduce the effects of stress.

Changes in Therapy through Cooperative Goal-Setting

Work mutually with the patient and family to encourage adherence to the treatment as prescribed. The need for long-term treatment should be discussed if appropriate to the circumstances.

When the patient feels that a change should be made in a treatment plan, encourage discussion with the physician.

Written Record

Enlist the patient's and family's aid in developing and maintaining a written record (Table 8.7) of monitoring parameters (e.g., blood pressure, pulse, degree of socialization and interaction, general mood, judgments, memory; daily or weekly weights, if a problem exists) and response to prescribed therapies for discussion with the physician. Patients should be encouraged to bring this record with them on follow-up visits.

Table 8.7

Example of a Written Record for Patients Receiving Antianxiety Medication or Antidepressants

Medications	Color	To be taken

Name _____

Physician _____

Physician's phone _____

Next appt.* _____

Parameters	Day of discharge							Comments
Weight								
Blood pressure	AM / PM	AM / PM	AM / PM	AM / PM	AM / PM	AM / PM	AM / PM	
Resting pulse rate								
I would like to be alone? All the time — Some of the time — Not really / 10 5 1								
How I feel about my children? Too much work — Fun to be with / 10 5 1								
How I feel today? Poor — Fair — Okay / 10 5 1								
Appetite? Poor — Fair — Good / 10 5 1 B L D S								
Has family noted any problems: Judgment? Socialization?								
Does patient dress daily (Yes/No)?								
Does patient take pride in appearance (Yes/No)?								
Use of alcohol (Yes/No)? Amount (e.g., one drink)?	/	/	/	/	/	/	/	

*Please bring this record with you to your next appointment.
Use the back of this sheet for additional information.

166

Fostering Compliance

Throughout the hospitalization, discuss medication information and how it will benefit the course of treatment. Seek cooperation on and understanding of the following points so that medication compliance may be enhanced:

1. Name.
2. Dosage.
3. Route and administration times.
4. Anticipated therapeutic response.
5. Side effects to expect.
6. Side effects to report.
7. What to do if a dosage is missed.
8. When, how, or if to refill the medication.

Difficulty in Comprehension

If it is evident that the patient or family does not understand all aspects of continuing therapy being prescribed (e.g., administration and monitoring of medications, sedative effect, hypotensive episodes, need to monitor depressed patient's response), consider use of social service or visiting nurse agencies.

Associated Teaching

Always inform the physician or dentist of any prescription or over-the-counter medication being taken.

Over-the-counter medications should not be taken without discussion first with the physician or pharmacist.

Always report side effects of rash, itching, or hives immediately. Nausea, vomiting, or diarrhea should be reported for the physician's evaluation if it is a new symptom.

Take all of the medication as prescribed for the full course of treatment. Do not discontinue use when feeling improved; do not save for future use or give medicine to another individual. Sudden discontinuation of certain medications may produce harmful effects.

Keep all medications out of the reach of children.

If pregnancy is suspected, consult an obstetrician as soon as possible about continuation of medication therapy.

At Discharge

Items to be sent home with the patient should include the following:

1. Written instructions for the item's use.
2. Items labeled in a level of language and size of print appropriate for the patient.
3. If needed, include identification cards or bracelets.
4. Include a list of additional supplies to be purchased after discharge.
5. A schedule for follow-up appointments.

Antianxiety Agents

Anxiety

Anxiety is a normal human emotion, similar to fear. When it recurs too frequently or becomes uncontrollable, it is considered to be pathological. Its clinical manifestations include apprehension, irritability, nervousness, feelings of inadequacy, indecision, worry, tremor, insomnia, restlessness, headache, constipation, diarrhea, nausea, muscle tensions, and palpitations.

Anxiety is a primary symptom of many psychiatric disorders and a component of many medical and surgical conditions. When it is decided to treat the anxiety in addition to the other medical or psychiatric diagnoses, *antianxiety* medications, also known as *anxiolytics* or *minor tranquilizers*, are prescribed. It must be kept in mind that these agents are not cures for anxiety and should be used only for a short time to prevent the development of tolerance and dependence.

A greaty many medications have been used over the decades to treat anxiety. They range from the purely sedative effects of ethanol, bromides, chloral hydrate, and barbiturates to drugs with more specific antianxiety and less sedative activity, such as meprobamate, hydroxyzine, and the benzodiazepines.

Benzodiazepines

Benzodiazepines are most commonly used because they are more consistently effective, less likely to interact with other drugs, less likely to cause overdose, and have less potential for abuse than barbiturates and antianxiety agents. They now account for perhaps 75% of the 100 million prescriptions written annually for anxiety.

Over 2000 benzodiazepine derivatives have been identified, and over 100 have been tested for sedative-hypnotic or other activity. Seven benzodiazepine derivatives are used as antianxiety agents (see Table 8.8). Patients with anxiety reactions to recent events and patients with a treatable medical illness that induces anxiety respond most readily to benzodiazepine therapy. Since all the benzodiazepines have similar mechanisms of action, selection of the appropriate derivative is dependent on how the benzodiazepine is metabolized. In patients with reduced hepatic function or in the elderly, alprazolam, lorazepam, or oxazepam may be most appropriate, since they have a relatively short duration of action and have no active metabolites. Oxazepam has been the most thoroughly investigated. The other benzodiazepines all have active metabolites that significantly prolong the duration of action and may accumulate to the point of excessive side effects with chronic administration. The primary active ingredient of both prazepam and clorazepate is desmethyldiazepam; therefore similar activity and patient response should be expected. Halazepam and diazepam are therapeutically active, but their major metabolite is again desmethyldiazepam, so similar response should be expected with chronic administration. Oxazepam, chlordiazepoxide, diazepam, and clorazepate are all approved for use in treating the anxiety associated with alcohol withdrawal. Oxazepam is the drug of choice because it has no active metabolites. Its use is somewhat limited, however, in patients who cannot tolerate oral administration because of nausea and vomiting. Chlordiazepoxide or diazepam may be administered intramuscularly for this indication.

Side Effects

The more common side effects of benzodiazepines are extensions of their pharmacologic properties. Drowsiness, fatigue, lethargy, and "morning hangover" are relatively common, dose-related adverse effects.

Paradoxic reactions occasionally occur within the first few weeks of therapy. These reactions are manifested by increased anxiety, hyperexcitation, hallucinations, acute rage, and insomnia.

The habitual use of benzodiazepines may result in physical and psychological dependence. Rapid discontinuance of benzodiazepines after long-term use may result in symptoms similar to alcohol withdrawal. They may vary from weakness and anxiety to delirium and grand mal seizures. The symptoms may not appear for several days after discontinuation. Treatment consists of gradual withdrawal of benzodiazepines over a 2- to 4-week period.

Benzodiazepines should be administered with caution to patients with a history of blood dyscrasias or hepatic damage.

Availability

See Table 8.8.

Dosage and Administration

See Table 8.8.

Nursing Interventions

See also General Nursing Considerations for Patients Receiving Psychotropic Agents.

**PATIENT CONCERNS:
NURSING INTERVENTION/RATIONALE**

Side Effects to Expect

"Hangover," Sedation, Lethargy

Patients may complain of "morning hangover," blurred vision, and transient hypotension on arising.

Table 8.8
Benzodiazepines Used to Treat Anxiety

GENERIC NAME	BRAND NAME	AVAILABILITY	INITIAL DOSE (PO)	MAXIMUM DAILY DOSE (MG)
Alprazolam	Xanax	Tablets: 0.25, 0.5, 1 mg	0.25–0.5 mg 3 times daily	4
Chlorazepate	Tranxene	Tablets: 3.75, 7.5, 15 mg Capsules: 3.75, 7.5, 15 mg	10 mg 1–3 times daily	60
Chlordiazepoxide	Librium, A-poxide	Tablets: 5, 10, 25 mg Capsules: 5, 10, 25 mg	5–10 mg 3–4 times daily	300
Diazepam	Valium	Tablets: 2, 5, 10 mg	2–10 mg 2–4 times daily	—
Lorazepam	Ativan	Tablets: 0.5, 1, 2 mg	2–3 mg 2–3 times daily	10
Oxazepam	Serax	Tablets: 15 mg Capsules: 10, 15, 30 mg	10–15 mg 3–4 times daily	120
Prazepam	Centrax	Tablets: 10 mg Capsules: 5, 10, 20 mg	20 mg at bedtime	60

Explain to the patient the need for arising first to a sitting position, equilibrating, and then standing. Assistance with ambulation may be required.

If "hangover" becomes troublesome, there should be a reduction in the dosage or a change in the medication or both.

Persons who are working around machinery, driving a car, pouring and giving medicines, or performing other duties in which they must remain mentally alert should not take these medications while working.

Side Effects to Report

Excessive Use or Abuse

Assist the patient to recognize the abuse problem.

Identify underlying needs and plan for more appropriate management of those needs.

Discuss the case with the physician and make plans to cooperatively approach gradual withdrawal of the medications being abused.

Provide for emotional support of the individual; display an accepting attitude—be kind but firm.

Paradoxic Response

Report for further evaluation. Alternative therapy may be necessary.

Blood Dyscrasias

Routine laboratory studies (RBC, WBC, and differential counts) should be scheduled. Stress the patient's returning for this laboratory work.

Monitor for the development of a sore throat, fever, purpura, jaundice, or excessive and progressive weakness.

Hepatotoxicity

The symptoms of hepatotoxicity are anorexia, nausea, vomiting, jaundice, hepatomegaly, splenomegaly, and abnormal liver function tests (elevated bilirubin, SGOT, SGPT, alkaline phosphatase, prothrombin time).

Drug Interactions

Drugs That Increase Toxic Effects

Antihistamines, alcohol, analgesics, anesthetics, tranquilizers, narcotics, cimetidine, and other sedative-hypnotics.

Monitor the patient for excessive sedation and reduce the dosage of the benzodiazepine if necessary.

Smoking

Smoking enhances the metabolism of the benzodiazepines. Larger dosages may be necessary to maintain sedative effects in patients who smoke.

Other Antianxiety Agents

Meprobamate (mep-ro-bam'ate)
Equanil (ek'wa-nil)
Miltown (mil'-towhn)

Meprobamate acts on multiple sites within the central nervous system to produce mild sedation, antianxiety, and muscle relaxation. Meprobamate is used as an antianxiety agent and mild skeletal muscle relaxant for the short-term relief (less than 4 months) of anxiety and tension. It is of little use in the treatment of psychoses.

Side Effects

Psychologic and physiologic dependence may occur in patients taking doses of 3.3 to 6.4 g per day for 40 or more days. Symptoms of chronic use and abuse of high doses include ataxia, slurred speech, and dizziness. Withdrawal reactions such as vomiting, tremors, confusion, hallucinations, and grand mal seizures may develop within 12 to 48 hours after abrupt discontinuation. Symptoms usually decline within the next 12 to 48 hours. Withdrawal from high and prolonged dosages should gradually be completed over 1 to 2 weeks.

Meprobamate may cause seizures in patients with epilepsy.

Adverse effects to meprobamate are generally mild and dose related. They include dizziness, slurred speech, headache, paradoxic excitement, and allergic reactions that usually occur between the first and fourth dose in patients having no previous exposure to the drug.

Availability

PO—200, 400, and 600 mg tablets and capsules.

Dosage and Administration

Adult

PO—400 mg 3 to 4 times daily. Smaller doses may work well in elderly and debilitated patients. Maximum daily doses should not exceed 2400 mg.

Nursing Interventions

See also General Nursing Considerations for Patients Receiving Psychotropic Agents.

PATIENT CONCERNS: NURSING INTERVENTION/RATIONALE

Side Effects to Expect

Sedation

Persons who are working around machinery, driving a car, pouring and giving medicines, or performing other duties in which they must remain mentally alert should not take these medications while working.

Side Effects to Report

Slurred Speech, Dizziness

These are signs of excessive dosage. Report to the physician for further evaluation.
Provide for patient safety during these episodes.

Excessive Use or Abuse

Assist the patient to recognize the abuse problem.
Identify underlying needs and plan for more appropriate management of those needs.
Discuss the case with the physician and make plans to cooperatively approach gradual withdrawal of the medications being abused.
Provide for emotional support of the individual; display an accepting attitude—be kind but firm.

Orthostatic Hypotension (Dizziness, Weakness, Faintness)

Although this effect is infrequent and generally mild, meprobamate may cause some degree of orthostatic hypotension manifested by dizziness and weakness, particularly when therapy is being initiated.
Monitor the blood pressure daily in both the supine and standing positions.
Anticipate the development of postural hypotension and take measures to prevent an occurrence. Teach the patient to rise slowly from a supine or sitting position; encourage the patient to sit or lie down if feeling "faint."

Paradoxic Excitement, Arrhythmias

Withhold further doses, report for further evaluation.

Hives, Pruritus, Rash

Report symptoms for further evaluation by the physician.
Pruritus may be relieved by adding baking soda in the bath water.

Drug Interactions

Drugs That Increase Toxic Effects

Antihistamines, alcohol, analgesics, tranquilizers, narcotics, and other sedative-hypnotics.
Monitor the patient for excessive sedation and reduce the dosage of the meprobamate if necessary.

Hydroxyzine (hi-drox'ee-zeen)
Vistaril (vis-tar'il), **Atarax** (ah-tar-axe')

Defined strictly by chemical structure, hydroxyzine is an antihistamine. It acts within the central nervous system, however, to produce sedation, antiemetic, anticholinergic, antihistaminic, antianxiety, and antispasmodic activity. This variety of actions makes it somewhat of a multipurpose agent. It is used as a mild tranquilizer in psychiatric conditions characterized by anxiety, tension, and agitation. It is also routinely used as a preoperative or postoperative sedative to control vomiting, diminish anxiety, and reduce the amount of narcotics needed for analgesia. Hydroxyzine may also be used as an antipruritic agent to relieve the itching associated with allergic reactions.

Side Effects

The most common side effects are those associated with anticholinergic activity. These include dry mucous membranes, drowsiness, constipation, blurred vision, and nasal stuffiness.

Availability

PO—10, 25, 50, and 100 mg tablets and capsules, 10 mg/5 ml syrup, 25 mg/5 ml suspension.
IM—25 and 50 mg/ml.

Dosage and Administration

Adult

Antianxiety
PO—25 to 100 mg 3 to 4 times daily.
IM—50 to 100 mg every 4 to 6 hours.
Pre- and Postoperative
IM—25 to 100 mg.
Antiemetic
IM—25 to 100 mg.

Nursing Interventions

See also General Nursing Considerations for Patients Receiving Psychotropic Agents.

**PATIENT CONCERNS:
NURSING INTERVENTION/RATIONALE**

Side Effects to Expect

Blurred Vision, Constipation, Dryness of Mucosa of the Mouth, Throat, and Nose

These symptoms are the anticholinergic effects produced by hydroxyzine. Patients taking these medications should be monitored for the development of these side effects.

Dryness of the mucosa may be relieved by sucking hard candy or ice chips, or by chewing gum.

The use of stool softeners such as docusate may be required for constipation.

Caution the patient that blurred vision may occur and make appropriate suggestions for personal safety.

Sedation

Persons who are working around machinery, driving a car, pouring and giving medicines, or performing other duties in which they must remain mentally alert should not take these medications while working.

Side Effects to Report

Slurred Speech, Dizziness

These are signs of excessive dosage. Report to the physician for further evaluation.

Provide for patient safety during these episodes.

Drug Interactions

Drugs That Increase Toxic Effects

Antihistamines, alcohol, analgesics, anesthetics, tranquilizers, barbiturates, narcotics, and other sedative-hypnotics.

Monitor the patient for excessive sedation and reduce the dosage of the meprobamate if necessary.

Antidepressants

Tricyclic Antidepressants

The tricyclic antidepressants have become the most widely used medications in the treatment of depression. They produce antidepressant and mild tranquilizing effects. After 2 to 3 weeks of therapy, the tricyclic antidepressants elevate the mood, improve the appetite, and increase alertness in about 80% of patients with endogenous depression. Combination therapy with phenothiazine derivatives may be beneficial in the treatment of the depression of schizophrenia or moderate to severe anxiety and depression observed with psychosis or psychoneurosis.

The tricyclic antidepressants are equally effective in treating depression, assuming that appropriate dosages are used for an adequate duration of time. Consequently the selection of an antidepressant is based primarily on the characteristics of each individual agent. Sedation is more notable with amitriptyline, doxepin, and trimipramine, while protriptyline has no sedative properties and may actually produce mild stimulation in some patients. All tricyclic compounds display anticholinergic activity, with amitriptyline displaying the most and desipramine the least. This factor should be considered in patients with cardiac disease, prostatic hypertrophy, or glaucoma. Other factors to consider are that men tend to respond better to imipramine than women do, and the elderly tend to respond better to amitriptyline than do younger patients.

Side Effects

The most common side effects are those associated with anticholinergic activity. These include dry mucous membranes, constipation, blurred vision, nausea, and urinary retention.

About 10% of patients develop a fine rapid tremor of the hands. Occasionally, patients have reported numbness and tingling of arms and legs. Rarely, extrapyramidal side effects resembling parkinsonism develop.

Cardiovascular side effects such as arrhythmias, congestive heart failure, and tachycardia are rare, but orthostatic hypotension is fairly common with therapeutic dosages.

High doses of tricyclic antidepressants lower the seizure threshold. Seizures may occur in those with and without a history of seizure activity.

Availability

See Table 8.9.

Dosage and Administration

Adult
PO—see Table 8.9.

PATIENT CONCERNS: NURSING INTERVENTION/RATIONALE

Side Effects to Expect

Blurred Vision, Constipation, Urinary Retention, Dryness of Mucosa of the Mouth, Throat, and Nose

These symptoms are the anticholinergic effects produced by these agents. Patients taking these medications should be monitored for the development of these side effects.

Dryness of the mucosa may be relieved by sucking hard candy or ice chips, or by chewing gum.

The use of stool softeners such as docusate or the occasional use of a potent laxative such as bisacodyl may be required for constipation.

Caution the patient that blurred vision may occur and make appropriate suggestions for personal safety of the individual.

Orthostatic Hypotension

All tricyclic antidepressants may cause some degree of orthostatic hypotension manifested by dizziness and weakness, particularly when therapy is being initiated.

Monitor the blood pressure daily in both the supine and standing positions.

Anticipate the development of postural hypotension and take measures to prevent an occurrence. Teach the patient to rise slowly from a supine or sitting position; encourage the patient to sit or lie down if feeling "faint."

Sedative Effects

Tell the patient of sedative effects, especially during the onset of therapy. Single doses at bedtime may diminish or relieve the sedative effects.

Side Effects to Report

Tremor

About 10% of patients develop this adverse effect. The tremor can be controlled with small doses of propranolol.

Numbness, Tingling

Report for further evaluation.

Parkinsonian Symptoms

If these symptoms develop, the tricyclic antidepressant dosage must be reduced or discontinued.

Antiparkinsonian medications will not control symptoms induced by tricyclic antidepressants.

Arrhythmias, Tachycardia, Congestive Heart Failure

Report for further evaluation.

Seizure Activity

High doses of antidepressants lower the seizure threshold. Adjustment of anticonvulsant therapy may be required, especially in seizure-prone patients.

Suicidal Actions

Monitor the patient for changes in thoughts, feelings, and behaviors during the initial stages of therapy.

Dosage and Administration

PO

Dosage should be initiated at a low level and increased gradually, particularly in elderly or debilitated patients. Increases in dosage should be made in the evening because increased sedation is often present.

Observation

Symptoms of depression may improve within a few days (e.g., improved appetite, sleep, and psychomotor

Table 8.9

Tricyclic Antidepressants

GENERIC NAME	BRAND NAME	AVAILABILITY	INITIAL DOSE (PO)	DAILY MAINTENANCE DOSE (MG)	MAXIMUM DAILY DOSE (MG)
Amitriptyline	Amitril, Elavil, Endep	Tablets: 10, 25, 75, 100, 150 mg IM: 10 mg/ml in 10 ml vials	25 mg 3 times daily	150–250	300
Amoxapine	Ascendin	Tablets: 50, 100, 150 mg	50 mg 3 times daily	200–300	400 (outpatients) 600 (inpatients)
Desipramine	Norpramin, Pertofrane	Tablets: 25, 50, 75, 100, 150 mg Capsules: 25, 50 mg	25 mg 3 times daily	75–200	300
Doxepin	Adapin, Sinequan	Capsules: 10, 25, 50, 75, 100, 150 mg Oral concentrate: 10 mg/ml	25 mg 3 times daily	at least 150	300
Imipramine	Antipress, Presamine, Imavate, Janimine, Tofranil	Tablets: 10, 25, 50 mg IM: 25 mg/2 ml	30–75 mg daily	150–250	300
Nortriptyline	Aventyl, Pamelor	Capsules: 25, 50 mg	25 mg 3–4 times daily	50–75	100
Protriptyline	Vivactil	Tablets: 5, 10 mg	5–10 mg 3–4 times daily	20–40	60
Trimipramine	Surmontil	Capsules: 25–50 mg	25 mg 3 times daily	50–150	200 (outpatients) 300 (inpatients)

activity). The depression still exists, however, and it usually takes several weeks of therapeutic doses before improvement is noted. Suicide precautions should be maintained during this time.

Drug Interactions

Enhanced Anticholinergic Activity

The following drugs enhance the anticholinergic activity associated with tricyclic antidepressant therapy: antihistamines, phenuthiazines, trihexyphenidyl, benztropine, and meperidine.

The side effects are usually not severe enough to cause discontinuation of therapy, but stool softeners may be required.

Enhanced Sedative Activity

The following drugs enhance the sedative activity associated with tricyclic antidepressant therapy: ethanol barbiturates, narcotics, tranquilizers, antihistamines, anesthetics, and sedative-hypnotics.

See Drug Interactions. Concurrent therapy is not recommended.

Barbiturates

Barbiturates may stimulate the metabolism of tricyclic antidepressants. Dosage adjustments of the antidepressant may be necessary.

Methylphenidate, Thyroid Hormones

These agents may increase serum levels of the tricyclic antidepressants. This reaction has been advantageous in attempts to gain a faster onset of antidepressant activity, but an increased incidence of arrhythmias also has been reported.

Guanethidine, Clonidine

Tricyclic antidepressants inhibit the antihypertensive effects of these agents. Concurrent therapy is not recommended.

Monoamine Oxidase Inhibitors

Severe reactions including convulsions, hyperpyrexia, and death have been reported with concurrent use.

It is recommended that 2 weeks lapse between discontinuance of an MAO inhibitor and starting tricyclic antidepressants.

Phenothiazines

Concurrent therapy may increase serum levels of both drugs, causing an increase in anticholinergic and sedative activity. Dosages of both agents may be reduced.

Maprotiline Hydrochloride (ma-pro'til-een)
Ludiomil (lew-deo'mil)

Maprotiline is the first of the tetracyclic antidepressants to be released for clinical use. The tetracyclic agents are similar to the tricyclic antidepressants, but the frequency and severity of anticholinergic effects, cardiac arrhythmias, and orthostatic hypotension are reported to be lower with maprotiline. There is a slightly higher incidence of seizure activity and delirium associated with maprotiline therapy.

Side Effects

Maprotiline shares the same adverse effects as those of the tricyclic antidepressants. See Tricyclic Antidepressants.

Availability

PO—25, 50, and 75 mg tablets.

Dosage and Administration

Adult
PO—Initially, 75 mg daily. Increase in increments of 25 to 50 mg daily as needed and tolerated. The usual maintenance dose is 150 mg daily. The maximum dose is 300 mg daily.

Increases in dosage should be made in the evening because increased sedation is often present.

Note: Symptoms of depression may improve (e.g., improved appetite, sleep, and psychomotor activity) within a few days. The depression still exists, however, and it usually takes several weeks of therapeutic doses before improvement in the depression is noted. Suicide precautions should be maintained during this time.

Drug Interactions

See Tricyclic Antidepressants.

Nursing Interventions

See Tricyclic Antidepressants.

Trazodone Hydrochloride (traz-oh-doan')
Desyrel (dez-er'el)

Trazodone is the first of the triazolopyridine antidepressants to be released for clinical use. They are chemically unrelated to the tricyclic and tetracyclic antidepressants. Trazodone has been shown to be as effective in treating depression as amitriptyline and imipramine. Compared with other antidepressants, it has a low incidence of anticholinergic side effects, making trazodone particularly useful in patients whose antidepressant dosages are limited by anticholinergic side effects and in patients with severe angle-closure glaucoma, prostatic hypertrophy, organic mental disorders, and cardiac arrhythmias.

Side Effects

Drowsiness and decreased energy are the most commonly reported adverse effects. Other CNS effects reported are fatigue, light-headedness, dizziness, ataxia, mild confusion, and inability to think clearly.

Cardiovascular side effects reported are orthostatic hypotension, tachycardia, and palpitations.

Availability

PO—50 and 100 mg tablets.

Dosage and Administration

Adult
PO—Initially, 150 mg in 3 divided doses. Increase in increments of 50 mg daily every 3 to 4 days while monitoring clinical response. Do not exceed 400 mg daily in outpatients or 600 mg daily in hospitalized patients.

Nursing Interventions

See also General Nursing Considerations for Patients Receiving Psychotropic Agents.

PATIENT CONCERNS: NURSING INTERVENTION/RATIONALE

Side Effects to Expect and Report

Confusion

Perform a baseline assessment of the patient's degree of alertness and orientation to name, place, and time *prior* to initiating therapy. Make regularly scheduled subsequent evaluations of mental status and compare findings. Report development of alterations.

Dizziness, Light-headedness

Provide for patient safety during episodes of dizziness; report for further evaluation.

Drowsiness

Persons who are working around machinery, driving a car, pouring and giving medicines, or performing other duties in which they must remain mentally alert should not take these medications while working.

Orthostatic Hypotension

Although episodes are infrequent and generally mild, trazodone may cause some degree of orthostatic hypotension manifested by dizziness and weakness, particularly when therapy is being initiated.

Monitor the blood pressure daily in both the supine and standing positions.

Anticipate the development of postural hypotension and take measures to prevent an occurrence. Teach the patient to rise slowly from a supine or sitting position; encourage the patient to sit or lie down if feeling "faint."

Arrhythmias, Tachycardia

Report for further evaluation.

Dosage and Administration

PO

Dosage should be initiated at a low level and increased gradually, particularly in elderly or debilitated patients.

Increases in dosage should be made in the evening because increased sedation is often present.

Administer medication shortly after a meal or with a light snack to reduce adverse effects.

Observation

Symptoms of depression may improve (e.g., improved appetite, sleep, and psychomotor activity) within a few days. The depression still exists, however, and it usually takes several weeks of therapeutic doses before improvement is noted. Suicide precautions should be maintained during this time.

Drug Interactions

Enhanced Sedative Activity

The following drugs enhance the sedative effects associated with trazodone therapy: ethanol, barbiturates, narcotics, tranquilizers, antihistamines, anesthetics, and sedative-hypnotics. Concurrent therapy is not recommended.

Guanethidine, Clonidine

Trazodone inhibits the antihypertensive effects of these agents. Concurrent therapy is not recommended.

Antipsychotic Agents

Phenothiazines, Thioxanthenes, Haloperidol, Molindone, and Loxapine

Antipsychotic agents, also known as neuroleptic agents and major tranquilizers, are used to treat severe mental illnesses such as schizophrenia, mania, psychotic depression, and psychotic organic brain syndrome. Medications used to treat these disorders are grouped into two broad categories: the phenothiazines and the nonphenothiazines (thioxanthenes, haloperidol, molindone, and loxapine). Although each agent is from a distinctly different chemical class, all antipsychotic agents are similar in that they act by blocking the action of dopamine in the brain. Since they work at different sites within the brain, the side effects are observed on different systems throughout the body.

Side Effects

The extrapyramidal effects are the most troublesome side effects associated with antipsychotic therapy. They include the following:

1. Parkinsonian symptoms (4% to 40%) of tremor, muscular rigidity, masklike expression, shuffling gait, and loss or weakness of motor function. These symptoms are often controlled by anticholinergic antiparkinsonian agents. (Levodopa does not control these adverse effects.)
2. Dystonias and dyskinesias (2% to 10%) are spasmodic movements of the body and limbs (dystonias) and coordinated, involuntary rhythmic movements (dyskinesias). Acute dystonic reactions may be controlled by diphenhydramine or benztropine.
3. Akathisias (7% to 10%) consist of involuntary motor restlessness, constant pacing, and the inability to sit still; they are often accompanied by fidgeting, with lip and limb movements. Occasionally, sedatives may be required.

All antipsychotic agents have the potential to produce tardive dyskinesias. This drug-induced neurologic disorder is noted for such symptoms as facial grimaces and involuntary movement of the lips, tongue, and jaw, producing smacking and frequent, recurrent protrusions of the tongue. This adverse effect is usually irreversible and appears after several years of antipsychotic therapy. The frequency (15% to 45%) appears to be higher in patients taking both antiparkinsonian anticholinergic agents and antipsychotic agents together. It is thought that a fine tremor of the tongue may be an early indication of the disease. If the dosage is gradually reduced, where possible, the tardive dyskinesia may not develop.

Side effects frequently observed with antipsychotic therapy, especially when initiating therapy, are chronic drowsiness and fatigue, hypotension, blurred vision, nasal stuffiness, constipation, and dry mouth. Use antipsychotic therapy with caution in patients with glaucoma, prostatic hypertrophy, or urinary retention.

Antipsychotic agents may lower the seizure threshold in patients with seizure disorders.

Antipsychotic agents may produce myriad side effects other than those already listed. These include hepatotoxicity, blood dyscrasias, allergic reactions, endocrine disorders, skin pigmentation, and reversible effects in the eyes.

Availability

See Table 8.10.

Dosage and Administration

See Table 8.10.

Dosages must be individualized according to the degree of mental and emotional disturbance. It will often take several weeks for a patient to show optimal improvement and become stabilized on an adequate maintenance dosage. As a result of the cumulative effects of antipsychotic agents, patients must be re-evaluated periodically to determine the lowest effective dosage necessary to control psychiatric symptoms.

Nursing Interventions

See also General Nursing Considerations for Patients Receiving Psychotropic Agents.

PATIENT CONCERNS: NURSING INTERVENTION/RATIONALE

Side Effects to Expect

Chronic Fatigue, Drowsiness

Persons who are working around machinery, driving a car, pouring and giving medicines, or performing other duties in which they must remain mentally alert should not take these medications while working.

Orthostatic Hypotension

All antipsychotic agents may cause some degree of orthostatic hypotension manifested by dizziness and weakness, particularly when therapy is being initiated.

Monitor the blood pressure daily in both the supine and standing positions.

Anticipate the development of postural hypotension and take measures to prevent an occurrence. Teach the patient to rise slowly from a supine or sitting position; encourage the patient to sit or lie down if feeling "faint."

Blurred Vision, Constipation, Urinary Retention, Dryness of the Mucosa of the Mouth, Throat, and Nose

These symptoms are the anticholinergic effects produced by these agents. Patients taking these medications should be monitored for the development of these side effects.

Dryness of the mucosa may be relieved by sucking hard candy or ice chips, or by chewing gum.

The use of stool softeners such as docusate or the occasional use of a potent laxative such as bisacodyl may be required for constipation.

Table 8.10
Antipsychotic Agents

GENERIC NAME	BRAND NAME	AVAILABILITY	ADULT DOSAGE RANGE (MG)	MAJOR SIDE EFFECTS			
				SEDATION	EPS*	HYPOTENSION	ACE†
Phenothiazines							
Acetophenazine	Tindal	Tablets: 20 mg	60–120	+ +	+ + +	+	+ +
Carphenazine	Proketazine	Tablets: 25 mg	25–400	+ +	+ + +	+	+
Chlorpromazine	Thorazine, Promapar, Ormazine	Tablets: 10, 25, 50, 100, 200 mg Sustained release capsules: 30, 75, 150, 200, 300 mg Syrup: 10 mg/5 ml; 30, 100 mg/ml Injection: 25 mg/ml	30–1000	+ + +	+ +	+ + +	+ +
Fluphenazine	Prolixin, Permitil	Tablets: 0.25, 2.5, 5, 10 mg Elixir: 2.5 mg/5 ml Injection: 2.5 mg/ml	0.5–20	+	+ + +	+	+
Mesoridazine	Serentil	Tablets: 10, 25, 50, 100 mg Concentrate: 25 mg/ml Injection: 25 mg/ml	30–400	+ + +	+	+ +	+ +
Perphenazine	Trilafon	Tablets: 2, 4, 8, 16 mg Concentrate: 16 mg/5 ml Injection: 5 mg/ml	12–64	+	+ + +	+	+ +
Piperacetazine	Quide	Tablets: 10, 25 mg	20–160	+ +	+ +	+ +	+ +
Prochloraperazine	Chlorpromazine	Tablets: 5, 10, 25 mg Sustained release capsules: 10, 15, 30, 75 mg Syrup: 5 mg/5 ml Injection: 5 mg/ml	15–150	+	+ + +	+	+
Promazine	Sparine	Tablets: 10, 25, 50, 100 mg Syrup: 10 mg/5 ml Concentrate: 30 mg/ml Injection: 25, 50 mg/ml	40–1000	+ +	+ +	+ +	+ + +
Thioridazine	Mellaril, Millazine	Tablets: 10, 15, 25, 50, 100, 150, 200 mg Suspension: 25, 100 mg/5 ml Concentrate: 30, 100 mg/ml	150–800	+ + +	+	+ +	+ +
Trifluoperazine	Stelazine	Tablets: 1, 2, 5, 10 mg Concentrate: 10 mg/ml Injection: 2 mg/ml	2–40	+	+ + +	+	+
Triflupromazine	Vesprin	Suspension: 50 mg/5 ml Injection: 10, 20 mg/ml	60–150	+ + +	+ +	+ + +	+ +
Thioxanthenes							
Chlorprothixene	Taractan	Tablets: 10, 25, 50, 100 mg Concentrate: 100 mg/5 ml Injection: 12.5 mg/ml	75–600	+ + +	+ +	+ + +	+ +
Thiothixene	Navane	Capsules: 1, 2, 5, 10, 20 mg Concentrate: 5 mg/ml Injection: 2.5 mg/ml	6–60	+	+ + +	+	+
Haloperidol	Haldol	Tablets: 0.5, 1, 2, 5, 10, 20 mg	1–15	+	+ + +	+	+

(Table continues on p. 178.)

Table 8.10 (continued)

GENERIC NAME	BRAND NAME	AVAILABILITY	ADULT DOSAGE RANGE (MG)	MAJOR SIDE EFFECTS			
				SEDATION	EPS*	HYPOTENSION	ACE†
Loxapine	Loxitane	Concentrate: 2 mg/ml Injection: 5 mg/ml Capsules: 5, 10, 25, 50 mg Concentrate: 25 mg/ml	20–250	+ +	+ + +	+	+
Molindone	Moban	Injection: 50 mg/ml Tablets: 5, 10, 25, 50, 100 mg Concentrate: 20 mg/ml	15–225	+ +	+ +	+ +	+

Key to symbols: (+) low; (+ +) moderate; (+ + +) high.
* Extrapyramidal symptoms.
† Anticholinergic effects.

Caution the patient that blurred vision may occur and make appropriate suggestions for personal safety of the individual.

Side Effects to Report

Seizure Activity

Provide for patient safety during episodes of seizures; report for further evaluation. Adjustment of anticonvulsant therapy may be required, especially in seizure-prone patients.

Parkinsonian Symptoms

Report the development of drooling, cogwheel rigidity, shuffling gait, masklike expression, or tremors. Anticholinergic agents may be used to control these symptoms.

Tardive Dyskinesia

Report the development of fine tremors of the tongue. This is particularly important in patients who have been receiving antipsychotic agents and anticholinergic agents for several years.

Hepatotoxicity

The symptoms of hepatotoxicity are anorexia, nausea, vomiting, jaundice, hepatomegaly, splenomegaly, and abnormal liver function tests (elevated bilirubin, SGOT, SGPT, alkaline phosphatase, prothrombin time).

Blood Dyscrasias

Routine laboratory studies (RBC, WBC, and differential counts) should be scheduled.

Monitor for the development of sore throat, fever, purpura, jaundice, or excessive and progressive weakness.

Hives, Pruritus, Rash

Report symptoms for further evaluation by the physician.

Photosensitivity

The patient should be cautioned to avoid exposure to sunlight and ultraviolet light. Suggest wearing long-sleeved clothing, a hat, and sunglasses when going to be exposed to sunlight. Advise against using artificial "tanning" lamps. Notify the physician for the advisability of discontinuing therapy.

Dosage and Administration

Dosage Adjustment

Dosages must be individualized according to the degree of mental and emotional disturbance. It will often take several weeks for a patient to show optimal improvement and become stabilized on an adequate maintenance dosage.

Periodic evaluations should be made to make sure the patient is taking the smallest effective dose.

Drug Interactions

Drugs That Increase Toxic Effects

Antihistamines, alcohol, analgesics, anesthetics, tranquilizers, barbiturates, narcotics, and other sedative-hypnotics.

Monitor the patient for excessive sedation and reduce the dosage of the above agents if necessary.

Guanethidine

Antipsychotic agents may inhibit the antihypertensive effect of guanethidine. Concurrent therapy is not recommended.

Beta Adrenergic Blockers

Beta adrenergic blocking agents (propanolol, timolol, nadolol, pindolol, and others) will significantly enhance the hypotensive effects of antipsychotic agents. Concurrent therapy is not recommended.

Barbiturates

Barbiturates may stimulate the rate metabolism of phenothiazines. Dosage adjustments of the antipsychotic agent may be necessary.

Insulin, Oral Hypoglycemic Agents

Diabetic or prediabetic patients need to be monitored for the development of hyperglycemia, particularly during the early weeks of therapy.

Assess regularly for glycosuria and report if it occurs with any frequency.

Patients receiving oral hypoglycemic agents or insulin may require an adjustment in dosage.

Antimanic Agent

Lithium Carbonate (lith-e'um)
Eskalith (esk-ah'lith)

Lithium carbonate is used to prevent reoccurrences of manic depression. It has no sedative, depressant, or euphoric properties, thus separating it from all other psychiatric agents.

Side Effects

Side effects frequently include nausea, vomiting, anorexia, and abdominal cramps. During the first week of therapy, excessive thirst and urination and fine hand tremors may occur. Other side effects rarely reported include nephrotoxicity, hyperglycemia, generalized pruritus with and without rash, edematous swelling of the ankles and wrists, and metallic taste.

Lithium may enhance sodium depletion, and sodium depletion enhances lithium toxicity. Early signs of toxicity include nausea, vomiting, abdominal pain, diarrhea, lethargy, speech difficulty, mild dizziness, and tremor.

Rarely, long-term lithium therapy (longer than 6 months) produces hypothyroidism. The hypothyroidism is treated by thyroid replacement.

Availability

PO—300 mg tablets, 300 and 450 mg slow-release tablets, and 300 mg/5 ml syrup.

Dosage and Administration

Note: Before the initiation of lithium therapy, the following laboratory tests should be completed for baseline information: electrolytes, fasting blood glucose, BUN, serum creatinine, creatinine clearance, urinalysis, and thyroid function tests.

Serum lithium levels are monitored once or twice weekly during initiation of therapy and monthly while on a maintenance dose. The normal serum level is 0.9 to 1.5 mEq/L. Report serum levels above these values to the physician promptly.

Adult

PO—300 to 600 mg 3 to 4 times daily. Administer with food or milk. Adequate diet is important to maintain normal serum sodium levels and prevent the development of toxicity.

Nursing Interventions

See also General Nursing Considerations for Patients Receiving Psychotropic Agents.

**PATIENT CONCERNS:
NURSING INTERVENTION/RATIONALE**

Side Effects to Expect

Nausea, Vomiting, Anorexia, Abdominal Cramps

These side effects are usually mild and tend to resolve with continued therapy. Encourage the patient not to discontinue therapy without first consulting the physician.

If gastric irritation occurs, administer medication with food or milk. If symptoms persist or increase in severity, report for physician evaluation. These may also be early signs of toxicity.

Excessive Thirst and Urination, Fine Hand Tremor

These side effects are usually mild and tend to resolve within a week with continued therapy. Encourage the patient not to discontinue therapy without first consulting the physician.

If these symptoms persist or become severe, the patient should consult the physician.

Side Effects to Report

Progressive Fatigue, Weight Gain

These may be early signs of hypothyroidism. Report for further evaluation.

Pruritus, Ankle Edema, Metallic Taste, Hyperglycemia

These are all rare side effects from lithium therapy. Report for further evaluation.

Nephrotoxicity

Monitor urinalysis and kidney function tests for abnormal results. Report on increasing BUN and creatinine, decreasing urine output and/or decreasing specific gravity (despite amount of fluid intake), casts or protein in the urine, frank blood or smoky-colored urine, or RBCs in excess of 0 to 3 on the urinalysis report.

Dosage and Administration

PO

Nausea, vomiting, anorexia, and abdominal cramps are frequently reduced by administering medication with meals.

Good Nutrition

Lithium may enhance sodium depletion, and sodium depletion enhances lithium toxicity. It is very important that patients maintain a normal dietary intake of sodium with adequate maintenance fluids (10 to 12 8-ounce glasses of water daily), especially during the initiation of therapy, to prevent toxicity.

Drug Interactions

Reduced Serum Sodium Levels

Therapeutic activity and toxicity of lithium are highly dependent on sodium concentrations. Decreased sodium levels significantly enhance the toxicity of lithium.

Patients who are to initiate diuretic therapy, a low-sodium diet, or activities that will produce excessive and prolonged sweating should be observed particularly closely.

Methyldopa

Monitor patients on concurrent, long-term therapy for signs (nausea, vomiting, abdominal pain, diarrhea, lethargy, speech difficulty, mild dizziness, and tremor) of the development of lithium toxicity.

Indomethacin

Indomethacin reduces the renal excretion of lithium, allowing it to accumulate, potentially to toxic levels.

Anticonvulsant Agents

Seizure Disorders

Seizures are a symptom of an abnormality in the nerve centers of the brain. Seizures may result from a fever, a head injury, hypoglycemia, hypocalcemia, a drug overdose or withdrawal, or poisoning. It is estimated that 8% to 10% of all people will have a seizure during their lifetime. If the seizures are chronic and recurrent, the patient is diagnosed as having *epilepsy*. Epilepsy is the most common of all neurologic disorders. It is actually not a single disease but several different diseases that have one common characteristic: a sudden discharge of excessive electrical energy from nerve cells in the brain. An estimated 2 million Americans suffer from this disorder. The cause of epilepsy may be unknown (idiopathic epilepsy), or it may be the result of a head injury, a brain tumor, meningitis, or a stroke.

Epilepsy has been classified in several different ways. Traditionally, the most important subdivisions have been *grand mal, petit mal, psychomotor,* and *Jacksonian* types. An international commission has recently classified epilepsies into two broad categories based on their clinical and electroencephalographic (EEG) patterns. These broad categories are (1) generalized and (2) focal (localized). Generalized seizures are subdivided into convulsive and nonconvulsive types; focal seizures may be subdivided into elemental and complex symptom types. See Table 8·11 for a classification of epilepsies. Since the traditional terms are still frequently used, they have been included in the table in parentheses. Epilepsy is treated almost exclusively with medications (anticonvulsants).

Table 8.11
International Classification of Common Seizures

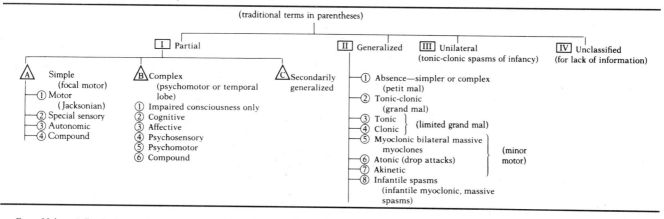

From Hahn, A.B.; Barkin, R.L., and Oestreich, S.J.: *Pharmacology in Nursing,* ed. 15, St. Louis, 1982, The C.V. Mosby Co.

Descriptions of Seizures

Generalized Tonic-Clonic (Grand Mal) Seizures. These sequences are the most common type. Patients suddenly lose consciousness and fall forcefully to the ground, experiencing generalized muscle spasms; the arms are flexed, the legs extended, and the eyes rolled upward. Respirations are temporarily suspended, the skin becomes cyanotic, perspiration and saliva flow, the patient may be incontinent of urine, and the tongue may be bitten if caught between the teeth. When the convulsions stop, the patient regains consciousness but remains confused and lethargic for a period of time (postictal state).

Absence (Petit Mal) Seizures. These seizures occur primarily in children and usually disappear at puberty, although the patient may develop a second type of seizure. Absence seizures consist of temporary lapses of consciousness that last for a few seconds. Patients appear to be staring into space and may exhibit a few rhythmic movements of the eyes or head. Falling does not occur, patients do not convulse, and they will have no memory of events occurring during the seizures. Consciousness returns rapidly and there is no postictal confusion.

Atonic of Akinetic Seizures. These seizures (drop attacks) are fairly uncommon, although they are seen frequently in mentally retarded patients. There is a sudden loss of consciousness and muscle tone that results in dramatic falls. Seated patients may slump forward violently. While unconscious, the patient has severe, rapid muscular contractions. The attacks are short, but there is frequent injury from the uncontrolled falls.

Partial Simple Motor (Jacksonian) Seizures. These seizures are focal in nature. A single body part, such as a finger or an extremity, may start jerking. The muscle spasm may end spontaneously or spread over the whole body. The patient does not lose consciousness unless the seizure develops into a generalized convulsion.

Partial Complex (Psychomotor) Seizures. These seizures are manifested by brief changes in consciousness; unusual and repeated chewing, lip smacking, or swallowing movements; confusion; and other inappropriate behavior, such as the tearing of clothes or aimless wandering. There are often brief periods of postictal confusion.

General Nursing Considerations for Patients with Seizure Disorders

Nurses may play an important role in the correct diagnosis of seizure disorders. Accurate seizure diagnosis is crucial to selecting the most appropriate medications for each individual patient. Because physicians are not always able to observe patient seizures directly, nurses should learn to observe and record these events objectively. It is important that the patient's behavior prior to the onset of the seizure be recorded. For example, did the patient complain of feeling ill or describe an unusual sensation? The onset, duration, and characteristics of the seizure should also be described as completely as possible. For example, did the eyes deviate to one side, or was spastic muscle activity localized to one area of the body? Another important factor is the patient's behavior after the seizure. For example, did the patient continue as though nothing had happened, or was the patient groggy and confused (postictal state)? Close, accurate observation of these factors will be a tremendous aid in the proper diagnosis and selection of therapy.

PATIENT CONCERNS: NURSING INTERVENTION/RATIONALE

History of Seizure Activity

What activities was the individual engaging in immediately prior to the latest seizure?

Has the individual noticed any particular activity that usually precedes attacks?

When was the last seizure before the current one?

Did the individual experience any changes in behavior prior to the onset (e.g., increasing anxiety or depression)?

Is the individual aware of a preseizure "aura" occurring (a particular feeling or odor that occurs prior to a seizure onset)?

Was there an "epileptic cry"?

Seizure Description

Record the exact time of seizure onset and duration of each phase, a description of the specific body parts involved, and any progression of the affected parts. Did the individual lose consciousness? Was stiffening and jerking present? Describe the course of progression to various body parts.

Describe automatic responses usually seen during the clonic phase—altered, jerky respirations or frothy salivation, dilated pupils and any eye movements, cyanosis, diaphoresis, incontinence.

Postictal Behaviors

Record the level of consciousness—orientation to time, place, and person.

Assess the degree of alertness, fatigue, or headache present.

Evaluate the degree of weakness, alterations in speech, and memory loss.

Patients frequently experience muscle soreness and extreme need for sleep. Record the time spent sleeping.

Evaluate any bodily harm that occurred during the seizure—bruises, cuts, lacerations.

Management of Seizure Activity

Assist the patient during a seizure by doing the following:

1. Protect the patient from further injury. Place padding around or under the head; do not try to restrain; loosen tight clothing. If in a standing position initially, lower the patient to a flat position.
2. If possible, place a soft object such as a face cloth between the patient's teeth to prevent accidental biting of the tongue or breakage of the teeth.
3. Once the patient enters into the relaxation stage, turn slightly on the side to allow secretions to drain out of the mouth.
4. Remain calm and quiet and give reassurance to the patient when the seizure is over.
5. Provide for a place for the patient to rest immediately after a seizure. Summon appropriate assistance so that the individual can get home.
6. If the patient starts into another seizure, immediately summon assistance; the patient may be going into status epilepticus.

Psychological Implications

Lifestyle

Encourage maintenance of a normal lifestyle. Provide for appropriate limitations (e.g., operating power equipment or a motor vehicle, swimming) to ensure patient safety.

Expression of Feelings

Allow for ventilation of feelings. Seizures may occur in public and may be accompanied by incontinence. Patients are usually very embarrassed about having a seizure in front of others.

Provide for ventilation of any discrimination the patient feels at the workplace.

School-age Children

Acceptance by peers can present a problem to the patient. The school nurse can help teachers and other children to understand seizures.

Denial

Be alert for signs of denial of the disease. An indication of this is increased seizure activity when the patient was previously well controlled. Question compliance with the drug regimen.

Compliance

Discuss underlying problems of noncompliance tactfully; kindly and firmly emphasize the need for adherence to a regular medication schedule.

Complications

Status Epilepticus

Status epilepticus is a rapidly recurring seizure that does not allow the individual to regain normal function between seizures.

Provide for patient protection and summon assistance for transportation of the patient to the emergency room.

Administer oxygen; have suction and resuscitation equipment available.

Establish an IV and have available drugs for treatment (e.g., phenytoin, phenobarbital, diazepam).

Monitor vital signs and neurologic status.

Insert a nasogastric tube if vomiting is present.

Patient Teaching Associated with

Anticonvulsant Therapy

PATIENT CONCERNS: NURSING INTERVENTION/RATIONALE

Communication and Responsibility

Encourage open communication with the patient concerning frustrations and anger as attempts are made to adjust to the diagnosis and need for treatment. The patient must be guided to gain insight into the disorder to assume the responsibility for the continuation of the treatment. Keep emphasizing those things the patient can do to alter the progression of disease, including maintenance of general health, nutritional needs, adequate rest and appropriate exercise, and continuation of prescribed medication therapy.

Expectations of Therapy

Discuss the expectations of therapy (e.g., level of seizure control, degree of lethargy, sedation, frequency of use of therapy, relief of symptoms, sexual activity, maintenance of mobility, ability to maintain activities of daily living and/or work, and limitations in operating power equipment or a motor vehicle).

Changes in Expectations

Assess changes in expectations as therapy progresses and the patient gains understanding and skill in the management of the diagnosis.

Stress that once seizures are controlled, medication must be continued.

Changes in Therapy through Cooperative Goal Setting

Work mutually with the patient to encourage adherence to the treatment prescribed. When the patient feels that a change should be made in a treatment plan, encourage discussion with the physician.

Written Record

Enlist the patient's aid in developing and maintaining a written record (Table 8.12) of monitoring parameters (e.g., degree of lethargy; sedation; oral hygiene for gum disorders; degree of seizure relief; nausea, vomiting, or anorexia present) and response to prescribed therapies for discussion with the physician.

Have others record the date, time, duration, and frequency of any seizure episodes. Also record the behavior immediately prior to and following seizures.

Patients should be encouraged to bring this record with them on follow-up visits.

Fostering Compliance

Throughout the hospitalization, discuss medication information and how it will benefit the course of treatment. Recognize that noncompliance may be a means of denial. Explore underlying problems in acceptance of disease and the need for strict compliance for maximum control. Seek cooperation and understanding of the following points so that medication compliance may be enhanced:

Table 8.12
Example of a Written Record for Patients Receiving Anticonvulsants

Medications	Color	To be taken

Name _____

Physician _____

Physician's phone _____

Next appt.* _____

	Parameters	Day of discharge							Comments
Previous seizure activity	Number / day?								
	Lasted how long?								
	Type, describe								
Present seizure activity	Number / day?								
	Lasted how long?								
	Type, describe								
	Slept after?								
Compliance	I take my medication as ordered.								
	Sometimes I forget.								
	I don't like to take medication.								
Drowsiness: Feel like sleeping all day / Feel like being active — 10 5 1									
Disease acceptance: I don't want people to know I have epilepsy / I have epilepsy and take medication — 10 5 1									
Oral hygiene: brushing and flossing teeth	3 times a day								
	2 times a day								
	1 time per day								
	I forgot								
Condition of gums?	No bleeding								
	Some bleeding (#) times / day								
	Bleeding every time I brush								
Nausea and vomiting	All day								
	Sometimes (when?)								

*Please bring this record with you to your next appointment.
Use the back of this sheet for additional information.

184

1. Name.
2. Dosage: Do not adjust the dosage without consulting the physician.
3. Route and administration times: If using the oral suspension, shake well and use an oral syringe for accurate measurement.
4. Anticipated therapeutic response: The eventual goal is to maintain the patient in a seizure-free state.
5. Side effects to expect: Drowsiness.
6. Side effects to report: Recurrence of seizures should always be reported. Other data to report are nausea and vomiting, sore throat, general malaise, mucosal ulcerations, gum swelling, lymph node swelling.
7. What to do if a dosage is missed; and when, how, or if to refill the medication: Always keep an adequate supply of medication on hand so that blood levels will be maintained by accurate, regular use.

Difficulty in Comprehension

If it is evident that the patient or family does not understand all aspects of continuing therapy being prescribed (e.g., administration and monitoring of medications, management of seizure activity when present, diets, follow-up appointments, and the need for lifelong management), consider use of social service or visiting nurse agencies.

Associated Teaching

Always inform the physician or dentist of any prescription or over-the-counter medication being taken.

Over-the-counter medications should not be taken without first discussing with the physician or pharmacist.

Always report side effects of rash, itching, or hives immediately. Nausea, vomiting, or diarrhea should be reported for the physician's evaluation if it is a new symptom.

Take all of the medication as prescribed for the full course of treatment. Do not discontinue use when feeling improved; do not save for future use or give medicine to another individual. Sudden discontinuation of certain medications may produce harmful effects.

Keep all medications out of the reach of children.

If pregnancy is suspected, consult an obstetrician as soon as possible about continuation of medication therapy.

The patient should carry an identification card or bracelet.

At Discharge

Items to be sent home with the patient should include the following:

1. Written instructions for the item's use.
2. Items labeled in a level of language and size of print appropriate for the patient.
3. If needed, include identification cards or bracelets.
4. Include a list of additional supplies to be purchased after discharge (e.g., oral syringes).
5. Schedule for follow-up appointments.

Barbiturates

The long-acting barbiturates (phenobarbital, mephobarbital, methabarbital, amobarbital) are very effective anticonvulsants. They may be used to treat grand mal, petit mal, myoclonic, and mixed seizures, usually in combination with other anticonvulsants (see Table 8.13). Barbiturates are discussed in greater detail elsewhere (see Index).

Benzodiazepines

The three benzodiazepines approved for use as anticonvulsants are diazepam, clonazepam, and clorazepate. Clonazepam is useful in the oral treatment of absence seizures in children. Diazepam must be administered intravenously to control seizures but is the drug of choice for treatment of status epilepticus. Clorazepate is used with other antiepileptic agents to control partial seizures.

Side Effects

The more common side effects of benzodiazepines are extensions of their pharmacologic properties. Drowsiness, fatigue, lethargy, and ataxia are relatively common, especially when other anticonvulsants with depressant effects are added to the therapy.

Behavioral disturbances such as aggressiveness and agitation have been reported, especially in patients who are mentally retarded or have psychiatric disturbances.

Rapid discontinuance of benzodiazepines after long-term use may result in symptoms similar to alcohol withdrawal. They may vary from weakness and anxiety

Table 8.13
Anticonvulsants

GENERIC NAME	BRAND NAME	AVAILABILITY	ADULT DOSAGE RANGE	USE IN SEIZURES
Barbiturates				
Mephobarbital	Mebaral	Tablets: 32, 50, 100, 200 mg	400–600 mg/day	Grand mal, petit mal
Metharbital	Gemonil	Tablets: 100 mg	Up to 600–800 mg/day	Grand mal, petit mal, myoclonic seizures, mixed seizures
Phenobarbital	Luminal, Solfoton, Barbita	Tablets: 8, 15, 30, 65, 100 mg Capsules: 16 mg Elixir: 20 mg/5 ml	100–300 mg/day	All forms of epilepsy
Benzodiazepines				
Clonazepam	Clonopin	Tablets: 0.5, 1, 2 mg	Up to 20 mg/day	Petit mal, myoclonic seizures
Clorazepate	Tranxene	Tablets: 3.75, 7.5, 11.25, 15, 22.5 mg Capsules: 3.75, 7.5, 15 mg	Up to 90 mg/day	Focal seizures
Diazepam	Valium	Tablets: 2.5, 10 mg IV: 5 mg/ml	Initially 5–10 mg, up to 30 mg	All forms of epilepsy; used in conjunction with other agents
Hydantoins				
Ethotoin	Peganone	Tablets: 250 mg	2–3 g/day	Grand mal, psychomotor seizures
Mephenytoin	Mesantoin	Tablets: 100 mg	200–600 mg/day	Grand mal, psychomotor seizures, focal seizures, Jacksonian seizures
Phenytoin	Dilantin	Tablets: 50 mg Capsules: 30, 100 mg Suspension: 30, 125 mg/5 ml	300–600 mg/day	Grand mal, psychomotor seizures
Succinimides				
Ethosuximide	Zarontin	Capsules: 250 mg Syrup: 250 mg/5 ml	1000–1250 mg/day	Petit mal
Methsuximide	Celontin	Capsules: 150, 300 mg	900–1200 mg/day	Petit mal
Phensuximide	Milontin	Capsules: 500 mg	1–2 g/day	Petit mal

to delirium and grand mal seizures. The symptoms may not appear for several days after discontinuation. Treatment consists of gradual withdrawal of benzodiazepines over a 2- to 4-week period.

Benzodiazepines should be administered with caution to patients with a history of blood dyscrasias or hepatic damage.

Availability

See Table 8.13.

Dosage and Administration

See Table 8.13.

Nursing Interventions

See also General Nursing Considerations for Patients with Seizure Disorders.

PATIENT CONCERNS: NURSING INTERVENTION/RATIONALE

Side Effects to Expect

Sedation, Drowsiness, Dizziness, Blurred Vision, Fatigue, Lethargy

These symptoms tend to disappear with continued therapy and possible readjustment of the dosage. Encourage the patient not to discontinue therapy without first consulting the physician.

Persons who are working around machinery, driving a car, or performing other duties in which they must remain mentally alert should be particularly cautious. Provide for patient safety during episodes of dizziness and ataxia; report for further evaluation.

Caution the patient that blurred vision may occur and make appropriate suggestions for personal safety of the individual.

Side Effects to Report

Behavioral Disturbances

Provide supportive physical care and safety during these responses.

Assess the level of excitement and deal calmly with the individual. During periods of excitement, protect persons from harm and provide for physical channeling of energy (e.g., walk with them).

Seek change in the medication order.

Blood Dyscrasias

Routine laboratory studies (RBC, WBC, and differential counts) should be scheduled.

Monitor for the development of sore throat, fever, purpura, jaundice, or excessive and progressive weakness.

Hepatotoxicity

The symptoms of hepatotoxicity are anorexia, nausea, vomiting, jaundice, hepatomegaly, splenomegaly, and abnormal liver function tests (elevated bilirubin, SGOT, SGPT, alkaline phosphatase, prothrombin time).

Administration

IV

Do not mix parenteral diazepam in the same syringe with other medications; do not add to other IV solutions because of precipitate formation.

Administer slowly at a rate of at least 5 mg per minute. If at all possible, give under ECG monitoring and observe closely for bradycardia. Stop boluses until the heart rate returns to normal.

Drug Interactions

Drugs That Increase Toxic Effects

Antihistamines, alcohol, analgesics, anesthetics, tranquilizers, narcotics, cimetidine, sedative-hypnotics, and other anticonvulsants.

Monitor the patient for excessive sedation, and eliminate the nonanticonvulsants if possible.

Smoking

Smoking enhances the metabolism of the benzodiazepines. Larger dosages may be necessary to maintain effects in patients who smoke.

Hydantoins

Hydantoins (phenytoin, ethotoin, and mephenytoin) are anticonvulsants used to control grand mal and psychomotor seizures. Mephenytoin may also be used to treat focal and Jacksonian seizures when less toxic anticonvulsants are unsuccessful. Phenytoin is by far the most commonly used anticonvulsant of the hydantoins.

Side Effects

Common adverse effects include nausea and vomiting, nystagmus, slurred speech, dizziness, gingival hyperplasia, insomnia, mental confusion, and transient nervousness.

Rarely, hydantoins may cause rashes, blood dyscrasias, and hepatitis.

Hydantoins may elevate blood sugar levels, especially if higher doses are used; patients with diabetes mellitus are more susceptible to hyperglycemia.

Availability

See Table 8.13.

Dosage and Administration

See Table 8.13.

Nursing Interventions

See also General Nursing Considerations for Patients with Seizure Disorders.

PATIENT CONCERNS: NURSING INTERVENTION/RATIONALE

Side Effects to Expect

Nausea, Vomiting, Indigestion

These effects are common during initiation of therapy. Gradual increases in therapy and administration with food or milk will reduce gastric irritation.

Sedation, Drowsiness, Dizziness, Blurred Vision, Fatigue, Lethargy

These symptoms tend to disappear with continued therapy and possible adjustment of dosage. Encourage the patient not to discontinue therapy without first consulting the physician.

Persons who are working around machinery, driving a car, or performing other duties in which they must remain mentally alert should be particularly cautious.

Provide for patient safety during episodes of dizziness; report for further evaluation.

Caution the patient that blurred vision may occur and make appropriate suggestions for personal safety of the individual.

Confusion

Perform a baseline assessment of the patient's degree of alertness and orientation to name, place, and time *prior* to initiating therapy. Make regularly scheduled subsequent evaluations of mental status and compare findings. Report development of alterations.

Gingival Hyperplasia

The frequency of gum overgrowth may be reduced by good oral hygiene including gum massage, frequent brushing, and proper dental care.

Side Effects to Report

Hyperglycemia

Particularly during the early weeks of therapy, diabetic or prediabetic patients need to be monitored for the development of hyperglycemia.

Assess regularly for glycosuria and report if it occurs with any frequency.

Patients receiving oral hypoglycemia agents or insulin may require an adjustment in dosage.

Blood Dyscrasias

Routine laboratory studies (RBC, WBC, and differential counts) should be scheduled.

Monitor for the development of sore throat, fever, purpura, jaundice, or excessive and progressive weakness.

Hepatotoxicity

The symptoms of hepatotoxicity are anorexia, nausea, vomiting, jaundice, hepatomegaly, splenomegaly, and abnormal liver function tests (elevated bilirubin, SGOT, SGPT, alkaline phosphatase, prothrombin time).

Dermatologic Reactions

Report a rash or pruritus immediately and withhold additional doses pending approval by the physician.

Dosage and Administration

PO

Administer medication with food or milk to reduce gastric irritation. If an oral suspension is used, shake well first. Encourage the use of an oral syringe for accurate measurement.

IM

If at all possible, avoid IM administration. Absorption is slow and painful.

IV

Do not mix parenteral phenytoin in the same syringe with other medications; because of precipitate formation, do not add to other IV solutions.

Administer slowly at a rate of 25 to 50 mg per minute. If at all possible, give under ECG monitoring and observe closely for bradycardia. Stop boluses until the heart rate returns to normal.

Drug Interactions

Drugs That Enhance Therapeutic and Toxic Effects

Warfarin, disulfiram, phenylbutazone, isoniazid, chloramphenicol, cimetidine, and sulfonamides.

Monitor patients with concurrent therapy for signs of phenytoin toxicity: nystagmus, sedation, lethargy. Serum levels may be ordered, and a reduced dosage of phenytoin may be required.

Drugs That Decrease Therapeutic Effects

Barbiturates, corbamazepine, folic acid, and antacids.

Monitor patients with concurrent therapy for increased seizure activity. Monitoring changes in serum levels should help warn of possible increased seizure activity.

Disopyramide, Quinidine

Phenytoin decreases serum levels of these agents. Monitor patients for redevelopment of arrhythmias.

Prednisolone, Dexamethasone

Phenytoin decreases serum levels of these agents. Monitor patients for reduced antiinflammatory activity.

Oral Contraceptives

Spotting or bleeding may be an indication of reduced contraceptive activity. Use of alternate forms of birth control is recommended.

Theophylline

Phenytoin decreases serum levels of theophylline derivatives. Monitor patients for a greater frequency of respiratory difficulty. The theophylline dose may have to be increased 50% to 100% to maintain the same therapeutic response.

Valproic Acid

This agent may increase or decrease the activity of phenytoin.

Monitor for increased frequency of seizure activity. Monitoring changes in serum levels should help warn of possible increased seizure activity.

Monitor patients with concurrent therapy for signs of phenytoin toxicity: nystagmus, sedation, lethargy. Serum levels may be ordered, and a reduced dosage of phenytoin may be required.

Succinimides

Succinimides (ethosuximide, methsuximide, and phensuximide) are used for the control of absence (petit mal) seizures.

Side Effects

Gastrointestinal symptoms of nausea, vomiting, indigestion, cramps, anorexia, diarrhea, and constipation occur frequently with this class of anticonvulsants.

As noted with other classes of anticonvulsants, drowsiness, ataxia, and dizziness are common side effects.

Availability

See Table 8.13.

Dosage and Administration

See Table 8.13.

Drug Interactions

The following drugs, when used concurrently with the succinimides, may enhance the toxic effects of the succinimides: antihistamines, alcohol, analgesics, anesthetics, tranquilizers, other anticonvulsants, and sedative-hypnotics.

Nursing Interventions

See also General Nursing Considerations for Patients with Seizure Disorders. See also Hydantoins.

Miscellaneous Agents

Carbamazepine (kar-bah-maz′e-peen)
Tegretol (teg′reh-tol)

Carbamazepine is an anticonvulsant frequently used in combination with other anticonvulsants to control grand mal seizures. It is not effective in the control of absence seizures. Carbamazepine has also been used successfully to treat the pain associated with trigeminal neuralgia (tic douloureux).

Side Effects

Side effects frequently seen when therapy is started are drowsiness, nausea, vomiting, and dizziness.

As a result of serious adverse reactions, the manufacturer recommends that the following baseline studies be repeated at regular intervals: complete blood count, liver function tests, urinalysis, BUN and serum creatinine, and ophthalmologic examination.

Side effects based on organ systems are as follows:
Cardiovascular: hypotension, hypertension, congestive heart failure, edema, and aggravation of coronary artery disease.
Neurologic: incoordination, nystagmus, visual hallucinations, and speech disturbances.
Dermatologic: pruritus, rashes, skin pigmentation, urticaria, and alopecia (loss of hair).

Availability

PO—100 and 200 mg tablets.

Dosage and Administration

Adult
PO—Initial dose is 200 mg 2 times daily in the first day. Increase gradually by 200 mg/day in divided doses at 6- to 8-hour intervals. Do not exceed 1200 mg daily.

Nursing Interventions

See also General Nursing Considerations for Patients with Seizure Disorders.

PATIENT CONCERNS: NURSING INTERVENTION/RATIONALE

Side Effects to Expect

Nausea, Vomiting, Drowsiness, Dizziness

These effects can be reduced by slowly increasing the dose.

These effects are usually mild and tend to resolve with continued therapy. Encourage the patient not to discontinue therapy without first consulting the physician.

Provide for patient safety during episodes of dizziness.

Persons who are working around machinery, driving a car, or performing other duties in which they must remain mentally alert should not take these medications while working.

Side Effects to Report

Orthostatic Hypotension, Hypertension

Monitor the blood pressure daily in both the supine and standing positions.

Anticipate the development of postural hypotension and take measures to prevent an occurrence. Teach the patient to rise slowly from a supine or sitting position; encourage the patient to sit or lie down if feeling "faint."

Dyspnea, Edema

If carbamazepine is used in patients with a history of congestive heart failure, monitor daily weights, lung sounds, and accumulation of edema.

Neurologic

Perform a baseline assessment of the patient's speech patterns and degree of alertness and orientation to name, place, and time *prior* to initiating therapy. Make regularly scheduled subsequent evaluations of mental status and compare findings. Report development of alterations.

Nephrotoxicity

Monitor urinalysis and kidney function tests for abnormal results. Report an increasing BUN and creatinine, decreasing urine output and/or decreasing specific gravity (despite amount of fluid intake), casts or protein in the urine, frank blood or smoky-colored urine, or RBCs in excess of 0 to 3 on the urinalysis report.

Hepatotoxicity

The symptoms of hepatotoxicity are anorexia, nausea, vomiting, jaundice, hepatomegaly, splenomegaly, and abnormal liver function tests (elevated bilirubin, SGOT, SGPT, alkaline phosphatase, prothrombin time).

Blood Dyscrasias

Routine laboratory studies (RBC, WBC, and differential counts) should be scheduled.

Monitor for the development of sore throat, fever, purpura, jaundice, or excessive and progressive weakness.

Dermatologic Reactions

Report a rash or pruritus immediately and withhold additional doses pending approval by the physician.

Drug Interactions

Isoniazid

Isoniazid inhibits the metabolism of carbamazepine. Monitor for signs of toxicity: disorientation, ataxia, lethargy, headache, drowsiness, nausea, and vomiting.

Propoxyphene

Propoxyphene increases serum levels of carbamazepine. Monitor for signs of toxicity: disorientation, ataxia, lethargy, headache, drowsiness, nausea, and vomiting.

Warfarin

Carbamazepine may diminish the anticoagulant effects of warfarin. Monitor the prothrombin time and increase the dosage of warfarin if necessary.

Phenobarbital, Phenytoin, Valproic Acid, Primidone

Carbamazepine enhances the metabolism of these agents. Monitor for increased frequency of seizure activity. Monitoring changes in serum levels should help warn of possible increased seizure activity.

Doxycycline

Carbamazepine enhances the metabolism of this antibiotic. Monitor patients for signs of continued infection.

Oral Contraceptives

Carbamazepine enhances the metabolism of estrogens. Spotting or bleeding may be an indication of reduced contraceptive activity. Use of alternate forms of birth control is recommended.

Primidone (prih′mih-doan) *Mysoline* (my′so-leen)

Primidone is structurally related to the barbiturates. It is metabolized into phenobarbital and phenylethylmalonamide (PEMA), both of which are active anticonvulsants. Primidone is used in combination with other anticonvulsants to treat grand mal and psychomotor seizures.

Side Effects

Common adverse effects include sedation, drowsiness, dizziness, blurred vision, and nystagmus.

Primidone may cause paradoxic excitability in children. Blood dyscrasias have rarely been reported with the use of primidone.

Availability

PO—50 and 250 mg tablets, and 250 mg/5 ml oral suspension.

Dosage and Administration

Adult

PO—250 mg daily, with weekly increases of 250 mg until therapeutic response or intolerance develops. Usual dose is 750 to 1500 mg daily. Do not exceed 2000 mg daily.

Nursing Interventions

See also General Nursing Considerations for Patients with Seizure Disorders.

PATIENT CONCERNS: NURSING INTERVENTION/RATIONALE

Side Effects to Expect

Sedation, Drowsiness, Dizziness, Blurred Vision

These symptoms tend to disappear with continued therapy and possible adjustment of dosage. Encourage the patient not to discontinue therapy without first consulting the physician.

Persons who are working around machinery, driving a car, or performing other duties in which they must remain mentally alert should be particularly cautious while working.

Provide for patient safety during episodes of dizziness; report for further evaluation.

Caution the patient that blurred vision may occur and make appropriate suggestions for personal safety of the individual.

Side Effects to Report

Blood Dyscrasias

Routine laboratory studies (RBC, WBC, and differential counts) should be scheduled.

Monitor for the development of sore throat, fever, purpura, jaundice, or excessive and progressive weakness.

Paradoxical Excitability

During a period of excitement, protect persons from harm and provide for physical channeling of energy (e.g., walk with them). Notify the physician for a possible change in medication.

Drug Interactions

Oral Contraceptives

Spotting or bleeding may be an indication of reduced contraceptive activity. Use of alternate forms of birth control is recommended.

Phenytoin

Phenytoin may increase the phenobarbital serum levels when taken concurrently with primidone. Monitor patients for increased sedation.

Valproic Acid (val-pro'ik) *(Depakene)* (dep'ah-keen)

Valproic acid is an anticonvulsant structurally unrelated to any other agent used to treat seizure disorders. It is most effective in treating petit mal seizure activity; it may be effective in treating other types of seizures when used in combination with other agents.

Side Effects

Side effects include nausea, vomiting and indigestion, dizziness, blurred vision, nystagmus, and headache.

The manufacturer recommends that the following baseline studies be completed before therapy is initiated and at regular intervals thereafter: liver function tests, bleeding time determination, and platelet count.

One of the metabolites of valproic acid is a ketone. It is excreted in the urine and may produce a false-positive test (Ketostix, Acetest) for urine ketones.

Availability

PO—250 mg tablets and 250 mg/5 ml syrup.

Dosage and Administration

Adult

PO—5 mg/kg every 8 hours. Increase by 5 to 10 mg/kg/day at weekly intervals. The maximum daily dosage is 30 mg/kg/day.

Nursing Interventions

See also General Nursing Considerations for Patients with Seizure Disorders.

PATIENT CONCERNS: NURSING INTERVENTION/RATIONALE

Side Effects to Expect

Nausea, Vomiting, Indigestion

These effects are common during initiation of therapy. Gradual increases in therapy and administration with food or milk will reduce gastric irritation.

Sedation, Drowsiness, Dizziness, Blurred Vision

These symptoms tend to disappear with continued therapy and possible adjustment of dosage. Encourage

the patient not to discontinue therapy without first consulting the physician.

Persons who are working around machinery, driving a car, or performing other duties in which they must remain mentally alert should not take these medications while working.

Provide for patient safety during episodes of dizziness; report for further evaluation.

Caution the patient that blurred vision may occur and make appropriate suggestions for personal safety of the individual.

Side Effects to Report

Blood Dyscrasias

Routine laboratory studies (RBC, WBC, and differential counts) should be scheduled.

Monitor for the development of sore throat, fever, purpura, jaundice, or excessive and progressive weakness.

Hepatotoxicity

The symptoms of hepatotoxicity are anorexia, nausea, vomiting, jaundice, hepatomegaly, splenomegaly, and abnormal liver function tests (elevated bilirubin, SGOT, SGPT, alkaline phosphatase, prothrombin time).

Dosage and Administration

PO

Administer medication with food or milk to reduce gastric irritation.

An enteric-coated tablet is available for those patients having persistent difficulty.

Drug Interactions

Enhanced Sedation

CNS depressants, including sleeping aids, analgesics, tranquilizers, and alcohol, will enhance the sedative effects of valproic acid. Persons who are working around machinery, driving a car, or performing other duties in which they must remain mentally alert should not take these medications while working.

Phenobarbital, Phenytoin, Carbamazepine

Monitor for increased frequency of seizure activity. Monitoring changes in serum levels should help warn of possible increased seizure activity.

Drugs Used for Motion Sickness

Nausea and vomiting associated with motion are thought to result from stimulation of the labyrinth system of the ear, with subsequent transmission of this stimulus to the vestibular network located near the vomiting center. When there is strong or frequent stimulation, such as from a rocking ship or airplane, the vestibular network is bombarded with an abnormally high number of impulses that radiate by cholinergic nerve impulses to the adjacent vomiting center. Thus drugs that inhibit the cholinergic nerve impulses from the vestibular network to the vomiting center should be effective in the treatment of motion sickness.

Agents used to reduce nausea and vomiting from motion sickness are chemically related to antihistamines. The effectiveness of antihistamines in motion sickness probably results from their anticholinergic properties, not their ability to block histamine. See Table 8.14.

Side Effects

The most common side effect of antihistamines used to control motion sickness is drowsiness. With prolonged therapy, most patients acquire a tolerance to this adverse effect. Reduction in dosage or a change to another antihistamine may occasionally be necessary.

The anticholinergic effects that are being capitalized on for the treatment of motion sickness also cause dry mouth, stuffy nose, blurred vision, constipation, and urinary retention. Patients with asthma, prostatic enlargement, or glaucoma should take antihistamines only under a physician's supervision. The drying effects may also make respiratory mucus more viscous and tenacious.

Availability

See Table 8.14.

Table 8.14
Antihistamines Used for Motion Sickness

GENERIC NAME	BRAND NAME	AVAILABILITY	ADULT DOSAGE	PEDIATRIC DOSAGE
Buclizine	Bucladin-S Softabs	Tablets: 50 mg	PO: 50 mg, repeated in 4–6 hours. Do not exceed 150 mg daily.	Not approved for use by children.
Cyclizine	Marezine	Tablets: 50 mg Inj: 50 mg/1 ml	PO: 50 mg, repeated in 4–6 hours. Do not exceed 200 mg daily. IM: 50 mg every 4–6 hours.	PO: 6–12 years: 25 mg up to 3 times daily.
Dimenhydrinate	Dramamine, Motion-Aid, Dramaban	Tablets: 50 mg Inj: 50 mg/ml Liquid: 12.5 mg/4 ml	PO: 50–100 mg every 4–6 hours. Do not exceed 400 mg in 24 hours. IM: 50 mg, as needed.	PO: 6–12 years: 25–50 mg every 6–8 hours; do not exceed 150 mg in 24 hours. 2–6 years: up to 25 mg every 6–8 hours; do not exceed 75 mg in 24 hours.
Diphenhydramine	Benadryl, Noradryl, Bendylate	Tablets: 50 mg Capsules: 25, 50 mg Elixir: 12.5 mg/5 ml Syrup: 12.5, 13.3 mg/5 ml Inj: 10, 50 mg/ml	PO: 25–50 mg 3 or 4 times daily. IM: 10–50 mg. Do not exceed 400 mg in 24 hours.	PO: Over 20 lbs: 12.5–25 mg 3 or 4 times daily (5 mg/kg/24). Do not exceed 300 mg/24 hours. IM: 5 mg/kg/24 hours, in 4 divided doses. Do not exceed 300 mg in 24 hours.
Hydroxyzine	Atarax, Durrax, Vistaril	Tablets: 10, 25, 50, 100 mg Capsules: 25, 50, 100 mg Syrup: 10 mg/5 ml Oral Suspension: 25 mg/5 ml Inj: 25, 50 mg/ml	PO: 25–100 mg 3–4 times daily. IM: As for PO.	PO: Over 6 years: 10–25 mg every 4–6 hours. Under 6 years: 10 mg every 4–6 hours. IM: As for PO.
Meclizine	Antivert, Bonine	Tablets: 12.5, 25 mg	PO: 25–50 mg. May be repeated every 24 hours.	PO: Not approved for use by children.

Dosage and Administration

It is essential that the patient take the medication 30 to 60 minutes prior to the activity that is likely to produce motion sickness.

**PATIENT CONCERNS:
NURSING INTERVENTION/RATIONALE**

Side Effects to Expect

Sedative Effects

Tolerance may develop over a period of time, thus diminishing the effect.

The operation of power equipment or the ability to operate a motor vehicle may prove hazardous. Caution patients to provide for their personal safety in these situations.

Fluid Intake

Maintain fluid intake at 8 to 12 8-ounce glasses daily.

Blurred Vision, Constipation, Urinary Retention, Dryness of Mucosa of the Mouth, Throat, and Nose

These symptoms are the anticholinergic effects produced by these agents. Patients taking these medications should be monitored for the development of these side effects.

Dryness of the mucosa may be relieved by sucking hard candy or ice chips, or by chewing gum.

The use of stool softeners such as docusate or the occasional use of a potent laxative such as bisacodyl may be required for constipation.

Caution the patient that blurred vision may occur and make appropriate suggestions for personal safety of the individual.

Patients who develop urinary hesitancy should discontinue the medication and contact their physician for further evaluation.

Dosage and Administration

PO

Administer 30 to 60 minutes prior to the activity that is likely to produce motion sickness.

Drug Interactions

Enhanced Sedation

CNS depressants, including sleeping aids, analgesics, tranquilizers, and alcohol, will enhance the sedative effects of the antihistamines. Persons who are working around machinery, driving a car, or performing other duties in which they must remain mentally alert should not take these medications while working.

Analgesics

Analgesics are drugs that relieve pain without producing loss of consciousness or reflex activity. Pain is an unpleasant sensation that is part of a larger experience called "pain experience." The pain experience includes all the emotional sensations (attention, anxiety, fatigue, suggestion, prior conditioning) for a particular person under a certain set of circumstances. This accounts for the wide variation in individual responses to the sensation of pain.

The search for an ideal analgesic continues, but it is difficult to find one that does all that is desired of it. It should (1) be potent, so that it will afford maximum relief of pain; (2) not cause dependence; (3) exhibit a minimum of side effects such as constipation, hallucinations, respiratory depression, nausea, and vomiting; (4) not cause tolerance to develop; (5) act promptly and over a long period of time with a minimum amount of sedation so that the patient is able to remain conscious and responsive; and (6) be relatively inexpensive. Needless to say, no present-day analgesic has all these qualifications, so the search must continue.

Classification and Terminology

There is, at present, no completely satisfactory classification of analgesics. Historically, we have categorized them based on potency (e.g., mild, moderate, and strong analgesics), by origin (e.g., opium, semisynthetic, synthetic, coal-tar derivatives), or by addictive properties (e.g., narcotic and nonnarcotic agents).

Research into the control of pain over the past decade has given new insight into pathways of pain within the nervous system and a better understanding of precise mechanisms of action of analgesic agents. The new nomenclature for analgesics stems from these recent discoveries into mechanisms of actions. In this section the medications have been divided into (1) opiate agonists; (2) opiate partial agonists, opiate antagonists; (3) nonsteroidal antiinflammatory agents; and (4) miscellaneous analgesic agents.

The term *opiate* was once used to refer to drugs derived from opium, such as heroin and morphine. It has been found that many other analgesics, not related to morphine, act at the same sites within the brain. It is now understood that when we refer to "opiate agonists" or "opiate antagonists," we are referring to drugs that act at the same site as morphine to either stimulate analgesic effects (opiate agonists) or block the effects of opiate agonists (opiate antagonists).

Another outdated word is *narcotic*. Originally it referred to medications that induced a stupor or sleep. Over the past 80 years it has gradually come to refer to addictive, morphinelike analgesics. The Harrison Narcotic Act of 1914, which placed morphinelike products under governmental control, helped foster this association. With the development in recent years of analgesics that are as potent as morphine but that do not have the sedative or addictive properties of morphine, the word narcotic should be abandoned in exchange for "opiate agonists" and "opiate partial agonists."

General Nursing Considerations for the Patient Experiencing Pain

Nurses need to assist the patient in the management of pain. The first vital step in this process is to believe the patient's description of the pain being experienced. Pain brings with it a variety of feelings, such as anxiety, anger, loneliness, frustration, and depression. Part of the patient's response is tied to past experiences, sociocultural factors, current emotional state, and beliefs regarding pain.

Psychological, physical, and environmental factors all need consideration in the management of the pain. Never overlook the value of general comfort measures such as a back rub, repositioning, and the use of hot or cold applications. Psychologically the use of a variety of relaxation techniques may prove beneficial. Measures to decrease environmental stimuli and thereby provide for successful periods of rest are essential.

PATIENT CONCERNS: NURSING INTERVENTION/RATIONALE

The Patient's Perception

Have the patient describe his or her perception of the pain being experienced. Whenever possible, chart the description in the patient's exact words.

Onset

When was the pain first noticed? When was the most recent attack? Is the onset slow or abrupt? Is there any particular activity that starts the pain?

Location

What is the exact location of the pain being experienced?

Quality

What is the actual sensation felt when the pain is present—stabbing, dull, cramping, sore, burning, other? Is the pain always in the same place and of the same intensity?

Duration

Is the pain continual or intermittent? How often does it occur, and once felt, how long does it last?

Relief

Is there anything specific that relieves the pain?

Nonverbal Observations

Note the patient's general body position during an episode of pain. Be particularly observant about subtle clues such as facial grimaces, immobility of a particular part, holding or resisting movement of an extremity.

Physical Data

Gather data concerning the vital signs: pupil dilation, presence of nausea and vomiting, skin color, muscle tension, diaphoresis.

Examine the affected part for any alterations in appearance, change in sensation, or limitation in mobility or range of motion.

Behavior Response

What is the patient's response to pain—crying, anger, withdrawal, depression, anxiety, fear, hopelessness?

Comfort Measures

Provide for the patient's basic hygiene and comfort. Utilize such techniques as back rubs, massage, hot and cold applications, or warm baths, as ordered.

Ask the patient what measures have been successful in the past in providing pain relief.

Relieve pain by doing any or all of the following, as appropriate:

- Support an affected part during movement.
- Provide appropriate assistance during movement or activities.
- Apply binders or splint an incisional area prior to initiating activities such as deep breathing and coughing.
- Give analgesics in advance of undertaking painful activities and plan for the activity to take place during the peak action of the medication given.

Environmental Control

Provide for a quiet environment with as little distraction as possible during periods of rest. Modify hospital schedules such as routine vital signs and specimen collection so that the individual is not disturbed once asleep.

Provide for mental stimulation through the appropriate use of television, visitors, card games, and other patients to take the patient's mind off the pain.

Relaxation Techniques

Institute relaxation techniques to assist the patient to relax. Try implementing these techniques at the same time the analgesic is administered to maximize the outcome.

Involve the patient's family or support group in the plan for relief of chronic pain.

Medication Administration

Note the intensity and duration of the pain being experienced and then administer an analgesic of the correct type.

If the patient is not nauseated, utilize oral medications first. With nausea, the rectal route may be tried as an alternate to parenteral administration.

During the immediate postoperative period, assess all complaints thoroughly so that complications (e.g., wound dehiscence, heart attack) are not overlooked or masked. During the first 24 to 48 hours, the pain may be severe, and the patient will respond best to liberal medication so that rest, deep breathing and coughing, and ambulation can be accomplished effectively. (Plan these activities when the pain medication is at a peak.)

Anticipate the patient's needs for pain relief and do not make the patient wait unnecessarily. Recognize that some individuals will not ask for pain relievers.

Record the degree and duration of pain relief achieved. Report poor control to the physician for further evaluation.

Patient Teaching Associated with Pain Therapy

PATIENT CONCERNS: NURSING INTERVENTION/RATIONALE

Communication and Responsibility

Encourage open communication with the patient concerning frustrations and anger as attempts are made to adjust to the diagnosis and need for prolonged treatment. The patient must be guided to gain insight into the disorder to assume the responsibility for the continuation of the treatment. Keep emphasizing those things the patient can do to alter progression of the disease, including maintenance of general health, nutritional needs, adequate rest and appropriate exercise, and continuation of prescribed medication therapy.

Nutritional Aspects

The patient should eat a diet that is well balanced and high in B-complex vitamins; should limit or eliminate sugar, nicotine, caffeine, and alcoholic intake; and should drink 8 to 10 8-ounce glasses of water per day and maintain normal elimination patterns.

Exercise and Activity

Unless contraindicated, moderate exercise should be encouraged.

Many times, pain causes the individual not to move the affected part or to position it in a manner that provides relief. Stress the need to prevent complications by utilizing a passive range of motion.

Relaxation

Teach the patient relaxation techniques and encourage use of the techniques simultaneously with the medication regimen.

Visualization techniques and biofeedback are also being utilized with some success.

Establish a schedule that provides for sufficient rest. Fatigue and anxiety may increase the perception of pain. Decrease noise; provide for a quiet environment.

Medication

Encourage use of the analgesic before the pain becomes severe. Give the smallest dose necessary to control the pain.

Physical Relief

Utilize hot or cold applications, massage, and warm baths.

Expectations of Therapy

Discuss the expectations of therapy (e.g., level of exercise attainable without severe pain, degree of pain relief, frequency of use of therapy, sexual activity, maintenance of mobility, ability to maintain activities of daily living and/or work).

Pain control without addiction is a goal for most patients, but for the terminally ill, comfort is the major priority. Concern for addiction is not a consideration.

Changes in Expectations

Assess changes in expectations as therapy progresses and the patient gains understanding and skill in the management of the diagnosis.

In terminal illnesses, increasing pain needs careful management. The duration and intensity of the pain should be constantly reported to the physician for appropriate modifications of the medication regimen.

Assist the patient to learn to cope effectively with the pain. Include family members in discussion of pain

management. Give praise when techniques are tried and success is achieved.

Changes in Therapy through Cooperative Goal-Setting

Work mutually with the patient to encourage adherence to the treatment as prescribed. When the patient feels that a change should be made in a treatment plan, encourage discussion first with the physician.

Written Record

Enlist the patient's aid in developing and maintaining a written record (Table 8.15) of monitoring parameters (e.g., frequency of pain attacks, activity being performed when pain occurs, techniques being used to control pain, degree of pain relief, exercise tolerance) and response to prescribed therapies for discussion with the physician. Patients should be encouraged to bring this record with them on follow-up visits.

Fostering Compliance

Throughout the hospitalization, discuss medication information and how it will benefit the course of treatment. Seek cooperation and understanding of the following points so that medication compliance may be enhanced:

1. Name.
2. Dosage.
3. Route and administration times.
4. Anticipated therapeutic response.
5. Side effects to expect.
6. Side effects to report.
7. What to do if a dosage is missed.
8. When, how, or if to refill the medication.

Difficulty in Comprehension

If it is evident that the patient or family does not understand all aspects of continuing therapy being prescribed (e.g., administration and monitoring of medications, exercises, diets, follow-up appointments), consider use of social service or visiting nurse agencies.

Table 8.15

Example of a Written Record for Patients Receiving Analgesics

Medications	Color	To be taken

Name _____

Physician _____

Physician's phone _____

Next appt.* _____

Parameters		Day of discharge								Comments
Pain: onset:	Example: 8AM 3PM / 9PM									
duration:	Before taking medication									
relief:	Example: 6hrs / 3hrs									
Describe pain	Location									
	Check one: C = Constant I = Intermittent	C __ I __	C __ I __	C __ I __	C __ I __	C __ I __	C __ I __	C __ I __		
	Record: sharp, dull, throbbing									
Pain after medication. No relief 10 — Better 5 — Much better 1	Time: e.g., 8AM = 4 9PM = 8 2AM = 1									
Sleep. No sleep 10 — Fair 5 — Slept well 1										
Appetite. Poor 10 — Decreased 5 — Normal 1										
I enjoy life? Yes 10 — only when not in pain 5 — No 1										

*Please bring this record with you to your next appointment.
Use the back of this sheet for additional information.

Associated Teaching

Always inform the physician or dentist of any prescription or over-the-counter medication being taken.

Over-the-counter medications should not be taken without first discussion with a physician or pharmacist.

Always report side effects of rash, itching, or hives immediately. Nausea, vomiting, or diarrhea should be reported for the physician's evaluation if it is a new symptom.

Take all of the medication as prescribed for the full course of treatment. Do not discontinue use when feeling improved; do not save for future use or give medicine to another individual. Sudden discontinuation of certain medications may produce harmful effects.

Keep all medications out of the reach of children.

If pregnancy is suspected, consult an obstetrician as soon as possible about continuation of medication therapy.

At Discharge

Items to be sent home with the patient should include the following:

1. Written instructions for the item's use.
2. Items labeled in a level of language and size of print appropriate for the patient.
3. If needed, include identification cards or bracelets.
4. Include a list of additional supplies to be purchased after discharge (e.g., syringes, dressings).
5. A schedule of follow-up appointments.

Opiate Agonists

Opiate agonists are a group of naturally occurring, semisynthetic, and synthetic drugs that have the capability to relieve severe pain without the loss of consciousness. These agents also have the ability to produce physical dependence and are thus considered controlled substances under the Federal Controlled Substances Act of 1970.

These agents can be subdivided into three groups: the morphine-like derivatives, the meperidine-like derivatives, and the methadone-like derivatives (see Table 8.16). Administration of these agents causes primary effects on the central nervous system; there are also significant effects on the respiratory, cardiovascular, gastrointestinal, and urinary tracts.

The opiate agonists are used to relieve acute or chronic moderate to severe pain such as that associated with acute injury, postoperative pain, renal or biliary colic, myocardial infarction, or terminal cancer. These agents may be used to provide preoperative sedation and supplement anesthesia. In patients with acute pulmonary edema, small doses of the opiate agonists are used to reduce anxiety and produce positive cardiovascular effects to control edema.

Side Effects

The most frequently observed adverse reactions include light-headedness, dizziness, sedation, nausea, vomiting, and sweating. These effects generally occur more frequently in standing patients receiving parenteral administration and those not suffering severe pain.

The actions of the opiate antagonists on the central nervous system are analgesia, suppression of the cough reflex, respiratory depression, drowsiness, sedation, mental clouding, euphoria, nausea, and vomiting.

The opiate agonists may produce orthostatic hypotension caused by peripheral vasodilation. This usually does not occur in patients who are supine, but it is commonly observed in ambulatory patients, particularly with the first dose.

Gastrointestinal effects include nausea and vomiting (usually limited to the first dose if it occurs) and constipation (with multiple doses). All opiate agonists may produce an increased pressure and spasm of the biliary tract, but the action depends somewhat on the agonist and the patient. Morphine appears to have the greatest effect, with meperidine and codeine having lesser effects. Nevertheless, the opiate agonists are frequently administered to patients with acute, painful, biliary colic because the spasm does not occur in all patients with therapeutic doses, and the sedation produced may contribute to the relief of pain.

Opiate agonists may produce spasms of the ureters and bladder, causing urinary retention. Patients may also have difficulty in starting the stream for urination.

With continued, prolonged use, opiate derivatives may produce tolerance or psychological and physical dependence (addiction). Tolerance is said to occur when a patient requires increases in dosages to receive the same analgesic relief. Development of tolerance seems to depend on the extent and duration of CNS depression. Patients who have prolonged depression by the continued use of opiate agonists have a higher incidence of developing tolerance. Patients who have developed tolerance to one opiate agonist usually require increased doses of all opiate agonists.

Physical and psychological dependence may develop with prolonged use and higher dosages of the opiate agonists. Patients who are physically dependent on opiate agonists remain asymptomatic as long as they are able to maintain their daily opiate agonist requirement. Addiction may develop after 3 to 6 weeks of continuous use of the opiate agonists. Early signs of withdrawal are restlessness, perspiration, gooseflesh, lacrimation, runny nose, and mydriasis. Over the next 24 hours, these symptoms intensify, and the patient develops muscular spasms; severe aches in the back, abdomen, and legs; abdominal and muscle cramps; hot and cold flashes; insomnia; nausea, vomiting, and diarrhea; severe sneezing; and increases in body temperature, blood pressure, respiratory rate, and heart rate. These symptoms reach a peak at 36 to 72 hours after discontinuation of the medication and disappear over the next 5 to 14 days.

Patients do not have to undergo the symptoms of withdrawal to be treated for addiction. Patients may be treated by gradual reduction of daily opiate agonist dosages. If withdrawal symptoms become severe, the patient may receive methadone. Temporary administration of tranquilizers and sedatives may aid in reducing patient anxiety and craving for the opiate agonist.

Availability

See Table 8.16.

Administration and Dosage

See Table 8.16.

Antidote

Naloxone.

Nursing Interventions

See also General Nursing Considerations for the Patient Experiencing Pain.

PATIENT CONCERNS: NURSING INTERVENTION/RATIONALE

Side Effects to Expect

Light-headedness, Dizziness, Sedation, Nausea, Vomiting, Sweating

These effects tend to occur most frequently with the initial dosage. Symptoms can be reduced by keeping the patient supine. Provide for patient safety, assurance, and comfort.

Orthostatic Hypotension

Orthostatic hypotension, manifested by dizziness and weakness, occurs particularly when therapy is being initiated in a patient not in a supine position. Monitor blood pressure closely, especially if the patient complains of dizziness or faintness. Do not allow the patient to sit up.

Constipation

Continued use may cause constipation. Maintain the patient's state of hydration and obtain an order for stool softeners or bulk-forming laxatives if necessary. Encourage the inclusion of sufficient roughage, fresh fruits, vegetables, and whole-grain products in the diet.

Confusion, Disorientation

Perform a baseline assessment of the patient's degree of alertness and orientation to name, place, and time *prior* to initiating therapy. Make regularly scheduled subsequent evaluations of mental status and compare findings. Report development of alterations. Provide for patient safety during these episodes.

Side Effects to Report

Respiratory Depression

Opiate agonists make the respiratory centers less sensitive to carbon dioxide, causing respiratory depression. This may occur before either the reduction in respiratory rate or tidal volume is noticeable. Check the respiratory rate and depth frequently. Have equipment for respiratory assistance available.

Urinary Retention

If the patient develops urinary hesitancy, assess for distension of the bladder. Report to the physician for further evaluation. Try to stimulate urination by running water or placing hands in water; if permitted, have male patients stand to void; female patients should sit on a bedpan or toilet with receptacle.

Excessive Use or Abuse

Evaluate the *patient's* response to the analgesic and suggest a change to a milder analgesic when indicated.

Table 8.16

Opiate Agonists

GENERIC NAME	BRAND NAME	AVAILABILITY	INITIAL ADULT DOSE	DURATION (HOURS)	DOSE EQUAL TO MORPHINE (10 MG)	
					IM (MG)	ORAL (MG)
1. Morphine-like derivatives						
Codeine	Codeine Sulfate Codeine Phosphate	Tablets: 15, 30, 60 mg Inj: 30, 60 mg	PO, SC, IM, IV: Analgesic: 15–60 mg every 4–6 hours. Antitussive: 10–20 mg every 4–6 hours.	4–6	130	200
Hydromorphone	Dilaudid	Tablets: 1, 2, 3, 4 mg Suppositories: 3 mg Inj: 1, 2, 3, 4 mg/ml	PO: 2 mg every 4–6 hours. SC, IM: 2 mg every 4–6 hours. Rectal: 3 mg every 6–8 hours.	4–5	1.5	7.5
Levorphanol	Levo-Dromoran	Tablets: 2 mg Inj: 2 mg/ml	PO: 2 mg. SC, IM, IV: 2 mg.	4–8	2	4
Morphine	Roxanol, Morphine Sulfate	Tablets: 10, 15, 30 mg Solution: 10, 20 mg/5 ml; 20 mg/10 ml; 20 mg/ml Suppositories: 5, 10, 20 mg Inj: 2, 4, 5, 8, 10, 15 mg/ml	PO: 10–30 mg every 4 hours. SC, IM: 10 mg/70 kg. IV: 4–10 mg slowly. Rectal: 10–20 mg every 4 hours.	up to 7	10	60
Oxycodone	Pecodan (with aspirin)	Tablets: 5 mg Solution: 5 mg/ml	PO: 5 mg every 6 hours.	4–5	15	30
Oxymorphone	Numorphan	Inj: 1 mg/ml Suppositories: 5 mg	IV: 0.5 mg. SC, IM: 1–1.5 mg every 4–6 hours. Rectal: 5 mg every 4–6 hours.	3–6	1	6
2. Meperidine-like derivatives						
Alphaprodine	Nisentil	Inj: 40, 60 mg/ml	SC: 0.4–1.2 mg/kg. IV: 0.4–0.6 mg/kg. Do not exceed 30 mg IV or 60 mg SC; or 240 mg in 24 hours.	0.5–2	45	—
Fentanyl	Sublimaze	Inj: 0.05 mg/ml	IM: 0.05–0.1 mg.	1–2	0.1	—
Meperidine	Demerol	Tablets: 50, 100 mg Syrup: 50 mg/5 ml Inj: 25, 50, 75, 100 mg/1 ml	PO, SC, IM: 50–150 mg every 3–4 hours. IV: 25–100 mg very slowly.	2–4	75	300
3. Methadone-like derivatives						
Methadone	Methadone, Dolophine	Tablets: 5, 10 mg Solution: 5, 10 mg/5 ml Inj: 10 mg/ml	Analgesia: PO, SC, IM: 2.5–10 mg every 3–4 hours. Maintenance: PO: 20–40 mg; up to 120 mg daily.	4–6	10	20

Assist the patient to recognize the abuse problem. Identify underlying needs and plan for more appropriate management of those needs.

Discuss the case with the physician and make plans to cooperatively approach gradual withdrawal of the medications being abused.

Provide for emotional support of the individual; display an accepting attitude—be kind but firm.

Drug Interactions

CNS Depressants

The following drugs may enhance the depressant effects of the opiate agonists: general anesthetics, phenothiazines, tranquilizers, sedative-hypnotics, tricyclic antidepressants, antihistamines, and alcohol.

Respiratory depression, hypotension, and profound sedation or coma may result from this interaction unless the dose of the opiate agonist has been reduced appropriately (usually by one third to one half the normal dose).

Phenobarbital, Phenytoin, Rifampin, Chlorpromazine

These enzyme-inducing agents may enhance the metabolism of meperidine to normeperidine. Patients receiving long-term, large oral doses of meperidine, those with renal impairment, and those with a highly acidic urine are predisposed to accumulating normeperidine. Evidence of toxic levels of normeperidine are seizures, tremors, and excitation.

Opiate Partial Agonists

Opiate partial agonists (butorphanol, nalbuphine, and pentazocine) are an interesting class of drugs in that their pharmacologic actions depend on whether an opiate agonist has been administered previously and the extent to which physical dependence has developed to that opiate agonist. When used without prior administration of opiate agonists, the opiate partial agonists are quite effective analgesics. Their potency with the first few weeks of therapy is similar to morphine; however, after prolonged use, tolerance may develop. Increasing the dosage does not significantly increase the analgesia but definitely increases the incidence of side effects. This is called a "ceiling effect" in that, contrary to the action of the opiate agonists, a larger dose does not produce a significantly higher analgesic effect.

If an opiate partial agonist is administered to a patient addicted to an opiate agonist such as morphine or meperidine, the opiate partial agonist will induce withdrawal symptoms from the opiate agonist. If the patient is not addicted to the opiate agonist, there is no interaction and the patient will be relieved of pain.

Opiate partial agonists may be used for the short-term relief (up to 3 weeks) of moderate to severe pain associated with cancer, burns, renal colic, preoperative analgesia, and obstetric and surgical analgesia.

Side Effects

The most commonly reported adverse effects to the opiate partial agonists are sedation, nausea, a clammy and sweaty sensation, dizziness, dry mouth, and headache.

The opiate agonists may cause respiratory depression. Dosage adjustments should be made in patients with bronchial asthma, obstructive respiratory conditions, cyanosis, or other respiratory depression from any other cause.

Butorphanol and pentazocine, and nalbuphine to a lesser degree, may produce hallucinations. Patients may complain of seeing multicolored flashing patterns or animals, with and without sound, or may have very vivid dreams. These adverse effects have been reported after only one or two doses of medication and may occur in as many as one third of the patients taking butorphanol or pentazocine.

Repeated use may lead to tolerance, dependence, and addiction. Abrupt discontinuance following extended use may result in withdrawal symptoms. The withdrawal symptoms may be treated by restarting the partial agonist and then gradually reducing the dosage over the next several days to weeks to prevent recurrences and stop the addiction.

Opiate partial agonists have weak antagonist activity. When administered to patients who have been receiving opiate agonists such as morphine or meperidine on a regular basis, it may precipitate withdrawal symptoms.

Availability

See Table 8.17.

Dosage and Administration

See Table 8.17.

Antidote

Naloxone.

Nursing Interventions

See also General Nursing Considerations for the Patient Experiencing Pain.

PATIENT CONCERNS: NURSING INTERVENTION/RATIONALE

Side Effects to Expect

Clamminess, Dizziness, Sedation, Nausea, Vomiting, Dry Mouth, Sweating

These effects tend to occur most frequently with the initial dosage. Symptoms can be reduced by keeping

Table 8.17
Opiate Partial Agonists

GENERIC NAME	BRAND NAME	AVAILABILITY	ADULT DOSAGE	DURATION (HOURS)	DOSE EQUAL TO MORPHINE 10 MG
Butorphanol	Stadol	Inj: 1, 2 mg in 1, 2, 10 ml vials	IM: 2 mg, repeated in 3–4 hours. Do not exceed single doses of 4 mg. IV: 1 mg, repeated in 3–4 hours.	(IM) 3–4	(IM) 2–3 mg
Nalbuphine	Nubain	Inj: 10 mg/ml in 1, 2, 10, ml vials	SC, IM, IV: 10 mg/70 kg, repeat every 3–6 hours. Do not exceed 160 mg daily.	3–6	10 mg
Pentazocine	Talwin, Talwin Nx*	Tablets: 50 mg Inj: 30 mg/ml in 1, 2, 10 ml vials	PO: 50–100 mg every 3–4 hours. Do not exceed 600 mg daily. SC, IM, IV: 30 mg every 3–4 hours. Do not exceed 360 mg daily.	2–3	30–60 mg

* Tablets contain naloxone to prevent abuse.

the patient supine. Provide for patient safety, assurance, and comfort.

Constipation

Continued use may cause constipation. Maintain the patient's state of hydration and obtain an order for stool softeners or bulk-forming laxatives if necessary. Encourage the inclusion of sufficient roughage, fresh fruits, vegetables, and whole-grain products in the diet.

Side Effects to Report

Confusion, Disorientation, Hallucinations

Perform a baseline assessment of the patient's degree of alertness and orientation to name, place, and time *prior* to initiating therapy. Make regularly scheduled subsequent evaluations of mental status and compare findings. Report development of alterations. Provide for patient safety during these episodes. If recurring, seek a change in the medication order.

Respiratory Depression

Opiate partial agonists make the respiratory centers less sensitive to carbon dioxide, causing respiratory depression. This may occur before either the reduction in respiratory rate or tidal volume is noticeable. Check the respiratory rate and depth frequently.

Excessive Use or Abuse

Evaluate the patient's response to the analgesic and suggest a change to a milder analgesic when indicated.

Assist the patient to recognize the abuse problem.

Identify underlying needs and plan for more appropriate management of those needs.

Discuss the case with the physician and make plans to cooperatively approach gradual withdrawal of the medications being abused.

Provide for emotional support of the individual; display an accepting attitude—be kind but firm.

Drug Interactions

CNS Depressants

The following drugs may enhance the depressant effects of the opiate partial agonists: general anesthetics, phenothiazines, tranquilizers, sedative-hypnotics, tricyclic antidepressants, antihistamines, and alcohol.

Respiratory depression, hypotension, and profound sedation or coma may result from this interaction unless the dose of the opiate partial agonist has been reduced appropriately (usually by one third to one half the normal dose).

Opiate Antagonist

Naloxone (nal-oks'own) *Narcan* (nar'can)

Naloxone is a so-called pure opiate antagonist because it has no effect of its own other than its ability to reverse the CNS depressant effects of opiate agonists, opiate partial agonists, and propoxyphene. When administered to patients who have not recently received opiates, there is no respiratory depression, psychomimetic effect, circulatory changes, or other pharmacologic activity. If administered to a person addicted to the opiate agonists or the opiate partial agonists, withdrawal symptoms may be precipitated. Naloxone is not effective in CNS depression induced by tranquilizers or sedative-hypnotics. Naloxone is a drug of choice for treatment of respiratory depression when the causative agent is unknown.

Side Effects

Naloxone rarely manifests any side effects. The following adverse effects have been reported very rarely when very high doses have been used: mental depression, apathy, inability to concentrate, sleepiness, irritability, anorexia, nausea, and vomiting. These adverse effects usually occurred in the first few days of treatment and dissipated rapidly with continued therapy.

Naloxone should be used with caution following the use of opiates during surgery because it may result in excitement, an increase in blood pressure, and clinically important reversal of analgesia. The early reversal of opiate effects may induce nausea, vomiting, sweating, and tachycardia.

Naloxone should be given with caution to patients known or suspected to be physically dependent on opiates (including neonates born to women who are opiate dependent) because the drug may precipitate severe withdrawal symptoms. The severity of the symptoms depends on the dose of the naloxone and the degree of dependence.

Availability

Injection—0.05 mg/ml (for neonatal use) and 0.4 mg/ml.

Dosage and Administration

Adult
IV—Postoperative opiate depression: 0.1 to 0.2 mg every 2 to 3 minutes until the desired response is achieved.
Opiate overdose: 0.4 to 2 mg every 2 to 3 minutes. If no response is seen after 10 minutes, the depressive condition may be caused by a drug or disease process not responsive to naloxone.

Drug Interactions

There are no drug interactions other than that of the antagonist activity toward opiate agonists, opiate partial agonists, and propoxyphene.

Nursing Interventions

See also General Nursing Considerations for the Patient Experiencing Pain.

Antiinflammatory Agents
Salicylates

The salicylates are the most common analgesics used for the relief of slight to moderate pain. The salicylates were introduced into medicine in the late nineteenth century because of their three primary pharmacologic effects as analgesic, antipyretic, and antiinflammatory agents.

Although the mechanisms of action are not fully known, it appears that most of the activity of the salicylates comes from inhibition of prostaglandin synthesis. Salicylates inhibit the formation of prostaglandins that sensitize pain receptors to stimulation (causing pain); they inhibit the prostaglandins that produce the signs and symptoms of inflammation (redness, swelling, warmth); and they inhibit the synthesis and release of prostaglandins in the brain that cause the elevation of body temperature. A major benefit of the salicylates is that they do not dull the conscious level and do not cause mental sluggishness, memory disturbances, hallucinations, euphoria, or sedation.

The combination of pharmacologic effects makes the salicylates the drugs of choice for symptomatic relief of discomfort and pain associated with bacterial and viral infections, headache, muscle aches, and rheumatoid arthritis. Salicylates can be taken to relieve pain on a chronic basis without inducing drug dependence. Many patients have difficulty accepting aspirin as an acceptable approach to a serious disorder such as rheumatoid arthritis. Recurrent teaching may be necessary to foster compliance.

Side Effects

As beneficial as the salicylates are, they are not without adverse effects. In normal therapeutic doses, salicylates may produce gastrointestinal irritation, occasional nausea, and gastric hemorrhage. Extreme caution should be used with administration to those patients with a history of peptic ulcer, liver disease, or coagulation disorders.

Patients receiving higher dosages on a continuing basis are susceptible to developing salicylate intoxication (salicylism). Symptoms include tinnitus (ringing in the ears), impaired hearing, dimness of vision, sweating, fever, lethargy, dizziness, mental confusion, nausea, and vomiting. This condition is reversible on reduction of the dosage. Massive overdoses may lead to respiratory depression and coma. There is no antidote; primary treatment is discontinuation of the drug, gastric lavage, forced IV fluids, and alkalinization of the urine with IV sodium bicarbonate.

Ingestion of 8 to 18 of the 325 mg tablets of aspirin daily may result in false-positive Clinitest and false-negative Tes-Tape urine glucose determinations.

Availability

See Table 8.18.

Dosage and Administration

See Table 8.18.

Nursing Interventions

See also General Nursing Considerations for the Patient Experiencing Pain.

PATIENT CONCERNS: NURSING INTERVENTION/RATIONALE

Side Effects to Expect

Gastric Irritation

If gastric irritation occurs, administer medication with food, milk, antacids (1 hour later), or large amounts of water. If symptoms persist or increase in severity, report for physician evaluation. Aspirin is available in enteric-coated form to reduce gastric irritation.

Side Effects to Report

Gastrointestinal Bleeding

Observe for the development of dark tarry stools and bright red or "coffee-ground" emesis.

Test any suspicious stools or emesis for presence of occult blood.

Salicylism

Patients who develop signs of salicylate toxicity should be reevaluated for other underlying disease and the possibility that other medication would be more effective.

Drug Interactions

Sulfinpyrazone, Probenecid

Salicylates inhibit the excretion of uric acid by these agents. Although an occasional aspirin will not be sufficient to interfere with the effectiveness of these agents, regular use of salicylates or products containing salicylate should be discouraged. If analgesia is required, suggest acetaminophen.

Warfarin

The salicylates may enhance the anticoagulant effects of warfarin. Observe for the development of petechiae, ecchymoses, nosebleeds, bleeding gums, dark tarry stools, and bright red or "coffee-ground" emesis. Monitor the prothrombin time and reduce the dosage of warfarin if necessary.

Phenytoin

Monitor patients with concurrent therapy for signs of phenytoin toxicity: nystagmus, sedation, lethargy. Serum levels may be ordered, and a reduced dosage of phenytoin may be required.

Oral Hypoglycemic Agents

The salicylates may enhance the hypoglycemic effects of these agents. Monitor for hypoglycemia: headache, weakness, decreased coordination, general apprehension, diaphoresis, hunger, blurred or double vision.

The dosage of the hypoglycemic agent may need to be reduced. Notify the physician if any of the above symptoms appear.

Methotrexate

Monitor for methotrexate toxicity: bone marrow suppression, decreased WBCs, RBCs, sore throat, fever, lethargy.

Corticosteroids

Although frequently used together, salicylates and corticosteroids may produce gastrointestinal ulceration. Monitor for signs of gastrointestinal bleeding: observe

Table 8.18
Nonsteroidal Antiinflammatory Agents

GENERIC NAME	BRAND NAME	AVAILABILITY	USES AND DOSAGES	MAXIMUM DAILY DOSE (MG)
1. SALICYLATES				
Aspirin	Ecotrin, Zorprin, A.S.A., Bayer, Empirin	Tablets: 65, 81, 325, 487.5, 650 mg Capsules: 325, 500 mg Suppositories: 60, 130, 195, 300, 325, 600, 625, 1200 mg	Minor aches and pains: 325–600 mg every 4 hours Arthritis: 2.6–5.2 g/day in divided doses Acute rheumatic fever: 7.8 g/day	—
Choline Salicylate	Arthropan	Liquid: 870 mg/5 ml	Mild pain: 870 mg every 3–4 hours (fewer GI side effects)	7000
Diflunisal	Dolobid	Tablets: 250, 500 mg	Mild to moderate pain: Initially, 1000 mg, then 500 mg every 8 hours Osteoarthritis: 250–500 mg 2 times daily	1500
Magnesium Salicylate	Magan, Efficin, Mobidin	Tablets: 325, 480, 500, 545, 600, 650 mg	Mild aches and pains: 500–650 mg 3 or 4 times daily	9600
Salicylamide	Uromide, Salicylamide	Tablets: 325, 667 mg	Minor aches and pains: 325–667 mg 3 or 4 times daily (less effective than equal doses of aspirin)	4000
Salsalate	Disalcid Arthra-G	Tablets: 500, 750 mg Capsules: 500 mg	Mild pain: 500–750 mg 4–6 times daily	3000
Sodium Salicylate	Uracel 5, Sodium Salicylate	Tablets: 325, 650 mg Enteric-coated tablets: 325, 650 mg	Mild analgesia: 325–650 mg every 4–8 hours (less effective than equal doses of aspirin)	3900
Sodium Thiosalicylate	Arthrolate, Nalate, Thiosol	Inj: 50 mg/ml in 2, 20 and 30 ml vials	Acute gout: IM: 100 mg every 3–4 hours for 2 days, then 100 mg/day Rheumatic fever: IM: 100–150 mg every 4–6 hours for 3 days, then 100 mg twice daily	—
2. NONSALICYLATE ANTIINFLAMMATORY AGENTS				
Fenoprofen	Nalfon	Capsules: 200, 300 mg	Rheumatoid and osteoarthritis: 300–600 mg 3 or 4 times daily Mild to moderate pain: 200 mg every 4–6 hours	3200
Ibuprofen	Motrin Rufen	Tablets: 300, 400, 600 mg	Rheumatoid and osteoarthritis: 300–600 mg 3–4 times daily Mild to moderate pain: 400 mg every 4–6 hours Primary dysmenorrhea: 400 mg every 4 hours	2400
Indomethacin	Indocin	Capsules: 25, 50 mg Sustained release capsules: 75 mg	Rheumatoid and osteoarthritis, ankylosing spondylitis: 25–50 mg 3–4 times daily Acute painful shoulder: 25–50 mg 2–3 times daily Acute gouty arthritis: 50 mg 3 times daily	200
Meclofenamate	Meclomen	Capsules: 50, 100 mg	Rheumatoid and osteoarthritis: 200–400 mg daily in 3–4 equal doses	400
Mefenamic Acid	Ponstel	Capsules: 250 mg	Moderate pain or primary dysmenorrhea: Initially 500 mg, then 250 mg every 6 hours	1000
Naproxen	Naproxyn	Tablets: 250, 375, 500 mg	Rheumatoid and osteoarthritis, ankylosing spondylitis: 250–375 mg 2 times daily Acute gout: 750–825 mg initially, followed by 250–275 mg every 8 hours	1000
Naproxen Sodium	Anaprox	Tablets: 275 mg		1100

Table 8.18 (continued)

GENERIC NAME	BRAND NAME	AVAILABILITY	USES AND DOSAGES	MAXIMUM DAILY DOSE (MG)
Phenylbutazone	Butazolidin Azolid	Tablets: 100 mg Capsules: 100 mg	Moderate pain, primary dysmenorrhea, acute tendonitis, bursitis: 500–550 mg followed by 250–275 mg. Rheumatoid and osteoarthritis, ankylosing spondylitis: 100 mg 4 times daily. Acute gout: 400 mg initially, followed by 100 mg every 4 hours	600
Piroxicam	Feldene	Capsules: 10, 20 mg	Rheumatoid and osteoarthritis: 20 mg 1 time daily	20
Sulindac	Clinoril	Tablets: 150–200 mg	Rheumatoid and osteoarthritis, ankylosing spondylitis: 150 mg 2 times daily. Acute painful shoulder: 200 mg 2 times daily	400
Tolmetin	Tolectin	Tablets: 200 mg Capsules: 400 mg	Rheumatoid and osteoarthritis: 400–600 mg 3 times daily	2000
Zomepirac	Zomax	Tablets: 100 mg	Mild to moderately severe: 100 mg every 4–6 hours	600

for the development of dark tarry stools and bright red or "coffee-ground" emesis.

Ethanol

Patients should avoid aspirin within 8 to 10 hours of heavy alcohol use. Small amounts of gastrointestinal bleeding often occur. If aspirin therapy is absolutely necessary, an enteric-coated product should be used.

Clinitest

This drug may produce false-positive Clinitest results. Blood glucose measurements may be required for an accurate reading.

Nonsalicylate Antiinflammatory Agents

The nonsteroidal antiinflammatory drugs (NSAIDs) are also known as "aspirin-like" drugs. They are chemically unrelated to the salicylates but are prostaglandin inhibitors and share many of the same therapeutic actions and side effects. They all have, to varying degrees, analgesic, antipyretic, and antiinflammatory activity. The antipyretic activity is low enough that they are not used clinically for the control of fever. In clinical studies, all these agents (see Table 8.18) are superior to placebos, and approach aspirin in effectiveness, but none is superior to aspirin. Depending on the agent used, the dosage, and the patient, the side effects of therapy tend to be somewhat less than those associated with salicylate therapy. The cost of therapy with NSAIDs is considerably higher than with aspirin treatment. Thus these agents are most effectively used as alternates for patients who do not tolerate aspirin. These agents are used to relieve the pain and inflammation of rheumatoid arthritis, osteoarthritis, ankylosing spondylitis, and gout. Certain agents are also approved for use to control the discomfort of primary dysmenorrhea. See Table 8.18.

Side Effects

The most frequent adverse effects associated with NSAID therapy are gastrointestinal complaints. Symptoms include nausea, abdominal pain, diarrhea, indigestion, constipation, and flatulence. The development of ulcers and gastrointestinal bleeding has been reported with all these agents.

Dizziness, lethargy, and headache may occur in up to 10% of patients taking these agents.

Other adverse effects that have been attributed to these agents include tinnitus, drowsiness, mental confusion, vision disturbances, and various rashes.

Many other side effects may be caused rarely by these agents. They include blood dyscrasias, such as anemia, thrombocytopenia, and agranulocytosis; various dermatoses, such as urticaria, purpura, pruritus, and rashes; and hepatotoxicity and renal toxicity. Therapy should be discontinued if these complications develop.

Availability

See Table 8.18.

Dosage and Administration

Note: Do not administer to patients who are allergic to aspirin. See Table 8.18.

Nursing Interventions

See also General Nursing Considerations for the Patient Experiencing Pain.

PATIENT CONCERNS: NURSING INTERVENTION/RATIONALE

Side Effects to Expect

Gastric Irritation

If gastric irritation occurs, administer medication with food, milk, antacids, or large amounts of water. If symptoms persist or increase in severity, report for physician evaluation.

Constipation

The use of stool softeners or bulk-forming laxatives may be necessary. Maintain the patient's state of hydration. Encourage the inclusion of sufficient roughage, fresh fruits, vegetables, and whole-grain products in the diet.

Dizziness

Provide for patient safety during episodes of dizziness.

Drowsiness

Persons who are working around machinery, driving a car, or performing other duties in which they must remain mentally alert should not take these medications while working.

Side Effects to Report

Gastrointestinal Bleeding

Observe for the development of dark tarry stools and bright red or "coffee-ground" emesis.

Confusion

Perform a baseline assessment of the patient's degree of alertness and orientation to name, place, and time *prior* to initiating therapy. Make regularly scheduled subsequent evaluations of mental status and compare findings. Report development of alterations.

Hives, Pruritus, Rash

Report symptoms for further evaluation by the physician.

Nephrotoxicity

Monitor urinalysis and kidney function tests for abnormal results. Report an increasing BUN and creatinine, decreasing urine output and/or decreasing specific gravity (despite amount of fluid intake), casts or protein in the urine, frank blood or smoky-colored urine, or RBCs in excess of 0 to 3 on the urinalysis report.

Hepatotoxicity

The symptoms of hepatotoxicity are anorexia, nausea, vomiting, jaundice, hepatomegaly, splenomegaly, and abnormal liver function tests (elevated bilirubin, SGOT, SGPT, alkaline phosphatase, prothrombin time).

Blood Dyscrasias

Routine laboratory studies (RBC, WBC, and differential counts) should be scheduled.

Monitor for the development of sore throat, fever, purpura, jaundice, or excessive and progressive weakness.

Drug Interactions

Warfarin

The NSAIDs may enhance the anticoagulant effects of warfarin. Observe for the development of petechiae, ecchymoses, nosebleeds, bleeding gums, dark tarry stools and bright red or "coffee-ground" emesis. Monitor the prothrombin time and reduce the dosage of warfarin if necessary.

Phenytoin

Monitor patients with concurrent therapy for signs of phenytoin toxicity: nystagmus, sedation, lethargy. Serum levels may be ordered, and a reduced dosage of phenytoin may be required.

Miscellaneous Analgesics

Acetaminophen (a-seet-a-min′o-fen) **Tylenol** (ty′le-nol), **Datril** (day′tril), **Tempra** (tem′prah′)

Acetaminophen is a synthetic nonopiate analgesic used in the treatment of mild to moderate pain. Its antipyretic effectiveness and analgesic potency are similar to that of aspirin in equal doses. This drug has no antiinflammatory activity and is therefore ineffective (other than as an analgesic) in the relief of symptoms of rheumatoid arthritis or other inflammation.

It is an effective analgesic-antipyretic for fever and discomfort associated with bacterial and viral infections, headache, and conditions involving musculoskeletal pain. It is a good substitute for patients who cannot take products containing aspirin because of allergic reactions, hypersensitivities, anticoagulant therapy, or possible bleeding problems from gastric or duodenal ulcers, gastritis, and hiatus hernia.

Side Effects

When used as directed, acetaminophen is essentially free of side effects.

During the past decade, acetaminophen has often been recommended as the drug of choice for the relief of mild pain and fever. Its acquisition does not require a prescription, and its use has climbed steadily. Unfortunately, overdosage due to acute and chronic ingestion has risen dramatically in the last few years. Severe, life-threatening hepatotoxicity has been reported in patients who either ingest 5 to 8 g daily for several weeks or attempt suicide by consuming large quantities at one time.

Early indications of toxicity include anorexia, nausea, and vomiting—symptoms often attributed to other causes. A few days later, the patient develops jaundice, and the SGOT and SGPT levels and prothrombin time rise dramatically. If acetaminophen toxicity is suspected, consult the manufacturer, a university drug information center, or a poison-control center for the most current recommendations for therapy.

Blood dyscrasias are rare side effects that may occur from prolonged administration of large doses.

Availability

PO—80, 325, 500, and 650 mg tablets; 500 mg capsules; 120 mg/5 ml, 160 mg/5 ml, 325 mg/5ml elixir; 100 mg/ml, 120 mg/2.5 ml solution; 165 mg/5ml liquid. Rectal—120, 125, 325, 650 mg suppositories.

Dosage and Administration

Adult
PO—300 to 650 mg every 4 hours. Doses up to 100 mg may be given 4 times daily for short-term therapy. Do not exceed 2.6 g daily.
Pediatric
PO—Doses may be repeated 4 or 5 times daily, not to exceed 5 doses in 24 hours.

0–3 months: 40 mg
4–11 months: 80 mg
12–24 months: 120 mg
2–3 years: 160 mg
4–5 years: 240 mg
6–8 years: 320 mg
9–10 years: 400 mg
11–12 years: 480 mg
Rectal—as for oral doses.

Drug Interactions

There are no clinically significant drug interactions reported involving acetaminophen.

Nursing Interventions

See also General Nursing Considerations for the Patient Experiencing Pain.

Propoxyphene (pro-poxs'ee-feen) *(Darvon)* (dar'von)

Propoxyphene is an effective, well-tolerated, synthetic nonopiate analgesic similar to aspirin in potency and duration of analgesic effect. It is used for the relief of mild to moderate pain associated with muscular spasms, premenstrual cramps, bursitis, minor surgery and trauma, headache, and labor and delivery. Greater pain relief may be attained when used in combination with aspirin or acetaminophen.

Side Effects

Side effects of propoxyphene include gastrointestinal disturbance, headache, dizziness, somnolence, and skin rashes. Tolerance and addiction have been reported.

Symptoms of acute overdose are coma, respiratory depression, pulmonary edema, and seizures. Symptoms of propoxyphene overdose may be complicated by salicylism, which may also develop as a result of an overdose of combination products containing both propoxyphene and aspirin.

Availability

PO—32 and 65 mg capsules, 100 mg tablets, and 10 mg/ml suspension. (The 65 mg capsules and the 100 mg tablets are equal in analgesic potency.)

Dosage and Administration

Adult
PO—65 mg (capsules) or 100 mg (tablets) every 4 hours as needed. Do not exceed 390 mg (capsules) or 600 mg (tablets) daily.

Antidote

Naloxone.

Nursing Interventions

See also General Nursing Considerations for the Patient Experiencing Pain.

PATIENT CONCERNS: NURSING INTERVENTION/RATIONALE

Side Effects to Expect

Gastric Irritation

If gastric irritation occurs, administer medication with food or milk. If symptoms persist or increase in severity, report for physician evaluation.

Sedation

This side effect is usually mild and tends to resolve with continued therapy.

Dizziness

Provide for patient safety during episodes of dizziness.

Side Effects to Report

Excessive Use or Abuse

Assist the patient to recognize the abuse problem.

Identify underlying needs and plan for more appropriate management of those needs.

Discuss the case with the physician and make plans to cooperatively approach gradual withdrawal of the medications being abused.

Provide for emotional support of the individual; display an accepting attitude—be kind but firm.

Skin Rashes

Report for further evaluation.

Dosage and Administration

PO

If gastric irritation occurs, administer medication with food or milk.

Drug Interactions

Orphenadrine

Combined use with propoxyphene is not recommended. Cases of mental confusion, anxiety, and tremors have been reported.

Cerebrospinal Stimulant

Caffeine (ka-feen') *NoDoz, Vivarin*

Caffeine may be one of the most frequently used drugs in the world because it is a natural ingredient in coffee, tea, cocoa, and cola beverages. The average cup of coffee contains 100 to 150 mg per cup, depending on the strength of the brew. Caffeine has several pharmacologic actions. It stimulates the central nervous system; the respiratory center, causing more rapid, deeper respirations; the heart, bringing about an increase in both cardiac rate and cardiac output; the secretion of hydrochloric acid in the stomach; and it has weak diuretic activity. With chronic ingestion, tolerance to the cardiovascular, CNS, and diuretic effects develop. Caffeine is sold as an aid in staying awake and for restoring mental alertness.

Side Effects

The adverse effects of caffeine are extensions of the pharmacologic effects of the drug. Overdose can cause nervousness, tremulousness (caffeine jitters), insomnia, heart palpitations, headache, nausea, stomach pains, and minor dehydration due to the diuretic effects.

Caffeine has minor "addictive" properties. Persons who regularly consume over 500 to 600 mg daily may develop headache, anxiety, and muscle tension about 18 hours after the last ingestion if consumption is suddenly stopped. A conscientious effort to gradually reduce the daily intake of caffeine will reduce these symptoms.

Availability

PO—65, 100, 150, and 200 mg tablets.

Dosage and Administration

Adult

PO—100 to 200 mg every 4 hours, as needed.

Chapter 9

The Autonomic Nervous System

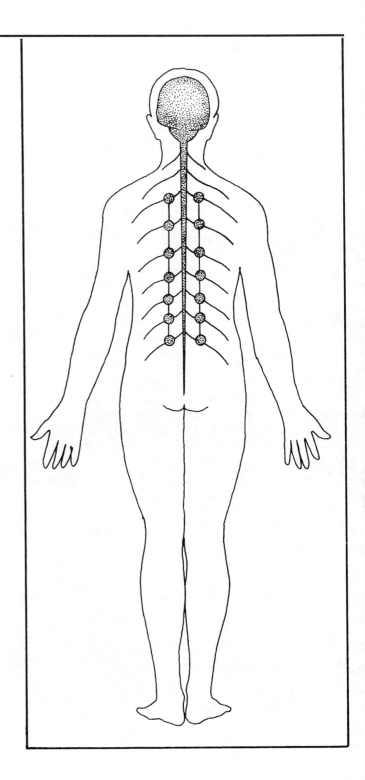

Objectives

After completing this chapter, the student should be able to do the following:

1. Explain the functions of the sympathetic and the parasympathetic nervous systems.
2. Identify the main actions (effects) of the adrenergic, cholinergic, antiadrenergic, and anticholinergic agents.
3. Describe patient data collection as it relates to each group of agents studied.
4. State important aspects of patient teaching associated with each drug classification group studied.

General Nursing Considerations for Patients Receiving Autonomic Agents

See also General Nursing Considerations for Patients with Cardiovascular Disease; General Nursing Considerations for Patients with Disorders of the Eyes; General Nursing Considerations for Patients with Disorders of the Urinary System Disease; General Nursing Considerations for Patients with Respiratory Disease.

The Autonomic Nervous System

The brain and the spinal cord make up the central nervous system. Nerves that leave the central nervous system to conduct signals to other parts of the body (efferent nerves) and nerves that transmit signals from other parts of the body to the brain and spinal cord (afferent nerves) make up the *peripheral nervous system*. The peripheral nervous system further subdivides into the *motor nervous system* and the *autonomic nervous system*. The autonomic nervous system is an efferent motor system which means that it relays information from the central nervous system to the rest of the body.

The autonomic nervous system controls the function of all tissues with the exception of striated muscle. This nervous system helps control blood pressure, gastrointestinal motility and secretion, urinary bladder function, sweating, and body temperature; in general it maintains a constant, internal environment (homeostasis) and responds to emergency situations. The word *autonomic* means "self-governing" or "automatic"; thus the autonomic nervous system has also been called the *involuntary* nervous system because we have little or no control over it. The *motor* nervous system controls skeletal muscle, and we can exercise control over much of it.

Studies have shown that the transmission of nerve impulses occurs because of the activity of chemical substances called *neurotransmitters* ("transmitters of nerve impulses"). A neurotransmitter is liberated at the end of one neuron, activating the next neuron in the chain, or at the end of the nerve chain, stimulating the "end organ" (the heart, smooth muscle, or gland). The two

major neurotransmitters are *norepinephrine* and *acetylcholine*. The nerve endings that liberate acetylcholine are called *cholinergic* fibers, the ones that secrete norepinephrine are called *adrenergic* fibers. Most organs are innervated by both adrenergic and cholinergic fibers, but they produce opposite responses. Examples of these opposing actions are in the heart, where adrenergic agents increase the heart rate and cholinergic agents slow the heart rate, and in the eyes, where adrenergic agents cause pupillary dilation and cholinergic agents cause pupillary constriction.

Drugs that cause effects in the body similar to those produced by acetylcholine are called *cholinergic* drugs because they mimic the action produced by stimulation of the parasympathetic division of the autonomic nervous system. Drugs that cause effects similar to those produced by the adrenergic neurotransmitter are called *adrenergic*, or sympathomimetic, drugs. Agents that block or inhibit cholinergic activity are called *anticholinergic agents*, and agents that inhibit the adrenergic system are referred to as *adrenergic blocking agents*. See Fig. 9.1 for a diagram of the autonomic system and representative stimulants and inhibitors.

Adrenergic Agents

The adrenergic nervous system may be stimulated by two broad classes of drugs: catecholamines and noncatecholamines. The naturally occurring catecholamines that are neurotransmitters in the human body are norepinephrine, epinephrine, and dopamine. Norepinephrine is secreted primarily from nerve terminals, epinephrine primarily from the adrenal medulla, and dopamine at selected sites within the brain, kidneys, and gastrointestinal tract. All three agents are synthetically manufactured and may be administered to produce the same effects as naturally secreted neurotransmitters. The noncatecholamines (see Table 9.1) have somewhat similar actions as the catecholamines but are more selective for certain types of receptors, are not quite as fast acting, and have a longer duration of action.

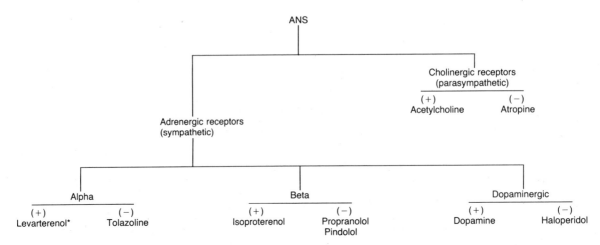

Fig. 9.1. The autonomic nervous system. (+) stimulates receptors; (−) inhibits receptors; asterisks indicate representative examples only.

As illustrated in Fig. 9.1, the autonomic nervous system can be subdivided into the alpha, beta, and dopaminergic receptors. These are specific types of receptors that, when stimulated by chemicals of certain shapes, produce a very specific action on that tissue. In general, stimulation of alpha receptors causes vasoconstriction of blood vessels; stimulation of beta receptors causes relaxation of smooth muscles in the bronchi, uterus, and gastrointestinal tract and stimulation of the heart rate. Stimulation of the dopaminergic receptors improves the symptoms associated with Parkinson's disease; increases urine output; and increases the force of contraction of the heart, making it a more effective pump. As noted in Table 9.1, many drugs act on more than one type of adrenergic receptor. Fortunately each agent acts to varying degrees, allowing a certain agent to be used for a specific purpose without many adverse effects. If recommended dosages are exceeded, however, certain receptors may be stimulated excessively, causing serious adverse effects. An example of this could be illustrated with terbutaline, which is primarily a beta stimulant. With normal doses, ter-

Table 9.1
Adrenergic Agents

GENERIC NAME	BRAND NAME	AVAILABILITY	ADRENERGIC RECEPTOR	ACTION	CLINICAL USE
Albuterol*	Proventil	Aerosol: 90 mcg per puff Tablets: 2, 4 mg	beta	bronchodilator	asthma, emphysema
Dopamine	Intropin	IV: 40, 80, 160 mg/ml in 5 ml ampules	alpha, beta, dopaminergic	vasopressor	shock, hypotension, inotropic agent
Dobutamine	Dobutrex	IV: 250 mg/20 ml vials	beta	cardiac stimulant	inotropic agent
Ephedrine*	Ephedrine	SC, IM, IV: 25, 50 mg/ ml in 1 ml ampules	alpha, beta	bronchodilator, vasoconstrictor	nasal decongestant, hypotension
Epinephrine*	Adrenalin	IV: 1:1000 in 1 and 2 ml ampules: 1:10,000 in 10 ml vials	alpha, beta	allergic reactions, vasoconstrictor, bronchodilator, cardiac stimulant	anaphylaxis, cardiac arrest, topical vasoconstrictor
Isoetharine*	Bronkosol	Nebulization: 0.125, 0.2, 0.25, 0.5, 1% solution	beta	bronchodilator	inhalation therapy

Table 9.1 (*continued*)

GENERIC NAME	BRAND NAME	AVAILABILITY	ADRENERGIC RECEPTOR	ACTION	CLINICAL USE
Isoproterenol	Isuprel	SC, IM, IV: 1:5000 solution, 1, 5, 10 ml vials Nebulization: 0.25, 0.5, 1% solution Aerosol: 0.2, 0.25% solution Sublingual tablets: 10, 15 mg	beta	bronchodilator, cardiac stimulant	shock, digitalis toxicity
Metaraminol	Aramine	SC, IM, IV: 10 mg/ml in 10 ml vials	alpha	vasoconstrictor	shock, hypotension
Norepinephrine (levarterenol)	Levophed	IV: 1 mg/ml in 4 ml ampules	alpha	vasoconstrictor	shock, hypotension
Phenylephrine†	NeoSynephrine	SC, IM, IV: 1% in 1 ml ampules Ophthalmic drops: 0.08, 0.12, 2.5, 10%	alpha	vasoconstrictor	shock, hypotension, nasal decongestant, ophthalmic vasoconstrictor, mydriatic
Phenylpropa-nolamine†		Tablets: 25, 50 mg Elixir: 20 mg/ 5 ml Syrup: 12.5 mg/5 ml	alpha	vasoconstrictor	nasal decongestant, anorectic
Terbutaline*	Brethine, Bricanyl	Tablets: 2.5, 5 mg SC: 1 mg/ml in 1 ml ampules	beta	bronchodilator, uterine relaxant	emphysema, asthma, premature labor

* See also Bronchodilators.
† See also Decongestants.

butaline is an effective bronchodilator. In addition to bronchodilation, terbutaline in higher doses causes central nervous system stimulation, resulting in insomnia and wakefulness. See Table 9.1 for clinical uses of the adrenergic agents.

Side Effects

Side effects associated with the use of adrenergic agents are usually dosage related and resolve when the dosage is reduced or discontinued. Palpitations, tachycardia, tremors, dizziness, and flushing of the skin are relatively common side effects when adrenergic agents are administered systemically. More serious adverse effects include arrythmias, hypotension, severe hypertension, anginal pain, nausea, vomiting, and weakness. Reduce or discontinue therapy if these symptoms develop.

Patients who are potentially more sensitive to adrenergic agents are those with impaired hepatic function, thyroid disease, hypertension, and heart disease. Patients with diabetes mellitus may also have increased frequency of episodes of hyperglycemia.

Availability

See Table 9.1.

Nursing Interventions

See also General Nursing Considerations for Patients with Respiratory Tract Disease; Nursing Interventions for Bronchodilators; Nursing Interventions for Decongestants.

PATIENT CONCERNS: NURSING INTERVENTION/RATIONALE

Side Effects to Expect

Palpitations, Tachycardia, Skin Flushing, Tremors

These side effects are usually mild and tend to resolve with continued therapy. Encourage the patient not to discontinue therapy without first consulting the physician.

Orthostatic Hypotension

Although infrequent and generally mild, adrenergic agents may cause some degree of orthostatic hypotension manifested by dizziness and weakness, particularly when therapy is being initiated.

Monitor the blood pressure daily in both the supine and standing positions.

Anticipate the development of postural hypotension and take measures to prevent an occurrence. Teach the patient to rise slowly from a supine or sitting position; encourage the patient to sit or lie down if feeling "faint."

Side Effects to Report

Arrhythmias, Chest Pain, Severe Hypotension, Hypertension, Nausea, and Vomiting

Discontinue therapy immediately and notify the physician.

Dosage and Administration

See manufacturer's literature for each agent.

Drug Interactions

Agents That May Increase Therapeutic and Toxic Effects

Monoamine oxidase inhibitors (isocarboxazid, pargyline, tranylcypromine); tricyclic antidepressants (ami-triptyline, imipramine, others); guanethidine, atropine, and cyclopropane or halothane anesthesia.

Monitor patients for tachycardia, serious arrhythmias, hypotension, hypertension, chest pain.

Agents That Inhibit Therapeutic Activity

Beta adrenergic blocking agents (propranolol, nadolol, timolol, pindolol, atenolol, metoprolol); alpha adrenergic blocking agents (phenoxybenzamine, phentolamine, tolazoline); guanethidine, reserpine, bretylium tosylate.

Concurrent use of these agents with adrenergic agents is not recommended.

Adrenergic Blocking Agents

Alpha Adrenergic Blocking Agents

The alpha adrenergic blocking agents act by plugging the alpha receptors, which prevents other agents, usually the naturally occurring catecholamines, from stimulating the alpha receptors. Since a primary action of the alpha receptor stimulants is vasoconstriction, we would expect that alpha blocking agents would be indicated in patients with diseases associated with vasoconstriction. Indeed, phenoxybenzamine and tolazoline are used as vasodilators in peripheral vascular diseases such as Raynaud's phenomena and Buerger's disease. (See Chapter 10, Cardiovascular Agents, for the clinical use of these agents.) Phentolamine is used in the diagnosis and treatment of pheochromocytoma, a tumor that secretes epinephrine.

Beta Adrenergic Blocking Agents

The beta adrenergic blocking agents (beta blockers) are used extensively in the treatment of hypertension, angina pectoris, cardiac arrhythmias, symptoms of hyperthyroidism, and "stage fright." Beta blockers act by plugging beta adrenergic receptors so that beta receptor stimulants, usually the naturally occurring norepinephrine and epinephrine cannot make contact with the receptor, thus preventing beta stimulation.

Side Effects

Most of the adverse effects associated with beta adrenergic blocking agents are dosage related. Potential side effects categorized by organ system are as follows:

- Cardiovascular—bradycardia, peripheral vascular insufficiency (Raynaud's phenomena).

- Gastrointestinal—diarrhea, nausea, vomiting, constipation, abdominal discomfort, anorexia, and flatulence.
- Central nervous system—dizziness, insomnia and fatigue. Sedation, hallucinations, changes in behavior and mental depression have been rarely reported.
- Hematologic—agranulocytosis and thrombocytopenic purpura have been reported very rarely.
- Allergic—rash, fever combined with aching and sore throat, laryngospasm, and respiratory distress.
- Other adverse effects—headache, dry mouth, eyes or skin; impotence or decreased libido, nasal stuffiness, sweating, tinnitus, and blurred vision.

Beta blockers must be used with extreme caution in patients with respiratory conditions such as bronchitis, emphysema, asthma, or allergic rhinitis. Beta blockage will produce severe bronchoconstriction and may aggravate wheezing, especially during the pollen season.

Use beta blockers with caution in diabetic patients and patients susceptible to hypoglycemia. The beta blockers will induce further hypoglycemic effects of insulin and will reduce the release of insulin in response to hyperglycemia. All beta blockers will mask most of the signs and symptoms of acute hypoglycemia.

Beta adrenergic blocking agents should be used in patients with controlled congestive heart failure. Further hypotension, bradycardia, and/or congestive heart failure may develop.

Availability

See Table 9.2.

Dosage and Administration

See Table 9.2.

There is great interpatient variation in response to given dosages of the beta blockers. Dosages must be individualized according to the pathologic condition being treated and the response of the patient.

It is extremely important that beta blocker therapy not be discontinued abruptly, especially in patients who are being treated for angina pectoris. Sudden discontinuation may result in an increased frequency of angina and possibly a myocardial infarction.

Nursing Interventions

See also General Nursing Considerations for Patients with Antiarrhythmic Therapy; General Nursing Considerations for Patients with Hypertension.

**PATIENT CONCERNS:
NURSING INTERVENTION/RATIONALE**

Side Effects to Expect or Report

See introductory text above for adverse effects associated with specific organ systems.

Response by individual patients is highly variable. Many of these side effects may occur but may be tran-

Table 9.2
Beta Adrenergic Blocking Agents

GENERIC NAME	BRAND NAME	AVAILABILITY	CLINICAL USES	DOSAGE RANGE
Atenolol	Tenormin	Tablets: 50, 100 mg	Hypertension	PO: Initial—50 mg daily Maintenance—Up to 100 mg daily
Metoprolol	Lopressor	Tablets: 50, 100 mg	Hypertension	PO: Initial—100 mg daily Maintenance—100–450 mg daily
Nadolol	Corgard	Tablets: 40, 80, 120, 160 mg	Angina pectoris, hypertension	PO: Initial—40 mg once daily Maintenance—80–320 mg daily Maximum—640 mg/day
Pindolol	Visken	Tablets: 5, 10 mg	Hypertension	PO: Initial—10 mg twice daily Maximum—60 mg/day
Propranolol	Inderal	Tablets: 10, 20, 40, 60, 80, 90 mg Capsules: 80, 120, 160 mg IV: 1 mg/ml in 1 ml capsules	Arrhythmias, hypertension, angina pectoris, myocardial infarction, migraine	PO: Initial—40 mg 2 times daily Maintenance—120–640 mg daily IV: 1–3 mg under very close ECG monitoring
Timolol	Blocadren	Tablets: 5, 10, 20 mg	Hypertension, myocardial infarction	PO: Initial—10 mg twice daily Maintenance—Up to 30 mg twice daily

sient. Stongly encourage patients to see their physician before discontinuing therapy. Minor dosage adjustment may be all that is required for most side effects.

Bronchospasm, Wheezing

Withhold additional doses until the patient has been evaluated by a physician.

Diabetic Patients

Monitor for hypoglycemia: headache, weakness, decreased coordination, general apprehension, diaphoresis, hunger, or blurred or double vision. Many of these symptoms may be masked by the beta adrenergic blocking agents. Notify the physician if you suspect that any of the above symptoms are appearing intermittently.

Congestive Heart Failure

Monitor patients for an increase in edema, dyspnea, rales, bradycardia, and orthopnea. Notify the physician if these symptoms are developing.

Dosage and Administration

Individualization of Dosage

Although the onset of activity is fairly rapid, it may often take several days to weeks for a patient to show optimal improvement and become stabilized on an adequate maintenance dosage. Patients must be periodically reevaluated to determine the lowest effective dosage necessary to control the disorder being treated.

Sudden Discontinuation

Sudden discontinuation of therapy has resulted in an exacerbation of anginal symptoms followed in some cases by myocardial infarction. When discontinuing chronically administered beta blockers, the dosage should be gradually reduced over a period of 1 to 2 weeks with careful monitoring of the patient. If anginal symptoms develop or become more frequent, beta blocker therapy should at least temporarily be restarted.

Compliance

Patients must be counseled against poor compliance or sudden discontinuation of therapy without a physician's advice.

Drug Interactions

Antihypertensive Agents

All the beta blocking agents have hypotensive properties that are additive with antihypertensive agents (guanethidine, methyldopa, hydralazine, clonidine, prazosin, minoxidil, captopril, saralasin and reserpine).

If it is decided to discontinue therapy in patients receiving beta blockers and clonidine concurrently, the beta blocker should be withdrawn gradually and discontinued several days before the gradual withdrawal of the clonidine.

Beta Adrenergic Agents

Depending on the dosages used, the beta stimulants (isoproterenol, metaproterenol, terbutaline, albuterol, and ritodrine) may inhibit the action of the beta blocking agents, and vice versa.

Lidocaine, Procainamide, Phenytoin, Disopyramide

Although these drugs are occasionally used concurrently, monitor patients very carefully for additional arrhythmias, bradycardia, and signs of congestive heart failure.

Enzyme-inducing Agents

Enzyme-inducing agents such as (cimetidine, phenobarbital, Nembutal, and phenytoin) enhance the metabolism of propranolol, metoprolol, pindolol, and timolol. This reaction probably does not occur with nadolol or atenolol since they are not metabolized, but excreted unchanged. The dosage of the beta blocker may have to be increased to provide therapeutic activity. If the enzyme-inducing agent is discontinued, the dosage of the beta blocking agent will also require reduction.

Indomethacin

Indomethacin and possibly other prostaglandin inhibitors inhibit the antihypertensive activity of propranolol and pindolol, resulting in loss of hypertensive control.

The dosage of the beta blocker may need to be increased to compensate for the antihypertensive inhibitory effect of indomethacin and perhaps other prostaglandin inhibitors.

Cholinergic Agents

Cholinergic agents, also known as parasympathomimetics, produce effects that are similar to those of acetylcholine. Some cholinergic agents act by directly stimulating the parasympathetic nervous system, whereas other agents act by inhibiting *acetylcholinesterase*, the enzyme that metabolizes acetylcholine once it is released by the nerve ending. These latter agents are known as *indirect-acting cholinergic agents*. Some of the cholinergic actions observed are the following: slowing of the heart, increased gastrointestinal motility and secretions, increased contractions of the urinary bladder with relaxation of muscle sphincter, increased secretions and contractility of bronchial smooth muscle, sweating, miosis of the eye reducing intraocular pressure, increased force of contraction of skeletal muscle, and sometimes a rise in blood pressure. See Table 9.3.

Side Effects

Since cholinergic fibers innervate the entire body, we can expect to see effects in most systems of the body. Fortunately all receptors do not respond to the same dosage, so all adverse effects are not seen at all times. The higher the dosages used, however, the greater the likelihood for more adverse effects. Cholinergic side effects that may be observed are nausea, vomiting, diarrhea, abdominal cramping, increased bronchial secretions, bradycardia, sweating, and possible hypotension.

Availability

See Table 9.3.

Nursing Interventions

See also General Nursing Considerations for Patients with Disorders of the Eyes; General Nursing Considerations for Patients with Glaucoma; General Nursing Considerations for Patients with Urinary System Disease; General Nursing Considerations for Patients with Respiratory Tract Disease.

PATIENT CONCERNS:
NURSING INTERVENTION/RATIONALE

Side Effects to Expect

Flushing of the Skin, Headache

A pharmacological property of cholinergic agents that arises from vasodilation of blood vessels.

Side Effects to Expect and Report

Nausea, Vomiting, Diarrhea, Abdominal Cramping

A pharmacological property of cholinergic agents. Encourage the patient not to discontinue the medication without seeing a physician. A dosage adjustment may control these adverse effects.

Table 9.3
Cholinergic Agents

GENERIC NAME	BRAND NAME	AVAILABILITY	CLINICAL USE
Ambenonium	Mytelase	Tablets: 10 mg	Treatment of myasthenia gravis
Bethanechol	Urecholine		See Chapter 14, *Drugs Affecting the Urinary System*
Edrophonium	Tensilon	Inj: 10 mg/ml in 1 and 10 ml vials	Diagnosis of myasthenia gravis Reverse nondepolarizing muscle relaxants such as tubocurarine
Neostigmine	Prostigmine	Tablets: 15 mg Inj: 1:1000, 1:2000, 1:4000	Treatment of myasthenia gravis Reverse nondepolarizing muscle relaxants such as tubocurarine
Physostigmine	Mestinon Regonol	Tablets: 60 mg Syrup: 60 mg/5 ml Inj: 5 mg/ml in 2 ml ampules	Reverse toxicity of overdoses of anticholinergic agents (e.g., pesticides, insecticides) Treatment of myasthenia gravis Reverse nondepolarizing muscle relaxants such as tubocurarine
Pilocarpine	Isopto-Carpine, Pilocel, Pilocar, Absorbocarpine		See Chapter 17, *Drugs Affecting the Eye*
Pyridostigmine	Eserine, Isopto-Eserine		See Chapter 17, *Drugs Affecting the Eye*

Bronchospasm, Wheezing, Bradycardia

Withhold the next dose until the patient is evaluated by a physician.

Drug Interactions

Atropine, Antihistamines

Atropine, other anticholinergic agents and most antihistamines antagonize the effects of the cholinergic agents.

Anticholinergic Agents

Anticholinergic agents, also known as cholinergic blocking agents or parasympatholytic agents, block the action of acetylcholine in the parasympathetic nervous system. These drugs act by occupying receptor sites at parasympathetic nerve endings, preventing the action of acetylcholine. The parasympathetic response is reduced depending on the amount of anticholinergic drug blocking the receptors. Inhibition of cholinergic activity (anticholinergic effects) include mydriasis of the pupil with increased intraocular pressure in patients with glaucoma; dry, tenacious secretions of the mouth, nose, throat, and bronchi; decreased secretions and motility of the gastrointestinal tract; increased heart-rate; decreased sweating. The anticholinergic agents are used clinically in gastrointestinal and ophthalmic disorders, bradycardia, Parkinson's disease, and genitourinary disorders; as a preoperative drying agent; and to prevent vagal stimulation from skeletal muscle relaxants or placement of an endotracheal tube. See Table 9.4.

Side Effects

Since cholinergic fibers innervate the entire body, we can expect to see effects from blocking this system throughout most systems in the body. Fortunately all receptors do not respond to the same dosage, so all adverse effects are not seen to the same degree with all cholinergic blocking agents. The higher the dosages, however, the greater the likelihood for more adverse effects. Anticholinergic side effects that may be observed are: dryness and soreness of the mouth and tongue, blurring of vision, mild nausea, and nervousness. Other side effects include constipation, urinary hesitancy or retention, tachycardia, palpitation, mydriasis, muscle cramping, mental dullness, loss of memory, and mild and transient postural hypotension. Psychiatric disturbances such as mental confusion, delusions, night-

mares, euphoria, paranoia, and hallucinations may be indications of overdosage.

All patients should be screened for the presence of closed-angle glaucoma. Anticholinergic agents may precipitate an acute attack of angle-closure glaucoma. Patients with open-angle glaucoma can safely use anticholinergic agents in conjunction with miotic therapy.

Availability

See Table 9.4.

Nursing Interventions

See also General Nursing Considerations for Patients with Parkinson's Disease; General Nursing Considerations for Patients with Disorders of the Eyes; Nursing Interventions for Antihistamines.

**PATIENT CONCERNS:
NURSING INTERVENTION/RATIONALE**

Side Effects to Expect

Blurred Vision, Constipation, Urinary Retention, Dryness of the Mucosa of the Mouth, Nose, and Throat

These symptoms are the anticholinergic effects produced by these agents. Patients taking these medications should be monitored for the development of these side effects.

Dryness of the mucosa may be alleviated by sucking hard candy or ice chips, or by chewing gum.

If patients develop urinary hesitancy, assess for distension of the bladder. Report to the physician for further evaluation.

Give stool softeners as prescribed. Encourage adequate fluid intake and foods to provide sufficient bulk.

Caution the patient that blurred vision may occur and make appropriate suggestions for personal safety of the individual.

Side Effects to Report

*Confusion, Depression,
Nightmares, Hallucinations*

Perform a baseline assessment of the patient's degree of alertness and orientation to name, place, and time *prior* to initiating therapy. Make regularly scheduled

Table 9.4

Anticholinergic Agents

GENERIC NAME	BRAND NAME	AVAILABILITY	CLINICAL USES
Anisotropine	Valpin		See Chapter 13, *Drugs Affecting the Digestive System*
Atropine	Atropine Sulfate	Inj: 0.05, 0.1, 0.3, 0.4, 1.2 mg/ml Tablets: 0.4 mg	Presurgery—reduce salivation and bronchial secretions Treatment of pylorospasm and spastic conditions of the GI tract Treatment of urethral and biliary colic
Belladonna	Belladonna Extract Belladonna Tincture	Tablets: 15 mg Tincture: 30 mg/100 ml	Indigestion, peptic ulcer Dysmenorrhea Nocturnal enuresis Parkinsonism
Clidinium bromide	Quarzan	Capsules: 2.5, 5 mg	Peptic ulcer diseases
Dicyclomine	Bentyl Antispas Dibent	Tablets: 20 mg Capsules: 10, 20 mg Syrup: 10 mg/5 ml Inj: 10 mg/ml	Irritable bowel syndrome Infant colic
Glycopyrrolate	Robinul	Tablets: 1, 2 mg Inj: 0.2 mg/ml	Peptic ulcer disease Presurgery—reduce salivation and bronchial secretions
Isopropamide	Darbid	Tablets: 5 mg	Peptic ulcer disease
Mepenzolate	Cantil	Tablets: 25 mg	Peptic ulcer disease
Methantheline	Banthine	Tablets: 50 mg	Peptic ulcer disease
Oxyphencyclimine	Daricon	Tablets: 10 mg	Peptic ulcer disease
Propantheline	Probanthine, Norpanth	Tablets: 7.5, 15 mg	Peptic ulcer disease
Trihexethyl chloride	Pathilon	Tablets: 25 mg	Peptic ulcer disease

subsequent evaluations of mental status and compare findings. Report development of alterations.

Provide for patient safety during these episodes.

Reduction in the daily dosage may control these adverse effects.

Orthostatic Hypotension

Although the instance is infrequent and generally mild, all anticholinergic agents may cause some degree of orthostatic hypotension manifested by dizziness and weakness, particularly when therapy is being initiated.

Monitor the blood pressure daily in both the supine and standing positions.

Anticipate the development of postural hypotension and take measures to prevent an occurrence. Teach the patient to rise slowly from a supine or sitting position; and encourage the patient to sit or lie down if feeling "faint."

Palpitations, Arrhythmias

Report for further evaluation.

Dosage and Administration

Glaucoma

All patients should be screened for the presence of angle-closure glaucoma *prior* to the initiation of therapy.

Patients with open-angle glaucoma can safely use anticholinergic agents. Monitoring of intraocular pressures should be performed on a regular basis.

PO

Administer medications with food or milk to minimize gastric irritation.

Drug Interactions

Amantadine, Tricyclic Antidepressants, Phenothiazines

These agents may potentiate the anticholinergic side effects. Developing confusion and hallucinations are characteristic of excessive anticholinergic activity.

Chapter 10

Cardiovascular Agents

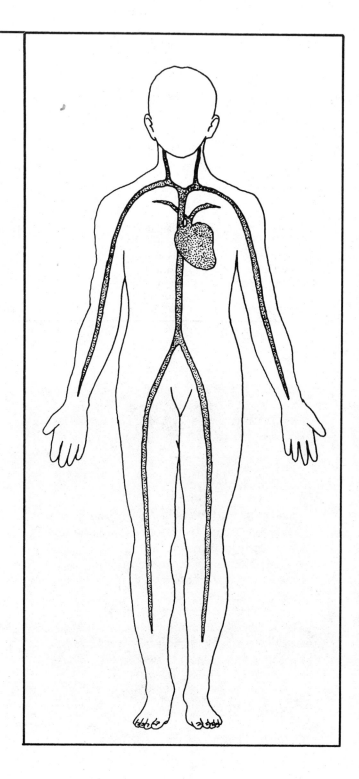

Objectives

After completing this chapter, the student should be able to do the following:

1. Explain the major actions and effects of drugs used to treat cardiovascular disorders.
2. Identify baseline data the nurse should collect on a continuous basis for comparison and evaluation of drug effectiveness.
3. Identify important nursing assessments and interventions associated with drug therapy and treatment of cardiovascular disorders.
4. Identify health teaching essential for a successful treatment regimen.

General Nursing Considerations for Patients with Cardiovascular Disease

The information the nurse assesses relative to the cardinal signs of cardiovascular disease can provide a basis for subsequent evaluation of the patient's response to the therapeutic modalities prescribed. Not all cardiovascular disorders exhibit every symptom.

PATIENT CONCERNS: NURSING INTERVENTION/RATIONALE

Cardinal Signs of Cardiovascular Disease

Dyspnea (Difficulty in Breathing)

If you are unfamiliar with the patient, first determine whether he or she has inhaled a foreign object.

Record if dyspnea is occurring upon exertion or while resting. Gather data relative to how the patient has been coping with any orthopneic problems.

Chest Pain

Record data relative to the time of onset, frequency, duration, and quality of the chest pain.

Specifically note any conditions the patient has found that either aggravate or relieve the chest pain.

Fatigue

Determine whether fatigue occurs only at specific times of the day, such as toward evening.

Ask the patient if fatigue decreases in relation to a decrease in activity level.

Edema

Chart the time of day that the edema is present, such as when arising in the morning, and the specific parts on the body where present.

Always perform daily weights:

1. Using the same scale
2. In approximately the same weight of clothing
3. At the same time of day

Syncopy

Elicit from the patient conditions surrounding any episodes of syncopy. Record the degree of presenting symptoms such as general muscle weakness, inability to stand upright, a feeling of "faintness," or loss of consciousness, and what activities, if any, bring on these syncopal episodes.

Palpitations

Record the patient's description of palpitations, such as "my heart skips some beats" or "it began to feel like it was racing." Ask if these conditions are preceded by strenuous or mild exercise, and how long the palpitations last.

Indications of Alterations in Cardiovascular Function

Skin color

Note the color of the skin, mucous membranes, tongue, earlobes, and nailbeds. Chart the exact location of any cyanosis present.

Clubbing

Inspect the fingernails for clubbing and perform the blanching test on both the fingernails and toenails.

Neck Vein Distension

Record any neck vein distension present.

Respirations

Observe and chart the rate and depth of respirations.

Edema

Record the presence or absence and location of edema and any measures the patient has employed in an attempt to bring relief.

Pulse

Assess bilaterally the rhythm, quality, equality, and strength of the pulses (carotid, brachial, radial, femoral, popliteal, posterior tibial, and dorsalis pedis). If any pulse is diminished or absent, record the level where initial changes are noted. The usual words to describe the pulse are *absent, diminished*, or *average, full and brisk*, or *full bounding, frequently visible*.

Auscultation and Percussion

Nurses with advanced skills can perform auscultation and percussion to note changes in heart size and heart and lung sounds. (See a medical-surgical nursing text for details of performing these advanced skills.)

Blood Pressure

Blood pressure readings should be performed at least two times daily in stable cardiac patients and more frequently if indicated by the patient's symptoms or the physician's orders. Be sure to use the proper sized blood pressure cuff and have the patient's arm at heart level.

Initially record the blood pressure in both arms. A systolic pressure variance of 5–10 mm Hg is normal; readings reflecting a variance of more then 10 mm Hg should be reported for further evaluation. ALWAYS REPORT A NARROWING PULSE PRESSURE (difference between systolic and diastolic readings).

Laboratory

Review laboratory tests and report abnormal results to the physician promptly. Such tests as serum electrolytes, especially potassium, SGOT, CPK, LDH, urinalysis, and electrocardiogram reports are an important means of monitoring the patient's response to therapy.

Perform hourly monitoring of I/O. Report outputs that are less than intake for evaluation.

Anxiety Level

Patients experiencing cardiac disorders usually exhibit varying degrees of anxiety. Act in a calm manner when dealing with the person experiencing anxiety. Remember that hostility and anger are frequently employed as a means of dealing with loss of personal control of one's life.

It is essential that the nurse establish a trusting relationship with the patient and that he or she listen to the patient's concerns.

Work cooperatively with the patient to establish mutual goals that can effectively deal with expressed problems or needs. Be readily available to the patient and encourage discussion of personal *feelings*.

Administer appropriate medications and treatments that can best alleviate the patient's presenting symptoms and provide the maximum level of comfort.

Other Health Care Measures

Prevention of Skin Breakdown

Many cardiovascular disorders require bedrest. Therefore, develop and follow a regular turning schedule that changes the patient's position every 2 hours around the clock.

Inspect pressure areas on the body for signs of skin breakdown each time you position the patient. Remember, when skin redness is seen and it does not subside rapidly, tissue damage is already extending into deeper tissue.

Facilitation of Breathing

If the patient is experiencing dyspnea, position the patient in a semi-Fowler's to full Fowler's position to improve lung expansion. Always maintain good body alignment.

Oxygen may be administered by various methods (cannula, tent, mask) as ordered by the physician. Specific oxygen levels are monitored by measuring arterial blood gases (ABGs).

Elimination Needs

Tell the patient to let the nurse know if he or she is experiencing constipation. It is extremely important that patients with cardiovascular disease not strain at stool. The physician usually orders a bulk laxative or stool softener to be taken on a scheduled basis.

Patient Teaching Associated with Cardiovascular Disease

Communication and Responsibility

Encourage open communication with the patient concerning frustrations and anger as the patient attempts to adjust to the diagnosis and need for prolonged treatment. The patient must be guided to gain insight into the condition in order to assume the responsibility for the continuation of treatment. Keep reemphasizing those factors the patient can control to alter the disease process.

SMOKING

Smoking causes vasonconstriction of the vessels; therefore, drastic reduction and preferably total abstinence from smoking should be encouraged.

HYPERTENSION

If the disease process is accompanied by hypertension, stress the importance of following prescribed emotional, dietary, and medicinal regimens to control the disease.

NUTRITION

The physician usually prescribes dietary modifications aimed at decreasing the cholesterol level and a reducing program designed to maintain an ideal weight range.

Caffeine consumption should be drastically reduced or discontinued. Introduce the patient to decaffeinated products that can be substituted for previously used caffeine-containing foods.

Expectations of Therapy

Discuss expectations of therapy with the patient.

ACTIVITIES AND EXERCISE

Activities of daily living need to be resumed within the boundaries set by the physician. (Such activities as regular, moderate exercise, meal preparation, resumption of usual sexual activities, and social interaction all need to be fostered.)

ENVIRONMENT

Tell the patient the importance of dressing warmly, avoiding cold winds, and the need to use a face mask in these conditions to prewarm inhaled air.

PAIN RELIEF

The degree of anginal pain relief with and without activity needs to be discussed.

STRESS MANAGEMENT

Some stressors may be within the work environment; therefore, involvement of the industrial nurse along with a thorough exploration of work factors that precipitate anginal attacks may be appropriate.

Teach the patient relaxation techniques and personal comfort measures such as a warm bath to alleviate stress.

Referral for mastery of biofeedback or other techniques may be necessary to alter stress levels substantially.

Stress produced within the dynamics of the family may require professional counseling.

Encourage the patient to openly express *feelings* about this chronic illness. The adjustment to this situation involves working through great personal fears, frustrations, hostilities, and resentments associated with the loss of personal control within one's life.

SEXUAL ACTIVITY

Encourage the patient to resume sexual activity. Discuss the use of medication or other adjustments for anginal pain before this activity.

Changes in Expectations

Assess changes in expectations as therapy progresses and the patient gains understanding and skill in management of the diagnosis.

Changes in Therapy through Cooperative Goal-Setting

Work with the patient to encourage adherence to the prescribed treatment. When the patient feels that a change should be made in a treatment plan, encourage a discussion first with the physician.

WRITTEN RECORD

Enlist the patient's aid in developing and maintaining a written record of the monitoring parameters (i.e., blood pressure, pulse, daily weights, degree of pain relief, exercise tolerance) and response to prescribed therapies for discussion with the physician. Patients should be encouraged to take this record to follow-up visits.

FOSTERING COMPLIANCE

Throughout the hospitalization, discuss medication information and how it will benefit the patient's course of treatment. Seek cooperation and understanding of the following points, so that medication compliance may be enhanced.

1. Name
2. Dosage
3. Route and administration times
4. Anticipated therapeutic response
5. Side effects to expect
6. Side effects to report
7. What to do if a dosage is missed
8. When, how, or if to refill the medication prescription

If it is evident that the patient and/or family does not understand all aspects of continuing therapy being prescribed (i.e., administration and monitoring of medications, exercises, diets, follow-up appointments), consider the use of social service or visiting nurse agencies.

ASSOCIATED TEACHING

Give patients the following instructions:

Always inform the physician or dentist of any prescription or over-the-counter medication being taken. Over-the-counter medications should not be taken without first consulting the physician or pharmacist.

Always report side effects of rash, itching, or hives immediately. Nausea, vomiting, or diarrhea should also be reported for the physician's evaluation if it is a new symptom.

Take all of the medication as prescribed for the full course of treatment. Do not discontinue use when feeling improved; do not save for future use; do not give your medicine to another individual. Sudden discontinuation of certain medicines may produce harmful effects.

Keep all medications out of the reach of children.

If pregnancy is suspected, consult an obstetrician as soon as possible about continuation of medication therapy.

At Discharge

Items to be sent home with the patient should:

1. Have written instructions for use.
2. Be labeled in a level of language and size of print appropriate for the patient.

3. If needed, include identification cards or bracelets.
4. Include a list of additional supplies to be purchased after discharge (i.e., syringes, dressings).
5. Include a schedule for follow-up appointments.

Digitalis Glycosides

The digitalis drugs are among the oldest and most effective therapeutic agents for the treatment of congestive heart failure. They are also used in the treatment of atrial fibrillation, atrial flutter, and paroxysmal tachycardia. Their use in medicine dates to the eighteenth century. In 1785 William Withering, the English physician and botanist, published excellent observations on the treatment of various ailments with digitalis. Once derived naturally from the dried leaves of *Digitalis purpurea*, or purple foxglove, the drug is now synthetically prepared.

Digitalis glycosides have two primary actions on the heart: (1) digitalis increases the force of contraction (positive inotropy), and (2) slows the heart rate (negative chronotropy). The exact mechanisms of these actions are unknown, but the net result is that the heart is able to fill and empty more completely, thus improving circulation. With improved circulation, there is a reduction in systemic and pulmonary congestion, a reduction in heart size toward normal, and a reduction in peripheral edema due to better perfusion of blood through the kidneys.

The treatment goal of heart failure is to give adequate doses of digitalis so that the best cardiac effects are achieved and most of the signs and symptoms (dyspnea, orthopnea, edema, etc.) disappear. The patient is often given a loading dose of the drug over a period of hours or days necessary to produce the desired cardiac effect. This is known as *digitalizing* the patient. A maintenance dose is then given, usually once daily. Many patients must continue to take digitalis preparations for the remainder of their lives.

Side Effects

Common side effects of digitalis include weakness, fatigue, vomiting, diarrhea, arrhythmias, and pulse rate below 60 beats a minute (bradycardia). Headache, visual disturbances, and restlessness may also occur.

Adverse effects of digitalis may also be induced by electrolyte imbalance, resulting in hypokalemia, hypomagnesemia, and hypocalcemia. (See Drug Interactions for agents that may induce electrolyte imbalance.)

The patient's other clinical conditions may also induce digitalis intoxication. Patients who suffer from hypothyroidism, acute myocardial infarction, renal disease, severe respiratory disease, or far advanced heart failure may require lower than normal doses of the digitalis glycosides. It is important to remember that it is essential to treat the patient and the clinical symptomatology and that individual variation is frequently observed with the digitalis glycosides.

Nursing Interventions

See General Nursing Considerations for Patients with Cardiovascular Disease.

See also Nursing Interventions for digoxin and digitoxin.

PATIENT CONCERNS: NURSING INTERVENTION/RATIONALE

Side Effects to Report

Digitalis Toxicity

CARDIAC EFFECTS

Always observe your patient for the development of a pulse deficit, bradycardia, tachycardia, or bigeminy. These may be signs of developing heart block. Whenever the individual is attached to a monitor, the pattern should be closely watched for any type of abnormal cardiac arrthythmia.

In children, digitalis toxicity is usually detected by the development of atrial arrhythmias.

NONCARDIAC EFFECTS

Noncardiac symptoms of digitalis toxicity are often quite vague and are difficult to separate from symptoms of the heart disease. Any patient who is taking digitalis products who develop loss of appetite, nausea, extreme fatigue, weakness of the arms and legs, psychiatric disturbances (nightmares, agitation, listlessness, or hallucinations), or visual disturbances (hazy or blurred vision, difficulty in reading, and difficulty in red–green color perception) should be evaluated for digitalis toxicity.

OTHER DISEASES

Other diseases such as hypothyroidism, myocardial infarction, renal disease, or pulmonary disease may increase the potential for digitalis toxicity. Monitor closely.

Electrolyte Balance

Monitor lab reports and notify the physician of deviations from the normal range of 4 to 5.4 mEq/liter of potassium. Always monitor the pulse carefully if potassium level is abnormal. Hypokalemia is especially likely to occur when the patient exhibits nausea, vomiting, diarrhea, or heavy diuresis.

Dosage and Administration

Digitalization

Digitalization is the administration of a larger dose of a digitalis preparation for an initial period of 24 to 48 hours. Following this initial "loading" period, the patient is switched to a daily maintenance dose. Be sure to monitor the patient carefully for signs of digitalis toxicity.

Pulse Variations

Always take the apical pulse 1 *full* minute *before* administering any digitalis preparation. Do not administer the drug when the pulse rate in an adult is below 60 beats per minute until the physician is consulted. In a child report findings below 90 beats per minute. The physician may decide to withhold the medication.

Accurate Identification

Digitalis glycosides are frequently given in minute amounts. *Always* have mathematical computations checked by another professional nurse.

Use the correct type of syringe to facilitate accuracy in dosage measurement.

Always question any order that is unusual *before* administration. Read the medication label carefully; *digoxin* and *digitoxin* are *not* the same.

Serum Levels

Serum levels of digitalis are performed to measure the amount of digitalis in the bloodstream. Blood should be drawn prior to the daily dose of medication, or at least 6 hours after administration. It is important to be consistent in the time of drawing the blood and administering the dose if more than one serum level is to be drawn in the same patient.

Oral Administration

Give digitalis glycosides after meals to minimize gastric irritation.

Drug Interactions

Drugs That Enhance Therapeutic and Toxic Effects

Verapamil, beta adrenergic blocking agents (e.g., atenolol, timolol, nadolol, propranolol, others), succinylcholine, calcium gluconate, and calcium chloride: Monitor for signs and symptoms of digitalis toxicity.

Drugs That Reduce Therapeutic Effects

Cholestyramine: Watch for an increase in the patient's disease symptomatology.

Drugs That May Alter Electrolyte Balance, Altering Digitalis Response

Drugs that may alter digitalis response and the incidence of any of the side effects by alteration of electrolyte imbalance include the following:

Hypokalemia
- Amphotericin B (Fungizone)
- Bumetanide (Bumex)
- Chlorthalidone (Hygroton)
- Corticosteroids
- Ethacrynic acid (Edecrin)
- Furosemide (Lasix)
- Metolazone (Zaroxolyn)
- Thiazide diuretics

Hyperkalemia
- Amiloride (Midamor)
- Beta adrenergic blockers
- Heparin
- Mannitol infusions
- Potassium chloride
- Potassium gluconate
- Potassium penicillin G
- Potassium supplements (K-Lyte, Kaon, K-Lore, others)
- Salt substitutes
- Succinylcholine

Hypomagnesemia
- Chlorthalidone (Hygroton)
- Ethacrynic acid (Edecrin)
- Ethanol
- Furosemide (Lasix)
- Metolazone (Zaroxolyn)
- Neomycin (Mycifradin)
- Thiazide diuretics

See the individual agents for drug interactions specific to digoxin and digitoxin.

Digitalis Preparations

Digitoxin (dij-i-tok′sin) ***(Crystodigin)*** (kris-to-dij′in), ***(Purodigin)*** (pu-ro-dij′in)

Availability

PO—0.05, 0.1, 0.15, and 0.2 mg tablets.
IV—0.2 mg/ml.

Dosage and Administration

Note: A baseline ECG is recommended before initiation of therapy. Assuming the patient has not ingested a digitalis preparation in the preceding 3 weeks the following dosages apply:

Adult
PO—1. Digitalizing: 0.6 mg initially followed by 0.2 mg at intervals of 4 to 6 hours.
2. Maintenance: 0.05 to 0.3 mg once daily. The average dose is 0.1 to 0.15 mg daily.
IV—1. Digitalizing: 0.6 mg initially followed by 0.4 mg 4 to 6 hours later, then followed by 0.2 mg every 4 to 6 hours thereafter until therapeutic effects are apparent. These effects are usually observed within 8 to 12 hours.
2. Maintenance: Same as for PO maintenance therapy.
Pediatric
PO—1. Digitalizing
a. Premature, full-term, and infants with impaired renal function: 0.022 mg/kg.
b. Ages 2 weeks to 1 year: 0.045 mg/kg
c. Over 2 years of age: 0.03 mg/kg
Note: Divide total digitalizing dose into 3 or more doses, administered at lease 6 hours apart.
2. Maintenance: Give one-tenth the total digitalizing dose daily.
IV—As for PO therapy.

Nursing Interventions

See General Nursing Considerations for Patients with Cardiovascular Disease.
See also Nursing Interventions for digitalis glycosides.

Digoxin (di-joks'in) *(Lanoxin)* (lah-noks'in)

Digoxin is the most commonly used member of the digitalis glycoside family. It digitalizes more rapidly than digitoxin. Oral administrations may digitalize within a few hours and IV injections within a few minutes.

Availability

PO—0.125, 0.25, and 0.5 mg tablets; 0.05, 0.1, and 0.2 mg Gelcaps; pediatric elixir, 0.05 mg/ml.
IV—0.25 mg/ml in 1 and 2 ml vials and ampules, and 0.1 mg/ml in 1 ml ampules.

Dosage and Administration

Note: A baseline ECG is recommended before initiation of therapy. Assuming the patient has not ingested a digitalis preparation in the preceding 2 weeks the following dosages apply:

Adult
PO—1. Digitalizing: 0.50 to 0.75 mg initially followed by 0.25 mg every 6 hours until adequate digitalization is achieved.
  2. Maintenance: 0.125 to 0.25 mg daily. Some patients may require 0.375 to 0.5 mg daily.
IV—1. Digitalizing: 0.25 to 0.5 mg initially followed by 0.25 mg every 6 hours until adequate digitalization is achieved. Administer at a rate of 0.5 to 1 ml/minute.
  2. Maintenance: Same as for PO administration.

Pediatric
Premature:
IM or IV—1. Digitalizing: 0.015 to 0.02 mg/kg initially followed by 0.01 mg every 6 to 8 hours for 2 doses (total digitalizing dose: 0.03 to 0.05 mg/kg).
  2. Maintenance: 0.003 to 0.006 mg/kg every 12 hours.

Ages 2 weeks to 2 years:
PO—1. Digitalizing: 0.03 to 0.04 mg/kg initially followed by 0.02 mg/kg every 6 to 8 hours for 2 doses (total digitalizing dose: 0.06 to 0.08 mg/kg).
  2. Maintenance: 0.006 to 0.01 mg/kg every 12 hours.
IM or IV—1. Digitalizing: 0.02 to 0.03 mg/kg initially, followed by 0.01 to 0.015 mg/kg every 6 to 8 hours for 2 doses (total digitalizing dose: 0.04 to 0.06 mg/kg).
  2. Maintenance: 0.003 to 0.006 mg/kg every 12 hours.

Over 2 years of age:
PO—1. Digitalizing: 0.02 to 0.03 mg/kg initially, followed by 0.01 to 0.015 mg every 6 to 8 hours for 2 doses (total digitalizing dose: 0.04 to 0.06 mg/kg).
  2. Maintenance: 0.004 to 0.009 mg/kg every 12 hours.
IM or IV—1. Digitalizing: 0.01 to 0.02 mg/kg initially followed by 0.005 to 0.01 mg/kg every 6 to 8 hours for 2 doses (total digitalizing dose: 0.02 to 0.04 mg/kg).
  2. Maintenance: 0.002 to 0.004 mg/kg every 12 hours.

Nursing Interventions

See General Nursing Considerations for Patients with Cardiovascular Disease.
See also Nursing Interventions for digitalis glycosides.

Drugs That Reduce Therapeutic Effects

Neomycin and antacids:
Monitor patient symptoms for response to therapy; recurrence or intensification of the patient's disease should be reported to the physician.

Antiarrhythmic Agents

Any patient with heart disease or a disease that affects cardiovascular function may experience arrhythmias. *Arrhythmias* are any heart rate and rhythm other than normal sinus rhythm. The more common causes of arrhythmias include electrolyte and acid-base imbalance, emotional stress, hypoxia, and congestive heart failure.

Patients may "sense" that they are having arrhythmias because they can feel the heart "flip-flop" or "race." Nurses may also suspect that a patient is having arrhythmias because of an irregular pulse. Arrhythmias, however, must be identified with the aid of an electrocardiogram (ECG), which provides a tracing of the electrical activity of the heart. When an arrhythmia is suspected, a patient is frequently admitted to a coronary care unit where wire leads are placed in appropriate locations to provide continuous ECG monitoring. A combination of the physical examination, patient history, and ECG pattern are used to diagnose the underlying cause of the arrhythmia. The goal of treatment is to restore normal sinus rhythm and normal cardiac function and to prevent recurrence of life-threatening arrhythmias.

The beginning nurse is not routinely assigned patients in a coronary care unit because advanced training in the interpretation of data from ECG monitors and in drug therapy used in the management of life-threatening arrhythmias is required. However, the information nurses assess relative to the cardinal signs of cardiovascular disease can provide a basis for subsequent evaluation of the patient's response to the therapeutic modalities prescribed.

General Nursing Considerations for Patients Receiving Antiarrhythmic Therapy

---

PATIENT CONCERNS: NURSING INTERVENTION/RATIONALE

Baseline Assessment

Vital Signs

Vital signs should be taken as often as necessary to monitor the patient's status.

Chest Pain

Not all patients with arrhythmias will have chest pain, but for those who do, record the time of onset, frequency, duration, and quality of the chest pain.

Specifically note any conditions the patient has found that either aggravate or relieve chest pain.

Mental Status and Anxiety Level

Perform a baseline assessment of the patient's degree of anxiety, alertness, and agitation. Subsequent, regular observations of this data should be made so that apparent improvement or deterioration can be assessed.

Patients experiencing cardiovascular disorders frequently exhibit varying degrees of anxiety. Act in a calm manner when dealing with the patient experiencing anxiety. Remember that hostility and anger are frequently employed as a means of dealing with loss of personal control of one's life.

It is essential that the nurse establish a trusting relationship with the patient and that he or she listen to the patient's concerns.

Arrhythmias

Arrhythmias are initially assessed by electrocardiographic monitoring. (Refer to a general medical-surgical text for details of arrhythmias.)

Cardinal Signs of Cardiovascular Disease

See above, General Nursing Considerations for Patients with Cardiovascular Disease.

Patient Teaching Associated with Antiarrhythmic Therapy

Communication and Responsibility

Encourage open communication concerning frustrations and anger as the patient attempts to adjust to the diagnosis and need for prolonged treatment. The patient must be guided to gain insight into the condition in order to assume responsibility for the continuation of treatment. Keep emphasizing those factors the patient can control to alter the disease process, including maintenance of general health, elimination of smoking, meeting nutritional needs, adequate rest, and appropriate exercise, and continuation of prescribed medication therapy.

Expectations of Therapy

Discuss expectations of therapy with the patient (i.e., level of exercise, degreee of pain relief, frequency of use of therapy, sexual activity, maintenance of mobility, ability to maintain activities of daily living and/or work).

Changes in Expectations

Assess changes in expectations as therapy progresses and the patient gains understanding and skill in management of the diagnosis.

Changes in Therapy through Cooperative Goal-Setting

Work with the patient to encourage adherence to the prescribed treatment. When the patient feels that a change should be made in a treatment plan, encourage discussion first with the physician.

WRITTEN RECORD

Enlist the patient's aid in developing and maintaining a written record of monitoring parameters (i.e., blood pressure, pulse, daily weights, degree of pain relief, exercise tolerance) and response to prescribed therapies for discussion with the physician. Patients should be encouraged to take this record on follow-up visits.

FOSTERING COMPLIANCE

Throughout the hospitalization, discuss medication information and how it will benefit the course of treatment. Seek cooperation and understanding of the following points so that medication compliance may be enhanced:

1. Name
2. Dosage
3. Route and administration times
4. Anticipated therapeutic response
5. Side effects to expect
6. Side effects to report
7. What to do if a dosage is missed
8. When, how, or if to refill the medication prescription

DIFFICULTY IN COMPREHENSION

If it is evident that the patient and/or family does not understand all aspects of continuing therapy being prescribed (i.e., administration and monitoring of medications, exercises, diets, follow-up appointments),

consider the use of social service or visiting nurse agencies.

ASSOCIATED TEACHING

Give patient the following instructions.

Always inform the physician or dentist of any prescription or over-the-counter medication being taken. Over-the-counter medications should not be taken without first consulting the physician or pharmacist.

Always report side effects of rash, itching, or hives immediately. Nausea, vomiting, or diarrhea should also be reported for the physician's evaluation if it is a new symptom.

Take all of the medication as prescribed for the full course of treatment. Do not discontinue use when feeling improved; do not save for future use; do not give your medicine to another individual. Sudden discontinuation of certain medications may produce harmful effects.

Keep all medications out of reach of children.

If pregnancy is suspected, consult an obstetrician as soon as possible about continuation of medication therapy.

At Discharge

Items to be sent home with the patient should:

1. Have written instructions for use.
2. Be labeled in a level of language and size of print appropriate for the patient.
3. If needed, include identification cards or bracelets.
4. Include a list of additional supplies to be purchased after discharge.
5. Include a schedule for follow-up appointments.

Bretylium tosylate (bre-til′ee-um tahs′e-layt) *(Bretylol)* (bre′ti-lol)

Bretylium, an adrenergic blocking agent, inhibits the release of norepinephrine. It is used to supress life-threatening ventricular arrhythmias, primarily tachycardia and fibrillation, that have not responded to other widely used antiarrhythmic drugs. Bretylium is not a cardiac depressant, so it is particularly useful in patients with poor myocardial contractility and low cardiac output.

Side Effects

Side effects include postural hypotension in most patients and often nausea and vomiting after rapid IV infusion. Other symptoms that may occur include vertigo, light-headedness, slow heart rate, syncope, increased premature ventricular contractions, increased arrhythmias, transient hypertension, substernal discomfort, anginal attacks, abdominal pain, diarrhea, renal dysfunction, hiccups, rash, hyperthermia, flushing, confusions, lethargy, anxiety, psychosis, shortness of breath, sweating, and nasal stuffiness.

Availability

IV—50 mg/ml in 10 ml ampules.

Disopyramide (die-so-peer′ah-myd) (Norpace) (nor′pace)

Disopyramide is effective in the treatment of primary cardiac arrhythmias and those that occur in association with organic heart disease, including coronary artery disease. It may be used in both digitalized and nondigitalized patients. It is usually a useful drug as an alternative to quinidine or procainamide when patients develop an intolerance to or serious side effects from these agents.

Side Effects

The more common adverse effects of therapy include dry mouth, nose, and throat, urinary hesitancy and retention, constipation with bloating and gas, and occasional diarrhea.

The myocardial toxicities of disopyramide may be manifested by premature ventricular contractions, bradycardia, atrioventricular block, ventricular tachycardia, ventricular fibrillation, or an increase in congestive heart failure.

Disopyramide generally has fewer side effects than quinidine and is comparable to quinidine in treatment of atrial and ventricular arrhythmias.

Availability

PO—100 and 150 mg capsules.

Dosage and Administration

PO—Dosage is individualized. Recommended adult dosage schedule is 150 mg every 6 hours. If body weight is less than 110 pounds (50 kg), the recommended dose is 100 mg every 6 hours.

Nursing Interventions

See also General Nursing Considerations for Patients with Cardiovascular disease.

See also General Nursing Considerations for Patients Receiving Antiarrhythmic Therapy.

PATIENT CONCERNS: NURSING INTERVENTION/RATIONALE

Side Effects to Expect

Dry Mouth, Nose, Throat

Suggest frequent mouth rinses or sucking on ice chips or hard candy to relieve symptoms.

Side Effects to Report

Myocardial Toxicity

Report bradycardia or increasing signs of congestive heart disease.

Monitoring of the ECG for various types arrhythmias may be indicated as ordered by the physician.

Urinary Hesitancy

Tell the patient that hesitancy in starting to urinate may occur. Suggest running tap water or immersing hands in water as means to stimulate urination. Report decreased urinary output and bladder distention.

In the hospitalized patient, record I/O. Palpate the area of the symphysis pubis to assess for actual distention.

Constipation with Distension and Flatus

Report difficulties in defecation to the physician. Assess distension by measuring abdominal girth, as appropriate. Assess ability to expell flatus.

Drug Interactions

Drugs That Enhance Therapeutic and Toxic Effects

Procainamide, quinidine, digitalis, and beta adrenergic blocking agents (propranolol, atenolol, timolol, others): Monitor for increases in severity of drug effects such as bradycardia and hypotension.

Drugs That Reduce Therapeutic Effects

Phenytoin, barbiturates, gluthimide, primidone, and rifampin.

Monitor for an increase in frequency of the patient's arrhythmias.

Drugs That Increase Hypotensive Effects

Diuretics and antihypertensive agents.
Instruct patients to rise slowly from a supine position. If symptoms become more severe, report to the physician.

Lidocaine (li′do-kayn) *(Xylocaine)* (zi′lo-kayn)

Lidocaine has become one of the most frequently used drugs in the treatment of ventricular arrhythmias. It is the drug of choice for the treatment of ventricular arrhythmias associated with acute myocardial infarction and ventricular tachycardia.

Side Effects

Side effects tend to be dose-related and are usually fairly minor. Adverse effects include light-headedness, tinnitus, muscle twitches, and blurred or double vision. When higher doses are used, patients may develop CNS stimulation, hypotension, restlessness, euphoria, and, rarely, convulsions. These side effects may be controlled by reducing the dosage.

Availability

IM—300 mg/3 ml; 10% (100 mg/ml) in 5 ml ampules.
Direct IV—1% (10 mg/ml) in 5 and 10 ml disposable syringes; 2% (20 mg/ml) in 5 ml disposable syringes and ampules.
IV Admixtures—4% (40 mg/ml) in 25 and 50 ml vials and additive syringes; 20% (200 mg/ml) in 5 ml and 10 ml additive syringes.
IV Infusion—0.2% (2 mg/ml) in 500 ml of 5% dextrose; 0.4% (4 mg/ml) in 500 ml of 5% dextrose.

Dosage and Administration

Note: Lidocaine should not be used in patients with complete heart block.
Adult
IM—200 to 300 mg in the deltoid muscle.
IV—The initial dose (bolus) is 50 to 100 mg (1 mg/kg) at a rate of 25 to 50 mg/minute. Boluses of 50 to 100 mg may be given every 3 to 5 minutes until the desired effect is achieved or side effects appear. Do not exceed 300 mg by intermittent bolus. To maintain the antiarrhythmic effect, an IV infusion must be initiated. The usual rate of administration is 1 to 4 mg/minute. For routine lidocaine administration for cardiac arrhythmias, add 50 ml of 40 mg/ml (2 g) of lidocaine to dextrose 5%.

Pediatric
IV—Initial bolus: 1 mg/kg up to 15 mg if under 25 kg (55 pounds); up to 25 mg if over 25 kg (55 pounds). Continous infusion: 20 to 40 μg/kg/minute (maximum total dose 5 mg/kg).

Nursing Interventions

See also General Nursing Considerations for Patients with Cardiovascular Disease.
See also General Nursing Considerations for Patients Receiving Antiarrhythmic Therapy.

**PATIENT CONCERNS:
NURSING INTERVENTION/RATIONALE**

Side Effects to Report

Light-headedness, Muscle Twitching, Hallucinations, Agitation, Euphoria

Monitor patients carefully for progressive symptoms of restlessness, agitation, anxiety, hallucinations, and euphoria.
Act calmly with the excited, anxious, or euphoric patient. Provide for safety and fulfillment of patient's needs. Report patient's alteration in response to the physician as soon as possible.

Respiratory Depression

Observe the rate and depth of respiratory effort. Monitor for cyanosis and increasing frequency of arrhythmias.

Dosage and Administration
IV

Lidocaine for IV use for arrhythmias is *different* from lidocaine used as a local anesthetic. For use with arrhythmias, check the label carefully to be certain it says: "Xylocaine for Arrhythmias" or "Lidocaine without Preservatives." Severe arrhythmias could result if "Lidocaine with Preservatives" or "Lidocaine with Epinephrine" were accidentally administered to these patients.

IM

Intramuscular injections of lidocaine should be given in the deltoid. The IM route should only be used in emergency situations until an IV can be established.

Drug Interactions

Drugs That Enhance Therapeutic and Toxic Effects

Phenytoin and beta adrenergic blocking agents (nadolol, atenolol, timolol, propranolol, others).
Monitor for an increase in severity of side effects such as bradycardia and hypotension.

Neuromuscular Blocking Action

When lidocaine is administered in conjunction with succinylcholine, observe for respiratory depression. Patients who are on respirators may require additional time to be weaned off ventilatory assistance.

Nadolol (na-doe'lol) *(Corgard)* (core-guard)

Another widely used antiarrhythmic agent is nadolol. It inhibits cardiac response to sympathetic nerve stimulation by blocking the beta receptors. As a result, it slows the heart rate and has an antiarrhythmic effect almost as potent as that of propranolol. Nadolol is effective in the treatment of various ventricular arrhythmias, sinus tachycardia, paroxysmal atrial tachycardia, premature ventricular contractions, and tachycardia associated with atrial flutter or fibrillation, because it inhibits atrioventricular conduction, thus slowing the ventricular rate.

Nadolol is discussed in detail elsewhere in the text (see Index).

Phenytoin (fen'i-toe-in) *(DPH), (Dilantin)* (di-lan'tin)

Phenytoin was introduced about 45 years ago for the treatment of epilepsy, but it is also effective in controlling ventricular arrhythmias, particularly those induced by digitalis toxicity. (For use in seizure disorders, see Index.)

Availability

PO—30, 100 mg capsules, 50 mg chewable tablets; oral suspension: 30, 125 mg/5 ml;
IV—50 mg/ml in 2 and 5 ml ampules, 2 ml syringes.

Procainamide hydrochloride (pro'kane'ah-myd) *(Pronestyl)* (pro-nes'til)

Procainamide is an effective synthetic antiarrhythmic agent that has many cardiac effects similar to those of quinidine, but generally with fewer side effects. It is used to treat a wide variety of ventricular and supraventricular arrhythmias, atrial fibrillation, and flutter. It is usually not as effective in the last two disorders as quinidine.

Side Effects

When taken orally, the most common side effects include anorexia, nausea, vomiting, bitter taste, flushing, and diarrhea.

Hypotension may be observed while therapy is being initiated, particularly by the intravenous route.

Hypersensitivity reactions including chills, fever, joint and muscle pain, pruritus, urticarial or maculopapular skin rashes, photosensitivity, and anaphylaxis have been reported.

Availability

PO—250, 375, 500 mg tablets and capsules; 250, 500 mg sustained release tablets and capsules.
IV—100 mg/ml in 10 ml ampules, 500 mg/ml in 2 ml ampules.

Dosage and Administration

Note: Do not use in complete atrioventricular block, and use with extreme caution in partial atrioventricular block.

Adult

PO—Loading dose: 1 to 1.25 g. Follow with 750 mg 1 hour later if the arrhythmia is still present. Maintain the dosage at 0.5 to 1 g every 4 to 6 hours. Some patients may require maintenance doses every 3 to 4 hours to maintain adequate control of arrhythmias.

IM—0.5 to 1 g every 6 hours until PO therapy is possible.

IV—100 mg every 5 minutes at 25 to 50 mg/minute until arrhythmias are suppressed, a maximum of 1 g has been administered, or side effects develop. Once arrhythmias are suppressed, a continuous infusion may be started at 25 to 30 μg/kg/minute. If arrhythmias recur, suppress the arrhythmias with bolus therapy as above and increase the rate of infusion.

Nursing Interventions

See also General Nursing Considerations for Patients with Cardiovascular disease.

See also General Nursing Considerations for Patients Receiving Antiarrhythmic Therapy.

**PATIENT CONCERNS:
NURSING INTERVENTION/RATIONALE**

Side Effects to Expect

Drowsiness, Sedation, Dizziness

Tell patients they may experience these symptoms early in therapy, as the dosage is being adjusted. Use caution in operating power equipment or driving.

Hypotension

Hypotension is usually transient. Patients can avoid this complication by rising slowly from supine and sitting positions.

Side Effects to Report

*Fever, Chills, Joint and Muscle Pain,
Skin Eruptions*

Tell patients to report the development of these symptoms.

Monitor laboratory reports for leukocyte counts and the antinuclear antibody (ANA) titer.

Dosage and Administration

Oral

Administer in divided doses around the clock.

If gastric irritation is a problem administer with food or milk.

IV

Patients should have ECG and blood pressure monitoring when receiving intravenous doses of procainamide.

Serum Levels

Serum levels of procainamide are performed to measure the amount of digitalis in the bloodstream. Blood should be drawn prior to the daily dose of medication, or at least 6 hours after administration. It is important to be consistent in the time of drawing the blood and administering the dose if more than one serum level is to be drawn in the same patient.

Drug Interactions

*Drugs That Enhance Therapeutic
and Toxic Effects*

Digitalis, quinidine, and beta adrenergic blocking agents (timolol, nadolol, propranolol, and others): Monitor for an increase in severity of side effects such as bradycardia and hypotension.

*Neuromuscular Blockage,
Respiratory Depression*

Surgical muscle relaxants (tubocurarine, succinylcholine, gallamine triethiodide) and aminoglycoside antibiotics (gentamicin, streptomycin, amikacin kanamycin, netilmycin, others): Monitor the patient's respiratory rate and depth. Observe for signs of cyanosis and additional arrhythmias.

Patients who are on respirators may require additional time to be weaned off ventilatory assistance.

Hypotension

Diuretics and antihypertensive agents: Instruct patients to rise slowly from a supine position. If symptoms are becoming more recurrent, report to the physician.

Propranolol (pro-pran'o-lol) *(Inderal)* (in'der-ahl)

Another widely used antiarrhythmic agent is propranolol. It inhibits cardiac response to sympathetic nerve stimulation by blocking the beta receptors. As a result, it slows the heart rate and has an antiarrhythmic effect. Propranolol is effective in the treatment of various ventricular arrhythmias. Propranolol has also been found to be effective in the treatment of certain digitalis-induced arrthythmias.

Propranolol is discussed in detail elsewhere in the text (see Index).

Quinidine (kwin'i-din)

Quinidine, originally obtained from cinchona bark, has been used as an antiarrhythmic agent for several decades. It works on the muscle of the heart, stabilizing the rate of conduction of impulses. It slows the heart and changes a rapid, irregular pulse to a slow, regular pulse. Quinidine is used most frequently to suppress atrial fibrillation, atrial flutter, paroxysmal supraventricular and ventricular tachycardia, and premature ventricular contractions. Use with extreme caution in patients with digitalis intoxication or heart block.

Side Effects

The most common side effects are diarrhea, nausea, and vomiting. Other side effects include hypotension, headache, facial flushing, hypersensitivity manifested by rash and fever, and arrhythmias.

Cinchonism (quinidine toxicity) is dose-related and will subside with reduction in dosage. It is manifested by salivation, tinnitus, vertigo, headache, visual disturbances, and confusion.

Availability

Quinidine sulfate:
PO—100, 200, 300 mg tablets; 200, 300 mg capsules; 300 mg sustained release tablets
IM, IV—200 mg/ml in 1 ml ampules.
Quinidine gluconate:
PO—324 mg, 330 mg sustained release tablets.
IM, IV—80 mg/ml in 10 ml vials.

Dosage and Administration

Adult
PO—Quinidine sulfate: 200 to 400 mg 3 to 5 times daily. Higher doses may be used, but the maximum single dose should not exceed 600 to 800 mg.
IM—Quinidine gluconate: 600 mg initially, then 400 mg every 2 hours as needed.
IV—Quinidine gluconate: 800 mg diluted to 40 ml with dextrose 5% and infused at a rate of 1 ml/minute.
Note: IV administration is extremely hazardous. Blood pressure and ECG readings should be monitored continuously as hypotension and arrhythmias may occur.

Pediatric
PO—Quinidine sulfate: 30 mg/kg/24 hours divided into 4 to 6 doses.
IM—Quinidine gluconate: As for PO administration.

Nursing Interventions

See also General Nursing Considerations for Patients with Cardiovascular disease.

See also General Nursing Considerations for Patients Receiving Antiarrhythmic Therapy.

PATIENT CONCERNS: NURSING INTERVENTION/RATIONALE

Side Effects to Expect
Diarrhea

Diarrhea is fairly common during initiation of therapy. It usually subsides, but occasionally a patient will have to change to another medication due to this adverse effect.

Chart the frequency and consistency of the diarrhea, and monitor the patient for dehydration and electrolyte imbalance.

Dizziness, Faintness

This may occur, particularly during initiation of therapy. It usually subsides within a few days.

Instruct patient to rise slowly from a supine position. Monitor the patient's blood pressure.

Side Effects to Report
Cinchonism

Monitor patients for signs of cinchonism and report the development of rash, chills, fever, ringing in the ears, and increasing mental confusion.

Dosage and Administration
Identification and Accuracy

Read labels carefully. Quinidine and quinine are *not* the same.

Gastric Irritation

Administer with food or milk if gastric irritation develops.

Serum Levels

Serum levels of quinidine are performed to measure the amount of digitalis in the bloodstream. Blood should be drawn prior to the daily dose of medication, or at least 6 hours after administration. It is important to be consistent in the time of drawing the blood and administering the dose if more than one serum level is to be drawn in the same patient.

Drug Interactions

Drugs That Enhance Therapeutic and Toxic Effects

Cimetidine, phenothiazines, procainamide, digitalis, and beta adrenergic blocking agents (propranolol, atenolol, timolol, others): Monitor for increases in severity of drug effects such as bradycardia, tachycardia, and hypotension.

Drugs That Reduce Therapeutic Effects

Rifampin: Monitor for an increase in the patient's arrhythmias.

Other Interactions

NEUROMUSCULAR BLOCKAGE, RESPIRATORY DEPRESSION

Surgical muscle relaxants (tubocurarine, succinylcholine, gallamine triethiodide) and aminoglycoside antibiotics (gentamicin, streptomycin, kanamycin, netilmycin, others): Monitor the patient's respiratory rate and depth. Observe for signs of cyanosis and additional arrhythmias.

Patients who are on respirators may require additional time to be weaned off ventilatory assistance.

DIGITALIS

Quinidine may increase the effects of digitalis.

Monitor the patient for symptoms of anorexia, nausea, vomiting, headaches, blurred or colored vision, and bradycardia. A digitalis serum level and quinidine serum level may be ordered by the physician.

BLEEDING

Quinidine may increase the anticoagulant effects of warfarin.

Monitor for signs of increased bleeding: bleeding gums, increased menstrual flow, petechiae, bruises.

Monitor the laboratory report and notify the physician immediately if the prothrombin time is abnormally high.

HYPOTENSION

Diuretics and antihypertensive agents: Instruct the patient to rise slowly from a supine position. If symptoms become excessive, report to the physician.

Timolol (tim'o-lol) *(Blocadren)* (blak'a-dren)

Another widely used antiarrhythmic agent is timolol. It inhibits cardiac response to sympathetic nerve stimulation by blocking the beta receptors. As a result, it slows the heart rate and has an antiarrhythmic effect. Timolol is approved for use as an antihypertensive agent and is the first beta adrenergic blocking agent to be approved for use to reduce the long-term risk of arrhythmias that may cause reinfarction and death in stabilized survivors of acute myocardial infarction. Timolol is discussed in detail elsewhere in the text (see Index).

Calcium Ion Antagonists

This class of chemicals represents a new approach to controlling heart disease. These agents are known variously as *calcium antagonists, slow channel blockers*, and *calcium ion influx inhibitors*. Regardless of their names, they all share the ability to inhibit the movement of calcium ions across a cell membrane. This results in fewer arrhythmias, a slower rate of contraction of the heart, and relaxation of smooth muscle of blood vessels, resulting in vasodilation.

Diltiazem hydrocholoride (dil'ty'az-em) *(Cardizem)* (kar'dih-zem)

Diltiazem is a calcium antagonist chemically unrelated to other members of this class of therapeutic agents. Its mechanisms of action are unknown, but it slows the heart rate and causes vasodilation of coronary and peripheral blood vessels, improving oxygenation to these tissues. Diltiazem is currently being used to treat angina pectoris in patients who do not receive therapeutic relief from nitrates or beta adrenergic blocker therapy.

Side Effects

The following side effects, although relatively infrequent (less than 3%), have been reported: nausea, swelling and edema, arrhythmias, headache, rash, and fatigue. Bradycardia, hypotension, congestive heart failure, mental depression, confusion, hallucinations, pruritus, petechiae, urticaria, photosensitivity, and paresthesias have all been reported but with an incidence of less than 1%.

Availability

PO—30 and 60 mg tables.

Dosage and Administration

Adult

PO—Initially 30 mg 4 times daily before meals and at bedtime. The dosage is gradually increased to 60 mg 4 times daily at 1 to 2 day intervals.

Note: Patients may continue nitroglycerin therapy for acute anginal attacks while being stabilized on diltiazem therapy.

Nursing Interventions

See also General Nursing Considerations for Patients with Cardiovascular disease.

See General Nursing Considerations for Patients Receiving Calcium Ion Antagonists.

Nifedipine (ny-fed′i-peen)
(Procardia) (pro-kar′dee-ah)

Nifedipine is a calcium ion antagonist structurally unrelated to other calcium antagonists available. Its mechanisms of action are unknown, but it is a potent vasodilator of coronary and peripheral arteries. It reduces peripheral vascular resistance, thus reducing systolic and diastolic blood pressure, and improves blood flow and oxygenation to the coronary tissues. Nifedipine is currently being used to treat patients with angina pectoris who do not respond adequately to nitrates or beta adrenergic agents. Nifedipine has an advantage in that since it does not slow the heart rate, it can be used more effectively in patients with a reduced heart rate and in combination with digitalis and beta adrenergic blocking agents.

Side Effects

When starting therapy or increasing doses, patients report an increased frequency of angina pectoris. The cause of this is unknown. Sublingual nitroglycerin therapy should be continued until the dosage is stabilized.

The following are the most common side effects and occur in about 10% of patients: dizziness, light-headedness, peripheral edema, nausea, weakness, headache, and flushing. Transient hypotension develops in about 5%, palpitations in 2%, and syncope in 0.5% of patients. Hypotension and peripheral edema occur more frequently in patients receiving higher dosages of nifedipine.

Other adverse effects that develop in less than 2% of patients include nasal and chest congestion, constipation, cramps, fever and chills, sweating, urticaria, pruritus, nervousness, and sleep disturbances.

Availability

PO—10 mg capsules.

Dosage and Administration

Adult

PO—Initially 10 mg 3 times daily. Adjust the dosage upward over the next 7 to 14 days to balance between antianginal and hypotensive activity. The usual effective dose is 10 to 20 mg 3 times daily. Dosages above 180 mg are not recommended. Sublingual nitroglycerin therapy may be continued for acute anginal attacks, especially during adjustment of dosages.

Nursing Interventions

See also General Nursing Considerations for Patients with Cardiovascular Disease.

See General Nursing Considerations for Patients Receiving Calcium Ion Antagonists.

Verapamil hydrochloride (ver-ap′a-mil)
(Calan, Isoptin) (ka′lan; ice-op′tin)

Verapamil is a calcium ion antagonist structurally unrelated to other calcium antagonists available. Its mechanisms of action are unknown, but it slows electrical conduction across the atrioventricular node, reducing rapid ventricular rate caused by atrial flutter or atrial fibrillation. It also produces coronary and peripheral arterial vasodilation, resulting in improved myocardial oxygenation. Verapamil is currently being used to treat angina pectoris and arrhythmias that are initiated within atrial tissue.

Side Effects

The following side effects have been reported with oral verapamil therapy: constipation (6.3%), dizziness (3.6%), hypotension (2.9%), headache (1.8%), peripheral edema (1.7), nausea (1.6%), fatigue (1.1%), bradycardia (1.1%), and complete atrioventricular heart block (0.8%).

The following side effects have been reported with IV verapamil therapy: hypotension (1.5%), bradycardia (1.2%), dizziness and headache (1.2%), severe tachycardia (1.0%), nausea (0.9%), and abdominal discomfort (0.6%).

Availability

PO—80 and 120 mg tablets.
IV—2.5 mg/ml in 2 ml ampules.

Dosage and Administration

Adult

PO—Initially 80 mg 3 to 4 times daily. Increase weekly until an optimal clinical response is achieved. The total daily dose ranges from 240 to 480 mg. Most patients will require 320 to 480 mg daily.

IV—Initially 5 to 10 mg administered over 2 to 3 minutes with continuous ECG monitoring. Additional doses of 10 mg every 30 minutes may be administered if therapeutic activity has not been achieved. Administer each dose over 3 minutes.

Note: Sublingual nitroglycerin therapy may be continued for acute anginal attacks.

Pediatric

IV—Newborn to 1 year of age: 0.1 to 0.2 mg/kg over 2 minutes with continuous ECG monitoring. 1 to 15 years of age: 0.1 to 0.3 mg/kg over 2 minutes with continuous ECG monitoring. Do not exceed 5 mg. Repeat above doses 30 minutes after the first dose if the initial response is not adequate.

Nursing Interventions

See also General Nursing Considerations for Patients with Cardiovascular disease.

See General Nursing Considerations for Patients Receiving Calcium Ion Antagonists

General Nursing Considerations for Patients Receiving Calcium Ion Antagonists

PATIENT CONCERNS: NURSING INTERVENTION/RATIONALE

Side Effects to Report

Anginal Attacks

Monitor patients taking calcium ion antagonists for an increase in anginal attacks during initiation of the medication or during dosage adjustments. Reduce patients' fears by assuring them that once the dosage is stabilized, the frequency of these attacks will subside.

Assess for frequency, location, duration, and intensity of anginal pain and have the patient *continue* to take the nitroglycerin sublingually when attacks occur.

Hypotension and Syncopy

Caution the patient that for the first week or so, the patient may experience hypotension and syncopy. These side effects decline once the dosage is stabilized.

Take blood pressure reading every shift in the hospitalized patient and stress the need for the patient to monitor it after discharge.

Prevent hypotensive episodes by having the patient rise slowly from a supine or sitting position and perform exercises to prevent blood pooling when standing or sitting in one position for prolonged periods. If the patient feels "faint," have him or her sit or lie down.

Edema

Assess the patient for development of edema. Perform daily weights:

1. At the same time
2. In similar clothing
3. On the same scale

Report increases in weight to the physician for further evaluation.

Dosage and Administration

Dosage Adjustments

See individual drugs for dosage parameters.

Adjustments are made based upon the individual patient's response to therapy.

Remember that anginal attacks may increase during dosage adjustments; sublingual nitroglycerin should be continued for these episodes.

Drug Interactions

Drugs That Enhance Therapeutic and Toxic Effects

Beta adrenergic blocking agents (i.e., propranolol, atenolol, nadolol, pindolol, others): Assess the patient for hypotension, light-headedness, dizziness, and bradycardia.

Provide for patient safety; prevent falls.

Other Interactions

DIGITALIS GLYCOSIDES

Calcium ion antagonists may increase serum levels of digitalis glycosides.

Monitor the patient for symptoms of anorexia, nausea, vomiting, headaches, blurred or colored vision, and bradycardia. The physician may order a digitalis serum level.

ANTIHYPERTENSIVE AGENTS

The vasodilating action of the calcium ion antagonists and antihypertensive agents may result in excessive hypotensive effects. Assess blood pressure at regular intervals to monitor the combined effects.

GLUCOSE METABOLISM

The dosage of oral hypoglycemic agents may require adjustment in non-insulin-dependent diabetes mellitus (NIDDM) patients.
Assess for signs of hyperglycemia.
Perform urine testing for glucose 4 times per day; report results 1% or above.

VERAPAMIL AND DISOPYRAMIDE

DO NOT administer disopyramide 48 hours before or 24 hours after the administration of verapamil.

Coronary Vasodilators

Vasodilators are drugs that cause dilation of blood vessels. The nitrites (organic nitrites and nitrates) have long been used in medicine as vasodilators. The nitrites have a direct action that causes relaxation of most smooth muscles in the body, including the bronchial, gastrointestinal, biliary, and uterine smooth muscle. The most important pharmacologic effects are on the smooth muscle of the blood vessels. Nitrites are used extensively for patients with angina pectoris, and the rapid-acting nitrites remain the drug of choice for this condition.

Side Effects

The side effects of the nitrites result from the vasodilator action. They include flushing of the skin, severe headache, nausea and vomiting, hypotension, and vertigo.

Tolerance to the "long-acting" nitrites develops easily, but usually does not develop with nitroglycerin. The smallest dose to give satisfactory results should be used so that the dose may be increased as tolerance develops. Tolerance can appear within a few days and may be well established within a few weeks. Tolerance is broken by withdrawal of the drug for a short period.

Drug Interactions

When used concurrently with the nitrites, alcohol may enhance the therapeutic and toxic effects of the nitrites.

General Nursing Considerations for Patients with Angina Pectoris

The patient experiencing anginal episodes is apprehensive and frequently becomes discouraged if unable to tolerate exercise or participate in activities of daily living at a pre-illness level. Appropriate use of medications can help these patients approach this goal.

The nurse must carefully perform a baseline assessment of the individual's pattern of anginal pain and the responses exhibited to medical management. Fostering compliance with the patient's total treatment plan is essential to his or her attainment of optimal response. (See General Nursing Considerations for Patients with Cardiovascular Disease for further details of assessment.)

PATIENT CONCERNS: NURSING INTERVENTION/RATIONALE

Degree of Anginal Pain Relief

Monitor and record the following data relative to the pain relief achieved from the medication:

1. Number of pain attacks per day (per shift while hospitalized).
2. Length of time between taking the medication and relief of anginal symptoms.
3. Degree of pain relief achieved (partial or complete).
4. Number of times sublingual doses were repeated before relief was achieved.
5. Record any particular activities that usually precipitate the anginal pain; suggest taking sublingual nitroglycerin, if ordered, prior to undertaking the activity.

Patient Teaching Associated with Coronary Vasodilator Therapy

Communication and Responsibility

Encourage open communication concerning frustrations and anger as the patient attempts to adjust to the diagnosis and need for prolonged treatment. The patient must be guided to gain insight into the condition in order to assume responsibility for the continuation of treatment. Keep emphasizing those factors the patient can control to alter progression of the disease.

SMOKING

Smoking causes vasoconstriction; therefore, encourage drastic reduction and preferably total abstinence from smoking.

HYPERTENSION

If the disease process is accompanied by hypertension, stress the importance of following prescribed emotional, dietary, and medicinal regimens to control the disease.

NUTRITION

The physician usually prescribes dietary modifications aimed at decreasing the cholesterol level and a reducing program to maintain an ideal weight.

Caffeine consumption should be drastically reduced or discontinued. Introduce the patient to decaffeinated products that can substitute for foods containing caffeine.

Expectations of Therapy

Discuss expectations of therapy with the patient:

ACTIVITIES AND EXERCISE

The patient must resume activities of daily living *within the boundaries* set by the physician. (Such activities as regular, moderate exercise, meal preparation, resumption of usual sexual activities, and social interaction all need to be fostered.)

Individuals who are unable to attain the degree of activity they hoped the drug would allow them to achieve may become frustrated.

Caution the patient *not* to attempt more exercise than recommended once pain relief is attained.

ENVIRONMENT

Tell the patient the importance of dressing warmly, avoiding cold winds, and the need to use a face mask in these conditions to prewarm inhaled air.

PAIN RELIEF

The degree of anginal pain relief with and without activity needs to be discussed.

SEXUAL ACTIVITY

Encourage the patient to resume sexual activity. Discuss the use of medication or other adjustments for anginal pain before this activity.

Changes in Expectations

Assess changes in expectations as therapy progresses and the patient gains understanding and skill in the management of the diagnosis.

Changes in Therapy through Cooperative Goal-Setting

Work with the patient to encourage adherence to the prescribed treatment. When the patient feels that a change should be made in a treatment plan, encourage discussion first with the physician.

WRITTEN RECORD

Enlist the patient's aid in developing and maintaining a written record (Table 10.1, page 242) of monitoring parameters (i.e., blood pressure, pulse, degree of pain relief, exercise tolerance, and side effects experienced), and response to prescribed therapies for discussion with the physician. Patients should be encouraged to take this record on follow-up visits.

FOSTERING COMPLIANCE

Throughout the hospitalization, discuss medication information and how it will benefit the course of treatment. Seek cooperation and understanding of the following points so that medication compliance may be enhanced:

1. Name.
2. Dosage.
3. Route and administration times.
4. Anticipated therapeutic response: Relief of anginal pain.
5. Side effects to expect: flushing of the face and neck, transient throbbing headache.

    Hypotension: Have the patient rise slowly from a sitting and/or lying position. Weakness, dizziness, or "faintness" can usually be relieved by increasing muscular activity or by sitting or lying down. Resting for 10 to 15 minutes after taking medication may also assist in management of the hypotension.
6. Side effects to report: Always report poor response to medication. The patient may exhibit tolerance to the medication, may need further evaluation of the progression of the disease, or re-education on the proper use of the medication (i.e., proper application of ointment, use of sublingual nitroglycerin prior to undertaking an activity known to precipitate an anginal attack).

Table 10.1

Example of a Written Record for Patients Receiving Cardiovascular Agents

Medications	Color	To be taken

Name _____

Physician _____

Physician's phone _____

Next appt.* _____

Parameters		Day of discharge								Comments
Weight	AM / PM	/	/	/	/	/	/	/	/	
Blood pressure	AM / PM	/	/	/	/	/	/	/	/	
Pulse	AM / PM	/	/	/	/	/	/	/	/	
Chest pain	Activity Lasting how long? How many nitroglycerin taken?									
Bowel movements	Normal (times) Diarrhea (times) Constipation									
Fatigue All day 10 After exercise 5 Normal 1										
Edema	Morning									
	Evening									
	Other									
	Can wear shoes, slippers?									
Visual changes	Clear, hazy, blurred, colored haloes?									
Fainting and dizziness	Standing, sitting, or lying									
Heart beat ("Skips a beat," "racing" feeling or irregular)	Times per day At rest Activity Asleep									
Difficulty breathing	Times per day At rest Activity Asleep (_#_) of pillows?									
Exercise: Degree of tiredness: Extremely 10 Very 5 Normal 1	Walk across room Walk (_#_) stairs Walk (_#_) blocks									
Sexual activity (Note pain experienced in comments at right side.) Very tired 10 Tired 5 Normal 1										

*Please bring this record with you to your next appointment.
Use the back of this sheet for additional information.

Report episodes of severe hypotension, prolonged headache, and blurred vision.
7. What to do if a dosage is missed
8. When, how, or if to refill the medication prescription.

If it is evident that the patient and/or family does not understand all aspects of continuing therapy being prescribed (i.e., administration and monitoring of medications, exercises, diets, follow-up appointments), consider the use of social service or visiting nurse agencies.

ASSOCIATED TEACHING

Give patients the following instructions:

Alway inform the physician or dentist of any prescription or over-the-counter medication being taken. Over-the-counter medications should not be taken without first discussing them with the physician or pharmacist.

Always report side effects of rash, itching, or hives immediately. Nausea, vomiting, or diarrhea should also be reported for the physician's evaluation if it is a new symptom.

Take all of the medication as prescribed for the full course of treatment. Do not discontinue use when feeling improved; do not save for future use; do not give your medicine to another individual. Sudden discontinuation of certain medications may produce harmful effects.

Keep all medications out of the reach of children.

If pregnancy is suspected, consult an obstetrician as soon as possible about continuation of medication therapy.

At Discharge

Items to be sent home with the patient should:

1. Have written instructions for use.
2. Be labeled in a level of language and size of print appropriate for the patient.
3. If needed, include identification cards or bracelets.
4. Include a list of additional supplies to be purchased after discharge (i.e., protective covering such as clear plastic, tape).
5. Include a schedule for follow-up appointments.

Vasodilator Preparations

Amyl nitrite (am′il ny′tryt)

Amyl nitrite is a volatile liquid, available in small glass ampules. The ampules are encased in a loosely woven material so that the ampule can be easily crushed under the patient's nostrils for inhalation. The onset of action is less than 1 minute, but the duration is only about 10 minutes.

The side effects of amyl nitrite are an extension of its pharmacologic activity. In addition to coronary vasodilation, it causes cutaneous vasodilation, marked lowering of systemic pressure, syncope, and tachycardia. Occasionally a patient will also suffer from a throbbing headache and nausea and vomiting. Consequently, amyl nitrite is no longer used frequently in the treatment of angina pectoris.

Availability

Inhalation—0.3 ml ampules in a woven sack for crushing.

Nursing Interventions

See also General Nursing Considerations for Patients with Cardiovascular Disease.

See also General Nursing Considerations for Patients with Angina Pectoris.

Erythrityl tetranitrate (e-rith′ri-til tet-rah-ny′trayt)
Cardilate (kar′di-layt)

Availability

PO—5, 10 mg oral/sublingual tablets; 10 mg chewable tablets.

Dosage and Administration

Adult

PO—Sublingual: 5 to 10 mg tablet placed under the tongue before anticipated physical or emotional stress. Oral: If the patient is able to swallow the tablet, therapy should be initiated with 10 mg before each meal, as well as midmorning and midafternoon if needed, and at bedtime for patients subject to nocturnal attacks. The dose may be increased or decreased as needed.

Dosage may be increased up to 100 mg daily, but temporary headache is more apt to occur with increasing doses. If headache occurs, the dose should be reduced for a few days.

Nusing Interventions

See also General Nursing Considerations for Patients with Cardiovascular Disease.

See also General Nursing Considerations for Patients with Angina Pectoris.

Isosorbide dinitrate (i-so-sor′byd) *(Isordil)* (i′sor-dil)

Availability

PO—2.5, 5 mg sublingual tablets; 5, 10, and 20 mg oral tablets; 5, 10 mg chewable tablets; and 40 mg long-acting oral tablets and capsules.

Dosage and Administration

Adult

PO—Sublingual: 5 to 10 mg every 3 hours.
Chewable: Initially 5 mg every 2 to 3 hours.
Oral: Initially 10 mg 4 times daily. Dosage may range up to 30 mg 4 times daily.
Long-acting: Initially 40 mg every 6 hours.

Nursing Interventions

See also General Nursing Considerations for Patients with Cardiovascular Disease.

See also General Nursing Considerations for Patients with Angina Pectoris.

Nitroglycerin (ny-tro-glis′er-in), *Glyceryl trinitrate* (glis′er-il try-ny′trayt)

Nitroglycerin is currently the drug of choice for treating angina pectoris. It is available in different dosages for adjustment to the patient's needs. Sublingual tablets dissolve quite rapidly and are used primarily for acute attacks of angina. The sustained release tablets and capsules, ointment, transmucosal tablets, and transdermal patches are used prophylactically to prevent anginal attacks.

Availability

Sublingual—0.15, 0.3, 0.4, and 0.6 mg tablets.
PO—2.5 and 6.5 mg tablets.
Ointment—2%.
Transmucosal—1 and 2 mg tablets.
Transdermal—5, 10, 15, 16, 20, 30, 32 mg patches.
Intravenous—5 mg/10 ml, 8 mg/10 ml, 25 mg/5 ml, and 50 mg/10 ml ampule.

Dosage and Administration

Sublingual. 0.15, 0.3, 0.4, or 0.6 mg for prophylactic use before the initiation of activity that may induce angina pectoris, or at the time of an acute anginal attack.

PO. Sustained release tablets or capsules: 1.3, 2.5, or 6.5 mg. 2 to 3 times daily at 8 and 12 hour intervals.

Transmucosal Tablets. 1 to 2 mg 3 to 6 times daily.

Topical Ointment. This dosage form is more suitable for patients who suffer from the fear of nocturnal attacks of angina pectoris. If the dosage is adjusted properly, the ointment may be used every 3 to 4 hours and at bedtime.

Topical Disks. This dosage form provides a controlled release of nitroglycerin through a semipermeable membrane for 24 hours when applied to intact skin. The dosage released is dependent upon the surface area of the disk. Therapeutic effect can be observed about 30 minutes after attachment, and is maintained for about 30 minutes after removal.

Intravenous. This dosage form is diluted and then administered by continuous infusion to treat high blood pressure during surgery, congestive heart failure associated with acute myocardial infarction, angina pectoris in patients who have not responded to other dosage forms of nitroglycerin, and to produce controlled hypotension during certain surgical procedures.

Nursing Interventions

See also General Nursing Considerations for Patients with Cardiovascular Disease.

See also General Nursing Considerations for Patients with Angina Pectoris.

PATIENT CONCERNS: NURSING INTERVENTION/RATIONALE

Side Effects to Report

Prolonged Headache, Excessive Hypotension, Tolerance (Increasing Doses to Attain Relief)

Report these adverse effects so that more appropriate dosage adjustment may be made.

Dosage and Administration

Sublingual

1. Have the patient sit or lie down at the first sign of an oncoming anginal attack.
2. Place a tablet under the tongue and allow it to dissolve; encourage the patient not to swallow the saliva immediately.
3. If more than 3 tablets within 15 minutes are required to control pain, the patient should seek medical attention.
4. One or two tablets may be taken prophylactically a few minutes before engaging in activities that may trigger an anginal attack.
5. Chart the patient's ability to place the sublingual medication under the tongue correctly.

MEDICATION DETERIORATION

Every 3 months, the nitroglycerin prescription should be refilled and the old tablets safely discarded. (Be sure the patient knows how to refill the prescription.)

MEDICATION STORAGE

Store nitroglycerin in the original, dark-colored glass container with a tight lid.

MEDICATION ACCESSIBILITY

Nonhospitalized patients should carry nitroglycerin with them at all times, but not in a pocket directly next to the body, because heat hastens the deterioration of the medication. When taken, the drug should produce a slight "stinging" or "burning" sensation, which usually indicates the drug is still potent.

Allow the hospitalized patient to keep the nitroglycerin at bedside, or on his or her person, if ambulatory. Check hospital policy to see if a fresh supply of medicine should be issued, rather than using the agents brought from home. (Remember, the nurse is still responsible for gathering and charting relevant data regarding all medication taken by the patient when the medication is left at bedside.)

Sustained Release Tablets

This type of nitroglycerin is best taken on an empty stomach every 8 to 12 hours, as prescribed.

If gastritis develops, it may be necessary to take the sustained release tablet with food.

Transmucosal Tablets

When placed under the upper lip or buccal pouch, it releases nitroglycerin for absorption by the oral mucosa over the next 3 to 5 hours.

Patients may eat, drink, and talk while the tablet is in place.

The usual initial dose is one tablet 3 times daily upon arising, after lunch, and after the evening meal.

Do not administer more than one tablet every 2 hours.

Development of headache, dizziness, and hypotension are indications of overdose.

Topical Ointment

1. Lay the dose-measuring applicator paper with the printed side down.
2. Squeeze the proper amount of ointment onto the applicator paper.
3. Place the measuring applicator on the skin, ointment down, spreading in a thin, uniform layer. Do not massage or rub in. Any area without hair may be used; however, many people prefer the chest, flank, or upper arm. (Because of the potential for skin irritation, do not shave an area to apply the medication.)
4. Help the patient develop a site rotation schedule to prevent skin irritation. Stress not applying the ointment to an area that still shows signs of irritation. Use of the applicator allows measuring of the proper dose and also prevents absorption through the fingertips.
5. Cover the area where the patch is placed with a clear plastic wrap and tape in place. (Caution the patient that the medication may discolor clothing.)
6. Close the tube tightly and store in a cool place.
7. When terminating the use of the topical ointment, gradually reduce the dose and frequency of application over 4 to 6 weeks.

Topical Disks

This dosage form provides a controlled release of nitroglycerin through a semipermeable membrane for 24 hours when applied to intact skin. The dosage released is dependent upon the surface area of the disk. Therapeutic effect can be observed in about 30 minutes after attachment, and continues for about 30 minutes after removal.

1. The disk should be applied to a hairless and clean-shaven area of skin on the upper chest or side, pelvis, or inner, upper arm. Avoid scars, skin folds, or wounds. Rotate skin sites daily. (Help the patient develop a rotation chart.)
2. Wash hands before applying and after removing the product.
3. Transderm-Nitro and Nitro-Dur may be worn while showering; Nitrodisc should be replaced after bathing.

4. If a disk becomes partially dislodged, discard it and replace with a new disk.
5. Sublingual nitroglycerin may be necessary for anginal attacks, especially while the dosage is being adjusted.

Intravenous Nitroglycerin

This drug is used in an intensive care setting and requires continuous monitoring of vital signs: blood pressure, pulse, respirations, and central venous pressure.

Use an infusion pump to monitor the precise delivery of the infusion. Dose is titrated to achieve the desired clinical response. Gradual weaning is needed under controlled conditions to prevent a rebound action.

This medication is never mixed with other medications and is administered only with administration sets made specially for nitroglycerin, since most plastic administration sets absorb the drug. See the manufacturer's literature for exact directions recommended for preparation and administration.

Drug Interactions

Alcohol

Alcohol accentuates the vasodilation and postural hypotension of the nitrates and nitrites. Patients should be warned that drinking alcohol while on therapy may cause hypotension.

Pentaerythritol tetranitrate (pen-tah-e-rith′ri-tol tet-rah-ny′trayt) **(Peritrate)** (per′i-trayt) **(Pentritol)** (pen′tri-tol)

Pentaerythritol tetranitrate is a nitrate derivative that is used for the relief of angina pectoris. It does not relieve the acute anginal episode, but is widely regarded as useful in the prophylactic treatment of angina pectoris.

Availability

PO—10, 20, 40 mg tablets; 80 mg sustained release tablet.

Dosage and Administration

Adult
PO—Initially 10 to 20 mg 4 times daily. Dosage may be adjusted up to 40 mg 4 times daily. Take one-half hour before meals. Tablets may be chewed or swallowed whole.

Alternatively, Peritrate SA (sustained action) can be administered every 12 hours. It should be taken on an empty stomach and *not* chewed.

Nursing Interventions

See also General Nursing Considerations for Patients with Cardiovascular Disease.
See also General Nursing Considerations for Patients with Angina Pectoris.

Peripheral Vasodilators

The use of vasodilating agents for chronic occlusive arterial disease or peripheral vascular disease has not been encouraging to date. However, several drugs have been used with some success in the treatment of these diseases.

General Nursing Considerations for Patients with Peripheral Vascular Disease

A baseline assessment of the individual patient should be completed. It should include the following data to evaluate the degree of oxygenation that exists in the extremities. Subsequent *regular* assessments should be performed for comparison and analysis of therapeutic effectiveness or lack of response to *all* treatment modalities instituted.

PATIENT CONCERNS: NURSING INTERVENTION/RATIONALE

Assessment of Tissue

Oxygenation

Observe the color of each hand, finger, leg, and foot; report cyanosis or reddish-blue locations.
Examine the skin of the extremities for any signs of ulceration.

Temperature

Feel the temperature in each hand, finger, leg, and foot. Report paleness and coldness. (Note that these symptoms will be increased if the limb is elevated above the level of the heart.)

Edema

Report edema and its extent, and whether relieved or unchanged when the limb is in a dependent position.

Peripheral Pulses

Record the pedal and radial pulses at least every 4 hours if circulatory impairment is found in that limb. Compare findings between each of the extremities; report diminished or absent pulses immediately.

Limb Pain

Monitor pain in the patient carefully. Pain upon exercise that is relieved by rest may be from claudication. Conversely, pain when the patient is at rest may be from sudden obstruction by a thrombus or embolus. Check pedal and radial pulses, vital signs, and the degree of apprehension of the patient, then notify the physician of the specific findings.

Patient Teaching for Patients with Peripheral Vascular Disease

Communication and Responsibility

Encourage open communication concerning frustrations and anger as the patient attempts to adjust to the diagnosis and need for prolonged treatment. The patient must be guided to gain insight into the condition in order to assume responsibility for the continuation of treatment. Keep emphasizing those factors that the patient can control to alter the progression of the disease, including:

SMOKING

Smoking causes vasoconstriction of the blood vessels. Therefore, encourage drastic reduction and preferably total abstinence from smoking.

PROMOTING PERIPHERAL CIRCULATION

Patients should be taught to maintain posture that will maximize peripheral circulation.

Encourage patients not to wear anything that constricts peripheral blood flow, such as tight-fitting anklets, socks, or garters. Always check with the physician before initiating elevation of the extremities. It is *contraindicated* in patients with *arterial* insufficiency. Tell the patient *not* to elevate the extremities above the level of the heart without specific orders to do so from the physician.

SITTING OR STANDING

Standing or sitting for prolonged periods should be avoided:

Persons who must sit for extended periods of time must have a properly fitting chair. The seat must be of the correct depth so that no pressure is exerted on the popliteal space.

Encourage individuals not to sit with knees or ankles crossed and to take frequent short breaks for walks.

Persons who must stand for long periods of time should seek aspects of the job that can be performed sitting down in a properly fitting chair or other alternatives.

For the hospitalized patient, do not place pillows in the popliteal space or flex the knee-rest on the bed.

LIMB PAIN

Meticulous foot and hand care are essential. The need to inspect the extremities for possible skin breakdown or signs of infection must be stressed. Notify the physician immediately of sudden changes in color, such as mottling or a more purplish color. Cold temperatures will increase pain or decrease sensations in the extremities.

Areas of discoloration in nails, cracking of skin, callouses, or blisters on the extremities need complete follow-up. Listen to the patient's description of changes he or she has noted. Tell the patient that going barefoot can be dangerous because of potential injuries to the feet.

Because of the possible decrease in sensation in the extremities, encourage the patient to test the water temperature prior to immersing the hands or feet. Following bathing, gently pat, do not vigorously rub, the feet and hands to dry them.

Patients should alternate pairs of shoes to allow for thorough drying between wearings, change socks or hose daily, and avoid rubber-soled shoes.

If the patient is hospitalized, use a cradle or footboard to prevent bedsheets from constricting the circulation. Show the patient or family how to improvise a footboard at home.

The physician may order the foot of the patient's bed elevated at night. Encourage the patient to maintain good posture and to sleep on a firm mattress.

UNABOOT or TED stockings may also be employed to promote circulation.

ACTIVITY AND EXERCISE

Maximum mobility should be maintained. Devise a daily activity plan that includes walks and usual activities of daily living, such as shopping and housework.

ENVIRONMENT

During periods of exposure to cold temperature, the patient should wear several layers of lightweight clothing. Caution needs to be exercised during exposure to the cold to avoid frostbite. Because of decreased sensations in the extremities, frostbite can occur without the patient's awareness.

PAIN RELIEF

Pain management and the psychological aspects of dealing with a prolonged illness with persistent symptoms are a major challenge to the patient and the nurse. (See Chapter 8 for pain management information.)

NUTRITIONAL STATUS

Dietary education is indicated in the treatment of peripheral vascular disease. It is particularly important to control obesity and cholesterol and triglyceride levels.

When ulcerations are present, encourage a high protein diet to promote the healing process.

Unless other medical conditions contraindicate, have the patient drink eight 8-ounce glasses of water daily to promote adequate hydration of body tissues. This will help reduce peripheral vasoconstriction.

Caffeine does not necessarily have to be limited unless other coexisting conditions warrant it.

Expectations of Therapy

Discuss expectations of therapy with the patient: degree of pain relief, ability to work, maintenance of mobility, and exercise tolerance that the drug regimen and preventive measures will permit.

Encourage the patient to express *feelings* with regard to this chronic illness. The adjustment to this situation involves working through great personal fears, frustrations, hostilities, and resentments associated with the loss of control within one's life.

Changes in Expectations

Assess changes in expectations as therapy progresses and the patient gains understanding and skill in the management of the diagnosis.

Changes in Therapy through Cooperative Goal-Setting

Work with the patient to encourage adherence to the prescribed treatment. When the patient feels that a change should be made in a treatment plan, encourage discussion first with the physician.

WRITTEN RECORD

Enlist the patient's aid in developing and maintaining a written record of monitoring parameters (Table 10.1, page 242) (i.e., degree of numbness, color, and temperature of extremities, degree of pain relief, exercise tolerance), and response to prescribed therapies for discussion with the physician. Encourage patients to take this record on follow-up visits.

FOSTERING COMPLIANCE

Throughout the hospitalization, discuss medication information and how it will benefit the course of treatment.

Stress the importance of all measures taught (stopping smoking, promotion of peripheral circulation, activity and exercise, and nutritional actions) to promote maximum peripheral vascular circulation and prevention of further tissue damage.

Seek cooperation and understanding of the following points so that medication compliance may be enhanced:

1. Name
2. Dosage
3. Route and administration times
4. Anticipated therapeutic response
5. Side effects to expect
6. Side effects to report
7. What to do if a dosage is missed
8. When, how, or if to refill the medication prescription

DIFFICULTY IN COMPREHENSION

If it is evident that the patient and/or family does not understand all aspects of continuing therapy being prescribed (i.e., administration and monitoring of medications, exercises, diets, follow-up appointments), consider the use of social service or visiting nurse agencies.

ASSOCIATED TEACHING

Give patients the following instructions:

Always inform the physician or dentist of any prescription or over-the-counter medication being taken. Over-the-counter medications should not be taken without first discussing them with the physician or pharmacist.

Always report side effects of rash, itching, or hives immediately. Nausea, vomiting, or diarrhea should also be reported for the physician's evaluation if it is a new symptom.

Take all of the medication as prescribed for the full course of treatment. Do not discontinue use when feeling improved; do not save for future use; do not give your medicine to another individual. Sudden discontinuation of certain medications may produce harmful effects.

Keep all medications out of the reach of children.

If pregnancy is suspected, consult an obstetrician as soon as possible about continuation of medication therapy.

At Discharge

Items to be sent home with the patient should:

1. Have written instructions for use.
2. Be labeled in a level of language and size of print appropriate for the patient.
3. If needed, include identification cards or bracelets.
4. Include a list of additional supplies to be purchased after discharge.
5. Include a schedule of appointments for follow-up visits.

Peripheral Vasodilating Agents

Cyclandelate (si-klan′de-layt)
(Cyclospasmol) (si-klo-spaz′mol)

Cyclandelate has a direct relaxation effect on the smooth muscles of peripheral arterial blood vessels, increasing circulation to the extremities. It is considered "possibly" effective in treating patients with intermittent claudication, arteriosclerosis obliterans, vasospasm associated with thrombophlebitis, nocturnal leg cramps, and Raynaud's disease.

Side Effects

Side effects include flushing, tingling, sweating, dizziness, headache, feeling of weakness, and tachycardia. These side effects tend to be more common during the first weeks of therapy, and resolve with continued therapy.

Since cyclandelate is a vasodilator, it should be used with caution in patients with glaucoma.

Availability

PO—100, 200, and 400 mg capsules.

Dosage and Administration

Adult
PO—It is often advantageous to initiate therapy at higher dosages: 1200 to 1600 mg daily in divided doses before meals and at bedtime. When a clinical response is noted, the dosage can be decreased in 200 mg increments until the maintenance dosage is reached. The usual maintenance dose is between 400 and 800 mg per day in 2 to 4 divided doses.

Nursing Interventions

See also General Nursing Considerations for Patients with Peripheral Vascular Disease.

**PATIENT CONCERNS:
NURSING INTERVENTION/RATIONALE**

Side Effects to Expect

Flushing, Tingling, Sweating

Explain to the patient that these side effects may occur during the initial phase of therapy; however, these symptoms resolve with continued therapy.

Dosage and Administration

PO

Administer at meals or with milk to decrease gastric irritation.

Drug Interactions

None specifically associated with cyclandelate have been reported.

Isoxsuprine hydrochloride (i-sok′su-preen)
(Vasodilan) (vas-o-dy′lan)

Isoxsuprine hydrochloride is a sympathomimetic agent that causes relaxation of the smooth muscles of the blood vessels. It is used to treat the symptoms of peripheral vascular spasm, cerebral vascular insufficiency, Raynaud's and Buerger's diseases, and arteriosclerosis obliterans.

Side Effects

Adverse effects are quite infrequent, but occasionally a patient may complain of flushing, hypotension, tachycardia, nausea, vomiting, dizziness, abdominal distress, or a severe rash. If a rash does appear, discontinue the medication. As the dosage is increased, more patients tend to complain of nervousness and weakness.

Dosage and Administration

Adult
PO—10 to 20 mg 3 or 4 times daily.
IM—5 to 10 mg 2 or 3 times daily. Intramuscular administration may be used initially in acute conditions.

Nursing Interventions

See also General Nursing Considerations for Patients with Peripheral Vascular Disease.

**PATIENT CONCERNS:
NURSING INTERVENTION/RATIONALE**

Side Effects to Expect

Flushing, Tingling, Sweating, Nausea, Vomiting

Explain to the patient that these side effects may occur during the initial phase of therapy; however, these symptoms resolve with continued therapy.

Side Effects to Report

Hypotension, Tachycardia

Monitor blood pressure and pulse throughout the course of therapy.
Prevent hypotensive episodes by having the patient rise slowly from a supine or sitting position, and perform exercises to prevent blood pooling when standing or sitting in one position for prolonged periods. Have the patient sit or lie down if feeling "faint."

Severe Rash

Discontinue medication if a severe rash develops. Notify the physician so that appropriate alternate agents may be prescribed.

Nervousness and Weakness

As therapy progresses, these symptoms may develop. Tell the patient to discuss them with the physician if they become a problem.

Drug Interactions

Drugs That Enhance Therapeutic and Toxic Effects

Antihypertensive agents:
The vasodilating action of isoxsuprine and antihypertensive agents may result in excessive hypotensive effects.
Assess the blood pressure at regular intervals to monitor the combined effects.
Monitor the patient for hypotension, light-headedness, dizziness, and tachycardia.
Provide for patient safety; prevent falls.

Drugs That Reduce Therapeutic Eeffects

Warn the patient against taking over-the-counter cough and cold preparations without first consulting the physician or pharmacist. Many of these products will counteract the effects of isoxsuprine.

Nicotinyl tartrate (nik-o-ti′nil tar′trayt) *(Roniacol)* (ro-ny′ah-kol)

Nicotinyl tartrate is the tartrate salt of nicotinyl alcohol. When ingested, it is converted to nicotinic acid, which produces direct peripheral vasodilation, primarily in the cutaneous vessels of the face, neck, and ears. There is very little vasodilation of the blood vessels of the lower extremities. This agent is used in the treatment of Raynaud's disease, Buerger's disease, vascular spasm, varicose ulcers, decubital ulcers, Ménière's syndrome, and vertigo.

Side Effects

Side effects are usually quite minor and do not require discontinuation of therapy. The most common side effects are transient flushing, nausea, vomiting, heartburn, tingling of the extremities, and minor rashes.

Higher dosages may cause dizziness, faintness, and hypotension.

Availability

PO—50 mg tablets; 150 mg sustained release tablets; 50 mg/5 ml elixir.

Dosage and Administration

Adult

PO—50 to 100 mg 3 times daily. Sustained release tablets: 150 to 300 mg every 12 hours.

Nursing Interventions

See also General Nursing Considerations for Patients with Peripheral Vascular Disease.

PATIENT CONCERNS:
NURSING INTERVENTION/RATIONALE

Side Effects to Expect

Flushing, Tingling, Sweating, Nausea, Vomiting

Explain to the patient that these side effects may occur during the initial phase of therapy; however, these symptoms resolve with continued therapy.

Side Effects to Report

Hypotension, Tachycardia

Monitor blood pressure and pulse throughout the course of therapy.

Prevent hypotensive episodes by having the patient rise slowly from a supine or sitting position, and perform exercises to prevent blood pooling when standing or sitting in one position for prolonged periods. Have the patient sit or lie down if feeling "faint."

Severe Rash

Discontinue medication if a severe rash develops. Notify the physician so that appropriate alternate agents may be prescribed.

Nervousness and Weakness

These symptoms may develop as therapy progresses. Tell the patient to discuss them with the physician if they become a problem.

Drug Interactions

Drugs That Enhance Therapeutic and Toxic Effects

Antihypertensive agents:

The vasodilating action of nicotinyl tartrate and antihypertensive agents may result in excessive hypotensive effects.

Assess the blood pressure at regular intervals to monitor the combined effects.

Monitor the patient for hypotension, light-headedness, dizziness, and tachycardia.

Provide for patient safety; prevent falls.

Drugs That Reduce Therapeutic Effects

Warn the patient against taking over-the-counter cough and cold preparations without first consulting the physician or pharmacist. Many of these products will counteract the effects of nicotinyl tartrate.

Papaverine hydrochloride (pah-pav′er-in)
(Pavabid) (pah-vah′bid)

Papaverine is a drug that has been tried for many illnesses for many years. Even so, there is very little objective evidence to indicate that it has any therapeutic value. Pharmacologically, it relaxes smooth muscle, vasodilates cerebral and coronary blood vessels, and inhibits atrial and ventricular premature contractions, and ventricular arrhythmias.

Papaverine is used orally as a smooth muscle relaxant to treat cerebral and peripheral ischemia associated with arterial spasm, and myocardial ischemia complicated by arrhythmias.

Side Effects

Side effects are usually quite mild and are dose related. Most common are facial flushing, sweating, nausea, abdominal distress, tachycardia, vertigo, drowsiness, headache, and sedation.

Availability

PO—30, 60, 100, 200, and 300 mg tablets; 150 and 300 mg timed release capsules; 200 mg timed release

tablets; 75 and 150 mg liquid filled capsules; 100 mg/
15 ml elixir.
IV—30 mg/ml in 2 ml ampules and 10 ml vials.

Dosage and Administration

Adult

PO—60 to 300 mg 1 to 5 times daily. Timed release
products: 150 mg every 12 hours. In difficult cases,
increase to 150 mg every 8 hours, or 300 mg every 12
hours.

Nursing Interventions

See also General Nursing Considerations for Patients
with Peripheral Vascular Disease.

**PATIENT CONCERNS:
NURSING INTERVENTION/RATIONALE**

Side Effects to Expect and Report

*Flushing, Sweating, Nausea, Abdominal
Distress, Tachycardia, Vertigo,
Drowsiness, Headache*

These side effects are usually quite mild and are
dose related.
Monitor vital signs (blood pressure, pulse, and respirations) and report deviations from baseline data for
the physician's evaluation.

Drug Interactions

*Drugs That Enhance Therapeutic
and Toxic Effects*

Antihypertensive agents:
The vasodilating action of papaverine and antihypertensive agents may result in excessive hypotensive
effects.
Assess the blood pressure at regular intervals to
monitor the combined effects.
Monitor the patient for hypotension, light-headedness,
dizziness, and tachycardia.
Provide for patient safety; prevent falls.

Drugs That Reduce Therapeutic Effects

Warn the patient against taking over-the-counter
cough and cold preparations without first consulting the
physician or pharmacist. Many of these products will
counteract the effects of papaverine.

Phenoxybenzamine hydrochloride (fe-nok-se-ben'zah-
meen) ***(Dibenzyline)*** (di-ben'zi-leen)

Phenoxybenzamine is an alpha adrenergic blocking
agent that relaxes the smooth muscle of blood vessels,
resulting in vasodilation and improved blood flow to
peripheral tissues. It is used in blood vessel disorders,
such as Raynaud's disease, leg ulceration, and the complications of frostbite.

Side Effects

Severity of side effects is usually dependent upon
the dosage administered. Common side effects include
nasal stuffiness, miosis, hypotension, and tachycardia.
Nausea and vomiting occasionally occur.

Availability

PO—10 mg capsules.

Dosage and Administration

Adult

PO—Initially 10 mg per day. After determining response
for 4 or more days, increase the dose by 10 mg increments
every few days to a maximum of 60 mg per day. Several
weeks of therapy are usually needed to observe full
therapeutic benefits.

Nursing Interventions

See also General Nursing Considerations for Patients
with Peripheral Vascular Disease.

**PATIENT CONCERNS:
NURSING INTERVENTION/RATIONALE**

Side Effects to Expect and Report

*Nasal Stuffiness, Miosis, Hypotension,
and Tachycardia*

Monitor blood pressure and pulse.
Prevent hypotensive episodes by having the patient
rise slowly from a supine or sitting position, and perform
exercises to prevent blood pooling when standing or
sitting in one position for prolonged periods. Have the
patient sit or lie down if feeling "faint."
Report increasing episodes so that dosage is adjusted
accordingly.

Drug Interactions

Drugs That Enhance Therapeutic and Toxic Effects

Antihypertensive agents and alcohol:
The vasodilating action of phenoxybenzamine and antihypertensive agents may result in excessive hypotension effects.
Assess the blood pressure at regular intervals to monitor the combined effects.
Monitor the patient for hypotension, light-headedness, dizziness, and tachycardia.
Provide for patient safety; prevent falls.

Drugs That Reduce Therapeutic Effects

Warn the patient against taking over-the-counter cough and cold preparations without first consulting the physician or pharmacist. Many of these products will counteract the effects of phenoxybenzamine.

Tolazoline hydrochloride (tol-az′o-leen) *(Priscoline)* (pris′ko-leen)

Tolazoline acts directly on the smooth muscle of the blood vessels to produce vasodilation and increased blood flow. It is used to improve the circulation of patients with diabetes, Raynaud's disease, chronic ulcers, gangrene, frostbite, and other spastic peripheral vascular diseases. It should be used cautiously in patients with ulcers, because it also causes stimulation of gastric secretions that might aggravate the ulcers.

Side Effects

Side effects are generally mild and usually decrease progressively during continued therapy. The most common response is flushing of the face, neck, chest, and back as a result of dilation of blood vessels. Other infrequent reactions include arrhythmias, tachycardia, anginal pain, nausea, vomiting, diarrhea, and, rarely, psychiatric reactions characterized by confusion or hallucinations.

Availability

Parenteral—25 mg/ml in 10 ml vials.

Dosage and Administration

Adult

IV, SC, IM—Dosage must be individualized. General dosage requirements are 10 to 50 mg 4 times daily. Start with lower dosages, increasing gradually until

therapeutic response (localized flushing) is observed. Keeping the patient warm will often increase effectiveness of the medication.

Nursing Interventions

See also General Nursing Considerations for Patients with Peripheral Vascular Disease.

PATIENT CONCERNS: NURSING INTERVENTION/RATIONALE

Side Effects to Expect

Flushing of the Face, Neck, Chest, and Back

Tell the patient to expect that these areas will become increasingly red; this is a desirable effect.
Keeping the patient warm enhances the effectiveness of the drug.

Tingling, Sweating, Nausea, Vomiting

Explain to the patient that these side effects may occur during the initial phase of therapy; however, these symptoms are self-limiting.

Side Effects to Report

Arrhythmias, Tachycardia, Anginal Pain

Monitor the pulse rate and report changes in rhythm.
Anginal pain should be reported and the time of onset, frequency, duration, and intensity documented in the nurse's notes for hospitalized patients.

Confusion, Hallucinations

These adverse effects are quite rare, but monitor patients carefully for progressive symptoms of restlessness, agitation, anxiety, hallucinations, and euphoria.
Act calmly with the excited, anxious, or euphoric patient. Provide safety and fulfillment of their needs.
Report this alteration in the patient's response to the physician as soon as possible.

Drug Interactions

Drugs That Enhance Therapeutic and Toxic Effects

Antihypertensive agents and alcohol:

> The vasodilating action of tolazoline and antihypertensive agents may result in excessive hypotensive effects.
>
> Assess the blood pressure at regular intervals to monitor the combined effects.
>
> Monitor the patient for hypotension, light-headedness, dizziness, and tachycardia.
>
> Provide for patient safety; prevent falls.
>
> ### Drugs That Reduce Therapeutic Effects
>
> Warn the patient against taking over-the-counter cough and cold preparations without first consulting the physician or pharmacist. Many of these products will counteract the effects of tolazoline.

Antihypertensive Agents

General Information on Treatment of Hypertension

Hypertension is a disease characterized by an elevation of the blood pressure above values considered normal for patients of similar racial backgrounds, age, and environment. Statistics in North America show that blood pressures above 140/90 to 150/90 mm Hg are associated with premature death, which results from accelerated vascular disease of the brain, heart, and kidneys.

Primary, or *essential*, hypertension accounts for 80% to 90% of all clinical cases of high blood pressure. The following stratification of hypertension by diastolic blood pressure has become standard:

- Mild—90 to 114 mm hg;
- Moderate—105 to 114 mm Hg;
- Severe—115 mm Hg or greater.

The etiology of hypertension is unknown. It is incurable at present, but it is certainly controllable. Thirty-five to forty million Americans have hypertension. The prevalence increases steadily with advancing age. In every age group, the incidence of hypertension is higher for black persons than for white persons of both sexes. Other factors associated with high blood pressure are a family history of hypertension, obesity, spikes of high blood pressure in young adult years, cigarette smoking, hyperglycemia, hypercholesterolemia, preexisting cardiovascular disease (angina, congestive heart failure), abnormal renal function, retinopathies, and a history of a previous stroke.

The goal of antihypertensive therapy is to prolong a useful life by preventing cardiovascular complications. To accomplish this goal, the blood pressure must be reduced and maintained at acceptable levels. Treatment schedules should interfere as little as possible with the patient's lifestyle. Nonpharmacologic therapy must include elimination of smoking, weight control, routine activity, and sodium control. If this therapy is successful in controlling high blood pressure, drug therapy is often not necessary.

Many drugs are used in the treatment of hypertension, but in general, there are only four classes of drugs used: (1) direct vasodilators, such as hydralazine, minoxidil, and prazosin; (2) diuretics, such as the thiazides, bumetanide, furosemide, and ethacrynic acid; (3) sympathetic nervous system stimulants and inhibitors, such as guanethidine, reserpine, methyldopa, the beta blocking agents, guanabenz, and clonidine; and (4) inhibitors of the renin-angiotensin system, such as captopril.

All these agents act either directly or indirectly to reduce the peripheral vascular resistance, therefore lowering blood pressure. It is routine practice to use two or more antihypertensive medications at a time; using drugs that act by different mechanisms to reduce peripheral vascular resistance provides the benefit of using lower doses of each drug, so that the patient suffers fewer side effects. This is known as the *stepped-care approach*, as recommended by the Joint National Committee on Detection, Evaluation, and Treatment of High Blood Pressure. The first step of treatment is the initiation of small doses of diuretics together with dietary and exercise instructions. The dose is gradually increased, and then other drugs are sequentially added until the hypertension is controlled. Addition of subsequent agents is often not necessary because 70% of the adult hypertensive population will respond to diuretics alone. See Table 10.2 for a list of the ingredients of the common antihypertensive combination products.

Patient education is vitally important in treating hypertension. This education should be emphasized and reiterated frequently by the physician, pharmacist, and nurse.

General Nursing Considerations for Patients with Hypertension: Patient Teaching Associated with Antihypertensive Therapy

---

PATIENT CONCERNS: NURSING INTERVENTION/RATIONALE

Communication and Responsibility

Encourage open communication concerning frustrations and anger as the patient attempts to adjust to the diagnosis and need for prolonged treatment.

Table 10.2
*Ingredients of Common Antihypertensive Combination Products**

PRODUCT	DIURETIC (mg)	ANTIHYPERTENSIVE (mg)	OTHER (mg)
Aldoclor-150	Chlorothiazide (150)	Methyldopa (250)	
Aldoril-15	Hydrochlorothiazide (15)	Methyldopa (250)	
Apresazide 25/25	Hydrochlorothiazide (25)	Hydralazine (25)	
Apresoline-Esidrix	Hydrochlorothiazide (15)	Hydralazine (25)	
Butiserpazide-25	Hydrochlorothiazide (25)	Reserpine (0.1)	Butabarbital (30)
Combipres 0.1	Chlorthalidone (15)	Clonidine (0.1)	
Combipres 0.2	Chlorthalidone (15)	Clonidine (0.2)	
Diupres-250	Chlorothiazide (250)	Reserpine (0.125)	
Diutensen-R	Methylclothiazide (2.5)	Reserpine (0.1)	
Enduronyl	Methylclothiazide (5)	Deserpidine (0.25)	
Hydropres-25	Hydrochlorothiazide (25)	Reserpine (0.125)	
Hydrotensin-25	Hydrochlorothiazide (25)	Reserpine (0.125)	
Naturetin W/K	Bendroflumethiazide (5)		Potassium chloride (500)
Oreticyl	Hydrochlorothiazide (25)	Deserpidine (0.125)	
Rautrax	Flumethiazide (400)	Rauwolfia (50)	Potassium chloride (400)
Regroton	Chlorthalidone (50)	Reserpine (0.25)	
Renese-R	Polythiazide (2)	Reserpine (0.25)	
Salutensin	Hydroflumethiazide (50)	Reserpine (0.125)	
Ser-Ap-Es	Hydrochlorothiazide (15)	Reserpine (0.1)	Hydralazine (25)
Serpesil-Apresoline		Reserpine 0.1	Hydralazine (25)
Timolide	Hydrochlorothiazide (25)		Timolol (10)
Unipres	Hydrochlorothiazide (15)	Reserpine 0.1	Hydralazine (25)

* This is a representative listing. Other strengths of these products, as well as products not listed, are available.

Since the disease process is frequently asymptomatic, the patient usually has difficulty accepting the diagnosis. The patient must be guided to insight into the condition in order to assume responsibility for the continuation of treatment. Keep emphasizing those factors the patient can control to alter the progression of the disease.

Smoking

Suggest that the patient stop smoking entirely. Explain the increased risk of coronary artery disease if the habit is continued. It may be necessary to settle for a drastic decrease in smoking in some persons, although total abstinence should be the goal.

Nutritional Status

Dietary counseling is essential in the treatment of hypertension. Control of obesity alone may be sufficient to alter the hypertensive condition. Most patients are placed on a reduced sodium and modified fat diet. Refer to Appendix K for foods high in potassium and/or low in sodium content if these alterations are part of the prescribed dietary modification needed.

Dietary planning should always involve the patient in menu planning so that personal preferences, availability of food products, and cost are discussed. Also include the person who actually purchases as well as prepares the meals in the dietary counseling.

Show the patient various food labels and explain which words to watch for that would indicate a high sodium content (i.e., salt, sodium, sodium chloride, sodium bicarbonate, sodium aluminum sulfate). Suggest the use of a variety of spices as substitutes for sodium when cooking. Explain which foods in large quantities should be avoided (i.e., bacon, smoked meats, crabmeat, tuna, crackers, processed cheeses, ham).

Stress Management

Identify stress-producing situations in the patient's life and seek means to significantly reduce these factors. In some cases, referral for training in stress management, relaxation techniques, meditation, or biofeedback may be necessary. If stress is produced in the work setting, it may be appropriate to involve the industrial nurse.

Stress within the family is often significant and may require professional counseling for the family and patient.

Exercise and Activity

Develop a plan for moderate exercise to improve the patient's general condition. Consult the physician for any individual modifications deemed appropriate.

Suggest including activities the individual finds that help reduce stress.

Blood Pressure Monitoring

Demonstrate the correct procedure for taking blood pressure. Validate the patient's and family's understanding by having them perform this task on several occasions under supervision.

Expectations of Therapy

Discuss expectations of therapy with the patient. Since the disease process is frequently asymptomatic, the patient usually has difficulty accepting the diagnosis.

Always suggest a hopeful course of treatment. Although there is no known cure at this point, there are several important treatments that are successful in the control of hypertension.

Changes in Expectations

Assess changes in expectations as therapy progresses and the patient gains understanding and skill in the management of hypertension.

Changes in Therapy through Cooperative Goal-Setting

Work with the patient to encourage adherence to the prescribed treatment. When the patient feels that a change should be made in a treatment plan, encourage discussion first with the physician.

Written Record

taining a written record (Table 10.3) of monitoring parameters (i.e., blood pressure, pulse, daily weights, exercise tolerance) and response to prescribed therapies for discussion with the physician. Patients should be encouraged to take this record on follow-up visits.

Fostering Compliance

Throughout the hospitalization, discuss medication information and how it will benefit the patient's course of treatment. Seek cooperation and understanding of the following points, so that medication compliance may be enhanced:

1. Name.
2. Dosage.
3. Route and administration times.
4. Anticipated therapeutic response.
   - Gradual reduction and maintenance of blood pressure at an optimal level for the individual.
5. Side effects to expect:
   - When initiating antihypertensive therapy in the hospitalized patient, protect from possible falls by assisting during ambulation and by carefully assessing for faintness. Take blood pressure in lying and standing positions to identify hypotensive responses.
   - Caution the patient that for the first 2 weeks of antihypertensive therapy, he or she may often experience drowsiness. Patients should be told that this side effect is self-limiting. They should be cautious in operating power equipment and driving as long as this symptom exists.
   - A common side effect of antihypertensive medications is hypotension. Have the patient rise slowly from a sitting or lying position. Tell him or her to avoid standing for long periods, especially within 2 hours of taking antihypertensive medication. Weakness, dizziness, or faintness can usually be relieved by increasing muscular activity or by sitting or lying down.
   - Have the person perform exercises that prevent blood pooling in the extremities when sitting or standing for long periods of time. These exercises include flexing the calf muscles, wiggling the toes, rising on the toes and then returning to the feet in a flat position.
6. Side effects to report:
   - See specific agents for further details.
   - The patient should always report a lack of response to the medications prescribed and/or a blood pressure that continues to rise after medications have been taken.
7. What to do if a dosage is missed:
   - Generally, the patient should not take an extra dose of medication if there is a question of a missed dose, but should resume a normal schedule.
   - If forgotten doses become a common occurrence, additional teaching aids should be provided to the patient.
   - Individual agents may require specific instructions.

Table 10.3

Example of a Written Record for Patients Receiving Vasodilators

Medications	Color	To be taken

Name _____

Physician _____

Physician's phone _____

Next appt.* _____

Parameters			Day of discharge							Comments
Weight										
Blood pressure										
Pulse (take for 1 full minute)										
Color of limbs	N = Normal P = Pale M = Mottled B = Blue	Left hand / Right hand Left foot / Right foot								
Pain in limb	Stress									
	Exercise									
	Resting									
	When cold									
	Dull ache									
	Sharp pain									

Intense ———— Moderate ———— Slight
10 ———— 5 ———— 1

Limb pulse	Feel every beat; can count									
	Feel beats; cannot count									
	No pulse felt									
Temperature in normal position										

Cold, pale ———— Cooler than rest of limb ———— Warm
10 ———— 5 ———— 1

Edema	More if hanging down									
	Present all the time									
Exercise	Normal Walk (_#_) stairs Walk (_#_) blocks									

*Please bring this record with you to your next appointment.
Use the back of this sheet for additional information.

8. When, how, or if to refill the medication prescription:
   - Stress that sudden discontinuation of medications can be dangerous. Have the patient explain to you how to refill the prescriptions.
   - You may want to determine if paying for medications is a problem; approach the issue with sensitivity. Also, try to find out if the person has insurance that may cover some of the medication costs. The patient may need assistance in filling out the insurance forms. Involve a social worker in this process if necessary.

Difficulty in Comprehension

If it is evident that the patient and/or family does not understand all aspects of continuing therapy being prescribed (i.e., administration and monitoring of medications, exercises, diets, follow-up appointments), consider the use of social service or visiting nurse agencies.

Associated Teaching

Give patients the following instructions:

Always inform the physician or dentist of any prescription or over-the-counter medication being taken. Over-the-counter medications should not be taken without first discussing them with the physician or pharmacist.

Always report side effects of rash, itching, or hives immediately. Nausea, vomiting, or diarrhea should also be reported for the physician's evaluation if it is a new symptom.

Take all of the medication as prescribed for the full course of treatment. Do not discontinue use when feeling improved; do not save for future use; do not give your medicine to another individual. Sudden discontinuation of certain medications may produce harmful effects.

Keep all medications out of reach of children.

If pregnancy is suspected, consult an obstetrician as soon as possible about continuation of medication therapy.

At Discharge

Items to be sent home with the patient should:

1. Have written instructions for use.

2. Be labeled in a level of language and size of print appropriate for the patient.
3. If needed, include identification cards or bracelets.
4. Include a list of additional supplies to be purchased after discharge.
5. Include a schedule of follow-up visits.

Sympathetic Nervous System Stimulants and Inhibitors

Atenolol (a-ten'o-lol) (Tenormin) (ten-or'-min)

Atenolol is a beta adrenergic blocking agent used in combination with other antihypertensive therapy to treat mild to severe hypertension. Atenolol is discussed in greater detail elsewhere (see Index).

Clonidine hydrochloride (klo'ni-deen) (Catapres) (cat'ah-pres)

Clonidine is a potent antihypertensive agent that acts within the central nervous system to reduce both cardiac output and peripheral vascular resistance, thus reducing both systolic and diastolic blood pressure. After prolonged therapy, the lowered blood pressure is a result mainly of reduced peripheral vascular resistance. Clonidine is now used in the treatment of mild to moderate hypertension. Its effectiveness is generally improved when used in combination with diuretics and other antihypertensive agents.

Side Effects

Patients must be warned of the need to continue this medication therapy. Abrupt discontinuities of clonidine may cause a rapid increase in diastolic and systolic blood pressure, nervousness, agitation, restlessness, tremor, headache, nausea, and increased salivation.

The most frequent adverse effects are dry mouth, drowsiness and sedation, constipation, headache, and dizziness.

Patients on long-term clonidine therapy should have periodic eye examinations. Laboratory animals have developed degenerative retinal changes, although none have been reported in humans.

Those patients having a diagnosis of mental depression may be more susceptible to further depressive activity.

Availability

PO—0.1, 0.2, 0.3 mg tablets.

Dosage and Administration

Adult

PO—Initially 0.1 mg twice daily. Maintenance dose: add 0.1 to 0.2 mg daily until desired effect is achieved. Average daily doses range from 0.2 to 0.8 mg in divided doses daily. Maximum recommended daily dose is 2.4 mg.

Clonidine may be administered together with other antihypertensive agents without interactions, but the antihypertensive effects of these agents will be enhanced, requiring careful adjustment of dosage.

Nursing Intervention

See also General Nursing Considerations for Patients with Hypertension.

PATIENT CONCERNS: NURSING INTERVENTION/RATIONALE

Side Effects to Expect

Drowsiness, Dry Mouth, Dizziness

Tell the patient these symptoms may occur but that they tend to be self-limiting. Tell him or her not to stop taking the medication, and to consult the physician if the side effects become an unacceptable problem.

Side Effects to Report

Depression

Assess the patient's affective (loneliness, sadness, anxiety, anger), cognitive (confusion, ambivalence, loss of interest), and other behavioral responses (agitation, irritability, altered activity level, withdrawal) before initiating therapy. After initiating therapy with clonidine, carefully monitor the patient for changes in usual response patterns. Assess otherwise normal emotions for an increase in duration or intensity.

Note the patient's degree of socialization, response to stimulation, and changes in interactions with others. All individuals taking this drug should be monitored for development of depression, especially those with a history of depression.

Dosage and Administration

Never suddenly discontinue the medication, as it may cause a rebound effect and a rapid increase in blood pressure, manifested by nervousness, agitation, restlessness, tremors, headache, nausea, and increased salivation.

Rebound symptoms are most pronounced after 1 to 2 months of therapy, and may begin to appear within a few hours of a missed dose. Within 8 to 24 hours, severe symptoms may develop.

When therapy is to be discontinued, a gradual reduction in dosage is necessary over 2 to 4 days, during which blood pressure must be carefully monitored.

Drug Interactions

Drugs That Enhance Therapeutic and Toxic Effects

Guanethidine, digitalis glycosides, barbiturates, tranquilizers, antihistamines, alcohol, and beta adrenergic blocking agents (such as propranolol, atenolol, pindolol, others) and other antihypertensive agents: Monitor the blood pressure response to the cumulative effects of antihypertensive agents. Take the blood pressures in supine and erect positions.

Monitor for an increase in severity of side effects such as sedation, hypotension, and bradycardia or tachycardia.

Drugs That Reduce Therapeutic Effects

Tricyclic antidepressants (amitriptyline, imipramine, desipramine) and trazodone: Monitor carefully for poor blood pressure control or a gradually increasing blood pressure.

Guanabenz (gwan-ah-benz) *(Wytensin)* (y-ten′sin)

Guanabenz is an alpha-2 adrenergic receptor stimulant that acts as an antihypertensive agent by reducing the outflow of sympathetic nervous system impulses to the peripheral blood vessels. This causes a drop in peripheal vascular resistance. It may be used alone or in combination with a diuretic.

Side Effects

The most common side effects are drowsiness and sedation. Other relatively common adverse effects reported include dry mouth, dizziness, weakness, and headache.

Patients must be warned to continue therapy. Abrupt discontinuance may result in a rapid increase in systolic and diastolic pressure. If therapy is to be discontinued, the patient's dose should be tapered down over 1 to 2 weeks, if possible.

Availability

PO—4 and 8 mg tablets.

Dosage and Administration

Adult
PO—Initially 4 mg twice daily. Doses may be increased every 1 to 2 weeks in increments of 4 to 8 mg daily. Maximum dose is 64 mg per day.

Nursing Interventions

See also General Nursing Considerations for Patients with Hypertension.

PATIENT CONCERNS:
NURSING INTERVENTION/RATIONALE

Side Effects to Expect

Drowsiness, Dry Mouth, Dizziness

Tell the patient these side effects may occur, but that they tend to be self-limiting. Tell the patient not to stop taking the medication and to consult the physician if side effects become an unacceptable problem.

Caution the patient against driving or performing hazardous tasks until adjusted to the sedative effects of the medication.

Dosage and Administration

Never suddenly discontinue the medication, as it may cause a rebound effect and a rapid increase in blood pressure, manifested by nervousness, agitation, restlessness, tremors, headache, nausea, and increased salivation.

When therapy is to be discontinued, a gradual reduction in dosage is necessary over 2 to 4 days, during which blood pressure must be carefully monitored.

Drug Interactions

Sedative Effects

Alcohol, barbiturates, phenothiazines, benzodiazepines, and antihistamines all potentiate the sedative effects of guanabenz. Patients should be warned that their tolerance to alcohol and other depressants may be diminished.

Guanadrel (gwan′a-drel) **(Hylorel)** (hi-lor′el)

Guanadrel is quite similar to guanethidine as an antihypertensive agent in that it causes a release and subsequent depletion of norepinephrine from adrenergic nerve endings. It is recommended for use in moderate to severe hypertension, usually in combination with a thiazide diuretic.

Side Effects

Orthostatic hypotension occurs frequently, especially with sudden changes in posture.

Some patients will develop significant salt and water retention, causing edema and congestive heart failure.

Sedation and lethargy commonly occur when guanadrel therapy is initiated or during adjustment to higher doses. These effects are most notable during the first few days and tend to dissipate with time.

Availability

PO—10 and 25 mg tablets.

Dosage and Administration

Adult
PO—Initially 10 mg daily in two divided doses. Adjust the dosages weekly to monthly until the therapeutic goal has been attained. The usual dosage range is 20 to 75 mg divided into 2 to 3 daily doses.

Nursing Interventions

See also General Nursing Considerations for Patients with Hypertension.

from postganglionic or adrenergic nerve endings. It is recommended for treatment of moderate to severe hypertension.

Side Effects

Side effects include fatigue, nausea, nasal stuffiness, abdominal distress, weight gain, bradycardia, diarrhea, and light-headedness and weakness, especially when first getting out of bed.

Availability

PO—10 and 25 mg tablets.

Dosage and Administration

Adult
PO—Initially 10 mg daily. Increase the dose 10 mg every 5 to 7 days, if the blood pressure measurements so indicate and side effects are tolerable. Maintenance doses range between 25 and 50 mg daily; however, much higher doses are occasionally required.

Nursing Interventions

See also General Nursing Considerations for Patients with Hypertension.

PATIENT CONCERNS: NURSING INTERVENTION/RATIONALE

Side Effects to Expect

Orthostatic Hypotension

This may occur, particularly during initiation of therapy. Patients can generally avoid this complication by rising slowly from supine and sitting positions.

Side Effects to Report

Edema

Salt and water retention may cause edema.
Weigh patients daily, using the same scale, at the same time of day, in similar clothing. Report increases of 2 pounds or more per week.
Report edema of the extremities, and increases in dyspnea, pallor, tachycardia, wheezing, and frothy or blood-tinged sputum.

Drug Interactions

Drugs That Enhance Therapeutic and Toxic Effects

Guanethidine, barbiturates, disopyramide, quinidine, diuretics, tranquilizers, antihistamines, alcohol, and beta adrenergic blocking agents (such as propanolol, atenolol, pindolol, others), diuretics, and other antihypertensive agents. Monitor the blood pressure response to the cumulative effects of antihypertensive agents. Take the blood pressures in supine and erect positions.
Monitor for an increase in severity of side effects such as sedation, hypotension, and bradycardia or tachycardia.

Drugs That Reduce Therapeutic Effects

Tricyclic antidepressants (amitriptyline, imipramine, others), amphetamines, ephedrine, phenothiazines, monoamine oxidase inhibitors, haloperidol: Monitor carefully for poor blood pressure control or a gradually increasing blood pressure.

Guanethidine sulfate (gwan-eth'i-deen)
(Ismelin) (is'meh-lin)

Guanethidine is an antihypertensive agent that causes a release and subsequent depletion to norepinephrine

---

PATIENT CONCERNS: NURSING INTERVENTION/RATIONALE

Side Effects to Expect

Light-headedness, Weakness

Guanethidine causes arteriolar and venous dilation that permits pools of blood to collect in the lower extremities, causing a reduction in cerebral blood flow. These symptoms often disappear during the day and can be lessened by rising slowly, sitting on the edge of the bed for a few minutes, and performing leg, foot, and toe exercises before standing.
These orthostatic effects are increased with alcohol consumption or prolonged standing with little movement.

Drug Interactions

Drugs That Enhance Therapeutic and Toxic Effects

Barbiturates, disopyramide, quinidine, diuretics, tranquilizers, antihistamines, alcohol, and beta adrenergic blocking agents (propranolol, atenolol, pindolol, others), and other antihypertensive agents: Monitor the blood pressure response to the cumulative effects of antihypertensive agents. Take the blood pressures in supine and erect positions.

Monitor for an increase in severity of side effects, such as sedation, hypotension, and bradycardia or tachycardia.

Drugs That Reduce Therapeutic Effects

Tricyclic antidepressants (amitriptyline, imipramine, others), amphetamines, ephedrine, phenothiazines, and haloperidol: Monitor carefully for poor blood pressure control or a gradually increasing blood pressure.

Other Interactions

INSULIN AND ORAL HYPOGLYCEMIC AGENTS

Guanethidine may increase the hypoglycemic effects of insulin and oral hypoglycemic agents.

Monitor these patients for headache, weakness, decreasing muscle coordination, diaphoresis. (Onset of hypoglycemic symptoms may be quite rapid.)

Give orange juice with two teaspoonfuls of sugar if the patient is still alert and responsive.

Methyldopa (meth′il-do′pah) *(Aldomet)* (al′do-met)

Methyldopa is an antihypertensive agent whose mechanism of action has never been fully determined. It is recommended for mild to moderate hypertension.

Side Effects

The most common side effects that occur with methyldopa are sedation, lethargy, and dizziness.

Methyldopa or its metabolites may discolor the urine, causing it to darken on exposure to air.

Methyldopa may cause a false-positive Clinitest reaction for urine glucose. It does not affect Tes-tape or Diastix, however.

Availability

PO—125, 250, and 500 mg tablets; 250 mg/5 ml suspension.
IV—250 mg/5 ml in 5 ml vials.

Dosage and Administration

Adult

PO—250 to 500 mg 3 times a day. Maximum recommended dose is 3 g daily.
IV—250 to 500 mg every 6 hours as needed. Add the desired dose of methyldopa to 100 ml of dextrose 5% and infuse IV over 30 to 60 minutes.

Nursing Interventions

See also General Nursing Considerations for Patients with Hypertension.

PATIENT CONCERNS: NURSING INTERVENTION/RATIONALE

Side Effects to Expect

Drowsiness, Dry Mouth, Dizziness

Tell the patient these side effects may occur, but that they tend to be self-limiting. Tell the patient not to stop taking the medication and to consult the physician if side effects become an unacceptable problem.

Altered Urine Color

Discoloration of the urine is to be expected and is not harmful. The darkened color usually occurs with prolonged exposure to air.

Altered Test Reactions

A false-positive urine glucose test may occur when using Clinitest; Diastix and Tes-tape are not affected by methyldopa.

Methyldopa may cause up to 20% of patients to develop a positive reaction to the direct Coomb's test. Less than 0.2% of these patients will develop hemolytic anemia, however. Blood counts should be determined annually during therapy to detect hemolytic anemia.

Side Effects to Report

Depression

Assess the patient's affective (loneliness, sadness, anxiety, anger), cognitive (confusion, ambivalence, loss of interest), and other behavioral responses (agitation, irritability, altered activity level, withdrawal) before initiating therapy. After initiating therapy with methyldopa, carefully monitor the patient for changes in usual response patterns. Assess otherwise normal emotions for an increase in duration or intensity.

Note the patient's degree of socialization, responses to stimulation, and changes in interactions with others. All individuals taking this drug should be monitored for development of depression, especially those with a history of depression.

Drug Interactions

Drugs That Enhance Therapeutic and Toxic Effects

Disopyramide, quinidine, procainamide, diuretics, levodopa, tranquilizers, phenothiazines, alcohol, and beta adrenergic blocking agents (propranolol, atenolol, pindolol, others), and other antihypertensive agents: Monitor the blood pressure response to the cumulative effects of antihypertensive agents. Take the blood pressures in supine and erect positions.

Monitor for an increase in severity of side effects such as sedation, lethargy, hypotension, and bradycardia or tachycardia.

Drugs That Reduce Therapeutic Effects

Tricyclic antidepressants (amitriptyline, imipramine, desipramine, doxepin, others): Monitor carefully for poor blood pressure control or a graduallly increasing blood pressure.

Other Interactions

TOLBUTAMIDE

Methyldopa may increase the hypoglycemic effects of tolbutamide.

Monitor these patients for headache, weakness, decreasing muscle coordination, diaphoresis. (Onset of hypoglycemic symptoms may be quite rapid.)

Give orange juice with two teaspoonfuls of sugar if the patient is still alert and responsive.

HALOPERIDOL

Methyldopa used concurrently with haloperidol may produce irritability, aggressiveness, assaultiveness, and dementia. Concurrent use is generally not recommended.

Metoprolol tartrate (meh-top'row-lol) *(Lopressor)* (lo-pres'or)

Metoprolol is a beta adrenergic blocking agent used in combination with other antihypertensive therapy

to treat mild to moderate hypertension. Metoprolol is discussed in greater detail elsewhere (see Index.)

Nadolol (na'doe-lol) *(Corgard)* (core-guard)

Nadolol is a beta adrenergic blocking agent used in combination with other antihypertensive therapy to treat mild to severe hypertension. Nadolol is discussed in greater detail elsewhere (see Index).

Pindolol (pin'doe-lol) *Visken* (viz'ken)

Pindolol is a beta adrenergic blocking agent used in combination with other antihypertensive therapy to treat mild to severe hypertension. Pindolol is discussed in greater detail elsewhere (see Index).

Propranolol (pro-pran'o-lol) *(Inderal)* (in'der-ahl)

Propranolol is a beta adrenergic blocking agent used in combination with other antihypertensive therapy to treat moderate to severe hypertension. Propranolol is discussed in greater detail elsewhere (see Index).

Timolol (tim'o-lol) *(Blocadren)* (blak-a'dren)

Timolol is a beta adrenergic blocking agent used in combination with other antihypertensive therapy to treat mild to severe hypertension. Timolol is discussed in greater detail elsewhere (see Index).

Reserpine (res'er-peen) *(Serpasil)* (ser'pah-sil)

Reserpine is an alkaloid obtained from the root of a certain species of *Rauwolfia*. It is one of the oldest antihypertensive agents available. Reserpine acts as an antihypertensive agent by reducing norepinephrine levels in peripheral nerve endings, thus reducing peripheral vascular resistance. Reserpine also depletes norepinephrine from various other organs, including the brain. Brain depletion of norepinephrine may be the cause of the sedative and depressive actions of reserpine. Reserpine is used to treat mild hypertension.

Side Effects

Side effects include nasal stuffiness, weight gain, diarrhea, dryness of the mouth, nosebleeds, itching, skin eruptions, insomnia, mental depression, and occasionally, gastric irritation and reactivation of old ulcers or formation of new ones.

Availability

PO—0.1, 0.25, 0.5, and 1 mg tablets; 0.5 mg sustained release capsules;
IM—2.5 mg/ml in 2 ml ampules and 10 ml vials.

Dosage and Administration

Adult

PO—Initially 0.5 mg daily for 1 to 2 weeks. Maintenance: 0.1 to 0.25 mg daily.
IM—Hypertensive crisis: Initially 0.5 to 1 mg, followed by 2 to 4 mg every 3 hours as needed.

Nursing Interventions

See also General Nursing Considerations for Patients with Hypertension.

PATIENT CONCERNS: NURSING INTERVENTION/RATIONALE

Side Effects to Expect

Nasal Stuffiness

Encourage the patient not to treat this symptom with over-the-counter nasal decongestants. (They aggravate the hypertension.) Fortunately, this side effect tends to be self-limiting, but have the patient consult the physician if it becomes a serious problem.

Diarrhea

Diarrhea and stomach cramps may be associated with depressed sympathetic activity. These side effects tend to be self-limiting, but if they persist, or if there is an increase in abdominal pain, the physician should be notified.

Side Effects to Report

Depression

Depression caused by this medication may progress to the point of the individual's becoming suicidal.

Assess the patient's affective (loneliness, sadness, anxiety, anger), cognitive (confusion, ambivalence, loss of interest), and other behavioral responses (agitation, irritability, altered activity level, withdrawal) before initiating therapy. After initiating medication therapy with reserpine, carefully monitor the patient for changes in usual response patterns. Assess otherwise normal emotions for an increase in duration or intensity.

Note the patient's degree of socialization, responses to stimulation, and changes in interactions with others. All individuals taking this drug should be monitored for development of depression, especially those with a history of depression.

Nightmares and Insomnia

If these symptoms occur, report them to the physician for evaluation. Drug therapy may need to be changed.

Gastric Symptoms

Patients experiencing gastric symptoms such as burning, pain, nausea, or vomiting should report them immediately since this medication can cause formation of new or exacerbation of old ulcers.

Drug Interactions

Drugs That Enhance Therapeutic and Toxic Effects

Phenothiazines, procainamide, disopyramide, thiothixene, quinidine, diuretics, tranquilizers, antihistamines, alcohol, and beta adrenergic blocking agents (propranolol, atenolol, pindolol, others), and other antihypertensive agents: Monitor the blood pressure response to cumulative effects of antihypertensive agents. Take the blood pressures in supine and erect positions.

Monitor for an increase in severity of side effects, such as sedation, hypotension, and bradycardia or tachycardia.

Drugs That Reduce Therapeutic Effects

Tricyclic antidepressants (amitriptyline, imipramine, doxepin, others): Monitor carefully for poor blood pressure control or a gradually increasing blood pressure.

Direct Vasodilators

Diazoxide (dy-az-ok'syd) *(Hyperstat IV Injection)*

Diazoxide is used for emergency reduction of blood pressure in hospitalized patients with severe hypertension. It is administered undiluted in a peripheral vein in a dosage of 300 mg in 30 seconds or less. The blood pressure must be continuously monitored.

Availability

IV—300 mg/20 ml ampule.

Hydralazine hydrochloride (hy-dral'ah-zeen) (Apresoline) (ah-pres'o-leen)

This antihypertensive agent is used to treat moderate to severe essential hypertension and hypertension associated with renal disease and toxemia of pregnancy. It acts directly on the smooth muscle of arteries and veins to cause vasodilation.

Side Effects

Early side effects that are sometimes observed and that usually disappear as the drug is continued include nausea, vomiting, dizziness, palpitations, tachycardia, numbness and tingling of legs and feet, nasal congestion, and postural hypotension. The nasal congestion can be treated with an antihistamine, such as pyribenzamine or diphenhydramine. If arthritic symptoms occur, the drug should be discontinued.

Availability

PO—10, 25, 50, and 100 mg tablets.
IV—20 mg/ml in 1 ml ampules.

Dosage and Administration

Adult
PO—Initially, 10 mg 4 times daily for the first 2 to 4 days, then 25 mg 4 times daily. The second week, increase the dosage of 50 mg 4 times daily as the patient tolerates the dosage and the blood pressure is brought under control.
IM, IV—20 to 40 mg repeated as necessary. Monitor blood pressure frequently. Results usually become evident within 10 to 20 minutes.

Nursing Intervention

See also General Nursing Considerations for Patients with Hypertension.

PATIENT CONCERNS: NURSING INTERVENTION/RATIONALE

Side Effects to Expect

Nausea, Dizziness, Palpitations, Tachycardia, Numbness and Tingling in the Legs, Nasal Congestion

Although these symptoms may be anticipated, they do require monitoring. If severe, they should be reported so that the dosage can be adjusted appropriately.

Orthostatic Hypotension

This may occur particularly during initiation of therapy. Patients can generally avoid this complication by rising slowly from supine and sitting positions.

Side Effects to Report

Fever, Chills, Joint and Muscle Pain, Skin Eruptions

Tell patients to report the development of these symptoms.
Monitor laboratory reports for leukocyte counts and the antinuclear antibody (ANA) titer.

Drug Interactions

Drugs That Enhance Therapeutic and Toxic Effects

Diuretics, alcohol, beta adrenergic blocking agents (propranolol, atenolol, pindolol, others), and other antihypertensive agents: Monitor the blood pressure response to the cumulative effects of antihypertensive agents. Take the blood pressures in supine and erect positions.
Monitor for an increase in severity of side effects, such as sedation, hypotension, and bradycardia or tachycardia.

Minoxidil (min-ox'i-dil) (Loniten) (lon'-i-ten)

Minoxidil acts by direct relaxation of the smooth muscle of arterioles, reducing peripheral vascular resistance. Due to the drop in peripheral vascular resistance, there is a compensatory increase in heart rate and sodium and water retention. For this reason, minoxidil is usually administered in conjunction with a beta adrenergic blocking agent and a potent diuretic such as furosemide or bumetanide. Minoxidil is used only for severely hypertensive patients who do not respond adequately to maximum therapeutic doses of a diuretic and two other antihypertensive agents.

Side Effects

Due to salt and water retention, about 10% of patients develop edema, tachycardia, and possible congestive heart failure.

Within 3 to 6 weeks after initiating therapy, about 80% of patients will start developing *hypertrichosis*— an elongation, thickening, and increased pigmentation of fine body hair. It is usually noticed first on the face and later extends to the back, arms, legs, and scalp.

Other adverse effects that have been reported include breast tenderness and gynecomastia, changes in skin pigmentation, polymenorrhea, thrombocytopenia, leukopenia, bullous lesions on the legs, and hypersensitivity rash.

Availability

PO—2.5 and 10 mg tablets.

Dosage and Administration

Adult
PO—Initially 5 mg daily. Dosage may be gradually increased after at least 3-day intervals to 10 mg, 20 mg, and then 40 mg daily in 1 to 2 doses. Maintenance dosage: 10 to 40 mg daily. Maximum dosage is 100 mg daily.

Nursing Interventions

See also General Nursing Considerations for Patients with Hypertension.

PATIENT CONCERNS: NURSING INTERVENTION/RATIONALE

Side Effects to Expect

Hair Growth

A gradual increase and thickening of body hair can be anticipated approximately 3 to 6 weeks after initiating therapy.

Growth may be controlled by shaving or by hair-removing creams. Upon discontinuation, new hair growth stops, but it may take up to 6 months for complete return to pretreatment appearance.

Side Effects to Report

Gynecomastia

Swelling or tenderness of the breasts may develop in men.

Salt and Water Retention

This drug is usually administered with a diuretic and a beta adrenergic blocking agent to reduce the incidence of fluid retention, and for additive antihypertensive effects.

Perform daily weights using the same scale, in similar clothing, and at approximately the same time of day. Report gains of more than 2 pounds per week, and swelling or puffiness of the face, ankles, or hands to the physician.

Increased Resting Pulse

Instruct and validate the patient's ability to take own pulse.

A resting pulse that increases 20 or more beats per minute above normal should be reported.

Light-headedness, Fainting, Dizziness

These symptoms require reporting to the physician. If possible, the individual's blood pressure during these episodes should be taken and reported.

Orthostatic Hypotension

This may occur, particularly during initiation of therapy. Patients can generally avoid this complication by rising slowly from supine and sitting positions.

Congestive Heart Failure

Assess for development of: dyspnea, orthopnea, edema, weight gain.

Drug Interactions

Drugs That Enhance Therapeutic and Toxic Effects

Diuretics, alcohol, beta adrenergic blocking agents (propanolol, atenolol, pindolol, others), guanethidine, guanadrel, and other antihypertensive agents: Monitor the blood pressure response due to the cumulative effects of antihypertensive agents. Take the blood pressures in supine and erect positions.

Monitor for an increase in severity of side effects, such as sedation, hypotension, and bradycardia or tachycardia.

Nitroprusside sodium (ny-tro-prus'yd)
(Nipride) (ny'pryd)

Nitroprusside is a potent vasodilator that acts directly on the smooth muscle of blood vessels to produce vasodilation. It is used in patients with sudden severe hypertensive crisis, and in those with refractory congestive heart failure.

Side Effects

Adverse effects are usually dose related and dissipate rapidly with dosage reduction. Side effects reported include nausea, retching, abdominal pain, diaphoresis, restlessness, apprehension, headache, muscle twitching, palpitations, and retrosternal discomfort. Keeping the patient in a supine position will also reduce the incidence of adverse effects.

Availability

IV—10 mg/ml in 5 ml vials.

Prazosin hydrochloride (pray'zo-sin)
(Minipress) (min'ee-pres)

Prazosin acts directly on the smooth muscle of arterioles to produce peripheral vasodilation and a reduction in diastolic blood pressure. Prazosin is used in combination with other antihypertensive agents in the treatment of mild to moderate hypertension.

Side Effects

The most common adverse effects reported with prazosin include dizziness, headache, drowsiness, nausea, weakness, and lethargy. All are transient and disappear with continued therapy.

Availability

PO—1, 2, and 5 mg capsules.

Dosage and Administration

Adult
PO—Initially 1 mg 3 times daily. Gradually increase until desired therapeutic response is achieved. The usual maintenance dose is 10 mg twice daily. Do not exceed 40 mg daily.

Note: The initial doses of praxosin may cause dizziness, tachycardia, and fainting, but these adverse effects occur in less than 1% of patients starting therapy. Symptoms occur 15 to 90 minutes after initial dosages and occur most frequently in patients who are already receiving propranolol (and presumably other beta adrenergic blocking agents). This effect may be minimized by giving the first doses with food and limiting the initial dose to 1 mg. Patients should be warned that this side effect may occur, that it is transient, and that they should lie down immediately if symptoms develop.

Nursing Interventions

See also General Nursing Considerations for Patients with Hypertension.

**PATIENT CONCERNS:
NURSING INTERVENTION/RATIONALE**

Side Effects to Expect

Drowsiness, Headache, Dizziness, Weakness, Lethargy

Tell the patient that these side effects may occur, but that they tend to be self-limiting. Tell the patient not to stop taking the medication and to consult the physician if they become an unacceptable problem.

Dosage and Administration

Dizziness, Tachycardia, and Fainting

These side effects occur in about 1% of patients when therapy is initiated. They develop 15 to 90 minutes after the first dosage is taken. To decrease their incidence, administer the first dose with food and limit the initial dose to 1 mg.

Tell the patient to lie down immediately if these symptoms occur.

Provide for your patient's safety.

Drug Interactions

Drugs That Enhance Therapeutic and Toxic Effects

Diuretics, tranquilizers, alcohol, barbiturates, antihistamines, beta adrenergic blocking agents (propranolol, atenolol, pindolol, others), and other antihypertensive agents: Monitor the blood pressure response to the cumulative effects of antihypertensive agents. Take the blood pressures in supine and erect positions.

Monitor for an increase in severity of side effects such as sedation, hypotension, and bradycardia or tachycardia.

Renin-Angiotensin Inhibitor

Captopril (kap-toe'pril)
(Capoten) (kap-o'ten)

Captopril represents a new class of agents used to control hypertension. Its exact mechanism of action is unknown, but it does inhibit angiotensin II, a potent vasoconstrictor. It has several side effects, so is recommended for use in mild to severe hypertension only after other multiple drug regimens have failed or are not tolerated.

Side Effects

About 1% of patients receiving captopril develop proteinuria during the first 8 months of therapy. About 25% of these patients develop nephrotic syndrome, a potentially fatal renal disease. Patients should have urinary protein determinations before initiation of therapy, and at monthly intervals for the first 9 months of treatment, and periodically thereafter.

Neutropenia and agranulocytosis due to drug-induced bone marrow suppression have been reported in less than 1% of patients receiving captopril.

About 10% of patients receiving captopril develop a rash in the first 4 weeks of therapy. The rash is often accompanied by pruritus and sometimes fever and eosinophilia.

About 7% of patients receiving captopril develop taste impairment manifested by loss of taste acuity, a metallic or salty taste, or loss of taste perception.

Many other side effects, including angina pectoris, palpitations, congestive heart failure, Raynaud's disease, headache, paresthesias, insomnia, gastric discomfort, constipation, and diarrhea have been infrequently reported.

Availability

PO—25, 50, and 100 mg tablets.

Dosage and Administration

Adult

PO—Initially 25 mg 3 times daily. Increase to 50 mg three times daily in 1 to 2 weeks. If therapeutic goals are not achieved in another 1 to 2 weeks, add a thiazide diuretic. If further antihypertensive activity is needed, continue the diuretic and increase the captopril first to 100 mg 3 times daily, then to 150 mg 3 times daily. Do not exceed 450 mg daily.

Nursing Interventions

See also General Nursing Considerations for Patients with Hypertension.

PATIENT CONCERNS: NURSING INTERVENTION/RATIONALE

Side Effects to Expect

Impaired Taste

Taste impairment develops within the first 3 months of therapy and resolves within 2 or 3 months of continued therapy. Encourage the patient not to discontinue therapy.

Side Effects to Report

Proteinuria

The nurse should check the urinalysis report before initiating therapy for evidence of protein in the urine. Report presence to the physician.

Continue regular checks of proteinuria once a month for at least the first 9 months of therapy, and periodically thereafter.

Nephrotic Syndrome

Assess the patient for the development of: proteinuria, hypotension, edema.

Neutropenia and Agranulocytosis

Neutropenia appears within the first 3 to 12 weeks and develops slowly over the next 10 to 30 days. The white count returns to normal in about 2 weeks after discontinuing captopril therapy.

Patients most susceptible are those with impaired renal function, serious autoimmune diseases (e.g., lupus erythematosis), or who are exposed to drugs known to affect the white cells or immune response (e.g., corticosteroids).

Patients at risk should have differential and total white cell counts before initiation of therapy, and then every 2 weeks thereafter for the first 3 months of therapy.

Tell patients to notify the physician promptly if any indication of infection, such as sore throat or fever, develops.

Rash, Pruritus, Fever, and Eosinophilia

The rash is usually mild and disappears a few days after dosage reduction, short-term treatment with an antihistaminic agent, and discontinuation of therapy. Remission may occur even if captropil is continued.

Drug Interactions

Drugs That Enhance Therapeutic and Toxic Effects

Diuretics, alcohol, beta adrenergic blocking agents (propranolol, atenolol, pindolol, others), and other antihypertensive agents: Monitor the blood pressure response to the cumulative effects of antihypertensive agents. Take the blood pressures in supine and erect positions.

Monitor for an increase in severity of side effects such as sedation, hypotension, and bradycardia or tachycardia.

Hyperkalemia

Captopril may cause small increases in potassium serum levels by inhibiting aldosterone secretion. Patients should not take dietary supplements of potassium or potassium-sparing diuretics (triamterene, spironolactone, amiloride) without specific approval from the physician.

If a patient has received spironolactone up to several months before captopril therapy, the serum potassium level should be monitored closely, because the potassium-sparing effect of spironolactone persists.

The Diuretics

The diuretics, including the thiazides, chlorthalidone, bumetanide, metolazone, furosemide, and ethacrynic acid, are mainstays in antihypertensive therapy. They have a low incidence of adverse effects, they potentiate the hypotensive activity of the nondiuretic antihypertensive agents, and they are often the least expensive of the antihypertensive agents.

The diuretics act as antihypertensive agents by causing volume depletion, sodium excretion, and direct vasodilation of peripheral arterioles. Diuretics are used to treat mild, moderate, and severe hypertension and are most effective when used in combination with other antihypertensive agents (see Table 10.2, page 255). The agents are discussed under the urinary system drugs (see Index).

Anticoagulants

Diseases associated with abnormal clotting within blood vessels are a frequent cause of death. Diseases caused by intravascular clotting are major causes of death from cardiovascular sources, such as coronary occlusion and thromboembolisms secondary to thrombophlebitis. Drugs that inhibit clotting are, therefore, most important.

Anticoagulant therapy is used during and after certain types of surgery, in the treatment of thrombophlebitis, in conjunction with hemodialysis, and in the management of certain heart valve disorders. Anticoagulants are used prophylactically; they cannot dissolve an existing clot! The primary purpose of anticoagulants is to prevent new clot formation or the extension of existing clots.

General Nursing Considerations for Patients Receiving Anticoagulant Therapy

PATIENT CONCERNS: NURSING INTERVENTION/RATIONALE

Patients at Risk

Patients at greater risk for clot formation are those with a history of clot formation, those with recent abdominal, thoracic, or orthopedic surgery, and those on prolonged bedrest.

Techniques for Preventing Clot Formation

Provide early, regular ambulation after surgery. Use active or passive leg exercises for patients on bedrest or restricted activity.

Develop and follow a specific turning schedule for persons on complete bedrest to prevent tissue breakdown and blood stasis. Implement good back care, deep breathing, and coughing exercises as part of general nursing care.

Do not flex the knees or place pressure against the popliteal space with pillows.

Do not allow the patient to stand or sit motionless for prolonged periods of time.

Use elastic hose, such as TED stockings. Remove stockings and inspect the skin on every shift. Make sure they are being worn properly and not becoming bunched around the knees or ankles.

Nutritional Status

The dietary regimen will depend on the individual's diagnosis and current clinical status.

Adequate hydration to promote fluidity of the blood is important. Unless coexisting diagnoses prohibit, give at least six to eight 8-ounce glasses of fluid daily.

Laboratory Data

Monitoring and reporting to the physician laboratory results is essential during anticoagulant therapy. Coagulation tests that might be ordered include the following: whole blood clotting time (WBCT); prothrombin time (PT); partial thromboplastin time (PTT); activated partial thromboplastin time (APTT); activated coagulation time (ACT). The prothrombin time (PT) is routinely used to monitor warfarin therapy, and the activated partial thromboplastin time (APTT) is most commonly used to monitor heparin therapy.

Never administer an anticoagulant without first checking the chart for the most recent laboratory results. Be certain that the anticoagulant to be administered has been ordered *since* the most recent results have been reported to the physician.

Patient Teaching Associated with Anticoagulant Therapy

Communication and Responsibility

Encourage open communication concerning frustrations and anger as the patient attempts to adjust to the diagnosis and need for treatment. The patient must be guided to gain insight into the condition in order to assume responsibility for the continuation of treatment. Keep emphasizing those factors the patient can control to alter the progress of the disease, including maintenance of general health, nuritional needs, adequate rest and appropriate exercise, and continuation of prescribed medication therapy.

Stress the need to prevent bodily injury: avoid use of power equipment; use care in stepping up or down from curbs; do not participate in contact sports; use only an electric razor, and brush teeth gently with a soft-bristled toothbrush.

Expectations of Therapy

Discuss expectations of therapy with the patient:

- Level of exercise specified by the physician.
- Ability to maintain activities of daily living and work.
- Pain relief, if appropriate to the etiology of clot formation.

Changes in Expectations

Assess changes in expectations as therapy progresses and the patient gains understanding and skill in the management of the diagnosis.

Changes in Therapy through Cooperative Goal-Setting

Work with the patient to encourage adherence to the prescribed treatment. When the patient feels that a change should be made in a treatment plan, encourage him or her to discuss it first with the physician.

WRITTEN RECORD

Enlist the patient's aid in developing and maintaining a written record of monitoring parameters (Table 10.4) (i.e., blood pressure, pulse, daily weights, degree of pain relief, exercise tolerance) and response to prescribed therapies for discussion with the physician. Patients should be encouraged to take this record on follow-up visits.

FOSTERING COMPLIANCE

Throughout the hospitalization, discuss medication information and how it will benefit the patient's course of treatment. Seek cooperation and understanding of the following points, so that medication compliance may be enhanced:

1. Name.
2. Dosage.
3. Route and administration times.
4. Anticipated therapeutic response.
5. Side effects to expect.
6. Side effects to report.
   - Nosebleeds, tarry stools, "coffee-ground" or blood-tinged vomitus; petechiae (tiny purple or red spots occurring in various sites on the skin); ecchymoses (bruises); hematuria (blood in the urine); or bleeding from the gums or any other body opening; cuts or injuries from which the bleeding is difficult to control. If a dressing is on, check periodically for bleeding.
   - Tell the patient that not all bleeding is clearly visible; therefore, report immediately a rapid, weak pulse; deep, rapid respirations; moist, clammy skin; and a general feeling of weakness of faintness.
7. What to do if a dosage is missed.
8. When, how, or if to refill the medication prescription.
   - Follow-up visits to the physician and laboratory are essential during anticoagulant therapy. Failure to keep these appointments may lead to serious complications.

DIFFICULTY IN COMPREHENSION

If it is evident that the patient and/or family does not understand all aspects of continuing therapy being

Table 10.4
Example of a Written Record for Patients Receiving Anticoagulants

Medications	Color	To be taken

Name _____

Physician _____

Physician's phone _____

Next appt.* _____

Parameters		Day of discharge							Comments
Weight									
Blood pressure									
Pulse									
Color of urine	Normal								
	Red								
	Orange								
Mouth	Gums bleed with brushing								
Shaving	Bleeding — difficulty stopping blood								
Bruising	Nosebleeds — (#) of times?								
	Bruising to light touch								
Pain relief	Name limb (e.g., left leg, right leg)								
	Color of limb								
	Temperature								
Activities of daily living	Able to do								
	Done with difficulty								
	Too difficult to do								
Bowel movements	Normal								
	Diarrhea								
	Color — normal or black, tarry								
	Smell — normal or foul								
Report immediately									
	Chest pain								
	Faintness								
	Dizziness								
	Red vomitus								
	Black stools								

*Please bring this record with you to your next appointment.
Use the back of this sheet for additional information.

prescribed (i.e., administration and monitoring of medications, exercises, diets, follow-up appointments), consider the use of social service or visiting nurse agencies.

ASSOCIATED TEACHING

Give patients the following instructions:

Always inform the physician or dentist of any prescription or over-the-counter medication being taken. While receiving anticoagulant therapy, no prescription or over-the-counter medications should be taken without first dicussing them with the physician or pharmacist.

Always report side effects of rash, itching or hives immediately. Nausea, vomiting, or diarrhea should also be reported for the physician's evaluation, if it is a new symptom.

Take all of the medication as prescribed for the full course of treatment. Do not discontinue use when feeling improved; do not save for future use; do not give your medicine to another individual. Sudden discontinuation of certain medications may produce harmful effects.

Keep all medications out of the reach of children.

If pregnancy is suspected, consult an obstetrician as soon as possible about continuation of medication therapy.

At Discharge

Items to be sent home with the patient should:

1. Have written instructions for use.
2. Be labeled in a level of language and size of print appropriate for the patient.
3. If needed, include identification cards or bracelets.
4. Include a list of additional supplies to be purchased after discharge.
5. Include a schedule for follow-up appointments.

Heparin (hep'ah-rin)

Heparin is a natural substance that is commercially extracted from gut and lung tissue of pigs and cattle. It acts directly on several plasma protein molecules within the blood to prevent coagulation. It is used to treat deep venous thrombosis, pulmonary embolism, cerebral embolism, and acute peripheral arterial embolism, and patients with a heart valve prosthesis. It is also used prophylactically before and during cardiovascular surgery and hemodialysis.

Side Effects

Adverse effects of heparin therapy are most commonly due to inappropriate administration technique or ov-

erdosage. Factors that can influence the incidence of complications include age, weight, sex, and recent trauma. The most common signs of overdosage are petechiae, hematomas, hematuria, bleeding gums, and melena.

Availability

SC, IV—1000, 5000, 10,000, 20,000, and 40,000 units/ml in various sizes of ampules and vials.

Dosage and Administration

Adult
SC—Prophylactic: 5000 units every 8 to 12 hours. Therapeutic: Initially 10,000 to 15,000 units. Maintenance: 6000 to 10,000 units every 8 to 12 hours (see Fig. 10.1).
IM—Not recommended because of the development of hematomas.
IV—Intermittent: Initially 10,000 unit bolus; maintenance: 5000 to 10,000 units every 4 to 6 hours.
IV—Continuous infusion: Initially 5000 unit bolus; Maintenance, 700 to 1200 units/hour. (Patient variation may require as little as 200 units/hour or as much as 2000 or more units/hour.)

Antidote

One mg of protamine sulfate will neutralize approximately 120 units of heparin. If protamine sulfate is given more than one-half hour after the heparin was administered, then give only one-half the dose of protamine sulfate. Excessive doses of protamine may

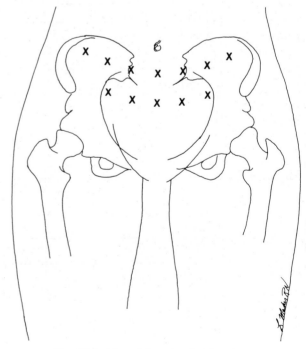

Fig. 10.1. *Sites of heparin administration.*

also cause excessive anticoagulation, so it must be used judiciously.

Nursing Interventions

See also General Nursing Considerations for Patients Receiving Anticoagulant Therapy.

PATIENT CONCERNS: NURSING INTERVENTION/RATIONALE

Side Effects to Expect

Hematoma Formation, Bleeding at Injection Site

Inappropriate administration techniques lead to hematoma formation at the site of injection. USE PROPER TECHNIQUE!

Side Effects to Report

Bleeding

Inspect the skin and mucous membranes for petechiae, ecchymoses, or hematomas. Also monitor for hematuria, bleeding gums, and melena.

Always monitor menstrual flow to be certain that it is not excessive or prolonged.

Assess and record vital signs at regular intervals. Report signs and symptoms of internal bleeding (decreasing blood pressure; increasing pulse; cold, clammy skin, feelings of faintness; or disoriented sensorium).

Check urine and stools for blood. Urine may appear red, smoke-colored, or brownish. Stools may appear to be dark and tarry. Perform a Hemocult test on the stool, if necessary.

Vomitus may contain bright red blood or may be coffee-ground in appearance.

Postoperative patients need assessment of dressings or drainage tubes for any signs of bleeding.

Dosage and Administration

Intramuscular Injections

DO NOT INJECT INTRAMUSCULARLY!

Dosage Adjustment

Blood samples for laboratory studies are usually drawn before each subcutaneous or intravenous dose, or every 6 to 8 hours during a continuous intravenous infusion.

Accuracy of Dose

Always confirm the dosage calculations with two nurses before subcutaneous or intravenous administration.

Be certain the strength is correct. There is a *drastic difference* in clinical response from 1 ml of 1:1,000 units and 1 ml of 1:10,000 units of heparin.

Subcutaneous Administration

Subcutaneous injection is usually made into the tissue over the abdomen, the upper arm, or lateral thigh (see Fig. 10.1).

Needle length and angle need to be adapted to the patient's size so that the drug will be deposited into the subcutaneous tissue. (Usually a 26 or 27 gauge, ½ inch needle is used.) The injection is usually made at a 90° angle to the skin.

Always use a tuberculin syringe so that the dosage can be accurately measured.

DO NOT aspirate, because this will increase local tissue damage and the possibility of hematoma formation.

DO NOT inject into a hematoma or an area with any infection present.

Follow a planned site rotation schedule.

After injection, apply gentle pressure for 1 to 2 minutes to control local bleeding.

Ice packs on the site following injection may be used; check your hospital policy. At this time, there is little documented evidence that ice packs prevent hematoma formation or affect drug absorption.

Intermittent Intravenous Administration

A heparin lock, consisting of a 22–25-gauge scalp vein needle attached to a 3½ inch tubing ending in a resealing rubber diaphragm, may be used to administer intermittent IV doses of heparin.

Advantages of a heparin lock are the mobility that it provides the patient and the fewer venipunctures.

After injecting a bolus of heparin through the rubber diaphragm, flush the line with 1 ml of a solution containing 10 units of heparin/ml of saline solution. The heparin flush solution ensures that the patient will receive the entire heparin bolus and it prevents the formation of a clot in the scalp vein needle.

Intravenous Infusion

Continuous infusions of heparin provide the advantage of steady heparin levels in the blood, but do require periodic dosage adjustment based upon the response of the patient.

When making a solution for infusion, always have two nurses confirm your calculations and the strength of the heparin to be used. As a safety measure, never make infusions to run more than 6 to 8 hours. This protects patients from receiving massive doses of heparin should the infusion "run away."

Always use an electronic control device for infusion, but also monitor the infusion rate regularly.

Drug Interactions

Increased Therapeutic and Toxic Effects

Concurrent use of aspirin, dipyridamole, and glyceryl guaiacolate may predispose the patient to hemorrhage.

Warfarin (war'fah-rin)
(Coumadin) (koo'mah-din), *(Panwarfin)* (pan-war'fin)

Warfarin is a very potent anticoagulant that acts by inhibiting the activity of vitamin K, which is required to produce certain blood coagulation factors in the blood. Warfarin is used to treat or prophylactically prevent venous thrombosis, atrial fibrillation with embolism, pulmonary embolism, and coronary occlusion.

Side Effects

Adverse reactions to warfarin, other than the possibility of hemorrhage due to overdosage, are quite rare. Evidence of hemorrhage is usually seen as petechiae, hematuria, bleeding gums, melena, or the development of hematomas after minor trauma.

Availability

PO—2, 2.5, 5, 7.5, and 10 mg tablets.
IV—50 mg vial with a 2 ml ampule of diluent.

Dosage and Administration

Adult

PO—10 to 15 mg daily for 3 days; maintenance: 2 to 15 mg daily as determined by the prothrombin time.
IV—As for PO administration; onset of action is similar to that of PO administration because of dependence on individual coagulation factor synthesis.

Nursing Interventions

See also General Nursing Considerations for Patients Receiving Anticoagulant Therapy.

PATIENT CONCERNS:
NURSING INTERVENTION/RATIONALE

Side Effects to Report

Bleeding

Inspect the skin and mucous membranes for petechiae, ecchymoses, or hematomas. Also monitor for hematuria, bleeding gums, and melena.

Always monitor menstrual flow to be certain that it is not excessive or prolonged.

Assess and record vital signs at regular intervals.
Report signs and symptoms of internal bleeding (de-

creasing blood pressure; increasing pulse; cold, clammy skin; feelings of faintness; or disoriented sensorium).

Check urine and stools for blood. Urine may appear red, smoke-colored, or brownish. Stools may appear to be dark and tarry. Perform a Hemocult test on the stool, if necessary.

Vomitus may contain bright red blood or may be coffee-ground in appearance.

Postoperative patients need assessment of dressings or drainage tubes for any signs of bleeding.

Dosage and Administration

Dosage Adjustment

Dosage during initial therapy is based on prothrombin times. The optimal dosage is that which maintains PT at 1½ to 2 times the control value.

When warfarin therapy is initiated, the patient should be monitored closely for evidence of hemorrhage, because of the drug's accumulative effects.

Stress the need to comply with the prescribed regimen and the need for laboratory data to determine the correct maintenance dose.

Tell the patient to resume a regular schedule if one dose is missed. If more than two doses are missed, he or she should consult the physician.

The following drugs, when used concurrently with warfarin, may enhance therapeutic and toxic effects of warfarin:

allpurinol	phenytoin	isoniazid
amiodarone	propoxyphene	meclofenamate
aminoglycoside	quinidine	mefenamic acid
antibiotics	chloral hydrate	metronidazole
anabolic steroids	chloramphenicol	meconazole
cephalosporins	cimetidine	nalidixic acid
disulfiram	clofibrate	salicylates
dextrothyronine	cotrimoxazole	sulfinpyrazine
eythromycin	danazol	sulindac
ethacrynic acid	diazoxide	sulfonamides
ethanol	diflunisal	tetracyclines
oxyphenbutazone	glucagon	thyroid hormones
phenylbutazone	indomethacin	vitamin E

The following drugs, when used concurrently with warfarin, may decrease the therapeutic activity of warfarin:

barbiturates	disopyramide	mercaptopurine
carbamazepine	ethchlorvynol	rifampin
cholestyramine	gluthethimide	spironolactone
cyclophosphamide	griseofulvin	vitamin K

All Prescription and Nonprescription Medications

Caution the patient *not* to take *any* over-the-counter or prescription medication without first discussing them with the physician or pharmacist.

Chapter 11

Drugs Affecting the
Respiratory System

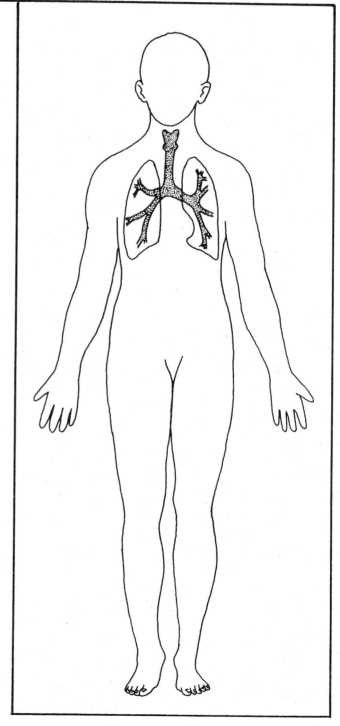

Objectives

After completing this chapter, the student should be able to do the following:

1. Explain the major action and effects of drugs used to treat disorders of the respiratory tract.
2. Identify baseline data the nurse should collect on a continuous basis for comparison and evaluation of drug effectiveness.
3. Identify important nursing assessments and interventions associated with the drug therapy and treatment of diseases associated with the respiratory tract.
4. Identify health teaching essential for a successful treatment regimen.

General Nursing Considerations for Patients with Respiratory Tract Disease

Nursing assessment of the signs of respiratory dysfunction can provide a baseline for subsequent evaluation of the patient's response to therapy. Assessment may range from the "common cold," of limited severity and duration, to chronic and progressively more debilitating disorders, such as emphysema.

Throughout the course of managing the respiratory disorder, adequate oxygenation of the individual body cells is essential to maintain the body functions. *Ventilation*, the movement of the air in and out of the lungs, is affected by a number of complex mechanisms. To be effective, air must reach the alveoli. This allows atmospheric air, with a fresh supply of oxygen, to be exchanged with carbon dioxide and "stale" air from the lungs by inspiration and expiration. Any blockage in the respiratory pathway prevents this process from occurring. Diseases that affect the tracheobronchial tree or the ability of the lungs to expand, can affect the ventilation process.

Blood flow through the pulmonary vessels, where gas exchange between the alveoli and pulmonary vessels occurs, is called *perfusion*. *Diffusion* is the point at which oxygen (O_2) enters and carbon dioxide (CO_2) leaves the cells. Blood circulation provides *distribution* of oxygen to the body's cells for the sustenance of life. Ventilation and perfusion must be equal to maintain homeostasis. Dysfunction of one or more of the processes that interfere with the gaseous exchange results in difficult breathing.

Oxygen is transported to the individual tissue cells either by combining with the hemoglobin or by dissolving in the blood plasma. Arterial blood gas (ABG) determinations indicate the effectiveness of pulmonary function. ABGs are a measurement for assessing ventilation and external respiratory effectiveness. They measure the amount of oxygen dissolved in blood plasma. ABGs are done to assist in the management of patients with acute and chronic pulmonary disorders.

Five main diagnostic tests are used to evaluate the patient's status. Beginning nurses need to know the normal range of the laboratory values and that reporting deviations is essential to effective management of the respiratory problem.

LABORATORY TEST	NORMAL VALUES	RESULTS		
pH	7.35–7.45	↑	=	alkalosis
		↓	=	acidosis
pCO_2	35 to 45 mmHg	↑	=	hypercapnea
		↓	=	hypocapnea
pO_2	80 to 100 mmHg	↓	=	hypoxemia
HCO_3	18 to 25 mEq/L			
SaO_2	97%			

PATIENT CONCERNS: NURSING INTERVENTION/RATIONALE

Normal Respiratory Activity

Respirations

RATE

Throughout the course of therapy, monitor the respiratory pattern at regularly scheduled intervals.

Normal values:

- Infants—26–34/minute
- Adults—14–25/minute

Report increasing or decreasing respiratory rate.

DEPTH

Shallow breathing may lead to hypercapnea, hypoxemia, hypoxia, and acidosis. Rapid, deep breathing (Kussmaul breathing) is one sign of metabolic acidosis.

Report *changes* in the patient's depth of respirations.

Indications of Respiratory Impairment

Dyspnea (Difficult or Labored Respirations)

Complete respiratory obstruction is evidenced by: inability to cough or speak, lack of chest movement, cyanosis; the patient may be clutching the throat in a state of panic.

Incomplete or partial respiratory obstruction is evidenced by: weak cough, cyanosis, shortness of breath, frequent respirations, and use of accessory muscles.

Always check the patient for possible inhalation of a foreign object if you are unfamiliar with the individual's diagnosis or the conditions surrounding the onset of respiratory difficulty.

Respiratory Distress

Assess the patient for the following:

Early signs and symptoms of respiratory distress include: increased blood pressure, pulse, and respiratory rate; anxiety; restlessness; headache; slight confusion or impaired judgment; possible sweating.

Late signs and symptoms include: flaring nostrils; cyanosis; dyspnea; use of accessory chest, abdominal and neck muscles; confusion progressing to coma; gradual reduction in pulse and blood pressure.

Cyanosis

Peripheral cyanosis is defined as a bluish coloring of an isolated area of the body (e.g., earlobes, toes, feet, fingers).

Central cyanosis indicates a general lack of oxygenated hemoglobin. The entire body has a slight bluish-white tinge. It is most readily observed on the lips and mucuous membranes of the mouth.

Muscle Involvement

Elevations of the shoulders, retraction of the neck and intercostal muscles, and use of the abdominal muscles is associated with advanced respiratory disease; report new observations immediately.

Changes in Mental Status

As the oxygen level in the body diminishes, the mental status will deteriorate from alertness to progressively lower levels of function (alert→anxious →restless→drowsy→unconscious→death).

Breath Sounds

Auscultation for rales, rhonchi, and lung clarity should be performed at appropriate intervals based on the patient's diagnosis and current status.

Posture

Dyspneic patients usually sit upright or lean forward from the waist, resting the elbows on the knees. Position patients experiencing dyspnea in the high Fowler's position, or place a pillow on table over the bed and allow them to rest with their head forward on the pillow.

Pain

Chest discomfort may result from lying on the affected side too long.

Chest Contour

Note changes in contour of the chest such as "barrel chest," kyphosis, or scoliosis.

Clubbing of Fingernails and Toenails

Assess for a decrease in the angle between the nailbeds and the fingers or toes.

Fatigue

Check for the degree of fatigue the patient is experiencing. Specifically question the individual regarding the correlation of the activity level with the onset and degree of fatigue.

Cough

Note whether a cough is productive or nonproductive. Record sputum color, consistency, amount, and any appearance or frothiness or blood (hemoptysis).

Patient Teaching Associated with Respiratory Therapy

Communication and Responsibility

Encourage open communication concerning frustrations and anger as the patient attempts to adjust to diagnosis and the need for prolonged treatment. The patient must be guided to gain insight into the condition in order to assume responsibility for the continuation of treatment. Keep emphasizing those factors the patient can control to alter the progression of the disease, including the following:

AVOIDING IRRITANTS

Smoking, pollen, and environmental pollutants frequently aggravate respiratory disorders.

ACTIVITY AND EXERCISE

Fatigue and resulting dyspnea may require alterations in physical activity and employment. Support the patient's concerns. Plan for rest periods to alternate with activity.

NUTRITIONAL STATUS

A well-balanced diet that avoids weight loss or excessive gains is important. Encourage patients with dyspnea to eat small bites, with several small servings throughout the day.

PREVENTING INFECTIONS

Encourage patients to do the following:

Avoid exposure to persons with infection; practice good hygiene, such as handwashing; get adequate rest; dispose of secretions properly. Seek medical attention at the earliest sign of suspected infection.

INCREASED FLUID INTAKE

Unless contraindicated, encourage patients to increase fluid intake. This will aid in decreasing the viscosity of secretions.

ENVIRONMENTAL ELEMENTS

People experiencing difficulty in breathing can benefit from proper temperature, humidification of the air, or ventilation of their immediate surroundings. Moist air from a humidifier or vaporizer can readily relieve dryness of the nose or throat.

BREATHING TECHNIQUES

If ordered by the physician, teach pursed-lip breathing or abdominal breathing and coughing, and postural drainage. Encourage the use of blow-bottles.

See a general medical-surgical nursing text for details of these treatment modalities.

Expectations of Therapy

Discuss expectations of therapy with the patient (e.g., level of exercise; degree of pain relief, if present; tolerance; frequency of use of therapy; relief of dyspnea; ability to maintain activities of daily living and work; and others as indicated by the underlying pathology).

Changes in Expectations

Assess changes in expectations as therapy progresses and the patient gains understanding and skill in the management of the diagnosis.

Changes in Therapy through Cooperative Goal-Setting

Work with the patient to encourage adherence to the prescribed treatment. When the patient feels that a change should be made in a treatment plan, encourage discussion first with the physician.

WRITTEN RECORD

Enlist the patient's aid in developing and maintaining a written record (see Table 11.1) of monitoring parameters (e.g., respirations, pulse, daily weights, degree of dyspnea relief, exercise tolerance, secretions being expectorated) and response to prescribed therapies for discussion with the physician. Patients should be encouraged to take this record with them on follow-up visits.

FOSTERING COMPLIANCE

Throughout the hospitalization, discuss medication information and how it will benefit the course of treatment. Seek cooperation and understanding of the following points so that medication compliance may be enhanced:

1. Name
2. Dosage
3. Route and administration times
4. Anticipated therapeutic response
5. Side effects to expect
6. Side effects to report
7. What to do if a dosage is missed
8. When, how, or if to refill the medication prescription

DIFFICULTY IN COMPREHENSION

If it is evident that the patient and/or family does not understand all aspects of the continuing therapy being prescribed (e.g., administration and monitoring of medications, exercise, diet, or follow-up appointments) consider the use of social service or visiting nurse agencies.

ASSOCIATED TEACHING

Give patients the following instructions:

Always inform the physician or dentist of any prescription or over-the-counter medication being taken.

Table 11.1
Example of a Written Record for Patients Receiving Respiratory Agents

Medications	Color	To be taken

Name _____

Physician _____

Physician's phone _____

Next appt.* _____

Parameters		Day of discharge							Comments
Blow bottles	AM # Liters								
	Noon								
	PM								
Postural drainage	Times of day performed (e.g., 8 AM, 2 PM)								
	Response: productive cough, non-productive								
Describe cough	Frequent, intermittent								
	Secretions: Color:								
	Thickness of secretions: thick, thin								
How do you feel today? (Record 2 times per day.) Awful 10 — Improving 5 — Good 1		AM / PM	AM / PM	AM / PM	AM / PM	AM / PM	AM / PM	AM / PM	
Exercise level: degree of tiredness with exercise. Extremely 10 — Moderate 5 — Normal 1									
Activities of daily living	Walk (#) of stairs								
	Walk (#) of blocks								
	Can or cannot perform daily activities Yes/No								
Pain pattern	Pain is on L (left) or R (right) side								
	Pain on inspiration = I Pain on expiration = E								
Difficulty breathing	Sleep with (#) pillows								
	Difficulty on exertion								
	Difficulty during stress								
	Difficulty when resting								
Appetite Poor 10 — Decreased 5 — Normal 1									

*Please bring this record with you to your next appointment.
Use the back of this sheet for additional information.

Over-the-counter medications should not be taken without first discussing them with a physician or pharmacist.

Always report side effects of rash, itching, or hives immediately. Nausea, vomiting, and diarrhea should also be reported for the physician's evaluation if it is a new symptom.

Take all of the medication as prescribed for the full course of treatment. Do not discontinue use when feeling improved; do not save for future use; do not give your medicine to another individual. Sudden discontinuation of certain medications may produce harmful effects.

Keep all medications out of reach of children.

If pregnancy is suspected, consult an obstetrician as soon as possible about continuation of medication therapy.

If medications are ordered for inhalation, be certain the individual understands the proper method of administration and operation of the nebulizer he or she will be using at home.

At Discharge

Items to be sent home with the patient should:

1. Have written instructions for use
2. Be labeled in language and size of print appropriate for the patient
3. If needed, include identification cards or bracelets
4. Include a list of additional supplies to be purchased after discharge (i.e., nebulizers, vaporizers)
5. Include a schedule for follow-up appointments.

Expectorant, Antitussive, and Mucolytic Therapy

Secretions of the Respiratory Tract

The fluids of the respiratory tract originate from specialized cells called *goblet cells* that line the respiratory tract and form the bronchial glands. The goblet cells produce a gelatinous mucus that forms a thin layer over the interior surfaces of the trachea, bronchi, and bronchioles. Factors that control the secretion of mucus from the goblet cells are not known, but exposure to irritants such as smoke, airborne particulate matter, and bacteria increases the mucus output of the cells. The bronchial glands are controlled by the cholinergic nervous system. When stimulated, the bronchial glands secrete a watery fluid to the interior surface of the

bronchial tract. There, the mucus secretions of the goblet cells and the watery secretions of the bronchial glands combine to form respiratory tract fluid.

Normally, respiratory tract fluid forms a protective layer over the trachea, bronchi, and bronchioles. Foreign bodies such as smoke particles and bacteria are caught in the respiratory tract fluid and are pushed upward by ciliary hairs that line the passages to the throat, where it is swallowed. This ciliary action cleanses the pulmonary system of foreign matter. The mucus becomes viscous, forming thick plugs in the bronchiolar airways, if too much mucus is secreted, the cilia are destroyed by chronic ingestion of smoke and alcohol, dehydration dries the mucus, or if anticholinergic agents inhibit watery secretions from the bronchial glands (Fig. 11.1). These thick plugs are quite difficult to eliminate. They allow the colonization of pathogenic microorganisms in the lower respiratory tract, causing additional mucus secretions and the possible development of pneumonia from trapped bacteria.

Cough

A cough is a reflex initiated by irritation of the airway. It is a protective, beneficial mechanism for

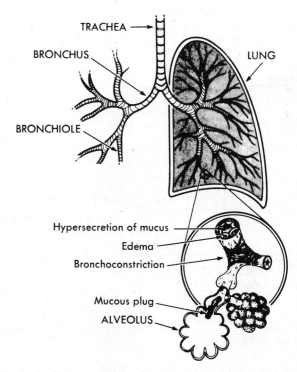

Fig. 11.1. *Factors restricting the airway. Major factors include hypersecretion of mucus, mucosal edema, and bronchoconstriction. Mucous plugs may form in the alveoli. (From Clark, J. B., Queener, S. F., and Karb, V. B.: Pharmacological Basis of Nursing Practice, p. 259. The C.V. Mosby Co., St. Louis, 1982.)*

Table 11.2

Antitussive Agents

GENERIC NAME	BRAND NAMES	AVAILABILITY	ADULT ORAL DOSAGE RANGE
Benzonatate	Tessalon Perles	Capsules: 100 mg	100 mg 3 times daily
Chlophedianol	Ulo	Syrup: 25 mg/5 ml	25 mg 3–4 times daily
Codeine*	—	Tablets: 15, 30, 60 mg	10–20 mg every 4–6 hours
Dextromethorphan	Sucrets, Romilar, Benylin DM	Lozenges: 7.5, 10 mg Syrup: 2.5, 5, 10, 15 mg/5 ml Liquid: 30 mg/5 ml	10–30 mg every 4–8 hours. Do not exceed 60–120 mg/24 hours
Diphenhydramine	Benylin, Diphen, Tusstat	Syrup: 12.5, 13.3 mg/5 ml	25 mg every 4 hours. Do not exceed 100 mg/24 hours.
Hydrocodone*	Dicodid	Tablets: 5 mg	5 mg every 4–6 hours
Levopropoxyphene	Novrad	Capsules: 100 mg	100 mg every 4 hours. Do not exceed 600 mg/24 hours
Noscapine	Tusscapine	Tablets: 15 mg Syrup: 15 mg/5 ml	15–30 mg every 4–6 hours. Do not exceed 120 mg/24 hours

* Often an ingredient in combination antitussive products.

clearing excess secretions from the tracheobronchial tree. The same irritants responsible for asthma or allergy may stimulate the cough receptors, or congestion of the nasal mucosa from a cold may cause a postnasal drip into the back of the throat, stimulating the cough.

A cough is "productive" if it helps remove accumulated secretions and phlegm from the tracheobronchial tree. A "nonproductive" cough results when irritants repeatedly stimulate the cough receptors, but are not removed by the coughing reflex. Excessive coughing, particularly if it is dry and nonproductive, is not only discomforting, but also tends to be self-perpetuating because the rapid air expulsion further irritates the tracheobronchial mucosa.

Treatment of the cough is of secondary importance; primary treatment is aimed at the underlying disorder. If the air is dry, a vaporizer may be used to liquefy the secretions so that they do not become irritating. A dehydrated state thickens respiratory secretions, so drinking plenty of fluids will help reduce the viscosity (thickness) of the secretions. Patients can also suck on hard candies to increase the flow of saliva to coat the throat, thus reducing irritation. If these simple measures do not reduce the frequency of the cough, expectorants or cough suppressants (antitussives) may be used. The therapeutic objective is to decrease the intensity and frequency of the cough yet permit adequate elimination of tracheobronchial secretions. In severe cases of pulmonary congestion, a mucolytic agent may be required.

Expectorants are agents that liquefy mucus by stimulating the secretion of natural lubricant fluids from the bronchial glands. This flow of natural secretions helps to liquefy thick mucous masses that may plug the narrow bronchioles. A combination of ciliary action and coughing will then expel the debris from the pulmonary system. Expectorants are used to treat nonproductive coughs, bronchitis, and pneumonia where mucus plugs inhibit the expulsion of irritants and bacteria causing the bronchitis or pneumonia.

Cough suppressants (antitussives) act by suppressing the cough center in the brain. They are used when the patient has a bothersome dry, hacking, nonproductive cough. These agents will not stop the cough completely, but should decrease the frequency of the cough and suppress the severe spasms which prevent adequate rest at night. Under normal circumstances, it is not appropriate to suppress a productive cough. See Table 11-2 for available antitussive agents.

Mucolytic agents reduce the thickness and stickiness of pulmonary secretions by acting directly on the mucous plugs to dissolve them. This eases the removal of the secretions by suction, postural drainage, or coughing. Mucolytic agents are most effective in removing mucous plugs obstructing the tracheobronchial airway. They are used in the treatment of patients with acute and chronic pulmonary disorders, as well as before and after bronchoscopy, following chest surgery, and as a part of the treatment of tracheostomy care.

Expectorants

Ammonium chloride (ah-mo'nee-um)

Ammonium chloride is believed to increase the amount of respiratory tract fluid by irritation of the gastric mucosa. Irritation of the gastric mucosa is thought to have a stimulating effect on the bronchial glands to increase secretions, thus decreasing the viscosity of the mucus. Ammonium chloride is a common ingredient in over-the-counter cough and cold preparations.

However, no well-controlled, double-blind studies have shown any expectorant effect over a placebo.

Guaifenesin (gwi-feh-neh'sin)
(Robitussin) (row-bih-tus'sin)

Guaifenesin, formerly known as glyceryl guaiacolate, is an expectorant that acts by enhancing the output of respiratory tract fluid. The increased flow of secretions promotes ciliary action and facilitates the removal of mucus. It is used for the symptomatic relief of conditions characterized by a dry, nonproductive cough, as well as to remove mucus plugs from the respiratory tract.

Guaifensin should not be used with a dry, persistent cough that lasts more than 1 week. The patient should seek medical attention if the cough does not subside.

Guaifenesin should be used with caution in patients with cardiovascular disorders, diabetes mellitus, hyperthyroidism, and people sensitive to sympathomimetic amines.

Side Effects

Side effects are infrequent, but gastrointestinal upsets, nausea, and vomiting have been reported.

Availability

PO—100 and 200 mg tablets, 200 mg capsules, 100 mg/5 ml syrup. It is also available in individual products in combination with pseudoephedrine, dextromethorphan, codeine phosphate, and phenylpropanolamine.

Dosage and Administration

Adult
PO—100 to 400 mg every 4 to 6 hours. Do not exceed 2400 mg/day.
Pediatric
PO—Ages 6 to 12: 50 to 100 mg every 4 to 6 hours. Do not exceed 600 mg/day. Ages 2 to 6: 50 mg every 4 hours. Do not exceed 300 mg/day.

Nursing Interventions

See also General Nursing Considerations for Patients with Respiratory Tract Disease.

PATIENT CONCERNS: NURSING INTERVENTION/RATIONALE

Side Effects to Expect

Gastrointestinal Upset, Nausea, Vomiting

Development of these side effects is rare.

Dosage and Administration

Fluid Intake

Maintain fluid intake at 8 to 12 8-ounce glasses daily.

Humidification

Suggest the concurrent use of a humidifier.

Drug Interactions

No significant drug interactions have been reported.

Iodine Products (SSKI, Potassium Iodide, others)

The iodides are the most commonly used expectorants. They act by stimulating increased secretions from the bronchial glands to decrease the viscosity of mucous plugs, making it easier for patients to cough up the dry, hardened plugs blocking the bronchial tubes. Iodides are used as expectorants in the symptomatic treatment of chronic pulmonary diseases where tenacious mucus is present.

Side Effects

Side effects are quite mild and infrequent. Oral and gastric irritation, with nausea, have been reported.

Patients with a hypersensitivity to iodides, hyperthyroidism, hyperkalemia, and acute bronchitis should not use iodide products. An early indication of hypersensitivity is development of a rash.

Long-term, chronic use may induce goiter, particularly in children with cystic fibrosis.

Availability

PO—liquids, tablets, syrups, and elixirs of varying strengths.

Dosage and Administration

Adult

PO—See individual products.

Nursing Interventions

See also General Nursing Considerations for Patients with Respiratory Tract Disease.

PATIENT CONCERNS: NURSING INTERVENTION/RATIONALE

Side Effects to Expect

Nausea

Symptoms are usually mild; if they become bothersome, report to a physician.

Dosage and Administration

Pregnancy

Ask if the patient is pregnant prior to administration. Excessive use of iodine-containing products may result in goiter in the newborn.

Thyroid Function Tests

Always inform the physician of the use of this product if thyroid function tests are to be scheduled.

Drug Interactions

Potassium Supplements, Salt Substitutes, Potassium-sparing Diuretics

DO NOT administer with potassium-sparing diuretics (amiloride, triamterene, spironolactone). Use potassium supplements or salt substitutes high in potassium because of potentially dangerous effects from hyperkalemia.

Lithium, Antithyroid Agents

Concurrent use with lithium and antithyroid medications (methimazole, propylthiouracil) may result in hypothyroidism.

Saline Solutions

Saline solutions of varying concentrations can be very effective expectorants when administered by nebulization. They act by hydrating mucus, reducing its viscosity. When administered by inhalation, hypotonic solutions (0.45% sodium chloride) are thought to provide deeper penetration into the more distant airways, while a hypertonic solution (1.8% sodium chloride) hydrates as well as stimulates a productive cough by irritating the respiratory passages. Isotonic saline solutions (0.9% sodium chloride), administered by nebulization, are used to hydrate respiratory secretions.

Saline nose drops are sometimes ordered for infants experiencing nasal congestion to clear the nasal passage and aid in breathing. Administration is usually immediately prior to giving them a bottle or breast feeding, since infants are nasal breathers.

Mucolytic Agents

Acetylcysteine (a-see'-til-cist-een)
(Mucomyst) (mu'-co-mist)

Acetylcysteine is currently the only mucolytic agent available that acts by dissolving chemical bonds within the mucus itself, thus causing it to separate and liquefy. It is used to dissolve abnormally viscous mucus secretions that may occur in chronic emphysema, emphysema with bronchitis, asthmatic bronchitis, and pneumonia.

Side Effects

The most common adverse effects of acetylcysteine are mouth and throat irritation, nausea, vomiting, chest tightness, bronchoconstriction and runny nose (rhinorrhea).

Availability

Inhalation—10% and 20% solutions in 4, 10 and 30 ml vials.

Dosage and Administration

Adult

Inhalation—The recommended dosage for most patients is 3 to 5 ml of the 20% solution 3 to 4 times daily. It may be administered by nebulization, direct application, or intratracheal instillation.

Note: After administration, the volume of bronchial secretions may increase. Some patients with inadequate cough reflex may require mechanical suctioning to maintain an open airway.

Nursing Interventions

See also General Nursing Considerations for Patients with Respiratory Tract Disease.

PATIENT CONCERNS: NURSING INTERVENTION/RATIONALE

Side Effects to Expect

Nausea, Vomiting

This drug has a pungent odor (similar to rotten eggs) which may cause nausea and vomiting. Have an emesis basin available in case vomiting should occur. (Do not, however, suggest it by having it in clear view.)

Side Effects to Report

Bronchospasm

This agent may occasionally cause bronchoconstriction and bronchospasm. Concurrent use of a bronchodilator may be necessary.

Dosage and Administration

Nebulizer

This solution tends to concentrate as the solution is used. When three-fourths of the original amount in the nebulizer is used, dilute the remaining solution with sterile water.

After therapy, wash the patient's face and hands because the drug is sticky and irritating. Thoroughly cleanse equipment used.

Storage

Store the opened solution of the drug in a refrigerator for up to 48 hours. Discard the unused portion after that time.

Discoloration

Use this medication only in plastic or glass containers. Contact with metals other than stainless steel can cause discoloration of the solution.

Drug Interactions

Antibiotics

Acetylcysteine inactivates most antibiotics. Do not mix together for aerosol administration. Schedule administration of inhalation antibiotics 1 hour after administration of acetylcysteine.

Bronchodilators

Bronchodilators are agents that relax the smooth muscle of the tracheobronchial tree. This allows an increase in the opening of the bronchioles and alveolar ducts and a decrease in resistance to airflow into the alveolar sacs.

Bronchodilators are used in patients with diseases that cause constriction of the tracheobronchial tree, obstructing the airways (see Fig. 11.1). Asthma and bronchitis are diseases that cause a reversible obstruction, while emphysema is a disease that has variable reversibility of airway constriction, depending on the severity and duration of the disease. The primary agents used in the treatment of airway-obstructive diseases include sympathomimetic agents and xanthine derivatives.

Sympathomimetic Bronchodilating Agents

Sympathomimetic agents are used as bronchodilators because they stimulate receptors within the smooth muscle of the tracheobronchial tree to relax, thus opening the airway passages to greater volumes of air. The primary sympathomimetic agents used as bronchodilators are listed in Table 11.3. They are used to reverse airway constriction caused by acute and chronic bronchial asthma, bronchitis, and emphysema.

Side Effects

Unfortunately, the receptors stimulated by sympathomimetic agents, causing relaxation of the smooth muscle in the tracheobronchial tree, are found in other tissues as well as the pulmonary system. The receptors are also found in the muscles of the heart, blood vessels, uterus, gastrointestinal, urinary and central nervous systems. They also help regulate fat and carbohydrate metabolism. For this reason, there are many side effects from these agents, particularly if used too frequently or in higher doses than recommended.

The most common side effects are dose related. These include tachycardia, tremor, nervousness, heart palpitations, and dizziness. Other, less frequent, side

Table 11.3

Bronchodilators

GENERIC NAME	BRAND NAMES	AVAILABILITY	ADULT DOSAGE RANGE
Sympathomimetics			
Albuterol	Proventil, Ventolin	Tablets: 2, 4 mg Aerosol: 90 mcg	PO: 2–4 mg 3–4 times daily Inhale: 2 inhalations every 4–6 hours
Ephedrine	Ephedrine	Tablets: 25 mg Capsules: 25, 50 mg Syrup: 11, 20 mg/5 ml Injection: 25, 50 mg/ml	PO: 25–50 mg every 3–4 hours SC, IM, IV: 25–50 mg
Epinephrine	Primatene, Vaponefrin, Bronkaid Mist	Nebulization: 1:100 Aerosol: 0.2, 0.25, 0.3 mg Injection: 1:200, 1:100	See Manufacturer's Recommendations
Ethylnorepinephrine	Bronkephrine	2 mg/ml	SC or IM: 0.5–ml
Isoetharine	Bronkosol, Beta-2, Bronkometer	Nebulization: 0.125, 0.2, 0.5, 1% Aerosol: 0.61%	See Manufacturer's Recommendations
Isoproterenol	Isuprel, Aerolone, Norisodrine	Nebulization: 0.25, 0.5, 1% Aerosol: 0.2, 0.25% Injection: 0.2 mg/ml SL: 10, 15 mg tabs	See Manufacturer's Recommendations
Metaproterenol	Alupent, Metaprel	Tablets: 10, 20 mg Syrup: 10 mg/5 ml Aerosol: 225 mg Nebulization: 5%	See Manufacturer's Recommendations
Terbutaline	Brethine, Bricanyl	Tablets: 2.5, 5 mg Injection: 1 mg/ml	PO: 5 mg every 6 hours SC: 0.25 mg; repeat, if needed, in 30 minutes
Xanthine Derivatives			
Aminophylline		Tablets: 100, 200 mg Elixir: 250 mg/15 ml Liquid: 105 mg/5 ml Suppositories: 250, 500 mg Injection: 250, 500 ml Others	See Manufacturer's Recommendations
Dyphylline	Dilor, Dyflex, Lufyllin	Tablets: 200, 400 mg Liquid: 100 mg/5 ml Elixir: 100, 160 mg/15 ml Injection: 250 mg/ml	PO: 15 mg/kg, 5 times daily IM: 250–500 mg slowly
Oxtriphylline	Choledyl	Tablets: 100, 200 mg Elixir: 100 mg/5 ml Syrup: 50 mg/5 ml	200 mg 4 times daily
Theophylline	Bronkodyl, Elixophyllin, Theolair, Others	Tablets: 125, 200, 225, 300 mg Capsules: 50, 100, 200, 250 mg Elixir: 80 mg/15 ml Liquid: 80 mg/15 ml Syrup: 80 mg/15 ml Suspension: 300 mg/15 ml Others	9–20 mg/kg/24 hours in 4 divided doses

effects may include nausea, vomiting, headache, restlessness, drowsiness, sweating, and tinnitus.

Patients who receive these medications by inhalation therapy may experience an unusual taste, heartburn, and dry throat leading to throat irritation.

Patients known to have hypertension, hyperthyroidism, diabetes mellitus, or cardiac disease with arrhythmias may be particularly sensitive to adverse reactions and must be observed closely.

Availability

See Table 11.3 for available sympathomimetic bronchodilator products and recommended dosage ranges.

Nursing Interventions

See also General Nursing Considerations for Patients with Respiratory Tract Disease.

PATIENT CONCERNS: NURSING INTERVENTION/RATIONALE

Side Effects to Report

Tachycardia, Palpitations

Since most symptoms are dose-related, alterations should be reported to the physician. Monitor the patient's heart rate and rhythm at regular intervals throughout therapy with bronchodilators.

Report heart rates significantly higher than baseline values.

Always report palpitations and suspected arrhythmias.

Tremors

Tell the patient to notify the physician if tremors develop after starting any of these medications. A dosage adjustment may be necessary.

Nervousness, Anxiety, Restlessness, Headache

Perform a baseline assessment of the patient's mental status—degree of anxiety, nervousness, alertness; compare subsequent, regular assessments to the findings obtained. Report escalation of tension.

Nausea, Vomiting

Monitor all aspects of the development of these symptoms. Question the patient concerning other medications being taken and any other symptoms that have also developed.

Administer the medication with food and a full glass of water or milk. Report if the symptoms are not relieved.

Dizziness

Provide for patient safety during episodes of dizziness; report for further evaluation.

Drug Interactions

Drugs That Enhance Toxic Effects

Tricyclic antidepressants (imipramine, amitriptyline, nortriptyline, doxepin, others), monoamine oxidase inhibitors (tranylcypromine, isocarboxazid, pargyline) and other sympathomimetic agents (metaproterenol, isoproterenol, others): Monitor for increases in severity of drug effects such as nervousness, tachycardia, tremors, and arrhythmias.

Drugs That Reduce Therapeutic Effects

Beta adrenergic blocking agents (propanolol, timolol, nadolol, pindolol, others): Higher doses, or use of another class of bronchodilator, may be required.

Antihypertensive Agents

Sympathomimetic agents may reduce the therapeutic effects of antihypertensive agents. Monitor blood pressure for an indication of loss of antihypertensive control.

Xanthine Derivative Bronchodilating Agents

Methylxanthines, more commonly known as the xanthine derivatives, act directly on the smooth muscle of the tracheobronchial tree to dilate the bronchi, thus increasing airflow in and out of the alveolar sacs. The primary xanthine derivatives used as bronchodilators are listed in Table 11.3. They are frequently used in combination with sympathomimetic bronchodilators to reverse airway constriction caused by acute and chronic bronchial asthma, bronchitis, and emphysema.

Side Effects

In addition to relaxing pulmonary smooth muscle, the xanthine derivatives stimulate the central nervous system, induce diuresis, increase gastric acid secretions, and stimulate the heart to beat more rapidly. Consequently, side effects associated with bronchodilator therapy, particularly in higher doses, include nervousness, agitation, insomnia, nausea, vomiting, abdominal cramps, epigastric pain, and tachycardia, possibly with arrhythmias. All of these side effects are dose-dependent, and may diminish with a reduction in dosage.

Xanthine derivatives should be administered cautiously to patients with congestive heart failure, chronic obstructive pulmonary disease, renal, or hepatic disease. These patients metabolize xanthine derivatives much more slowly and may develop toxicities more easily.

Xanthine derivatives should also be used with caution in patients with angina pectoris, peptic ulcer disease, hyperthyroidism, glaucoma, and diabetes mellitus.

Availability

See Table 11.3 for available xanthine derivative bronchodilator products and recommended dosage ranges.

Nursing Interventions

See also General Nursing Considerations for Patients with Respiratory Tract Disease.

PATIENT CONCERNS: NURSING INTERVENTION/RATIONALE

Side Effects to Report

Tachycardia, Palpitations

Since most symptoms are dose-related, alterations should be reported to the physician. Monitor the patient's heart rate and rhythm at regular intervals throughout therapy with bronchodilators.

Report heart rates significantly higher than baseline values.

Always report palpitations and suspected arrhythmias.

Tremors

Tell the patient to notify the physician if tremors develop after starting any of these medications. A dosage adjustment may be necessary.

Nervousness, Anxiety, Restlessness, Headache

Perform a baseline assessment of the patient's mental status—degree of anxiety, nervousness, alertness; compare subsequent, regular assessments to the findings obtained. Report escalation of tension.

Dosage and Administration

Nausea, Vomiting, Epigastric Pain, and Abdominal Cramps

These symptoms may occur from gastric irritation caused by increased gastric acid secretions stimulated by these agents.

If gastric irritation occurs, administer with food or milk. If symptoms persist or increase in severity, report for physician evaluation.

Plasma Levels

To maintain consistent plasma levels, administer the medication around the clock.

Drug Interactions

Drugs That Enhance Toxic Effects

Cimetidine, erythromycin, troleandomycin, thiabendazole, influenza vaccine, propranolol, and allopurinol: Monitor for increases in severity of drug effects such as nervousness, agitation, nausea, tachycardia, and arrhythmias.

Drugs That Reduce Therapeutic Effects

Tobacco or marijuana smoking. Higher doses of the bronchodilator may be required.

Lithium

Xanthine derivatives may increase the renal excretion of lithium carbonate. Higher doses of lithium are required to maintain therapeutic effects. Monitor for the return of manic or depressive activity. Enlist the aid of family and friends to help identify early symptoms.

Beta Adrenergic Blocking Agents

Xanthine derivatives and beta adrenergic blocking agents (propranolol, timolol, nadolol, atenolol, others) may be mutually antagonistic in their actions. Patients must be observed for inhibition of either drug.

Nasal Decongestants

Nasal stuffiness and congestion are caused by swelling of the nasal mucous membranes. Two major causes of a stuffy nose are *allergic rhinitis* (in which the nasal passages swell because of an allergic reaction, most commonly due to dust or pollen) and symptoms of the "common cold."

Symptomatic relief of nasal congestion is a result of reduced swelling of the nasal passages. Nasal decongestants stimulate the alpha adrenergic receptors of the vascular smooth muscle of the nasal passages, causing constriction of the blood vessels within the nasal passages. This constriction reduces blood flow in the engorged nasal area, resulting in shrinkage of the engorged membranes, thus promoting drainage, improving nasal air passage, and relieving the feeling of stuffiness.

The use of nasal decongestants provides temporary relief of the symptoms. Initially, the "stuffiness" or "blocked" sensation exhibits relief. However, as the constricting action diminishes, the symptoms return. Prolonged use can cause irritation of the nares; excessive use may result in a "rebound" effect caused by swelling of the nasal passages. Instill drops or sprays appropri-

Table 11.4
Nasal Decongestants

GENERIC NAME	BRAND NAMES	AVAILABILITY	ADULT DOSAGE RANGE
Ephedrine	Efedron, Vatronol	Solution: 0.5, 1, 3% Jelly: 0.6%	Nasal: 2–3 drops 2–3 times daily
Epinephrine	Adrenalin	Solution: 0.1%	Nasal: 1–2 drops in each nostril every 4–6 hours
Phenylephrine	Neo-Synephrine, Sinex	Solution: 0.125, 0.16, 0.2, 0.25, 0.5, 1% Jelly: 0.5%	Nasal: 0.25% every 3–4 hours
Phenylpropanolamine	Propadrine, Propagest	Tablets: 25, 50 mg Capsules: 25, 50 mg Syrup: 12.5 mg/5 ml Elixir: 20 mg/5 ml	PO: 25 mg every 3–4 hours or 50 mg every 6–8 hours. Do not exceed 150 mg daily
Pseudoephedrine	Sudafed, Neofed, Novafed	Tablets: 30, 60 mg Liquid: 30 mg/5 ml	PO: 60 mg every 6 hours. Do not exceed 240 mg/24 hours
Oxymetazoline	Afrin, Bayfrin, Duration	Solution: 0.025–0.05%	Nasal: 2–3 drops or sprays of 0.05% solution twice daily
Tetrahydrozoline	Tyzine	Solution: 0.05–0.1%	Nasal: 2–4 drops of 0.1% solution every 4–6 hours
Xylometazoline	Otrivin, Corimist	Solution: 0.05, 0.1%	Nasal: 2–3 sprays every 8–10 hours

ately. (See Administration by Inhalation in Chapter 7.)

Decongestant Products

All decongestants currently available are alpha adrenergic receptor stimulants that reduce nasal obstruction by constricting blood vessels in the nasal passages. They are used to open swollen nasal passages and relieve congestion caused by hay fever, allergic rhinitis, and the common cold (see Table 11.4).

Side Effects

Products used as nasal decongestants also have the ability to stimulate alpha receptors at other sites in the body as well. Therefore, they should be used with caution in patients with hypertension, hyperthyroidism, diabetes mellitus, cardiac disease, increased intraocular pressure, or prostatic hypertrophy.

It is important for the patient to carefully follow directions on the label. Misuse by patients, including excessive use or frequency of administration, may cause a "rebound" swelling of the nasal passages. This secondary congestion is thought to be caused by excessive vasoconstriction of the blood vessels and by direct irritation of the nasal membranes by the solution. When the vasoconstrictor effects wear off, the irritation causes excessive blood flow to the passages, causing them to swell and become engorged again; the nose feels more stuffy and congested than before treatment. Rebound effects are minimal if decongestants are used for only 3 to 5 days.

Availability

See Table 11.4 for available decongestant products.

Nursing Interventions

See also General Nursing Considerations for Patients with Respiratory Tract Disease.

PATIENT CONCERNS: NURSING INTERVENTION/RATIONALE

Side Effects to Expect

Mild Nasal Irritation

A burning or stinging sensation may be experienced. This may be alleviated by using a weaker strength of solution.

Drug Interactions

Drugs That Enhance Toxic Effects

Beta adrenergic blocking agents (e.g., propanolol, timolol, atenolol, nadolol, others) and monoamine oxidase inhibitors (tranylcypromine, isocarboxazid, pargyline).

Excessive use may result in significant hypertension.

Patients already receiving antihypertensive therapy should avoid the use of decongestants.

Methyldopa, Reserpine

Frequent use of decongestants inhibits the antihypertensive activity of these agents. Concurrent therapy is not recommended.

Antihistamines

Histamine is a compound derived from an amino acid called *histidine*. It is stored in small granules in most body tissues. Its physiologic functions are not completely known, but it is released in response to allergic reactions and tissue damage from trauma or infection. When histamine is released in the area of tissue damage or at the site of an antigen-antibody reaction (such as a pollen being inhaled into the nose of a patient allergic to that specific pollen) the following reactions take place: (1) arterioles and capillaries in the region dilate, allowing an increased blood flow to the area, resulting in redness; (2) capillaries become more permeable, resulting in the outward passage of fluid into the extracellular spaces and, thus, edema; this edema is manifested by congestion in the mucous membranes of the patient's nose and lungs; (3) nasal, lacrimal, and bronchial secretions are released, resulting in the running nose and eyes noted in patients with allergies.

When large amounts of histamine are released, such as in a severe allergic reaction, there is extensive arteriolar dilatation. The blood pressure drops (hypotension), and the skin becomes flushed and edematous with severe itching (urticaria). Constriction and spasm of the bronchial tubes makes respiratory effort more difficult (dyspnea), and copious amounts of pulmonary and gastric secretions are released.

Histamine response can be antagonized by two types of drugs, rapidly acting epinephrine and the more slowly acting group of antihistamines. Epinephrine is used only in severe, acute allergic reactions.

Antihistamines can reduce the severity of the symptoms observed in the allergic patient. *Antihistamines* are chemical agents that act by competing with the allergy-liberated histamine for receptor sites in the patient's arterioles, capillaries, and glands. Antihistamines do not prevent histamine release, but will reduce the symptoms of an allergic reaction if the concentration of the antihistamine at the receptor site exceeds the concentration of histamine at the receptors. Antihistamines are, therefore, more effective if taken when the symptoms are first appearing.

Antihistamines treat only the symptoms of allergy, and do not immunize the patient against allergic reactions. Relief of various allergic symptoms is obtained only while the drug is being taken. There is no cumulative action, so these drugs can be taken for prolonged periods of time. Some patients, requiring frequent antihistamine use, find that they do not obtain the same degree of relief after several weeks or months of therapy. If tolerance does develop, patients may easily switch to another antihistamine that does provide relief.

Side Effects

The most common side effect of many of the antihistaminic drugs is drowsiness. Most patients acquire a tolerance to this adverse effect with continued therapy. Reduction in dosage or a change to another antihistamine may occasionally be necessary, however.

All antihistamines display anticholinergic side effects, particularly when higher dosages are used. Symptoms include dry mouth, stuffy nose, blurred vision, constipation, and urinary retention. Patients with asthma, prostatic enlargement, or glaucoma should take antihistamines only under a physician's supervision. The drying effects may also make respiratory mucus more viscous and tenacious. Use antihistamines with caution in patients who have a productive cough. If the cough continues but becomes nonproductive, consider additional hydration of the patient and discontinuation of the antihistamine.

Availability

See Table 11.5 for available antihistamine products and recommended dosage ranges.

Nursing Interventions

See also General Nursing Considerations for Patients with Respiratory Tract Disease.

Since antihistamines are prescribed for a variety of symptoms such as hay fever, dermatological reactions, drug hypersensitivity, rhinitis, and transfusion reactions, it is necessary for the nurse to individualize the patient assessments with the underlying pathology. Identification of the trigger mechanism, or allergens, that initiate an allergic response is imperative to the patient's treatment. Repeated exposure to the conditions that precipitate an attack will again initiate an allergic response.

Table 11.5
*Antihistamines**

GENERIC NAME	BRAND NAMES	AVAILABILITY	ADULT DOSAGE RANGE	MAXIMUM DAILY DOSE (MG)
Brompheniramine maleate	Bromamine, Dimetane, Bromphen	Injection, tablets, elixir	4 mg three to six times daily	24
Chlorpheniramine maleate	Chlor-tab-4, Chlor-Trimeton, Trymegen	Tablets, capsules, syrup	4 mg three to six times daily	24
Cyproheptadine hydrochloride	Periactin, Cyprodine	Tablets, syrup	4 mg three times daily	32
Diphenhydramine hydrochloride	Benadryl, Bendylate, Nordryl	Injection, capsules, tablets, syrup, elixir	25–50 mg three or four times daily	300
Doxylamine succinate	Decapryn	Tablets, syrup	12.5–25 mg every 4–6 hours	150
Promethazine hydrochloride†	Phenergan, Remsed, Baymethazine	Injection, tablets, syrup, suppository	12.5–25 mg three or four times daily	100
Pyrilamine maleate	—	Tablets	25–60 mg four times daily	200
Tripelennamine	PBZ	Tablets, elixir	25–50 mg every 4–6 hours	300

* Many of these antihistamines are also available in combination with decongestants and analgesics for relief of cold and flu symptoms.
† Promethazine is a phenothiazine with antihistaminic properties.

PATIENT CONCERNS: NURSING INTERVENTION/RATIONALE

Side Effects to Expect

Sedative Effects

The types of antihistamines ordered can produce varying degrees of sedation. Tolerance may be produced over a period of time, thus diminishing the effect.

Operating power equipment or driving may be hazardous. Caution patients to provide for their personal safety in these situations.

Drying Effects

Monitor the patient's cough and degree of sputum production when antihistamines are administered. Because of their drying effects, antihistamines may impair expectoration.

Fluid Intake

Give adequate fluids concurrently with the use of antihistamines. Maintain fluid intake at 8 to 12 8-ounce glasses daily.

Blurred Vision, Constipation, Urinary Retention, Dryness of Mucosa of the Mouth, Throat, and Nose

These symptoms are the anticholinergic effects produced by antihistamines. Patients taking these medications should be monitored for the development of these side effects.

Dryness of the mucosa may be alleviated by sucking hard candy or ice chips, or chewing gum.

Caution the patient that blurred vision may occur and make appropriate suggestions for personal safety of the individual.

Drug Interactions

CNS Depressants

CNS depressants, including sleep aids, analgesics, tranquilizers, and alcohol will potentiate the sedative effects of antihistamines. People who work around machinery, drive a car, pour and give medicines, or perform other duties, in which they must remain mentally alert, should not take these medications while working.

Other Agents

Cromolyn Sodium (kro'mo-lin)
(Intal) (in-tahl')

Cromolyn sodium is a unique medication that is administered to prevent the release of histamine from its storage sites, the mast cells. It must be administered before the body receives a stimulus to release histamine, such as an antigen that initiates an antigen-antibody allergic reaction. Cromolyn is recommended for use in conjunction with other medications in the treatment of patients with severe bronchial asthma to prevent the release of histamine that results in asthmatic attacks.

Cromolyn has no direct bronchodilatory, antihistaminic, anticholinergic, or antiinflammatory activity. A 2- to 4-week course of therapy is usually required to determine clinical response. Therapy should only be continued if there is a decrease in the severity of asthmatic symptoms during treatment.

Side Effects

The most common side effect is irritation of the throat and trachea caused by inhalation of the dry powder. This irritation may be manifested by nasal itching and burning, nasal stuffiness, sneezing, coughing, and bronchospasm. Other side effects that infrequently arise are nausea, drowsiness, dizziness, and headache.

Availability

Inhalation—20 mg capsules, 20 mg/2 ml solution for nebulizer.

Dosage and Administration

Adult
PO—Patients must be advised that the capsules are not absorbed when swallowed and that the drug is inactive when administered by this route.
Inhalation—20 mg (1 capsule), via inhaler, 4 times daily.

Drug Interactions

No significant drug interactions have been reported.

Nursing Interventions

See also General Nursing Considerations for Patients with Respiratory Tract Disease.

PATIENT CONCERNS: NURSING INTERVENTION/RATIONALE

Side Effects to Expect

Oral Irritation, Dry Mouth

Start regular oral hygiene measures when the therapy is initiated. Suggest the use of 1 tsp of hydrogen peroxide in 6 to 8 ounces of water as a mouthwash. Commercial mouthwashes contain alcohol which may cause further drying and oral irritation.

Other measures to alleviate dryness include sucking on ice chips or hard candy.

Side Effects to Report

Bronchospasm, Coughing

Notify the physician if inhalation causes these symptoms.

Administration and Dosage

Inhalation

Inhalation during an acute asthma attack may aggravate symptoms since the powder form of the drug can increase the irritation in the respiratory passage causing more bronchospasm.

Proper technique is quite important to the success of therapy. Document and verify that the patient can do the following:

1. Load the inhaler with a capsule and pierce (only once) the capsule immediately before use.
2. Hold the inhaler away from the mouth and exhale, emptying as much air from the lungs as possible.
3. With the head tilted back and teeth apart, close lips around the mouthpiece.
4. Inhale deeply and rapidly through the inhaler with a steady, even breath.
5. Remove the inhaler and hold the breath for a few seconds, then exhale. (Do not exhale through the inhaler, because moisture from the breath will interfere with proper function of the inhaler.)
6. Repeat several times until the powder is inhaled. (A light dusting of powder remaining in the capsule is normal.)

Drug Interactions

No significant drug interactions have been reported.

Chapter 12

Drugs Affecting
the Muscular System

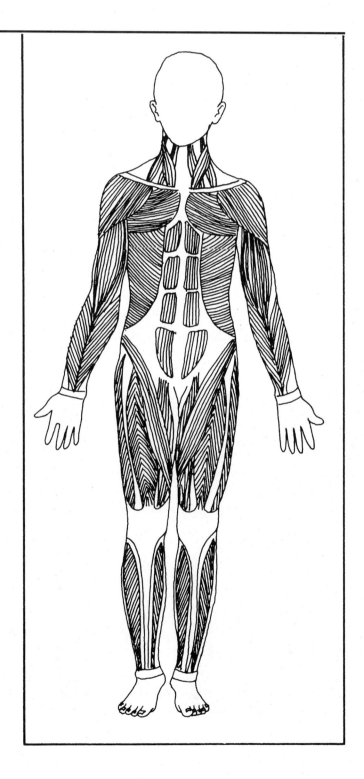

Objectives

After completing this chapter, the student should be able to do the following:

1. Explain the major actions and effects of drugs used to treat disorders of the muscular system.
2. Identify baseline data the nurse should collect on a continuous basis for comparison and evaluation of drug effectiveness.
3. Identify important nursing assessments and interventions associated with drug therapy and treatment of diseases associated with the muscular system.
4. Identify health teaching essential for a successful treatment regimen.

General Nursing Considerations for Patients Receiving Muscle Relaxants

Musculoskeletal disorders may produce varying degrees of pain, immobility, and impact on the individual's daily activities of living. The nursing assessments performed are individualized to the muscles affected and the disease processes involved.

PATIENT CONCERNS: NURSING INTERVENTION/RATIONALE

Assessment of Skeletal Muscle Disorders

Muscle Spasticity

Assess the extent of the spasticity and the muscle groups affected.

History

Obtain a brief history of injury and details of the areas involved.

Degree of Impairment

Seek information relative to the degree of impairment being experienced (strength, gait, conservation effect, compensatory action).

Activities of Daily Living

Determine which activities of daily living the individual can perform independently and those which require assistance.

Pain Level

Determine the pain level and extent, frequency of analgesic use, precipitating factors, and any measures the patient has identified that alleviate it.

Examination

Inspect the affected part for swelling, edema, bruises, redness, and localized tenderness. (Be gentle during the inspection.)

Patient Teaching Associated with Muscle Relaxants

Communication and Responsibility

Encourage open communication concerning frustrations and anger as the patient attempts to adjust to the diagnosis and need for prolonged treatment. The patient must be guided to gain insight into the condition in order to assume responsibility for continuation of treatment. Keep emphasizing those factors the patient can control to alter the progression of the disease, including the following measures:

HOT OR COLD APPLICATIONS

Provide specific instructions regarding the application of heat or cold. Generally, ice packs alleviate swelling immediately after muscle injury. Later in the course of treatment, application of heat provides comfort.

ELEVATION

Elevating the extremity immediately following injury decreases swelling and, to some degree, alleviates pain.

ACTIVITY AND EXERCISE

During the initial phase of treatment, immobilizing the affected part will decrease muscle spasms and thereby decrease pain. Various approaches may be used for immobilization: Ace bandages, splinting, casts, bedrest, or modified activity levels.

Range of motion exercises may be prescribed to maintain joint function and to prevent muscle atrophy and contractures. The activity plan prescribed will be individualized to the diagnosis and should be carefully followed for maximum effectiveness.

PAIN MANAGEMENT

Analgesic and antiinflammatory agents may be given, if appropriate to the underlying pathology, to relieve pain and reduce inflammation.

POSITIONING

Maintenance of proper alignment and immobility of the affected part will also relieve pain and swelling.

The following measures are appropriate for persons with lower back pain: (1) Bedrest with the head of the bed elevated 15–20° and the knees slightly flexed will provide relief to muscles of the lower back area. (2) Proper body alignment during sleep is important. (3) Maintenance of optimal body weight will prevent undue stress on lower back musculature. (4) Proper techniques of lifting to avoid future injury must be taught.

ANXIETY

Increased anxiety produces stress on the body's muscles. Implement measures to produce relaxation and provide for the psychological needs of the individual.

Expectations of Therapy

Discuss expectations of therapy with the patient.

ACTIVITIES AND EXERCISES

The patient must resume activities of daily living within the boundaries set by the physician. (Such activities as regular moderate exercise, meal preparation, resumption of usual sexual activities, and social interaction all need to be fostered once specific orders are obtained.)

PAIN RELIEF

The degree of musculoskeletal pain relief with and without activity needs to be discussed. Make modifications appropriate to the diagnosis and degree of impairment.

EMOTIONAL SUPPORT

For disorders of a chronic nature, encourage the patient to express feelings openly regarding chronic illness. The adjustment to this situation involves working through great personal fears, frustrations, hostilities, and resentments associated with the loss of personal control within one's life.

Changes in Expectations

Assess changes in expectations as therapy progresses and the patient gains understanding of the diagnosis. Areas to assess include pain relief, resumption of daily activities, and increasing mobility.

Changes in Therapy through Cooperative Goal-Setting

Work with the patient to encourage adherence to the prescribed treatment. When the patient feels that a change should be made in a treatment plan, encourage discussion first with the physician.

WRITTEN RECORD

Enlist the patient's aid in developing and maintaining a written record of monitoring parameters (Table 12.1) (i.e., level, location, duration of pain, areas or muscles affected, degree of impairment with improvement in mobility, exercise tolerance) and response to prescribed therapies for discussion with the physician. Patients should be encouraged to take this record on follow-up visits.

FOSTERING COMPLIANCE

Throughout hospitalization, discuss medication information and how it will benefit the course of treatment. Seek cooperation and understanding of the following points so that medication compliance may be enhanced:

1. Name
2. Dosage
3. Route and administration times
4. Anticipated therapeutic response; increased ability to participate in activities of daily living as a result of pain relief and increased degree of mobility; increased tolerance of exercise
5. Side effects to expect: sedation, weakness, lethargy, dizziness, light-headedness
6. Side effects to report
7. What to do if a dosage is missed
8. When, how, or if to refill medication prescription

Table 12.1

Example of a Written Record for Patients Receiving Muscle Relaxants

Medications	Color	To be taken

Name _____

Physician _____

Physician's phone _____

Next appt.* _____

Parameters			Day of discharge							Comments
Muscle areas affected	List areas:		AM	AM	AM	AM	AM	AM	AM	
	1.									
	2.									
	3.									
	4.									
	Example: 1. Arm, lower 2. Lower back 3. 4.	AM 1, 2 PM 1, 2	PM	PM	PM	PM	PM	PM	PM	
Chart areas affected 2 times per day										
Exercise and range of motion pain No improvement 10 Moderate improvement 5 Much improvement 1										
Pattern of pain	Location									
	Time of day pain occurs									
	Relieved by									
	Made worse by									
Impairment(s) and improvement	Example: Could not comb hair — can now. Could not turn head without pain — can now.									
Physical therapy prescribed	Example: Application of cold packs at 8 AM – 4 PM and bedtime	Therapy								
		Time of day								
		Feeling, response								

Please bring this record with you to your next appointment.
Use the back of this sheet for additional information.

DIFFICULTY IN COMPREHENSION

If it is evident that the patient and/or family does not comprehend all aspects of the prescribed continuing therapy (i.e., administration and monitoring of medications, exercises, diets, follow-up appointments), consider use of social service or visiting nurse agencies.

ASSOCIATED TEACHING

Give patients the following instructions:

Always inform the physician or dentist of any prescription or over-the-counter medication being taken.

Over-the-counter medications should not be taken without first discussing them with a physician or pharmacist.

Always report side effects of rash, itching, or hives immediately. Nausea, vomiting, or diarrhea should also be reported for the physician's evaluation if it is a new symptom.

Take all of the medication as prescribed for the full course of treatment. Do not discontinue use when feeling improved; do not save for future use; do not give your medicine to another individual. Sudden discontinuation of certain medications may produce harmful effects.

Keep all medications out of reach of children.

If pregnancy is suspected, consult an obstetrician as soon as possible about continuation of medication therapy.

At Discharge

Items to be sent home with the patient should:

1. Have written instructions for use.
2. Be labeled in language and size of print appropriate for the patient.
3. If needed, include identification cards or bracelets.
4. Include a list of additional supplies to be purchased after discharge (i.e., elastic bandages, dressings).
5. Include a schedule of follow-up appointments.

Centrally Acting Skeletal Muscle Relaxants

The centrally acting skeletal muscle relaxants are a class of compounds used to relieve acute muscle spasm. The exact mechanism of action of the centrally acting skeletal muscle relaxants is not known, except that they act by CNS depression. They do not have any direct effect on muscles, nerve conduction, or myoneural junctions. All of these muscle relaxants produce some degree of sedation, and most physicians think that the benefits of these agents come from their sedative effects rather than from actual muscle relaxation. These agents are used in combination with physical therapy, rest, and analgesics to relieve muscle spasm associated with acute, painful musculoskeletal conditions. They should not be used in muscle spasticity associated with cerebral or spinal cord disease since they may reduce the strength of remaining active muscle fibers and produce further impairment and debilitation. The centrally acting skeletal muscle relaxants are listed in Table 12.2.

Side Effects

These relaxants have many side effects. Mild symptoms include drowsiness, blurred vision, headache, dizziness, light-headedness, and feelings of weakness, lethargy, and lassitude. Abdominal distress, heartburn, diarrhea, and constipation are common.

Rarely, these centrally acting relaxants may produce hepatotoxicity or blood dyscrasias. Periodic laboratory tests, including blood counts and liver function tests, are recommended to avoid complications.

Availability

See Table 12.2 for available products and recommended dosage ranges.

Nursing Interventions

See also General Nursing Considerations for Patients Receiving Muscle Relaxants.

PATIENT CONCERNS: NURSING INTERVENTION/RATIONALE

Side Effects to Expect

Sedation, Weakness, Lethargy, Gastrointestinal Complaints

These side effects are usually mild and tend to resolve with continued therapy. Encourage the patient not to discontinue therapy without first consulting the physician.

Provide for patient safety for the duration of these symptoms. Patients must avoid operating power equipment or driving.

Table 12.2
Centrally Acting Muscle Relaxants

GENERIC NAME	BRAND NAME	ADULT DOSAGE (PO)	COMMENTS
Carisoprodol	Rela, Soma	350 mg 4 times daily	Onset of action—30 minutes; duration—4 to 6 hours
Chlorphenesin carbamate	Maolate	400–800 mg 3 to 4 times daily	Recommended only for short-term treatment (8 weeks) of muscle spasm induced by trauma or inflammation; may cause blood dyscrasias
Chlorzoxazone	Paraflex	250–750 mg 3 to 4 times daily	Commonly causes gastrointestinal discomfort; may be hepatotoxic
Cyclobenzaprine	Flexeril	10 mg 3 times daily; do not exceed 60 mg daily	Recommended only for short-term treatment (2 to 3 weeks) of painful musculoskeletal conditions
Metaxalone	Skelaxin	800 mg 3 to 4 times daily	Use with caution in patients with liver disease; causes false-positive Clinitest reaction
Methocarbamol	Robaxin, Delaxin	1–1.5 g 4 times daily	Parenteral forms also available
Orphenadrine citrate	Norflex, Flexon, Myolin	100 mg 2 times daily	Also has analgesic properties; do not use in patients with glaucoma or prostatic hypertrophy

Dizziness

Provide for patient safety during episodes of dizziness; report for further evaluation.

Side Effects to Report

Hepatotoxicity

The symptoms of hepatotoxicity are anorexia, nausea, vomiting, jaundice, hepatomegaly, splenomegaly, and abnormal liver function tests (elevated bilirubin, SGOT, SGPT, alkaline phosphatase, prothrombin time).

Blood Dyscrasias

Routine laboratory studies (RBC, WBC, and differential counts) are scheduled for patients taking these agents for 30 days or longer. Stress returning for this laboratory work.

Monitor for the development of sore throat, fever, purpura, jaundice, or excessive progressive weakness.

Drug Interactions

CNS Depressants

Alcohol, narcotics, barbiturates, anticonvulsants, sedative-hypnotics, tranquilizers, phenothiazines, antidepressants: Persons who are working around machinery, driving a car, pouring and giving medicines, or performing other duties in which they must remain mentally alert should not take these medications while working.

Baclofen (bak'lo-fen) ***(Lioresal)*** (ly-or'e-sahl)

Baclofen is a skeletal muscle relaxant that apparently acts somewhat differently from the centrally acting musculoskeletal agents. Its complete mechanism of action is unknown, although reflex activity at the spinal cord is partially inhibited. Baclofen is used in the management of spasticity resulting from multiple sclerosis, spinal cord injuries, and other spinal cord diseases. It is not recommended for use in spasticity associated with Parkinson's disease, cerebral palsy, stroke, or rheumatic disorders. Use with caution in patients who must use spasticity to maintain an upright posture and balance in moving.

Side Effects

The most common side effects associated with baclofen therapy are drowsiness, fatigue, nausea, mental depression, headache, and muscle weakness. These side effects are usually transient and may be minimized by starting therapy with low dosages. Increases in dosage should be made as tolerated.

Availability

PO—10 and 20 mg tablets

Dosage and Administration

Note: Do not abruptly discontinue therapy. Severe exacerbation of spasticity and hallucinations may result.
Adult
PO—Initially 5 mg 3 times daily. Increase the dosage by 5 mg every 3 to 7 days based on response. Optimum

effects are usually noted at dosages of 40 to 80 mg daily but may take several weeks to achieve.

Nursing Interventions

See also General Nursing Considerations for Patients Receiving Muscle Relaxants.

**PATIENT CONCERNS:
NURSING INTERVENTION/RATIONALE**

Side Effects to Expect

Nausea, Fatigue, Headache, Drowsiness

These side effects are usually mild and tend to resolve with continued therapy. Encourage the patient not to discontinue therapy without first consulting the physician.

Dizziness

Provide for patient safety during episodes of dizziness; report for further evaluation.

Drug Interactions

CNS Depressants

CNS depressants, including sleeping aids, analgesics, tranquilizers, and alcohol, will potentiate the sedative effects of baclofen. Persons who are working around machinery, driving a car, pouring and giving medicines, or performing other duties in which they must remain mentally alert should not take these medications while working.

Direct Acting Skeletal Muscle Relaxant

Dantrolene (dan'tro-leen)
(Dantrium) (dan'tree-um)

Dantrolene is a muscle relaxant that acts directly on skeletal muscle. It produces generalized mild weakness of skeletal muscles and decreases the force of reflex muscle contractions, hyperflexia, clonus, muscle stiffness, involuntary muscle movements, and spasticity. Dantrolene is used to control the spasticity of chronic disorders such as cerebral palsy, multiple sclerosis, spinal cord injury, and stroke syndrome.

Side Effects

Common side effects include muscle weakness, drowsiness, dizziness, light-headedness, and diarrhea. These effects occur early in treatment and may be prevented by initiating treatment with low doses. If symptoms persist or recur after temporary discontinuation of the drug, dantrolene may have to be permanently discontinued.

Dantrolene must not be used in patients whose spasticity is needed to obtain or maintain an upright posture and balance or body function.

Drug-induced photosensitivity may occur, so patients should refrain from excessive or unnecessary exposure to sunlight.

Dantrolene must be used with caution in patients with chronic lung disease, liver disease, or impaired myocardial function. Dantrolene has been implicated as a causative factor in reported cases of hepatitis.

Availability

PO—25, 50, 100 mg capsules; IV—0.32 mg/ml in 70 ml vials.

Dosage and Administration

Adult
PO—Initially 25 mg daily. Increase to 25 mg two, three, or four times daily at 4 to 7 day intervals, then gradually increase the dosage up to 100 mg two, three, or four times daily. A few patients may require 200 mg four times daily.

Nursing Interventions

See also General Nursing Considerations for Patients Receiving Muscle Relaxants.

**PATIENT CONCERNS:
NURSING INTERVENTION/RATIONALE**

Side Effects to Expect

Weakness, Diarrhea, Drowsiness

These side effects are usually mild and tend to resolve with continued therapy. Encourage the patient not to discontinue therapy without first consulting the physician.

Dizziness, Light-headedness

Provide for patient safety during episodes of dizziness; report for further evaluation.

Response to Therapy

Tell the patient that effectiveness of the drug may not be apparent for 1 week or longer. Encourage the patient not to discontinue therapy without first consulting the physician.

Side Effects to Report

Photosensitivity

The patient should be cautioned to avoid exposure to sunlight and ultraviolet light. Suggest wearing long-sleeved clothing, hat, and sunglasses while exposed to sunlight. The patient must not use artificial "tanning" lamps. The patient should not discontinue therapy without advising the physician.

Hepatotoxicity

The symptoms of hepatotoxicity are anorexia, nausea, vomiting, jaundice, hepatomegaly, splenomegaly, and abnormal liver function tests (elevated bilirubin, SGOT, SGPT, alkaline phosphatase, prothrombin time).

Drug Interactions

CNS Depressants

CNS depressants, including sleeping aids, analgesics, tranquilizers, and alcohol, will potentiate the sedative effects of dantrolene. Persons who are working around machinery, driving a car, pouring and giving medicines, or performing other duties in which they must remain mentally alert should not take these medications while working.

Skeletal Muscle Relaxants Used during Surgery

General Nursing Considerations for Patients Receiving Neuromuscular Blocking Agents

See also General Nursing Considerations for Patients with Respiratory Disease.

Assessment of the patient's vital signs, mental status, and in particular, respiratory function, is mandatory for persons having received neuromuscular blocking agents. The side effects associated with these drugs may occur 48 hours or more after their administration; therefore, close observation of respiratory function, ability to swallow (handle secretions), and cough reflex is necessary. Suction, oxygen, mechanical ventilators, and resuscitation equipment should be available in the immediate area.

PATIENT CONCERNS: NURSING INTERVENTION/RATIONALE

Detection of Respiratory Depression

Restlessness, Lethargy, Decreased Mental Alertness

Early signs of diminished ventilation are difficult to detect, particularly in the immediate postoperative period. Often the signs of restlessness, anxiety, decreased mental alertness, and headache are early, subtle clues to distress.

Blood Pressure, Pulse, and Respirations

Know the baseline readings of your patient's vital signs before administration of anesthetic and neuromuscular blocking agents.

Generally, *changes* from the baseline should be reported.

Monitor your patient closely for clinical signs (tachycardia, hypotension, cyanosis) of hypoxia and hypercapnia. Arterial blood gases (ABGs) may be drawn to accurately confirm your clinical observations.

Use of Accessory Muscles

Use of the abdominal, intercostal, or neck muscles is an indication of respiratory distress. Flaring of the nostrils may be present in severe cases.

Respiratory Rate, Depth

As respiratory distress progresses, respirations become shallow and rapid; assess for asymmetrical chest movements as well.

Cyanosis

The development of cyanosis is a late sign of respiratory complications. Respiratory distress should be detected early through close observation before cyanosis develops.

Ventilated Respirations

The use of various mechanical ventilators may be employed to improve alveolar ventilation and oxygenation of the patient. See a general medical-surgical nursing text for a detailed discussion of nursing care while the patient is on mechanical ventilation.

Nursing Measures Associated with Neuromuscular Blockade Therapy

Respiratory Secretions

The histamine release caused by these drugs may produce increased salivation. In patients who are paralyzed or who have incomplete return of control over swallowing, coughing, and deep breathing, these secretions may obstruct the airway.

Assess for dyspnea and loud or gurgling sounds with respirations. Suction secretions according to hospital policies and procedures. If qualified, palpate for coarse chest wall vibrations and listen for rales or rhonchi.

Cough Reflex

In order to cough effectively, the patient must be able to breathe deeply, contract the abdominal and diaphragmatic muscles, and control the closing and opening of the epiglottis so that air can be trapped in the lung and then forcefully expelled.

Deep Breathing

Deep breathing exercises can allow the opportunity to assess the patient's cough reflex. Assist the patient by splinting any abdominal or thoracic incisions. Have the patient take 3 or 4 deep breaths, then cough. During this process, assess the ability to breathe deeply. Cupping your hand and holding it a few inches from the mouth while the patient breathes allows you to feel the air being exhaled.

Positioning

Patients can usually cough better in a semi-Fowler's or high-Fowler's position; therefore, depending on the situation and stability of the patient's vital signs, elevating the head of the bed may assist coughing and breathing. For unconscious or semiconscious individuals, position them, using good body alignment, on the side. Keep the siderails up.

Pain Management

Persons still paralyzed by the effects of these agents may experience pain and be unable to speak to request medication. Make sure analgesics are scheduled on a regular basis and administered on time.

Anxiety

Deal calmly with the patient experiencing respiratory dysfunction. The inability to breathe may cause the patient to panic. Give reassurance while initiating measures to assist the patient.

Neuromuscular Blocking Agents

Neuromuscular blocking agents are important skeletal muscle relaxants. These agents are used to (1) produce adequate muscle relaxation during anesthesia to reduce the use (and side effects) of general anesthetics, (2) ease endotracheal intubation and prevent laryngospasm, (3) decrease muscular activity in electroshock therapy, and (4) aid in the muscle spasms associated with tetanus. The neuromuscular blocking agents are listed in Table 12.3.

Neuromuscular blocking agents act by interrupting transmission of impulses from motor nerves to muscles at the skeletal neuromuscular junction. Neuromuscular blocking agents have no effect on consciousness, memory, or the pain threshold. Reassurance by nursing personnel is essential to paralyzed patients (such as those on respirators), and analgesics must be administered on schedule. These patients may suffer extreme pain without being able to ask for analgesics.

Side Effects

Side effects shared by all neuromuscular blocking agents are residual muscle weakness, hypersensitivity reactions, and interference with respiratory function. They also cause histamine release which may cause bronchospasm, bronchial and salivary secretions, flushing, edema, and urticaria.

Patients with hepatic, pulmonary, or renal disease, or neurologic disorders such as myasthenia gravis, spinal cord injury, or multiple sclerosis must be fully evaluated to assess their ability to tolerate neuromuscular blocking agents. Much smaller doses are often necessary when these diseases are present. Neonates and elderly patients also require adjustments in dosage because of the insensitivity of their neuromuscular junction.

Table 12.3
Neuromuscular Blocking Agents

GENERIC NAME	BRAND NAME	AVAILABILITY
Atacurium besylate	Tracrium	10 mg/ml in 5 ml ampules
Gallamine triethiodide	Flaxedil	20 mg/ml in 10 ml vials
Metocurine iodide	Metubine Iodide	2 mg/ml in 20 ml vials
Pancuronium bromide	Pavulon	1 mg/ml in 10 ml vials; 2 mg/ml in 2 and 5 ml ampules
Succinylcholine	Anectine, Quelicin, Sux-Cert	20 mg/ml in 5 and 10 ml vials, 50 mg/ml in 10 ml ampules, 100 mg/ml in 10 ml vials and ampules
Tubocurarine chloride	Tubocurarine Chloride	3 mg/ml in 10 and 20 mg vials

Administration

These agents are usually given intravenously but may also be given intramuscularly. They are potent drugs, so they should be used only by persons thoroughly familiar with their effects, such as an anesthetist or anesthesiologist, and under conditions where the patient can receive constant, close attention for signs of respiratory failure. Adequate equipment for artificial respiration, antidotes, and other measures for prompt treatment of toxicity must be readily available.

Treatment of Overdose

Treatment of overdose includes artificial respiration with oxygen and antidotes such as neostigmine methylsulfate (Prostigmin), pyridostigmine bromide (Mestinon, Regonal), and edrophonium chloride (Tensilon). Atropine sulfate is usually administered with neostigmine or pyridostigmine to block bradycardia, hypotension, and salivation induced by these agents. There is no antidote for the early blockade induced by succinylcholine. Fortunately, it is of short duration and does not require reversal.

Nursing Interventions

See also General Nursing Considerations for Patients Receiving Neuromuscular Blocking Agents.

PATIENT CONCERNS: NURSING INTERVENTION/RATIONALE

Side Effects to Expect

Mild Discomfort

Mild to moderate discomfort, particularly in the neck, upper back, lower intercostal, and abdominal muscles, will be noted when first ambulating following use.

Side Effects to Report

Signs of Respiratory Distress

Monitor vital signs for a prolonged period following administration of neuromuscular blocking agents.

Diminished Cough Reflex, Inability to Swallow

Assess deep breathing and coughing at regular intervals. Have suction and oxygen equipment available and be familiar with emergency code practices at your hospital.

Drug Interactions

Drugs That Enhance Therapeutic and Toxic Effects

General anesthetics (ether, fluroxene, methoxyflurane, enflurane, halothane, cyclopropane), aminoglycoside antibiotics (kanamycin, gentamicin, neomycin, streptomycin, netilmycin, tobramycin, amikacin), quinidine, quinine, beta adrenergic blocking agents (propranolol, timolol, pindolol, nadolol, others), and agents that deplete potassium (thiozide diuretics, furosemide, bumetanide, ethacrynic acid, chlorthalidone, amphotericin B, corticosteroids), thus prolonging neuromuscular blockage.

Label charts of patients scheduled for surgery who are taking any of these agents. These combinations may potentiate repiratory depression. Check the anesthetist's records of surgical patients; monitor postoperative patients for a prolonged period for respiratory depression. This may occur 48 hours or more after drug administration.

Drugs That Reduce Therapeutic Effects

Neostigmine methylsulfate, pyridostigmine bromide, and edrophonium chloride.

These agents are used as antidotes in case of overdosage of the neuromuscular blocking agents.

Respiratory Depressants

Analgesics, sedatives, tranquilizers.

These agents, in combination with muscle relaxants, may potentiate respiratory depression. Check the anesthetist's records of surgical patients. Monitor postoperative patients for a prolonged period for respiratory depression. This may occur 48 hours or more after drug administration.

Chapter 13

Drugs Affecting the Digestive System

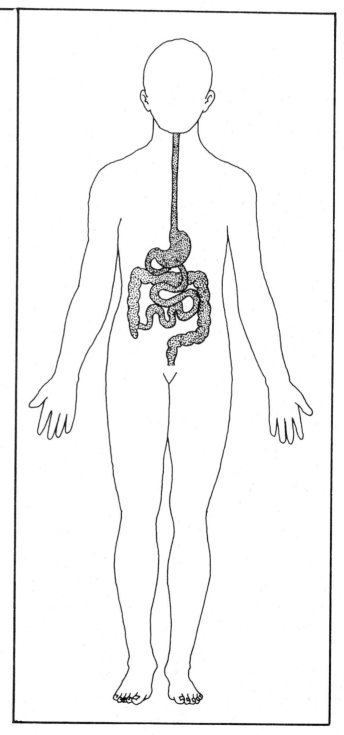

Objectives

After completing this chapter, the student should be able to do the following:

1. Explain the major action and effects of drugs used to treat disorders of the digestive tract.
2. Identify baseline data the nurse should collect on a continuous basis for comparison and evaluation of drug effectiveness.
3. Identify important nursing assessments and interventions associated with the drug therapy and treatment of diseases associated with the digestive system.
4. Identify health teaching essential for a successful treatment regimen.

General Nursing Considerations for Patients with Gastrointestinal Disorders

The nurse should assess the following areas to form a baseline for comparison with subsequent observations.

PATIENT CONCERNS: NURSING INTERVENTION/RATIONALE

Assessment of Patients with Gastrointestinal Disorders

Oral Cavity

Assessment of the mouth indicates the patient's ability to salivate, chew, and swallow, and provides signs of disease that can interfere with nutrition. Examine the tongue, lips, and mucous membranes for color, cyanosis, sores (describe location, size, and characteristics), moisture (dryness may indicate dehydration), swelling, or inflammation.

Assess for the presence of teeth, dental caries, plaque, inflamed or receding gums, and sores from poorly fitting dentures.

A foul odor to the breath may indicate poor dental hygiene or oral infection. Odors may occur after certain foods are consumed, such as garlic or alcohol, or with some systemic diseases (acetone for diabetes, ammonia for liver disease).

Esophagus, Stomach

Ask patients to describe any symptoms in their own words. Question in detail what is meant by their use of the terms *indigestion, heartburn, upset stomach, nausea,* or *pain.*

PAIN, DISCOMFORT

Have the patient give specific details of the onset, duration, location, and characteristics of pain or discomfort. Determine whether there is a relationship between ingestion of certain types of food or drinks,

and what the patient has done in the past to relieve the pain or discomfort.

EMESIS

Has the patient vomited? What is the frequency, color, consistency, and duration of current symptoms? Has there been any bright red or "coffee-ground" colored emesis? What initiates the vomiting episodes, and what causes them to stop? How many episodes of vomiting has the patient experienced over what time span?

In the postoperative patient always check the following: patency of the nasogastric tube; that the abdomen is splinted when vomiting; that dressings and wound sites are checked frequently for possible increases in drainage or wound dehiscence.

Prevent possible aspiration while a patient is vomiting by placing the person in a high Fowler's position and/or on the side, if not fully alert.

Always give regular oral hygiene to patients experiencing nausea and vomiting.

Bowels

Ask patients to describe any changes they have noted in their abdomen (e.g., distension, "swelling or bloating," loud gurgling sounds, or the presence of any lumps).

Using a stethoscope, listen for hyperresonance (loud tingling and rushing), absence of bowel sounds, or the presence of a bruit (similar to a systolic murmur).

Measure and record the abdominal girth. Continue measurements in the same location daily, especially if ascites or paralytic ileus are suspected.

Record any changes in abdominal contour (e.g., hernia, enlarged spleen or liver).

Record any sharp pain felt when fingers are withdrawn suddenly after palpation of the abdomen.

CONSTIPATION

Constipation is the formation of dry, hard stools that are difficult and sometimes painful to pass.

The underlying cause of constipation needs to be determined.

Elimination Pattern. Determine whether the onset of constipation is recent and can be associated with a change in diet or new environment (from travel or undue stress). Ask patients to describe their "normal" elimination pattern—number of stools per day, color, and consistency. Has there been any change in the "normal" pattern of bowel movements? It is important for patients to understand that not all people defecate daily; every 2 or 3 days is normal for some people.

Fluid Intake. Ask patients to describe fluid intake: how much water, coffee, tea, soft drinks, fruit juice, and alcoholic beverages are consumed daily?

Eating Pattern. Ask patients for a description of their diet over the past 24 hours. Evaluate the data for types of foods from each of the four food groups eaten, the quantity eaten, and the amount of time spent in eating. Ask if the eating pattern has changed over recent months and to what the patients attribute any identified changes.

Ask whether certain foods cause bloating, indigestion, or constipation, and how much seasoning and spices are put on foods.

Exercise. Ask the patient about exercise levels and activity. Does the patient play vigorous sports, take walks, jog, or have a sedentary job and hobby?

Nursing Measures. Explain the benefits of trying dietary and exercise modification to treat constipation, prior to initiating the use of laxatives.

Nurses may facilitate defecation in hospitalized patients by encouraging ambulation (if possible), providing privacy, and having the individual sit in an upright position. If possible, sitting on the actual toilet or bedside commode is best.

Encourage the patient to attempt to defecate as soon as the urge arises, and not to suppress this urge until a later time. The urge to defecate occurs most frequently following meals, particularly breakfast.

If an enema or laxative is ordered, explain the purpose to the patient and how long it will take before action is expected.

DIARRHEA

Diarrhea is an increased frequency and/or fluid content of bowel movements. Diarrhea may result from disturbances in either the small or large intestine caused by a change in the fecal contents or an increase in intestinal transit time, so that less fluid is reabsorbed. The result is passage of feces which are high in water content.

Since diarrhea is usually caused by a pathologic condition or is a side effect of medications, medical treatment usually consists of correcting the underlying cause.

History. Ask the patient experiencing diarrhea if there has been a recent change in eating habits, a change in water source, additional stress, or if medications (especially laxatives or antibiotics) are being taken.

Obtain a detailed history of the illness, including the onset and duration of the diarrhea, characteristics of the stool, and associated symptoms.

Dehydration and Electrolyte Imbalance. Monitor patients with prolonged or severe diarrhea for dehydration and electrolyte imbalance. (See Chapter 14, Drugs Affecting the Urinary System).

Skin Breakdown. Provide for protection of the tissue surrounding the anal area when the symptoms of diarrhea start, *prior to skin breakdown.* Cleanse the anal area thoroughly, dry gently, and apply protective products such as Desitin or A & D Ointment. Repeat this process after *every* defecation.

Patient Teaching Associated with Gastrointestinal Drug Therapy

Communication and Responsibility

Encourage open communication concerning frustrations and anger as the patient attempts to adjust to the diagnosis and need for prolonged treatment. The patient must be guided to gain insight into the disorder in order to assume responsibility for the continuation of the treatment. Keep emphasizing those factors the patient can control to alter the progress of the disease, including maintenance of general health, nutritional needs, adequate rest, appropriate exercise, and continuation of the prescribed medication therapy.

SELF-TREATMENT

Millions of patients treat their own gastrointestinal symptoms with over-the-counter products each year. Patients must understand that symptoms that are not relieved by self-treatment, usually within 1 to 2 weeks, require a physician's evaluation. Many people consider gastrointestinal symptoms to be minor and do not realize that chronic symptoms may be an indication of a serious underlying disease.

ALTERNATIVE THERAPIES

For Gastrointestinal Distress. Avoid foods known to cause gas such as cabbage, cauliflower, Brussels sprouts, and bran products.

Avoid irritating foods and beverages such as spices, alcohol, coffee, chocolate, citrus fruits, fried foods, and gravies. Occasionally, foods high in roughage (e.g., lettuce, celery, raw fruits, and vegetables) can aggravate an inflamed mucosa.

Elevation of the head of the bed at night may help patients who have developed a hiatus hernia, night regurgitation, or reflux esophagitis.

Antacids may be used to neutralize stomach acid, thus reducing gastric irritation, but continued use may mask a more serious underlying disorder.

Contrary to popular opinion, large glasses of milk or baking soda used as an antacid will actually stimulate more acid production, causing further gastric irritation. Occasional use of an antacid is more appropriate.

Other measures to reduce gastrointestinal distress include the ingestion of frequent, small feedings, taking a walk after meals, and remaining upright after meals rather than sitting or lying down.

For Nausea, Vomiting. Before using antiemetics, try more simple measures such as a cup of warm tea or carbonated beverages served at room temperature.

For Constipation. Before making any suggestions, the underlying cause of the constipation must be established. Determine whether the onset of constipation is recent, and if it can be associated with a change in diet or new environment from travel, or undue stress. Constipation from these causes is usually self-limiting and resolves with the one-time use of a mild laxative.

People with chronic constipation frequently drink an inadequate amount of water daily. Initially, encourage patients to drink 6 to 8 8-ounce glasses of water daily, gradually increasing to 8 to 12 glasses daily.

A regular diet containing sufficient roughage, in the form of fresh fruits and vegetables and whole grain breads and cereals, should be encouraged unless co-existing medical problems prohibit these foods.

A plan of regular exercise can be helpful, particularly if the person leads a sedentary lifestyle. Exercise promotes bowel activity and improves the abdominal muscle tone necessary for defecation. Straight-leg raises also promote increased abdominal muscle strength.

If the above measures fail, or if the patient has a medical indication to prevent straining at the stool, medications such as stool softeners or bulk-forming laxatives may be suggested. It is *essential* that *adequate water* be taken with these products.

Also stress personal hygiene by having patients wash their hands after each defecation and urination. For females, teach the importance of wiping from front to back (urethra to rectum) to prevent development of urinary tract infections.

For Diarrhea. Ask patients experiencing diarrhea if they have an idea of what is causing the diarrhea (e.g., a change in food, water sources, travel, recent undue stress, or the initiation of a new medication).

Explain what medications have been ordered, how often they are repeated, and when to discontinue therapy, in order to prevent constipation.

Initiate protection of the tissue surrounding the anal area when diarrhea symptoms start, *prior to skin breakdown.* Cleanse the anal area thoroughly, dry gently, and apply protective skin products such as Desitin or A & D Ointment. Repeat this procedure after *every* defecation.

Expectations of Therapy

Discuss the expectations of therapy: relief of heartburn, indigestion, nausea and vomiting, or diarrhea.

(Occasionally a patient may have the unrealistic expectation that a medication will change a lifelong pattern of defecation from every 3 to 4 days to a daily defecation, even though there was no change in dietary and fluid intake or activity.)

Changes in Expectations

Assess changes in expectations as therapy progresses and the patient gains understanding and skill in the management of the diagnosis.

Symptoms of recurrent gastrointestinal discomfort need thorough diagnosis to identify any underlying pathology.

Changes in Therapy through Cooperative Goal-Setting

Work with the patient to encourage adherence to the prescribed treatment. When the patient feels that a change should be made in a treatment plan, encourage discussion with the physician.

A definite plan to alleviate the gastrointestinal symptoms should be developed and the patient's response carefully evaluated.

Cooperatively explore any conditions the patient feels may be precipitating these episodes. Mutually set goals to eliminate underlying stressors. Simpler approaches such as dietary modification should be used *prior* to the initiation of medications.

WRITTEN RECORD

Enlist the patient's aid in developing and maintaining a written record of monitoring parameters (Table 13.1) (e.g., diet diary, onset of pain, nausea or vomiting in relation to mealtime or type of foods eaten, frequency and characteristics of stools during diarrhea) and response to prescribed therapies for discussion with the physician. Patients should be encouraged to take this record on follow-up visits.

FOSTERING COMPLIANCE

Throughout the hospitalization, discuss medication information and how it will benefit the course of treatment. Seek cooperation and understanding of the following points so that medication compliance may be enhanced:

1. Name.
2. Dosage (be certain specific instructions are given for each medication).
3. Route and administration times (if the patient is taking more than one medication, be sure that the patient knows when to take each one (e.g., with meals, one hour before or two hours after antacids).
   - For antidiarrheal medication, be sure that the patient understands how much and how often the prescription is to be taken, and when to discontinue the medication.
   - For constipation, stress the use of diet, exercise, and adequate fluid intake prior to the initiation of a laxative. Ensure that the individual understands that bulk forming laxatives and stool softeners must be taken with a full glass of water to be safe and effective.
4. Anticipated therapeutic responses include the following:
   - Antidiarrheal products: relief of diarrhea.
   - Antacids: relief of heartburn or pain.
   - Laxatives: relief of constipation.
   - Stool softeners: smooth, consistent bowel movement with no straining or gripping.
5. Side effects to expect: see individual product information.

6. Side effects to report: lack of improvement in the symptoms for which the medication was prescribed, or excessive therapeutic ability. Patients should be told to immediately report any vomitus that looks like "coffee grounds" or contains bright red blood; bloody or tarry-colored stools; or recurrent abdominal pains. Patients must not attempt to treat these symptoms by themselves.
7. When, how, or if to refill the medication.

DIFFICULTY IN COMPREHENSION

If it is evident that the patient and/or family does not understand all aspects of continuing therapy being prescribed (e.g., administration and monitoring of medications, exercises, diets, follow up appointments) consider the use of social service or visiting nurse agencies.

ASSOCIATED TEACHING

Give patients the following instructions:

Always inform the physician or dentist of any prescription or over-the-counter medication being taken. Over-the-counter medications should not be taken without first discussing them with the physician or pharmacist.

Always report side effects of rash, itching, or hives immediately. Nausea, vomiting, or diarrhea should also be reported for the physician's evaluation if it is a new symptom.

Take all of the medication, as prescribed, for the full course of treatment. Do not discontinue use when feeling improved; do not save for future use; do not give your medicine to another individual. Sudden discontinuation of certain medications may produce harmful effects.

Keep all medications out of reach of children.

If pregnancy is suspected, consult an obstetrician as soon as possible about continuation of medication therapy.

At Discharge

Items to be sent home with the patient should:

1. Have written instructions for use.
2. Be labeled in language and size of print appropriate for the patient.
3. If needed, include identification cards or bracelets.
4. Include a list of additional supplies to be purchased after discharge (i.e., syringes, dressings).
5. Include a schedule for follow-up appointments.

Table 13.1

Example of a Written Record for Patients Receiving Agents Affecting the Digestive System

Medications	Color	To be taken

Name _____

Physician _____

Physician's phone _____

Next appt.* _____

Parameters		Day of discharge							Comments
Bloating	Time it occurs — night, after eating, midday								
	Causes, eg., food eaten								
Pain: Severity of pain Severe 10 — Moderate 5 — Dull 0	Time—before/after meals								
	Location								
Nausea	Vomiting — describe amount, color, time of day								
	Nausea — no vomiting								
Bowels	Color?								
	No. of stools per day?								
	Soft, watery, or hard?								
Diet: List foods that cause problems									
Degree of relief from medications? Great 10 — Good 5 — Poor 1									
Appetite? Excellent 10 — Good 5 — Poor 1									

*Please bring this record with you to your next appointment.
Use the back of this sheet for additional information.

Drugs Affecting the Mouth: Mouthwashes and Gargles

A common personal need in the hospitalized patient is oral hygiene. The most effective treatment of oral discomfort is mechanical cleansing of the teeth with a toothbrush and dentifrice. However, this may not be possible for the patient who has undergone oral surgery or who has suffered facial trauma. Although mouthwashes and gargles cannot be used in strong enough concentrations to ensure germicidal effects, they may be temporarily effective in removing disagreeable tastes and reducing halitosis.

Cepacol mouthwash is used in many hospitals and is available commercially in liquid and lozenge form. It is used full strength. Chloraseptic mouthwash maintains oral hygiene and also provides surface anesthesia when needed to alleviate pharyngeal discomfort. It is diluted with equal parts of water or sprayed full strength.

Occasionally, certain mouthwashes are recommended for specific purposes. Products containing zinc chloride are used as astringents to temporarily decrease bleeding or irritation. A 0.9% solution of sodium chloride (normal saline) is an effective gargle. It can be used to provide temporary, soothing relief of pharyngeal irritation from nasogastric tubes, endotracheal tubes, sore throat, or oral surgery. Solutions containing hydrogen peroxide may be used to cleanse and debride minor lesions. However, their use should be limited to 7 to 10 days in order to prevent further tissue irritation. Mouthwashes containing 0.05% fluoride have been shown to significantly reduce tooth decay.

Drugs Affecting the Mouth: Dentifrices

The primary purpose for brushing teeth is to promote dental health. Dentifrices contain one or more mild abrasives, a foaming agent, and flavoring materials. They are available in powder or paste form and are used as an aid in the mechanical cleansing provided by a soft nylon toothbrush. The essential requirement of toothpaste or toothpowder is that it must not injure the teeth or surrounding tissues. For children and teenagers, who are most susceptible to tooth decay, the best dentifrices are those that contain fluoride. The American Dental Association recommends Crest, Colgate with MFP, Macleans Fluoride, Aim Fluoride, Aqua-Fresh Fluoride, and Gleem as the only toothpastes having proven caries-inhibiting properties.

Adults should use toothpastes that are the least abrasive to the teeth while controlling gum disease as well as decay. This is especially important to patients with receding gums. Colgate Regular and Peak tooth-

pastes are the least abrasive, while smokers' products such as Pearl Drops and Zact are the most abrasive. Baking soda is a very mild abrasive agent and can be very effective and inexpensive as a dentifrice. The only disadvantages to baking soda are its slightly bitter taste and lack of fluoride. Denquel is a mildly abrasive toothpaste that also contains a desensitizing agent. The American Dental Association states that it is the only toothpaste that "has been shown to be an effective desensitizing dentifrice that with regular brushing can be of significant value in relieving sensitivity to hot and cold in otherwise normal teeth."

Drugs Affecting the Stomach: Antacids

Antacids are chemical substances used in the treatment of hyperchlorhydria and peptic ulcer disease. Peptic ulcer disease is thought to be the result of several pathogenic processes. The control of hyperacidity is one of the therapeutic measures used in its treatment.

The main digestive substances secreted by the stomach are *hydrochloric acid* and *pepsin*. Hydrochloric acid activates the secretion of pepsin, and pepsin then begins protein digestion. Excess secretion of hydrochloric acid may result in erosion, ulceration, and possible perforation of the gastric walls. Antacids lower the acidity of gastric secretions by buffering the hydrochloric acid (normally pH 1 or 2) to a lower hydrogen ion concentration. Buffering hydrochloric acid to a pH of 3 or 4 is highly desired, since then the proteolytic action of pepsin is reduced, and the gastric juice loses its corrosive effect.

Antacid products account for one of the largest sales volumes of medication that may be purchased without prescription. Antacids are commonly used for treatment of heartburn, excessive eating and drinking, and peptic ulcer disease. However, nurses and patients must be aware that not all antacids are alike, and they should be used judiciously, particularly by certain types of patients. Long-term self-medication with antacids may also mask symptoms of serious underlying diseases, such as a bleeding ulcer.

The most effective antacids available are combinations of aluminum hydroxide, magnesium oxide or hydroxide, magnesium trisilicate, and calcium carbonate (Table 13.2). All act by neutralizing gastric acid. Combinations of these compounds must be used because any compound used alone in therapeutic quantities may also produce severe systemic side effects. Other ingredients found in antacid combination products include simethicone, oxethazaine, alginic acid, and bismuth. *Simethicone* is a defoaming agent that breaks up gas bubbles in the stomach, reducing stomach distension

Table 13.2
Ingredients of Commonly Used Antacids

PRODUCT	FORM	CALCIUM CARBONATE	ALUMINUM HYDROXIDE	ALUMINUM CARBONATE	MAGNESIUM OXIDE OR HYDROXIDE	MAGNESIUM TRISILICATE	MAGNESIUM CARBONATE	SODIUM BICARBONATE	SIMETHICONE	OTHER INGREDIENTS
Aludrox	Tablet, suspension		X		X					
Amphojel	Tablet, suspension		X							
Basaljel	Tablet, capsule, suspension			X						
BiSoDol	Tablet, powder	X			X	X	X			
Delcid	Suspension		X		X					
Di-Gel	Tablet, liquid		X		X		X		X	
Gelusil II	Tablet, suspension		X		X				X	
Kolantyl	Tablet, wafer, liquid									
Maalox	Tablet, suspension		X		X					
Maalox Plus	Tablet, suspension		X		X				X	
Mylanta	Tablet, suspension		X		X				X	
Mylanta II	Tablet, suspension		X		X				X	
Phillips' Milk of Magnesia	Tablet, suspension									
Phosphaljel	Suspension									Aluminum phosphate
Riopan	Tablet, suspension									Magaldrate
Riopan Plus	Tablet, suspension								X	Magaldrate
Rolaids	Tablet									Dihydroxyaluminum sodium carbonate
Titralac	Tablet, suspension	X								Glycine
Tums	Tablet	X								
WinGel	Tablet, suspension		X		X					

and heartburn. It is effective for use in patients who have overeaten or who suffer from heartburn, but it is not effective in the treatment of ulcer disease. *Oxethazaine* is a local anesthetic that has been used in combination with antacids. However, it requires a prescription and has no proven therapeutic benefit in the treatment of gastric disease. *Alginic acid* produces a highly viscous solution of sodium alginate that floats on top of the gastric contents. It may be effective only in the patient who suffers from esophageal reflux or hiatal hernia and should not be used in the patient with acute gastritis or ulcer disease. *Bismuth* compounds have little acid neutralizing capacity and are therefore poor antacids.

Nurses are frequently asked by patients and friends to recommend antacid products. Before recommending antacid therapy, several questions should be asked to help ascertain whether there is a serious underlying medical condition:

1. How long has the pain been present?
2. When and where does the pain occur? Immediately after meals, or several hours after meals?
3. Have you vomited blood or black "coffee grounds" material?
4. Have you noticed blood in the stool or have the stools been black?
5. Are you on any dietary restrictions, such as a low salt diet?
6. Are you under a physician's care?

If the answers to these questions suggest an underlying disease, patients should be referred immediately to a physician.

The following principles should be considered when antacid therapy is being planned:

1. For indigestion antacids should not be administered for more than 2 weeks. If, after this time, the pa-

tient is still experiencing discomfort, a physician should be contacted.

2. Patients with edema, congestive heart failure, hypertension, renal failure, pregnancy, or salt restricted diets should use low-sodium antacids. These products include Riopan, Maalox, and Mylanta II. Therapy should only continue on the recommendation of a physician.

3. Antacid tablets should be used only for the patient with an occasional case of indigestion or heartburn. Tablets *do not* contain enough antacid to be effective in treating peptic ulcer disease.

4. Excessive use of antacids frequently results in either constipation or diarrhea. If a patient experiences these symptoms and is still suffering from stomach discomfort, a physician should be consulted.

5. Effective management of ACUTE ulcer disease requires large volumes of antacids. The selection of an antacid, and the quantity to be taken, depend on the neutralizing capacity of the antacid. Any patient with "coffee-grounds" hematemesis, bloody stools, or recurrent abdominal pain should seek medical attention immediately and must not attempt to self-treat the disorder.

6. Most antacids have similar ingredients (see Table 13.2). Selection of an antacid for occasional use should be determined by quantity of each ingredient, cost, taste, and frequency of side effects. Patients may need to try more than one product while weighing the advantages and disadvantages of each product.

Side Effects

A common complaint of patients consuming large quantities of calcium carbonate or aluminum hydroxide is constipation, while excess magnesium results in diarrhea.

Calcium carbonate and sodium bicarbonate may cause rebound hyperacidity.

Patients with renal failure should not use large quantities of antacids containing magnesium. The magnesium ions cannot be excreted and may produce hypermagnesemia and toxicity.

Availability

See Table 13.2.

Dosage and Administration

Follow directions on the product container.

Drug Interactions

The absorption of tetracycline antibiotics, digoxin, digitoxin, and iron compounds is inhibited by antacids. These medications should be administered 1 hour before or 2 hours after the administration of antacids.

Levodopa absorption is increased by antacids. When antacid therapy is added, toxicity may result in the parkinsonian patient who is well controlled taking a certain dosage of levodopa. If the patient's parkinsonism is well controlled on levodopa *and* antacid therapy, withdrawal of antacids may result in a recurrence of parkinsonian symptomatology.

Frequent use of antacid therapy may result in increased urinary pH. Renal excretion of quinidine and amphetamines may be inhibited and toxicity may occur.

Nursing Interventions

See General Nursing Considerations for Patients with Gastrointestinal Disorders.

Drugs Affecting the Stomach: Histamine H₂ Antagonists

Cimetidine (si-met′i-deen) *(Tagamet)* (tag′ah-met)

Stimulation of H₂ receptors in the stomach by food, caffeine, histamine, and insulin causes gastric acid secretion. Cimetidine is a histamine H₂ antagonist, which decreases daytime and nighttime secretion of gastric acid. Cimetidine is now being extensively used to treat duodenal ulcers and pathologic hypersecretory conditions, such as Zollinger-Ellison syndrome, and for the prevention and treatment of stress ulcers.

Side Effects

Most side effects are quite mild and transient. About 1% of patients develop diarrhea, dizziness, headaches, or somnolence.

Mental confusion, slurred speech, disorientation, and hallucinations may occur if high doses are used in patients with hepatic or renal disease, and patients over 50 years of age.

Mild bilateral gynecomastia and breast soreness may occur with long-term use (greater than 1 month) but resolves after discontinuation of therapy.

Other rare adverse effects include transient hyperthermia, maculopapular rashes, urticaria, muscular pain, transient neutropenia, hypotension, and bradycardia.

Availability

PO—200 and 300 mg tablets, 300 mg/5 ml liquid.
Injection—300 mg/2 ml.

Dosage and Administration

Adult
PO—300 mg 4 times daily with meals and at bedtime.
Do not exceed 2400 mg daily. Antacid therapy may
be continued for relief of pain, but should be administered 1 to 2 hours before or after the cimetidine
dosage.
IV—300 mg every 6 hours.

Nursing Interventions

See also General Nursing Considerations for Patients
with Gastrointestinal Disorders.

**PATIENT CONCERNS:
NURSING INTERVENTION/RATIONALE**

Side Effects to Expect

Dizziness, Headaches, Diarrhea, Somnolence

These side effects are usually mild and resolve with
continued therapy. Encourage the patient not to discontinue therapy without consulting the physician.

Provide for patient safety during episodes of dizziness.

If patients develop somnolence and lethargy, encourage them to use caution when working around machinery or driving a car.

Side Effects to Report

Confusion, Disorientation, Hallucinations

Perform a baseline assessment of the patient's degree of alertness and orientation to name, place, and
time *before* initiating therapy. Make regularly scheduled
subsequent mental status evaluations and compare
findings. Report development of alterations.

*Gynecomastia, Rashes, Neutropenia,
Hypotension, Bradycardia*

Report for further observation and possible laboratory
tests.

Administration

PO

Administer with food.

Antacids

Since antacid therapy is often continued during early
therapy of ulcer disease, administer 1 hour before or
2 hours after the cimetidine dose.

IV

Dilute in 20 ml of saline solution or D_5W and administer
over 1 to 2 minutes *or* dilute in 100 ml of IV fluid and
infuse over 15 to 20 minutes.

Drug Interactions

Benzodiazepines

Cimetidine inhibits the metabolism and/or excretion
of the following benzodiazepines: chlordiozepoxide, diazepam, clorazepate, fluorazepam, halazepam, and
prazepam.

Patients taking cimetidine and a benzodiazepine
concurrently should be observed for increased sedation
and may require a reduction in dosage of the benzodiazepine. The metabolism of temazepam, prazepam,
and lorazepam do not appear to be affected.

Theophylline Derivatives

Cimetidine inhibits the metabolism and/or excretion
of the following xanthine derivatives: aminophylline, oxtryphylline, dyphylline, and theophylline.

Patients at greater risk include those receiving larger
doses of theophylline or those patients with liver disease.
Observe for restlessness, vomiting, dizziness, and cardiac arrhythmias. The dosage of theophylline may need
to be reduced.

Beta Adrenergic Blocking Agents

Beta adrenergic blocking agents (propranolol, metoprolol) may accumulate due to inhibited metabolism.
Monitor for signs of toxicity such as hypotension and
bradycardia.

Phenytoin

Cimetidine inhibits the metabolism of phenytoin.
Monitor patients undergoing concurrent therapy for
signs of phenytoin toxicity (e.g., nystagmus, sedation,

lethargy). Serum levels may be ordered, and a reduced dosage of phenytoin may be required.

Lidocaine, Quinidine, Procainamide

Cimetidine inhibits the metabolism and/or excretion of these agents.

Monitor patients for signs of toxicity (e.g., bradycardia, additional arrhythmias, hyperactivity, sedation) and reduce the dose if necessary.

Antacids

Administer 1 hour before or 2 hours after administration of cimetidine.

Warfarin

Cimetidine may enhance the anticoagulant effects of warfarin. Observe for the development of petechiae, ecchymoses, nosebleeds, bleeding gums, dark tarry stools, and bright red or "coffee-ground" emesis. Monitor the prothrombin time and reduce the dosage of warfarin if necessary.

Ranitidine (ran-it'ih-deen) *(Zantac)* (zahn-tack)

Ranitidine is another H₂ antagonist. It is similar, in action and use, to cimetidine, but has the apparent advantage of having fewer drug interactions.

Side Effects

Up to 1% of patients may develop mild and transient lethargy, dizziness, constipation, nausea, abdominal pain, and rash. About 3% of patients develop headaches with ranitidine therapy.

There have been cases of hepatitis associated with ranitidine.

Availability

PO—150 mg tablets

Dosage and Administration

Adult
PO—150 mg two times daily. Absorption is not affected by food and, thus, may be taken without regard to meals.

Drug Interactions

No clinically significant drug interactions have been reported.

Nursing Interventions

See General Nursing Considerations for Patients with Gastrointestinal Disorders.

PATIENT CONCERNS: NURSING INTERVENTION/RATIONALE

Side Effects to Expect

Dizziness, Headaches, Constipation, Lethargy

These side effects are usually mild and are resolved with continued therapy. Encourage the patient not to discontinue therapy without consulting the physician.

Provide for patient safety during episodes of dizziness.

If patients develop somnolence and lethargy, encourage them to use caution when working around machinery or driving a car.

Maintain the patient's state of hydration, and obtain an order for stool softeners or bulk-forming laxatives, if necessary. Encourage the inclusion of sufficient roughage, fresh fruits, vegetables, and whole grain products in the diet.

Side Effects to Report

Hepatotoxicity

The symptoms of hepatotoxicity are anorexia, nausea, vomiting, jaundice, hepatomegaly, splenomegaly, and abnormal liver function as indicated by the following tests: elevated bilirubin, SGOT, SGPT, alkaline phosphatase, and prothrombin time.

Drugs Affecting the Stomach: Coating Agent

Sucralfate (sook-rahl'fate) *(Carafate)* (kair-ah'fate)

Sucralfate is a new agent that, when swallowed, forms a complex that adheres to the crater of an ulcer, protecting it from aggravators such as acid, pepsin, and bile salts. Sucralfate does not inhibit gastric secretions (like the H₂ antagonists), or alter gastric pH (like antacids). It is used to treat duodenal ulcers, particularly in those patients who do not tolerate other forms of therapy.

Side Effects

Since there is very little absorption of sucralfate, there are very few side effects associated with its use. The most common complaints are constipation (2.2%) and dry mouth. Other very infrequently reported side effects are nausea, stomach discomfort, and dizziness.

Availability

PO—1 g tablets.

Dosage and Administration

Adult

PO—1 tablet before each meal and at bedtime, all on an empty stomach. Antacids may be used, but should not be administered within half an hour before, or after, sucralfate.

Nursing Interventions

See also General Nursing Considerations for Patients with Gastrointestinal Disorders

PATIENT CONCERNS: NURSING INTERVENTION/RATIONALE

Side Effects to Expect

Constipation, Dry Mouth, Dizziness

These side effects are usually mild and tend to resolve with continued therapy. Encourage the patient not to discontinue therapy without first consulting the physician.

Measures to alleviate dry mouth include sucking on ice chips or hard candy. Avoid mouthwashes that contain alcohol, since it causes further drying and irritation.

Maintain the patient's state of hydration, and obtain an order for stool softeners or bulk-forming laxatives, if necessary. Encourage the inclusion of sufficient roughage, fresh fruits, vegetables, and whole grain products in the diet.

Provide for patient safety during episodes of dizziness.

Administration

PO

Administer on an empty stomach.

Antacids

Administer antacids at least one half hour before or after sucralfate.

Drug Interactions

Tetracyclines

Sucralfate may interfere with the absorption of tetracycline.

Administer tetracyclines 1 hour before or 2 hours after sucralfate.

Drugs Affecting the Stomach: Gastric Stimulant

Metoclopramide (met-oh-klo′prah-myd) *(Reglan)* (reg′lan)

Metoclopramide is a gastric stimulant that has an unknown mechanism of action. It increases stomach contractions, relaxes the pyloric valve, and increases peristalsis in the gastrointestinal tract, resulting in an increased rate of gastric emptying and intestinal transit. Metoclopramide is used to relieve the symptoms of diabetic gastroparesis, as an antiemetic for vomiting associated with cancer chemotherapy, as an aid in small bowel intubation, and to stimulate gastric emptying and intestinal transit of barium after radiologic examination of the upper GI tract.

Side Effects

Common side effects are drowsiness, fatigue, and lethargy. Other less frequent adverse effects include insomnia, headache, dizziness, nausea, and bowel disturbances.

About 1 in 500 patients may develop extrapyramidal symptoms manifested by restlessness, involuntary movements, facial grimacing, and possibly oculogyric crisis, torticollis, or rhythmic protrusion of the tongue. Children and young adults are most susceptible as well as those receiving higher doses of metoclopramide as an antiemetic. Metoclopramide should not be used in patients with epilepsy or in patients receiving drugs that are likely to cause extrapyramidal reactions (e.g., phenothiazines), since the frequency and severity of seizures or extrapyramidal reactions may be increased.

Metoclopramide must not be used in patients when increased gastric motility may be dangerous, such as gastrointestinal perforation, mechanical obstruction, or hemorrhage.

Availability

PO—10 mg tablets and 5 mg/5 ml syrup.
Injection—5 mg/ml in 2 and 10 ml ampules.

Dosage and Administration

Adult

PO—Diabetic gastroparesis: 10 mg 30 minutes before each meal and at bedtime. Duration of therapy is dependent on response and continued well-being after discontinuation of therapy.
IV—Antiemesis: Initial 2 doses: 2 mg/kg. If vomiting is suppressed, follow with 1 mg/kg.

Note: Rapid IV infusion may cause sudden, intense anxiety and restlessness, followed by drowsiness.

Note: If extrapyramidal symptoms should develop, treat with diphenhydramine.

PATIENT CONCERNS: NURSING INTERVENTION/RATIONALE

Side Effects to Expect

Drowsiness, Fatigue, Lethargy, Dizziness, Nausea

These side effects are usually mild and tend to resolve with continued therapy. Encourage the patient not to discontinue therapy without first consulting the physician.

People who are working around machinery, driving a car, or performing other duties that require mental alertness should be particularly cautious.

Provide for patient safety during episodes of dizziness.

Side Effects to Report

Extrapyramidal Symptoms

Provide for patient safety, then report immediately.

Administration

IV

Dilute the dose in 50 ml of parenteral solution (D₅W, N.S. 0.9%, D₅/.45 N.S., Ringer's solution, or lactated Ringer's solution).

Infuse over at least 15 minutes, 30 minutes before beginning chemotherapy. Repeat every 2 hours for 2 doses, followed by 1 dose every 3 hours for 3 doses.

Drug Interactions

Drugs That Increase Sedative Effects

Antihistamine, alcohol, analgesics, tranquilizers, sedative-hypnotics.

Monitor the patient for excessive sedation, and reduce the dosage of the above agents, if necessary.

Drugs That Decrease Therapeutic Effects

Anticholinergic agents (atropine, benztropine, antihistamines, dicyclomine) and narcotic analgesics (meperidine, morphine, oxycodone, others). Try to avoid the use of these agents while using metoclopramide.

Altered Absorption

The gastrointestinal stimulatory effects of metoclopramide may alter absorption of food and drugs:

DIGOXIN

Monitor for signs of decreased activity, (e.g., return of edema, weight gain, congestive heart failure).

LEVODOPA

Monitor for signs of increased activity, (e.g., restlessness, nightmares, hallucinations, additional involuntary movements such as bobbing of head and neck, facial grimacing, and active tongue movements).

ALCOHOL

Monitor for signs of sedation, drunkenness with smaller amounts of alcohol.

INSULIN

The absorption of food may be altered, requiring an adjustment in timing or dosage of insulin in patients with diabetes mellitus.

Antispasmodic Agents

Drugs used as antispasmodic agents are actually anticholinergic agents. The gastrointestinal (GI) tract is heavily innervated by the cholinergic branch of the autonomic nervous system. Cholinergic fibers stimulate the gastrointestinal tract causing (1) secretion of saliva, hydrochloric acid, pepsin, bile, and other enzymatic fluids necessary for digestion; (2) relaxation of sphincter muscles; and (3) peristalsis to move the contents of the stomach and bowel through the GI tract. The antispasmodic agents act by preventing acetylcholine from attaching to the cholinergic receptors in the GI tract. The extent of reduction of cholinergic activity depends upon the amount of anticholinergic drug blocking the receptors. Inhibition of cholinergic nerve conduction results in decreased GI motility and reduced secretions.

Antispasmodic agents are used to treat irritable bowel syndrome, biliary spasm, mild ulcerative colitis, diverticulitis, pancreatitis, infant colic, and in conjunction with diet and antacids, to treat peptic ulcer disease. Due to the advent of the histamine H₂ antagonists, antispasmodic agents are used much less frequently in the treatment of ulcers.

Side Effects

Since cholinergic fibers innervate the entire body, and since these agents are not selective in their actions to the GI tract, we can expect to see the effects of blocking this system throughout the body. In order to provide adequate doses to inhibit gastrointestinal motility and secretions, we should also expect a reduction in perspiration and in oral and bronchial secretions; *mydriasis* (dilation of the pupils) with blurring of vision; constipation; urinary hesitancy or retention; tachycardia, possibly with palpitations; and mild, transient postural hypotension. Psychiatric disturbances such as mental confusion, delusions, nightmares, euphoria, paranoia, and hallucinations may be indications of overdosage.

All patients should be screened for the presence of closed-angle glaucoma. Anticholinergic agents may precipitate an acute attack of closed-angle glaucoma. Patients with open-angle glaucoma can safely use anticholinergic agents in conjunction with miotic therapy.

Availability

See Table 13.3.

Dosage and Administration

See Table 13.3.

Nursing Interventions

PATIENT CONCERNS: NURSING INTERVENTION/RATIONALE

Side Effects to Expect

Blurred Vision, Constipation, Urinary Retention, Dryness of the Mouth, Nose, and Throat

These symptoms are the anticholinergic effects produced by these agents. Patients taking these medications should be monitored for the development of these side effects.

Dryness of the mucosa may be alleviated by sucking hard candy or ice chips or by chewing gum.

If patients develop urinary hesitancy, assess for distension of the bladder. Report to the physician for further evaluation.

Give stool softeners as prescribed. Encourage adequate fluid intake and foods to provide sufficient bulk.

Caution the patient that blurred vision may occur and make appropriate suggestions for personal safety of the individual.

Side Effects to Report

Confusion, Depression, Nightmares, Hallucinations

Perform a baseline assessment of the patient's degree of alertness and orientation to name, place, and time *before* initiating therapy. Make regularly scheduled subsequent mental status evaluations and compare findings. Report development of alterations.

Provide for patient safety during these episodes.

Reduction in the daily dosage may control these adverse effects.

Orthostatic Hypotension

Although infrequent and generally mild, all antispasmodic agents may cause some degree of orthostatic hypotension. It is manifested by dizziness and weakness, particularly when therapy is being initiated.

Monitor the blood pressure daily in both the supine and standing positions.

Anticipate the development of postural hypotension and take meaures to prevent an occurrence. Teach the patient to rise slowly from a supine or sitting position, and encourage them to sit or lie down if feeling faint.

Table 13.3

Antispasmodic Agents

GENERIC NAME	BRAND NAME	AVAILABILITY	CLINICAL USES	INITIAL DOSAGE
Anisotropine	Valpin 50	Tablets: 50 mg	Peptic ulcer disease	PO: 50 mg 3 times daily
Atropine	Atropine Sulfate	Inj: 0.05, 0.1, 0.3, 0.4, 1.2 mg/ml Tablets: 0.4 mg	Treatment of pylorospasm and spastic conditions of the GI tract	PO: 0.4–0.6 mg
Belladonna	Belladonna Extract, Belladonna Tincture	Tablets: 15 mg Tincture: 30 mg/ 100 ml	Indigestion, peptic ulcer Nocturnal enuresis Parkinsonism	Extract—PO: 15 mg 3–4 times daily Tincture—PO: 0.6–1 mg 3–4 times daily
Clidinium bromide	Quarzan	Capsules: 2.5, 5 mg	Peptic ulcer disease	PO: 2.5–5 mg 3–4 times daily
Dicyclomine	Bentyl, Antispas, Dibent	Tablets: 20 mg Capsules: 10, 20 mg Syrup: 10 mg/5 ml Inj: 10 mg/ml	Irritable bowel syndrome Infant colic	Adults—PO: 10–20 mg 3–4 times daily Infants—PO: 5 mg 3–4 times daily
Glycopyrrolate	Robinul	Tablets: 1, 2 mg Inj: 0.2 mg/ml	Peptic ulcer disease	PO: 1 mg 2–3 times daily
Hexocyclium	Tral	Tablets: 25, 50 mg	Peptic ulcer disease	PO: 25 mg 4 times daily
Isopropamide	Darbid	Tablets: 5 mg	Peptic ulcer disease	PO: 5 mg every 12 hours
Mepenzolate	Cantil	Tablets: 25 mg	Peptic ulcer disease	PO: 25–50 mg 4 times daily
Methantheline	Banthine	Tablets: 50 mg	Peptic ulcer disease	PO: 50–100 mg every 6 hours
Methscopolamine	Pamine	Tablets: 2.5 mg	Peptic ulcer disease	PO: 2.5 mg 30 min before meals and 2.5–5 mg at bedtime
Oxyphencyclimine	Daricon	Tablets: 10 mg	Peptic ulcer disease	PO: 10 mg 2 times daily, morning and bedtime
Propantheline	Probanthine, Norpanth	Tablets: 7.5, 15 mg	Peptic ulcer disease	PO: 15 mg before meals and 30 mg at bedtime
Scopolamine	Scopolamine	Inj: 0.3, 0.4, 1 mg/ml Tablets: 0.4, 0.6 mg	GI hypermotility, pylorospasm, irritable colon syndrome	PO: 0.4–0.8 mg
Trihexethyl chloride	Pathilon	Tablets: 25 mg	Peptic ulcer disease	PO: 25–50 mg 3–4 times daily before meals and at bedtime

Palpitations, Arrhythmias

Report for further evaluation.

Dosage and Administration

Glaucoma

All patients should be screened for the presence of closed-angle glaucoma before the initiation of therapy.

Patients with open-angle glaucoma can safely use anticholinergic agents. Monitoring intraocular pressure should be performed on a regular basis.

PO

Administer with food or milk to minimize gastric irritation.

Drug Interactions

Amantadine, Tricyclic Antidepressants, Phenothiazines

These agents may potentiate the anticholinergic side effects. Developing confusion and hallucinations are characteristic of excessive anticholinergic activity.

Digestants

Digestants are combination products used to treat various digestive disorders and supplement deficiencies of natural digestive enzymes. They are taken orally to aid digestion and absorption of dietary carbohydrates, proteins, and fats.

These products usually contain a wide variety of ingredients, each supposedly serving a purpose. See Table 13.4 for a list of components and their intended purpose.

Dosage and Administration

Adult
PO—Take one or two tablets or capsule with, or after meals.

Drug Interactions

Concurrent administration of antacids containing calcium carbonate or magnesium hydroxide interferes with the action of the digestive enzymes.

Table 13.4
Digestants

INGREDIENT	PURPOSE
Bile extracts	Activation of lipase, emulsification of fats, absorption of food
Glutamic acid and betaine HCl	Acidifiers
Simethicone and ginger	Antiflatulents
Activated charcoal	Adsorbant
Calcium carbonate or sodium bicarbonate	Antacids
Dehydrocholic acid and desoxycholic acid	Increase secretion of bile and aid in digestion of fats
Digestive enzymes:	
pepsin, papain, protease	Digest protein
lipase, amylase	Digest starch, fat, protein
diastase	Digest starch
cellulase	Digest cellulose
Anticholinergic agents	Relieve spasm and reduce hypermotility
Barbiturates, antihistamines	Sedatives
Berberis and hydrastis	Astringents used in inflammation of the mucosa

Emetics

Ipecac Syrup (ip′e-kak)

Syrup of ipecac is used to induce vomiting in cases of ingested noncorrosive poisons. It probably acts by irritating the gastric mucosa and by stimulating the vomiting center in the brain. Vomiting usually occurs within 20 to 30 minutes.

Availability

PO—15 and 30 ml syrup.

Dosage and Administration

Note: Before giving a dose of ipecac to induce vomiting, *call a physician, poison control center, or hospital emergency room for advice!*

Do not use ipecac if any of the following have been ingested: corrosives, such as alkalies (lye) and strong acids; strychnine; petroleum distillates, such as gasoline, coal oil, fuel oil, kerosene, cleaning fluid, or paint thinner.

Adult

PO—15 to 30 ml, followed by 200 to 300 ml of water or fruit juice. Do not administer with milk or carbonated beverages.

Pediatric

PO—Over 1 year of age: 10 to 15 ml followed by 200 ml of liquid. Under 1 year of age: 5 to 10 ml followed by as much liquid as the patient will take.

The dosages may be repeated once after 20 minutes if the first dose is not effective. If vomiting does not occur within 30 minutes, gastric lavage should be performed.

Nursing Interventions

See Appendix J for a list of Poison Control Centers.

PATIENT CONCERNS: NURSING INTERVENTION/RATIONALE

Side Effects to Expect

Vomiting

Vomiting should appear within 20 minutes. Report failure to vomit after 20 additional minutes following a second dose.

Side Effects to Report

Cardiotoxic Effects, Shock, Arrhythmias

Monitor pulse, respirations, and blood pressure. Report alterations in vital signs or developing symptoms of shock or cardiac arrhythmias.

Dosage and Administration

PO

See above.
Read the label carefully. Syrup of ipecac is *not* the same as fluid extract of ipecac.

Antiemetics

Nausea is the sensation of abdominal discomfort that is intermittently accompanied by a desire to vomit. Vomiting is the forceful expulsion of gastric contents up the esophagus and out the mouth. Nausea may occur without vomiting, and sudden vomiting may occur without prior nausea, but the two symptoms often occur together.

Nausea and vomiting are common symptoms experienced by virtually everyone at one time or another. They are symptoms that accompany almost any illness. Nausea and vomiting may be due to a wide variety of causes:

- Infection
- Gastrointestinal disorders such as gastritis, liver, gallbladder, or pancreatic disease
- Overeating or irritation of the stomach by certain foods or liquids
- Motion sickness (see Chapter 8)
- Drug therapy; nausea and vomiting are the most common side effects of drug therapy
- Emotional disturbances and mental stress
- Pain and unpleasant sights and odors
- Radiation therapy

The physiologic mechanisms of nausea and vomiting are not well understood. It is known that the vomiting center in the brain transmits impulses after receiving certain stimuli such as those listed, and that the stomach and duodenum respond to these impulses in the form of nausea and vomiting.

Control of vomiting is important, not only to relieve the obvious distress associated with vomiting, but also to prevent aspiration of gastric contents into the lungs, dehydration, and electrolyte imbalance. Primary treatment of nausea and vomiting should be directed at the underlying cause. Since this is not always possible, treatment with both non-drug and drug measures is appropriate. Most drugs (antiemetics) used to treat nausea and vomiting act either by suppressing the action of the vomiting center or by inhibiting the impulses going to or coming from the center. These agents are generally more effective if administered before the onset of nausea, rather than after the vomiting has already started. The agents used as antiemetics (see Table 13.5) may be grouped into three therapeutic classifications: (1) phenothiazines, (2) antihistamines (see motion sickness), and (3) miscellaneous agents.

See also General Nursing Considerations for Patients with Gastrointestinal Disorders.

Laxatives

Constipation

Constipation is the infrequent, incomplete, or painful elimination of feces. It may result from decreased motility of the colon or from retention of feces in the lower colon or rectum. In either case, the longer the time that the feces remain in the colon, the greater

Table 13.5
Antiemetic Agents

GENERIC NAME	BRAND NAME	AVAILABILITY	ANTIEMETIC DOSAGE		COMMENTS
			ADULTS	CHILDREN	
Phenothiazines					**Comments for All Phenothiazines**
Chlorpromazine	Thorazine	Tablets: 10, 25, 50, 100, 200 mg Capsules: 30, 75, 150, 200, 300 mg Syrup: 10 mg/5 ml Concentrate: 30 100 mg/ml Suppositories: 25, 100 mg Injection: 25 mg/ml	PO: 10–25 mg every 4–6 hours Rectal: 50–100 mg every 6–8 hrs IM: 25 mg	PO: 0.25 mg/lb every 4–6 hrs Rectal: 0.5 mg/lb every 6–8 hrs IM: 0.25 mg/lb every 6–8 hrs (Maximum IM dose: up to age 5: 40 mg/day; ages 5–12: 75 mg/day)	Phenothiazines may suppress the cough reflex. Assure that the patient does not aspirate vomitus. Use with caution in patients, especially children, with undiagnosed vomiting. The phenothiazines can mask signs of toxicity of other drugs, or mask symptoms of other diseases such as brain tumor, Reye Syndrome, or intestinal obstruction. Use with extreme caution in patients with seizure disorders. Discontinue if rashes develop. May cause orthostatic hypotension. See Chapter 8, Drugs Affecting the Central Nervous System, for a complete listing of adverse effects, drug interactions, and nursing interventions.
Perphenazine	Trilafon	Tablets: 2, 4, 8, 16 mg Concentrate: 16 mg/5 ml Injection: 5 mg/ml	PO: 4 mg every 4–6 hrs IM: 5 mg	Not recommended	
Prochlorperazine	Compazine	Tablets: 5, 10, 25 mg Syrup: 5 mg/5 ml Suppositories: 2.5, 5, 25 mg	PO: 5–10 mg every 6–8 hrs Rectal: 25 mg 2 times daily IM: 5–10 mg	PO or Rectal: 20–29 lbs—2.5 mg 1–2 times daily 30–39 lbs—2.5 mg 2–3 times daily 40–85 lbs—2.5 mg 3 times daily IM: 0.6 mg/lb	
Triethylperazine	Torecan	Tablets: 10 mg Suppositories: 10 mg Injection: 5 mg/ml	PO, Rectal, IM: 10–30 mg daily in divided doses	Not recommended	
Triflupromazine	Vesprin	Suspension: 50 mg/5 ml Injection: 10–20 mg/ml	PO: 20–30 mg daily in divided doses IM: 5–15 mg every 4 hrs	PO: 0.2 mg/kg, up to 10 mg/day IM: 0.2–0.25 mg/kg up to 10 mg/day	
Antihistamines	(See Motion Sickness in Index)				
Miscellaneous Agents					
Benzquinamide	Emete-Con	Injection: 50 mg/vial	IM: 0.5–1 mg/kg; repeat in 1 hr, then every 3–4 hrs IV: 25 mg at a rate of 1 ml/min	Not recommended	Recommended for nausea and vomiting associated with anesthesia and surgery. Reconstitute with sterile water. IM route preferred.

320

Table 13.5 (*continued*)

GENERIC NAME	BRAND NAME	AVAILABILITY	ANTIEMETIC DOSAGE ADULTS	ANTIEMETIC DOSAGE CHILDREN	COMMENTS
Diphenidol	Vontrol	Tablets: 25 mg	PO: 25–50 mg every 4 hrs	PO: 0.4 mg/lb every 4 hrs. Do not exceed 2.5 mg/lb/ 24 hrs	Used in adults for dizziness, nausea, and vomiting. Use in children for nausea and vomiting only. May cause auditory and visual hallucinations within 3 days. Discontinue therapy.
Metoclopramide Trimethobenzamide	(See Index) Tigan	Capsules: 100, 250 mg Suppositories: 100, 200 mg Injection: 100 mg/ml	PO: 250 mg 3–4 times daily Rectal: 200 mg 3–4 times daily IM: 200 mg 3–4 times daily	PO: 30–90 lbs; 100–200 mg 3–4 times daily Rectal: <30 lbs: 3–4 times daily 30–90 lbs: 100–200 mg 3–4 times daily	Injectible form contains benzocaine. Do not use in patients allergic to benzocaine or local anesthetics. Inject in upper, outer quadrant of gluteal region. Avoid escape of solution along the route. May cause burning, stinging, pain, on injection.

the reabsorption of water and the drier the stool becomes. The stool is then more difficult to expel from the anus. Causes of constipation are (1) improper diet— too little residue, too little fluid, or not enough vitamins; (2) muscular weakness of the colon; (3) sedentary habits; (4) failure to respond to the normal defecation impulses; (5) diseases such as anemia and hypothyroidism; (6) addiction to heroin, morphine, or codeine; (7) tumors of the bowel or pressure on the bowel from tumors; (8) diseases of the rectum.

Occasional constipation is not detrimental to a person's health, although it can cause a feeling of general discomfort or abdominal fullness, anorexia, and anxiety in some persons. Habitual constipation leads to decreased intestinal muscle tone, increased straining at stool as the person bears down in the attempt to pass the hardened stool, and an increased incidence of hemorrhoids. The daily use of laxatives or enemas should be avoided, since these decrease the muscular tone and mucus production of the rectum and may result in water and electrolyte imbalance. They also become habit forming: the weakened muscle tone adds to the inability to expel the fecal contents, which leads to the continued use of enemas or laxatives.

Drugs have been used for centuries to overcome constipation. Today, many people believe that even occasional failure of the bowel to move daily should be treated with a laxative. Daily bowel movements are frequently not necessary. Many people have "normal" bowel habits even though they have one or two bowel movements per week. As long as the patient's health is good, and the stool is not hardened or impacted, this schedule is acceptable.

Types of Laxatives

Laxatives are chemicals that act to promote the evacuation of the bowel. They are usualy subclassified, based upon the mechanism of action:

Contact or Stimulant Laxatives. These agents act directly on the intestine, causing an irritation that promotes peristalsis and evacuation. If given orally, these agents act within 6 to 10 hours. If administered rectally, they act within 60 to 90 minutes. These products should only be used intermittently, because chronic use may cause loss of normal bowel function and dependency on the agent for bowel evacuation.

Saline Laxatives. These are hypertonic compounds that attract water into the intestine from surrounding tissues. The accumulated water affects stool consistency and distends the bowel, causing peristalsis. These agents usually act within 1 to 3 hours. Continued use of these products significantly alters electrolyte balance and may cause dehydration.

Lubricant or Emollient Laxatives. These lubricate the intestinal wall and soften the stool, allowing a smooth passage of fecal contents. Onset of action is 6 to 8 hours, but is highly dependent upon the individual patient's normal gastrointestinal transit time. Peristaltic activity does not appear to be increased. If used frequently, these oils may inhibit the absorption of fat-soluble vitamins.

Bulk-Producing Laxatives. These must be administered with a full glass of water. The laxative causes water to be retained within the stool, increasing bulk that stimulates peristalsis. Onset of action is usually 12 to 24 hours, but may be as long as 72 hours, depending upon the individual patient's gastrointestinal transit time. Bulk-forming agents are usually considered to be the safest of any laxative, even when taken routinely. Fresh fruits, vegetables, and cereals such as bran are natural bulk-forming products.

Fecal Softeners. These "wetting agents" draw water into the stool, causing it to soften. They do not stimulate peristalsis and may require up to 72 hours to aid in a soft bowel movement. Action from these agents depends upon the patient's state of hydration and the gastrointestinal transit time.

Indications

Laxatives may be indicated as follows: (1) contact or saline laxatives may be used to relieve acute constipation; (2) contact or saline laxatives are used to remove gas and feces before radiologic examination of the kidneys, colon, intestine, or gall bladder; (3) stool softeners are routinely used for prophylactic purposes to prevent constipation or straining at stool, for example, in patients recovering from myocardial infarction or abdominal surgery; (4) bulk-forming laxatives may be used in patients with irritable bowel syndrome to provide a softer consistency to the stools if a high-fiber diet is not adequate; and (5) bulk-forming laxatives are used to control certain types of diarrhea by absorbance of the irritating substance, thus allowing its removal from the bowel during defecation.

Side Effects

The most common adverse effects are excessive bowel stimulation resulting in gripping, diarrhea, nausea, vomiting, and rectal irritation. Patients who are severely constipated may develop abdominal cramps.

Obstruction within the gastrointestinal tract may result from a bulk laxative that forms a sticky mass. This is usually due to inadequate mixing with water before ingestion.

Mineral oil may cause lipid pneumonia if inhaled into the lungs. Do not administer to debilitated patients who are constantly in a recumbent position.

Do not administer laxatives to patients with undiagnosed abdominal pain, or patients with inflammation of the gastrointestinal tract such as gastritis, appendicitis, or colitis.

Do not administer when fecal impaction exists or when there is intestinal obstruction, hemorrhage, severe spasm, diarrhea, or intestinal perforation.

Availability

See Table 13.6.

Dosage and Administration

See product label.

Nursing Interventions

See also General Nursing Considerations for Patients with Gastrointestinal Disorders.

PATIENT CONCERNS: NURSING INTERVENTION/RATIONALE

Side Effects to Expect

Gripping, Minor Abdominal Discomfort

The patient should first experience the urge to defecate, then defecate and feel a sense of relief.

Side Effects to Report

Abdominal Tenderness, Pain, Bleeding, Vomiting, Diarrhea, Increasing Abdominal Girth

Failure to defecate or defecation of only a small amount may be an indication of an impaction. These symptoms may indicate an "acute abdomen."

Dosage and Administration

PO

Follow directions on the container. Be sure to give adequate water with bulk-forming agents to prevent esophageal, gastric, intestinal, or rectal obstruction.

Drug Interactions

Dulcolax

Do not administer with milk, antacids, cimetidine, or ranitidine. These products may allow the enteric coating

Table 13.6
Laxatives

PRODUCT	CONTACT	SALINE	BULK-FORMING	LUBRICANT	FECAL SOFTENER
Agoral	Phenolphthalein		Agar, Tragacanth, Acacia, Egg albumin	Mineral oil	
Colace					Docusate sodium
Dialose					Docusate potassium
Dialose Plus	Casanthranol				Docusate potassium
Doxidan	Danthron				Docusate calcium
Dulcolax	Bisacodyl				
Ex–lax	Phenolphthalein				
Haley's MO		Magnesium hydroxide		Mineral oil	
Metamucil			Psyllium hydrophilic mucilloid		
Modane	Danthron				
Peri–Colace	Casanthranol				Docusate sodium
Phillips' Milk of Magnesia		Magnesium hydroxide			
Phospho–Soda		Sodium phosphate			
Surfak					Docusate calcium
X–Prep	Senna concentrate				

to dissolve prematurely, causing nausea, vomiting, and cramping.

Psyllium

Do not administer products containing psyllium (Metamucil, Siblin, others) at the same time as salicylates, nitrofurantoin, or digitalis glycosides. The psyllium may inhibit absorption. Administer these tablets at least 1 hour before or 2 hours after the psyllium.

Mineral Oil

Daily administration of mineral oil for more than 1 to 2 weeks may cause a deficiency of the fat-soluble vitamins.

Docusate

Docusate enhances the absorption of mineral oil. Concurrent use is not recommended in order to prevent granuloma formation in the liver, lymph nodes, and intestinal lining.

Antidiarrheal Agents

Diarrhea

Diarrhea is an increase in the frequency and/or fluid content of bowel movements. Since normal patterns of defecation and the patient's perception of bowel function vary, a careful history must be obtained to determine the change in a particular patient's bowel elimination pattern. An important fact to remember about diarrhea is that diarrhea is a symptom, rather than a disease. It may be caused by any of the following:

- Intestinal infections. These are most frequently associated with ingestion of food contaminated with bacteria or protozoa (food poisoning), or eating or drinking water that contains bacteria that is foreign to the patient's gastrointestinal tract. People traveling, often to other countries, develop what is known as *traveler's diarrhea* due to ingestion of microorganisms that are pathogenic to their gastrointestinal tract, but not to the local residents.
- Spicy foods may produce diarrhea by irritating the lining of the gastrointestinal tract. Diarrhea occurs particularly frequently when the patient does not routinely eat spicy foods.
- Patients with deficiencies of digestive enzymes such as lactase or amylase have difficulty digesting foods. Diarrhea usually develops due to irritation from undigested food.
- Excessive use of laxatives.
- Drug therapy. Diarrhea is a common side effect, due to the irritation of the gastrointestinal lining by ingested medication. Diarrhea may also result from the use of antibiotics that may kill certain normal bacteria living in the gastrointestinal tract that help digest food.

Table 13.7
Antidiarrheal Agents

GENERIC NAME	BRAND NAME	AVAILABILITY	ADULT DOSAGE	COMMENTS
Systemic Action				
Diphenoxylate with atropine	Lomotil, Diphenatol, Lofene	Tablets: 2.5 mg diphenoxylate with 0.025 mg atropine Liquid: 2.5 mg diphenoxylate, with 0.025 mg atropine per 5 ml	PO: 5 mg 4 times daily	Inhibits peristalsis. Atropine added to minimize potential overdose or abuse. May cause drowsiness or dizziness. Use caution in performing tasks requiring alertness. Do not use in children less than 2 years of age.
Loperamide	Immodium	Capsules: 2 mg	PO: 4 mg initially, followed by 2 mg after each unformed movement. Do not exceed 16 mg/day.	Inhibits peristalsis. Used in acute nonspecific diarrhea, and to reduce the volume of discharge from ileostomy.
Camphorated tincture of opium	Paregoric	Liquid	PO: 5–10 ml 4 times daily	Inhibits peristalsis and pain of diarrhea. 5 ml of liquid = 2 mg morphine.
Local Action				
Kaolin/pectin	Kaopectate, K-P, K-Pek	Suspension	PO: 60–120 mg after each loose bowel movement	Used as adsorbent.
Attapulgite, pectin	Diar-Aid	Tablets	PO: 2 tablets after each loose bowel movement	Used as adsorbent.
Lactobacillus acidophilus	Lactinex, Bacid, Dofus	Capsules, Granules, Tablets	PO: 2–4 tablets or capsules, 2–4 times daily, with milk. Granules: 1 packet added to cereal, fruit juice, milk 3–4 times daily	Bacteria used to recolonize the gastrointestinal tract in an attempt to treat chronic diarrhea. Do not use in acute diarrhea.
Bismuth subsalicylate	Pepto-Bismol	Tablets, Suspension	PO: 30 ml or 2 tablets chewed every 30–60 minutes up to 8 doses	Used as adsorbent.
Combination Action				
Opium, kaolin, pectin	Parepectolin	Suspension	PO: 15–30 ml after each loose bowel movement	Opium inhibits peristalsis and pain of diarrhea. Kaolin and pectin act as adsorbents.
Kaolin, pectin, hyoscyamine, atropine, scopolamine	Donnagel, Quiagel	Suspension	PO: Initially, 30 ml, followed by 15 ml every 3 hours	Hyoscyamine, atropine and scopolamine are used to inhibit peristalsis and reduce gastrointestinal secretions. Kaolin and pectin act as adsorbents.
Kaolin, pectin, codeine, bismuth subsalicylate, carboxymethylcellulose	Kaodene with Codeine	Suspension	PO: Initially, 15 ml, followed by 10 ml every 30 min as needed	Codeine inhibits peristalsis and pain of diarrhea. Other ingredients act as adsorbents.

- Emotional stress. Diarrhea is a common symptom of stress and anxiety.
- Hyperthyroidism induces increased gastrointestinal motility, resulting in diarrhea.
- Inflammatory bowel diseases such as diverticulitis, ulcerative colitis, gastroenteritis, and Crohn's disease cause inflammation of the gastrointestinal lining, resulting in diarrhea.
- Surgical bypass procedures of the intestine often result in chronic diarrhea because of the decreased absorptive area remaining after surgery. Incompletely digested food and water rapidly pass through the gastrointestinal tract.

Types of Antidiarrheal Agents

Antidiarrheal agents include a wide variety of drugs, but they can be divided into two broad categories (1) locally acting agents and (2) systemic agents. Locally acting agents such as activated charcoal, kaolin, pectin, psyllium, and activated attapulgite adsorb excess water to cause a formed stool and to adsorb irritants or bacteria that are causing the diarrhea. The systemic agents act through the autonomic nervous system to reduce peristalsis and motility of the gastrointestinal tract, allowing the mucosal lining to absorb nutrients, water, and electrolytes, leaving a formed stool from the residue remaining in the colon. Representatives of the systemically acting agents are paregoric, diphenoxylate, loperamide, and certain anticholinergic agents (Table 13.7).

Diarrhea may be acute or chronic, mild or severe. Since diarrhea may be a defense mechanism to rid the body of infecting organisms or irritants, it is usually self-limiting. If severe or prolonged, diarrhea may cause dehydration, electrolyte depletion, and exhaustion. Specific antidiarrheal therapy depends on the cause of the diarrhea. Antidiarrheal products are usually indicated when:

- The diarrhea is of sudden onset, has lasted more than 2 or 3 days, and is causing significant fluid and water loss. Young children and elderly patients are more susceptible to rapid dehydration and electrolyte imbalance, and therefore should start antidiarrheal therapy earlier.
- Patients with inflammatory bowel disease develop diarrhea. Rapid treatment allows the patient to live a more normal lifestyle. Other agents such as adrenocortical steroids or sulfonamides may also be used to control the underlying bowel disease.
- Postgastrointestinal surgery patients develop diarrhea. These patients may require chronic antidiarrheal therapy to allow adequate absorption of fluids and electrolytes.
- The cause of the diarrhea has been diagnosed and the physician determines that an antidiarrheal product is appropriate for therapy. Since many cases of diarrhea are self-limiting, therapy may not be necessary.

Side Effects

The locally acting agents have essentially no adverse effects, but if used excessively, they may cause abdominal distension, nausea, and constipation.

The systemically acting agents are associated with more adverse effects (see Table 13.7). These agents should not be used to treat diarrhea caused by substances toxic to the gastrointestinal tract, such as bacterial contaminants or other irritants. Since these agents act by reducing GI motility, they tend to allow the toxin to remain in the GI tract longer causing further irritation.

Availability

See Table 13.7.

Dosage and Administration

See Table 13.7.

Nursing Interventions

See General Nursing Considerations for Patients with Gastrointestinal Disorders.

Chapter 14

Drugs Affecting
the Urinary System

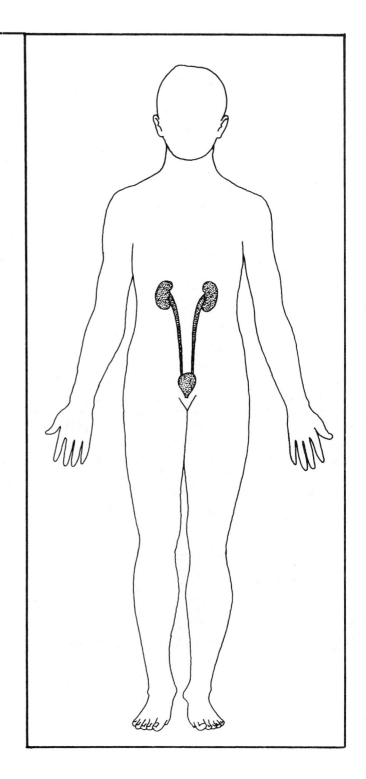

Objectives

After completing this chapter, the student should be able to do the following:

1. Explain the major actions and effects of drugs used to treat disorders of the urinary tract.
2. Identify baseline data the nurse should collect on a continuous basis for comparison and evaluation of drug effectiveness.
3. Identify important nursing assessments and interventions associated with drug therapy and treatment of diseases of the urinary tract.
4. Identify health teaching essential for a successful treatment regimen.

General Nursing Considerations for Patients with Urinary System Disease

The information the nurse assesses relative to the patient's general clinical symptoms is important to the physician when analyzing data for diagnosis. In addition to assessing overall clinical symptoms, the nurse should include the following data for subsequent evaluation of the patient's response to prescribed therapeutic modalities that act upon the urinary system.

PATIENT CONCERNS: NURSING INTERVENTION/RATIONALE

Alterations in Renal Function

Pattern of Pain

Record the details of any pain the patient describes: frequency, intensity, duration, and location. Pain associated with renal pathology usually occurs at the groin, flank, and suprapubic area, and on urination (dysuria).

Pattern of Urination

Ask the patient to describe his or her current urination pattern and to cite changes. Such details as frequency, dysuria, incontinence, changes in the stream, hesitancy in starting to void, hematuria, nocturia, and urgency are all of significance.

Intake and Output

Intake and output should be recorded accurately every shift and totaled every 24 hours for all patients having renal evaluations or receiving diuretics.

INTAKE

Measure and record *accurately* all fluids taken (oral, parenteral, rectal, and via tubes). Ice chips and foods such as Jell-O that turn to a liquid state need to be included. Irrigation solutions should be carefully measured so that the difference between that instilled and that returned can be recorded as intake.

Remember to enlist the patient, family, and other visitors' help in this process. Ask them to keep a record of how many water glasses, juice glasses, or coffee cups were consumed. You then convert the household measurements to milliliters.

OUTPUT

Record all output from the mouth, urethra, rectum, wounds, and tubes (surgical drains, nasogastric tubes, indwelling catheters).

Liquid stools should be recorded according to consistency, color, and quantity.

Urine output should include information on quantity, color, pH, odor, and specific gravity.

All other secretions should be characterized by color, consistency, volume, and changes from previous collections, if possible.

Daily output is usually 1200 to 1500 cc, or 30 to 50 cc per hour. Always report urine output below this hourly rate. Low hourly output may indicate dehydration, renal failure, or cardiac disease.

Keep the urinal or bedpan readily available.

Tell patients and their visitors the importance of not "helping" by dumping the bedpan or urinal, but rather to use the call light and allow the hospital personnel to empty and record all output.

States of Hydration

DEHYDRATION

Assess, report, and record significant signs of dehydration in the patient. Observe for poor skin turgor, sticky oral mucous membranes, a shrunken or deeply-furrowed tongue, crusted lips, weight loss, deteriorating vital signs, soft or sunken eyeballs, weak pedal pulses, delayed capillary filling, excessive thirst, high urine specific gravity (or no urine output), and possible mental confusion.

Skin Turgor. Check skin turgor by *gently* pinching the skin together over the sternum, forehead, or on the forearm.

Elasticity is present and the skin rapidly returns to a flat position in the well-hydrated patient. With dehydration, the skin will remain in a "peaked" or "pinched" position and returns very slowly to the flat, normal position.

Oral Mucous Membranes. With adequate hydration, the membranes of the mouth feel smooth and glisten. With dehydration, they appear dull and are sticky.

Laboratory Changes. The values of the hematocrit, hemoglobin, BUN, and electrolytes will appear to fluctuate, based on the state of hydration. When a patient is overhydrated, the values appear to drop due to "hemodilution." A dehydrated patient will show higher values due to "hemoconcentration."

OVERHYDRATION

Increases in abdominal girth, weight gain, neck vein engorgement, and circumference of the medial malleolus are indications of overhydration.

Measure the adominal girth daily at the umbilical level.

Measure the extremities bilaterally daily at a level approximately 5 cc above the medial malleolus.

Weigh the patient daily using the same scale, at the same time, in similar clothing.

EDEMA

Edema is a term used to describe excess fluid accumulation in the extracellular spaces.

Pitting Edema. Edema is considered "pitting" when an indentation remains in the tissue after pressure is exerted against a bony part such as the shin, ankle, or sacrum. The degree is usually recorded as 1+ (slight) to 4+ (deep).

Pale, cool, tight, shiny skin is another sign of edema.

Electrolyte Imbalance

Because the symptoms of most electrolyte imbalances are similar, the nurse should gather data relative to changes in the patient's mental status (i.e., alertness, orientation, confusion), muscle strength, muscle cramps, tremors, nausea, and general appearance.

SUSCEPTIBLE PERSONS

Those who are particularly susceptible to the development of electrolyte disturbances frequently have a history of renal or cardiac disease, hormonal disorders, massive trauma or burns, or are on diuretic or steroid therapy.

SERUM ELECTROLYTES

Monitor serum electrolyte reports; notify physicians of deviations from normal values.

HYPOKALEMIA

Serum potassium (K^+) levels below 3.5 mEq/liter.

Hypokalemia is especially likely to occur when a patient exhibits vomiting, diarrhea, or heavy diuresis. All diuretics, except the potassium-sparing type, are likely to cause hypokalemia.

HYPERKALEMIA

Serum potassium levels above 5.5 mEq/liter.

Hyperkalemia occurs most commonly when a patient is given excessive amounts of potassium supplementation, either intravenously or orally. It may also occur as an adverse effect of potassium-sparing diuretics.

HYPONATREMIA

Serum sodium (Na^+) below 135 mEq/liter.

Remember the phrase, "Where sodium goes, water goes." Since diuretics act by excreting sodium, monitor your patient for hyponatremia during and after diuresis.

HYPERNATREMIA

Serum sodium above 145 mEq/liter.

Hypernatremia occurs most frequently when a patient is given intravenous fluids in excess of that excreted.

Nutrition

EDEMA

Patients are routinely placed on a restricted sodium diet to help control edema associated with congestive heart failure.

RENAL DISEASE

Diet therapy for renal disease is directed at keeping a normal equilibrium of the body while decreasing the excretory load on the kidneys. See a nutrition text for modifications specific to acute and chronic renal failure.

Renal Diagnostics

Many laboratory tests are ordered throughout the treatment of renal dysfunction (BUN, serum creatinine,

Table 14.1

Urinalysis

	NORMAL DATA	ABNORMAL DATA
Color	Straw, clear yellow, or amber	Dark smoky color, reddish or brown may indicate blood. White or cloudy may indicate urinary tract infection or chyluria. Dark yellow to amber may indicate dehydration. Green, deep yellow or brown may indicate liver or biliary disease. Some drugs may also alter urine color: Pyridium—orange; methylene blue—blue.
Odor	Ammonialike on standing	Foul smell may indicate an infection. The dehydrated patient's urine is concentrated and the ammonia smell is apparent.
Protein	0	Foamy or frothy-appearing urine may indicate protein. Proteinuria is associated with kidney disease, toxemia of pregnancy, and may be present following vigorous exercise.
Glucose	0–trace	Presence is usually associated with diabetes mellitus or low renal threshold with glucose "spillage." Also seen at times of stress, such as major infection, or following a high carbohydrate meal.
pH	4.6–8.0	Medications can be prescribed to produce an alkaline or acid urine. pH of urine increases if urine is tested after standing four hours or more.
RBC	0–3	Indicative of bleeding at some location in the urinary tract: infection, obstruction, calculi, renal failure, or tumors. (Be sure urine is not contaminated by menses.)
Casts	Rare	May indicate dehydration, possible infection within renal tubules, or other types of renal disease.
WBC	0–4	An increase indicates infection somewhere in the urinary tract.
Specific gravity	1.003–1.030	Used as an indicator of the state of hydration (in absence of renal pathology). Above 1.018 is early sign of dehydration; below 1.010 is "dilute urine" and may indicate fluid accumulation. A fixed specific gravity at around 1.010 may indicate renal disease.

creatinine clearance, urine culture, serum osmolalities, and renal concentration tests).

Urinalysis

The urinalysis is the most basic test the nurse encounters and an understanding of the significant data this routine test can reveal is imperative to monitoring the patient. Refer to Table 14.1 for a description of the data. See a general medical-surgical text for details of collecting urine samples correctly.

Diuretic Agents

Diuretics are drugs that act to increase the flow of urine. The purpose of diuretics is to increase the net loss of water. To achieve this, they act on the kidneys in different locations to enhance the excretion of sodium. The xanthines increase glomerular filtration; spironolactone inhibits tubular reabsorption of sodium by inhibiting aldosterone; and the thiazides, furosemide, bumetanide, and ethacrynic acid act directly on the kidney tubules to inhibit the reabsorption of sodium and chloride from the lumen of the tubule. Sodium and chloride that are not reabsorbed are excreted into the collecting ducts and then into the ureters to the bladder, taking with them large volumes of water to be excreted from the body through urination (Fig. 14.1).

Side Effects

All diuretics may cause electrolyte abnormalities, including hyponatremia, hypochloremia, hyperkalemia and hypokalemia.

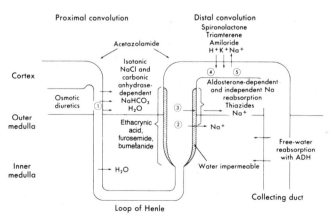

Fig. 14.1. *Sites of actions of diuretics. (Adapted from Melmon, K. L., and Morrelli, H. F., editors:* Clinical Pharmacology: Basic Principles in Therapeutics. *Macmillan Publishers, New York, 1972.)*

Diuretics should be administered with particular caution to the elderly, to any patients with impaired renal function, cirrhosis of the liver, or diabetes mellitus. These types of patients are at greater risk for developing hyperkalemia.

General Nursing Considerations for Patients Receiving Diuretic Therapy

See also General Nursing Considerations for Patients with Urinary System Disease.

Patient Teaching Associated with Diuretic Therapy

PATIENT CONCERNS: NURSING INTERVENTION/RATIONALE

Communication and Responsibility

Encourage open communication concerning frustrations and anger as the patient attempts to adjust to the diagnosis and need for treatment. The patient must be guided to gain insight into the condition in order to assume responsibility for the continuation of treatment. Keep emphasizing those factors the patient can control to alter the progression of the disease, including maintenance of general health, nutritional needs, adequate rest and appropriate exercise, and continuation of prescribed medication therapy.

Hypertension

If the disease process is hypertension, stress the importance of following prescribed ways to deal with emotions and the dietary and medicinal regimens that can control the disease. (See General Nursing Considerations for Patients with Hypertension in Chapter 10.)

Nutrition

The physician usually prescribes dietary modifications aimed at weight reduction, if necessary, and sodium restrictions.

Do not suggest salt substitutes without physician approval. See Appendix K for sodium and potassium contents of common salt substitutes.

Patients receiving potassium-sparing diuretics should be taught which foods are high in potassium content. These foods should be moderately restricted but not withheld from the diet.

Expectations of Therapy

Discuss expectations of therapy with the patient. This discussion needs to be individualized to the patient and to the underlying diagnosis for which diuretic therapy is prescribed (i.e., hypertension, congestive heart failure).

Changes in Expectations

Assess changes in expectations as therapy progresses and the patient gains understanding and skill in the management of the diagnosis.

Changes in Therapy through Cooperative Goal-Setting

Work mutually with the patient to encourage adherence to the prescribed treatment. When the patient feels that a change should be made in a treatment plan, encourage discussion first with the physician.

Written Record

Enlist the patient's aid in developing and maintaining a written record of monitoring parameters (Table 14.2) (i.e., blood pressure, pulse, daily weights, exercise tolerance, and urine glucose, if appropriate) and response to prescribed therapies for discussion with the physician. Patients should be encouraged to take this record on follow-up visits.

Fostering Compliance

Throughout the hospitalization, discuss medication information and how it will benefit the course of treatment. Seek cooperation and understanding of the following points so that medication compliance may be enhanced:

1. Name
2. Dosage
3. Route and administration times—Tell patients to take their diuretic in the morning so that the diuresis

Table 14.2
Example of a Written Record for Patients Receiving Diuretics or Urinary Antibiotics

Medications	Color	To be taken

Name _____

Physician _____

Physician's phone _____

Next appt.* _____

Parameters		Day of discharge							Comments
Weight									
Blood pressure									
Pulse									
Faintness, dizziness	At rest								
	On exertion								
	No. of occurrences								
Muscle weakness	With exertion								
	When at rest								
Pain pattern and severity Severe Moderate Low 10 5 1 Description: On urination Without urination Flank area Suprapubic area									
Voiding and frequency	# times voiding per day								
	# times voiding per hour								
Fluid intake	# glasses per day								
	# cups per day								
Urine	Color (check one)	Straw							
		Dark							
		Red							
	Odor: usual or unusual								

*Please bring this record with you to your next appointment.
Use the back of this sheet for additional information.

331

will not keep them up at night. They can reduce gastric irritation by taking it with food or milk.

4. Anticipated therapeutic response: When administered for edema: diuresis—During initial therapy, the individual can anticipate a 1 to 2 pound daily weight loss. Tell the patient who will be discharged with diuretics to weigh and keep a record of his or her weight at home and to report weight gains or losses of more than 2 pounds per week. When administered for hypertension: a gradual reduction in blood pressure toward mutually set goals.

5. Side effects to expect: Increased frequency and amount of urination; possible orthostatic hypotension, which can be avoided by rising slowly from supine and sitting positions.

6. Side effects to report: Tell the patient to notify the physician if experiencing changes in muscle strength, tremors, visible edema, nausea, vomiting, diarrhea, excessive thirst, or changes in normal behavior (progressively feeling more exhausted, becoming confused). Since so many electrolyte changes can be involved in diuretic therapy, it is best to use general terms when teaching the lay person.

7. What to do if a dosage is missed.

8. When, how, or if to refill the medication.

Difficulty in Comprehension

If it is evident that the patient and/or family does not understand all aspects of continuing therapy being prescribed (i.e., administration and monitoring of medications, exercises, diets, follow-up appointments), consider the use of social service or visiting nurse agencies.

Associated Teaching

Give the following instructions:

Always inform the physician or dentists of any prescription or over-the-counter medication being taken. Over-the-counter medications should not be taken without first discussing them with your physician or pharmacist.

Always report side effects of rash, itching, or hives immediately. Nausea, vomiting, or diarrhea should also be reported for the physician's evaluation if it is a new symptom.

Take all of the medication as prescribed for the full course of treatment. Do not discontinue use when feeling improved; do not save for future use; do not give your medicine to another individual. Sudden discontinuation of certain medications may produce harmful effects.

Keep all medications out of the reach of children.

If pregnancy is suspected, consult your obstetrician as soon as possible about continuation of medication therapy.

At Discharge

Items to be sent home with the patient should:

1. Have written instructions for use.

2. Be labeled in a level of language and size of print appropriate for the patient.

3. If needed, include identification cards or bracelets.

4. Include a list of additional supplies to be purchased after discharge.

Acetazolamide (ah-see-tah-zol′a-myd) *(Diamox)* (dy′ah-moks)

Acetazolamide is a rather weak diuretic that acts by inhibiting the enzyme carbonic anhydrase within the kidney, brain, and eye. As a diuretic, it promotes the excretion of sodium, potassium, water, and bicarbonate. This agent is infrequently used now as a diuretic due to the availability of more effective medications; however, it is used to reduce intraocular pressure in patients with glaucoma and to reduce seizure activity in patients with certain types of epilepsy (see Index).

Aminophylline (ah-mi-noff′ih-lin)

Aminophylline is a methylxanthine derivative used for its diuretic effects in cardiorenal disease and as a bronchodilator in patients with pulmonary disease. The methylxanthine derivatives include theophylline, caffeine, and theobromine, all of which display weak diuretic properties. All act by improving blood flow to the kidneys.

Aminophylline is rarely used now as a diuretic because of the availability of more effective diuretic agents. However, a diuresis is occasionally noted when aminophylline is used in the treatment of asthma. For discussion of aminophylline as a bronchodilator, see Index.

Bumetanide (bu-met'an-eyd) *(Bumex)* (bu'mex)

Bumetanide is the newest of the potent diuretics. Its diuretic activity starts within 30 to 60 minutes after administration, and lasts for about 4 hours. It is used to treat edema due to congestive heart failure, cirrhosis of the liver, and renal disease, including nephrotic syndrome.

Side Effects

If given in excessive dosages or to patients with massive fluid accumulation, treatment with bumetanide may lead to excessive diuresis and thus water dehydration and electrolyte imbalance.

The most common side effects are oral and gastric irritation, abdominal pain, upset stomach, and dry mouth. Other generalized side effects include muscle weakness, fatigue, dizziness, dehydration, hives, pruritus, and asterixis.

Availability

PO—0.5 and 1 mg tablets.
IV—0.25 mg/ml in 2 ml ampules.

Dosage and Administration

Adult
PO—Initially 0.5 to 2 mg is administered as a single, daily dose. If additional diuresis is required, additional doses may be administered at 4 to 5 hour intervals. Do not exceed a maximum daily dose of 10 mg.
IM or IV—Initially, 0.5 to 1 ml administered over 1 to 2 minutes. Additional doses may be administered at 2 to 3 hour intervals, as necessary. Do not exceed 10 mg per 24 hours.

Nursing Interventions

See also General Nursing Considerations for Patients Receiving Diuretic Therapy.

**PATIENT CONCERNS:
NURSING INTERVENTION/RATIONALE**

Side Effects to Expect

Oral Irritation, Dry Mouth

Start regular oral hygiene measures when the therapy is initiated. Suggest the use of 1 tsp of hydrogen peroxide in 6 to 8 ounces of water as a mouthwash. Commercial mouthwashes contain alcohol which may cause further drying and oral irritation.

Other measures to alleviate dryness include sucking on ice chips or hard candy.

Orthostatic Hypotension (Dizziness, Weakness, Faintness)

Although infrequent and generally mild, all diuretics may cause some degree of orthostatic hypotension manifested by dizziness and weakness, particularly when therapy is being initiated.

Monitor the blood pressure daily in both the supine and erect positions.

Anticipate the development of postural hypotension and take measures to prevent an occurrence. Teach the patient to rise slowly from a supine or sitting position, and encourage the patient to sit or lie down if feeling "faint."

Side Effects to Report

Gastric Irritation, Abdominal Pain

If gastric irritation occurs, administer with food or milk. If symptoms persist or increase in severity, report for physician evaluation.

Electrolyte Imbalance, Dehydration

The electrolytes most commonly altered are potassium (K^+), sodium (Na^+), and chloride (Cl^-). *Hypokalemia* is most likely to occur.

Many symptoms associated with altered fluid and electrolyte balance are subtle and interspersed with general symptoms of drug toxicity or the disease process itself.

Gather data relative to *changes* in the patient's mental status (i.e., alertness, orientation, confusion), muscle strength, muscle cramps, tremors, nausea, and general appearance.

Always check the electrolyte reports for early indications of electrolyte imbalance.

Keep accurate records of intake and output, daily weights, and vital signs.

Hives, Pruritus, Rash

Report symptoms for further evalaution by the physician.

Pruritus may be relieved by adding baking soda in the bath water.

Dosage and Administration

PO

Do not administer after midafternoon so the diuresis will not keep the patient awake at night.

Administer with food or milk to reduce gastric irritation.

Drug Interactions

Alcohol, Barbiturates, Narcotics

Orthostatic hypotension associated with bumetanide therapy may be aggravated by these agents.

Digitalis Glycosides

This diuretic may excrete excess potassium, leading to hypokalemia. If your patient is also receiving a digitalis glycoside, monitor closely for digitalis toxicity (anorexia, nausea, fatigue, blurred or colored vision, bradycardia, arrhythmias).

Aminoglycosides (Gentamicin, Amikacin, Netilmicin, Others)

The potential for ototoxicity from the aminoglycosides is increased. Assess the patient for gradual, often subtle changes in hearing. Note if the patient seems to speak more loudly, asks for statements to be repeated, and turns the TV or radio progressively louder.

Indomethacin

Indomethacin inhibits the diuretic activity of this agent. The dose of bumetanide may need to be increased, or indomethacin discontinued. Maintain accurate I/O records and monitor for a decrease in diuretic activity.

Corticosteroids (Prednisone, Others)

Corticosteroids may enhance the loss of potassium. Check potassium levels and monitor more closely for hypokalemia when these two agents are used concurrently.

Probenecid

Probenecid inhibits the diuretic activity of bumetanide. In general, do not use concurrently.

Ethacrynic acid (eth-ah-krin'ik) (Edecrin) (e'deh-krin)

Ethacrynic acid is another diuretic more potent than the thiazides. Its diuretic activity begins in about 30 minutes, and lasts 6 to 8 hours. Ethacrynic acid is used to treat edema due to congestive heart failure, cirrhosis of the liver, renal disease, malignancy, and for hospitalized pediatric patients with congenital heart disease.

Side Effects

If given in excessive dosages or to patients with massive fluid accumulation, treatment with ethacrynic acid may lead to excessive diuresis, and thus water dehydration and electrolyte imbalance.

Dizziness, deafness, ringing, and a sense of fullness in the ears may occur in patients with severe impairment of renal function.

Gastrointestinal bleeding has been reported, particularly in patients receiving intravenous dose.

Sudden profuse watery diarrhea has been reported. Discontinue therapy if the diarrhea becomes severe and monitor the patient's electrolytes and state of hydration.

Ethacrynic acid may induce hyperglycemia and aggravate preexisting diabetes mellitus. Dosages of oral hypoglycemic agents and insulin may need adjustment in patients with diabetes mellitus who also require diuretic therapy.

Availability

PO—25 and 50 mg tablets.
IV—50 mg per vial.

Dosage and Administration

Adult

PO—50 to 100 mg initially followed by 50 to 200 mg daily.

IV—50 mg or 0.5 to 1 mg/kg. Add 50 ml of dextrose 5% or saline solution to 50 mg of ethacrynic acid. This solution is stable for 24 hours.

- Administer over several minutes through the tubing of a running infusion, or by direct IV.
- Occasionally the addition of a diluent may result in an opalescent solution. These solutions should not be used. Do not mix with blood derivatives.

Pediatric

PO—Initially 25 mg daily. Increase the dosage in increments of 25 mg to the desired effects.

IV—1 mg/kg. Dilute with dextrose 5% and administer over 5 minutes through a running infusion.

Nursing Interventions

See also General Nursing Considerations for Patients Receiving Diuretic Therapy.

PATIENT CONCERNS: NURSING INTERVENTION/RATIONALE

Side Effects to Expect

Orthostatic Hypotension (Dizziness, Weakness, Faintness)

Although infrequent and generally mild, all diuretics may cause some degree of orthostatic hypotension manifested by dizziness and weakness, particularly when therapy is being initiated.

Monitor the blood pressure daily in both the supine and erect positions.

Anticipate the development of postural hypotension and take measures to prevent its occurrence. Teach the patient to rise slowly from a supine or sitting position, and encourage him or her to sit or lie down if feeling "faint."

Side Effects to Report

Electrolyte Imbalance, Dehydration

The electrolytes most commonly altered are potassium (K^+), sodium (Na^+), and chloride (Cl^-). *Hypokalemia* is most likely to occur.

Many symptoms associated with electrolyte imbalance are subtle and interspersed with general symptoms of drug toxicity or the disease process itself.

Gather data relative to *changes* in the patient's mental status (i.e., alertness, orientation, confusion), muscle strength, muscle cramps, tremors, nausea, and general appearance.

Always check the electrolyte reports for early indications of electrolyte imbalance.

Keep accurate records of intake and output, daily weights, and vital signs.

Gastrointestinal Bleeding

Observe for "coffee-ground" vomitus or dark tarry stools, particularly in patients receiving intravenous therapy.

Dizziness, Deafness, Tinnitus

Persons with impaired renal function may experience these symptoms. Assess the patient for gradual, often subtle changes in balance and hearing. Note if the patient seems more unsteady when standing, or speaks loudly, asks for statements to be repeated, and turns the TV or radio progressively louder.

Diarrhea

Diarrhea may become severe; report to the physician and monitor the patient for dehydration and fluid and electrolyte imbalance.

Hyperglycemia

Diabetic or prediabetic patients need to be monitored for the development of hyperglycemia, particularly during the early weeks of therapy.

Assess regularly for glycosuria and report if it occurs with any frequency.

Patients receiving oral hypoglycemia agents or insulin may require an adjustment in dosage.

Dosage and Administration

PO

Do not administer after midafternoon so the diuresis will not keep the patient awake at night.

Administer with food or milk to reduce gastric irritation.

IV

Always monitor vital signs and I/O at regular intervals when administering this agent intravenously. Report blood pressure that decreases steadily or a narrowing pulse pressure, which may indicate hypovolemia.

Do not use IV solution if it turns opalescent when the diluent is added.

Follow the manufacturer's recommended procedure for mixing the solution. It is stable for 24 hours.

Drug Interactions

Aminoglycosides (Gentamicin, Amikacin, Netilmicin, Tobramycin, Others)

The potential for ototoxicity from the aminoglycosides is increased. Assess the patient for gradual, often subtle changes in hearing.

Note if the patient seems to speak loudly, asks for statements to be repeated, or turns the TV or radio progressively louder.

Digitalis Glycosides

This diuretic may cause excess potassium excretion, leading to hypokalemia. If your patient is also receiving a digitalis glycoside, monitor closely for digitalis toxicity (anorexia, nausea, fatigue, blurred or colored vision, bradycardia, arrhythmias).

Warfarin

Ethacrynic acid may enhance the anticoagulant effects of warfarin. Monitor for the development of petechiae, ecchymosis, bleeding gums, nosebleeds, dark tarry stools.

Corticosteroids (Prednisone, Others)

Corticosteroids may enhance the loss of potassium. Check potassium levels and monitor more closely for hypokalemia when these two agents are used concurrently.

Furosemide (fu-ro'se-myd) (Lasix) (lay'siks)

Furosemide is one of the most potent and effective diuretics currently available. Maximum effect occurs within 1 hour after oral administration and lasts up to 4 hours. In addition to treating edema caused by congestive heart failure, renal disease, and cirrhosis of the liver, it may also be used for the treatment of hypertension, alone or in combination with other antihypertensive therapy.

Side Effects

The most common side effects are oral and gastric irritation, and constipation. Flushing, pruritus, postural hypotension, weakness, dizziness, blurred vision, and dermatitis may also occur.

If given in excessive dosages or to patients with massive fluid accumulation, treatment with furosemide may lead to excessive diuresis with water dehydration and electrolyte imbalance.

Patients who are allergic to sulfonamides may also be allergic to furosemide.

With long-term use, furosemide may inhibit the urinary secretion of uric acid, resulting in hyperuricemia. This may exacerbate an attack of gouty arthritis.

Furosemide may induce hyperglycemia and aggravate cases of preexisting diabetes mellitus. Dosages of oral hypoglycemia agents and insulin may need adjustment in patients with diabetes mellitus who also require diuretic therapy.

Availability

PO—20, 40, and 80 mg tablets; 10 mg/ml oral solution. IV—10 mg/ml in 2, 4, and 10 ml ampules, vials, and prefilled syringes.

Dosage and Administration

Adult
PO—20 to 80 mg as a single dose given preferably in the morning. If a second dose is necessary, administered 6 to 8 hours later.
IV—20 to 40 mg given over 1 to 2 minutes. Much larger doses are frequently administered IV. The rate of administration should not exceed 4 mg per minute.
Pediatric
PO—Initially 2 mg/kg. If the response is not satisfactory, increase by 1 to 2 mg/kg every 6 hours.
IV—Initially 1 mg/kg. If diuresis is not satisfactory, increase by 1 mg/kg every 2 hours to a maximum of 6 mg/kg.

Nursing Interventions

See also General Nursing Considerations for Patients Receiving Diuretic Therapy.

**PATIENT CONCERNS:
NURSING INTERVENTION/RATIONALE**

Side Effects to Expect

Oral Irritation, Dry Mouth

Start regular oral hygiene measures when therapy is initiated. Suggest the use of 1 tsp of hydrogen peroxide in 6 to 8 ounces of water as a mouthwash. Commercial mouthwashes contain alcohol and may cause further drying and oral irritation.

Other measures to alleviate dryness include sucking on ice chips or hard candy.

Orthostatic Hypotension (Dizziness, Weakness, Faintness)

Although infrequent and generally mild, all diuretics may cause some degree of orthostatic hypotension manifested by dizziness and weakness, particularly when therapy is being initiated.

Monitor the blood pressure daily in both the supine and erect positions.

Anticipate the development of postural hypotension and take measures to prevent an occurrence. Teach the patient to rise slowly from a supine or sitting position, and encourage the patient to sit or lie down if feeling "faint."

Side Effects to Report

Electrolyte Imbalance, Dehydration

The electrolytes most commonly altered are potassium (K^+), sodium (Na^+), and chloride (Cl^-). *Hypokalemia* is most likely to occur.

Many symptoms associated with altered fluid and electrolyte balance are subtle and interspersed with general symptoms of drug toxicity or the disease process itself.

Gather data relative to *changes* in the patient's mental status (i.e., alertness, orientation, confusion), muscle strength, muscle cramps, tremors, nausea, and general appearance.

Always check the electrolyte reports for early indications of electrolyte imbalance.

Keep accurate records of I/O, daily weights, and vital signs.

Hives, Pruritus, Rash

Report symptoms for further evaluation by the physician.

Pruritus may be relieved by adding baking soda to the bath water.

Hyperuricemia

This diuretic may inhibit the excretion of uric acid, resulting in hyperuricemia. Patients who have had previous attacks of gouty arthritis are particularly susceptible to additional attacks due to hyperuricemia.

Monitor the laboratory reports for early indications of hyperuricemia. Report to the physician, who may then add a uricosuric agent or allopurinol to the patient's medication regimen.

Hyperglycemia

Diabetic or prediabetic patients need to be monitored for the development of hyperglycemia, particularly during the early weeks of therapy.

Assess regularly for glycosuria and report if it occurs with any frequency.

Patients receiving oral hypoglycemic agents or insulin may require an adjustment in dosage.

Dosage and Administration

PO

Do not administer after midafternoon so that diuresis will not keep the patient awake at night.

Administer with food or milk to reduce gastric irritation.

IV

Always monitor vital signs and I/O at regular intervals with the IV administration of this agent. Report blood pressure that decreases steadily or a narrowing pulse pressure, which may indicate hypovolemia.

Administer at a rate no greater than 4 mg per minute.

Drug Interactions

Digitalis Glycosides

This diuretic may excrete excess potassium, leading to hypokalemia. If your patient is also receiving a digitalis glycoside, monitor closely for digitalis toxicity (anorexia, nausea, fatigue, blurred or colored vision, bradycardia, arrhythmias).

Propranolol

The action of propranolol may be increased. Monitor for hypotension and bradycardia. Dosage adjustment may be necessary.

Theophylline Derivatives

The action of theophylline derivatives may be increased. Assess patients for signs of theophylline toxicity (restlessness, irritability, insomnia, nausea, vomiting, tachycardia, arrhythmias). Serum levels of theophylline may be beneficial in dosage adjustment.

Aminoglycosides (Gentamicin, Amikacin, Netilmicin, Tobramycin, Others)

The potential for ototoxicity from the aminoglycosides is increased. Assess the patient for gradual, often subtle, changes in balance and hearing. Note if patient seems more unsteady when standing, or speaks loudly, asks for statements to be repeated, or turns the TV or radio progressively louder.

Salicylates

The potential for salicylate toxicity may be increased if taken concurrently for several days. Monitor patients for nausea, tinnitus, fever, sweating, dizziness, mental confusion, lethargy, and impaired hearing. Serum levels of salicylates may be beneficial in determining the amounts of salicylate dosage reduction.

Indomethacin

Indomethacin inhibits the diuretic activity of this agent. The dose of furosemide may need to be increased, or indomethacin discontinued. Maintain accurate I/O records and monitor for a decrease in diuretic activity.

Metolazone

When used concurrently, there is a considerably greater diuresis than when either agent is used alone. Monitor closely for dehydration and electrolyte imbalance.

Phenytoin

Phenytoin may inhibit the absorption of orally administered furosemide. The dosage of furosemide may need to be increased based upon the clinical response of the patient to normal doses.

Thiazides

The benzothiadiazides, better known as the thiazides, have been an important and useful class of diuretic and antihypertensive agents for the past two decades. As diuretics, thiazides act primarily on the distal tubules of the kidney to block the reabsorption of sodium and chloride ions from the tubule. The unreabsorbed sodium and chloride ions are passed into the collecting ducts, taking molecules of water with them, thus resulting in a diuresis. The thiazides are used as diuretics in the treatment of edema associated with congestive heart failure, renal disease, hepatic disease, pregnancy, obesity, premenstrual syndrome, and administration of adrenocortical steroids. The antihypertensive properties of the thiazides result from a direct vasodilatory action on the peripheral arterioles. (See Index for antihypertensive therapy.)

Side Effects

Mild side effects, such as gastrointestinal disorders, dizziness, weakness, fatigue, and rash may occur.

Use of thiazides may cause or aggravate electrolyte imbalance, so patients should be observed regularly for signs such as dry mouth, drowsiness, confusion, muscular weakness, and nausea. Hypokalemia is the most likely of the electrolyte imbalances to occur, and supplementary potassium is often prescribed to prevent or treat hypokalemia.

The thiazides may induce hyperglycemia and aggravate cases of preexisting diabetes mellitus. Dosages of oral hypoglycemic agents and insulin may need adjustment in patients with diabetes mellitus who also require diuretic therapy.

The plasma uric acid is frequently elevated by the thiazides. Patients prone to hyperuricemia and acute attacks of gouty arthritis should also be placed on thiazide therapy with caution.

Patients should be observed for rare occurrences of leukopenia, thrombocytopenia, agranulocytosis, and aplastic anemia.

The thiazide diuretics should be used with caution in pregnant patients, because depression of bone marrow and thrombocytopenia are possible effects on the newborn.

Availability

Tables 14.3 and 14.4 provide a list of thiazide diuretics and those diuretics chemically related to the thiazides. Most of the diuretics listed are administered in divided daily doses for the treatment of hypertension. However, single daily dosages may be most effective for mobilization of edema fluid.

Nursing Interventions

See also General Nursing Considerations for Patients Receiving Diuretic Therapy.

PATIENT CONCERNS: NURSING INTERVENTION/RATIONALE

Side Effects to Expect

Orthostatic Hypotension (Dizziness, Weakness, Faintness)

Although infrequent and generally mild, all diuretics may cause some degree of orthostatic hypotension

Table 14.3
Thiazide Diuretic Products

THIAZIDE	BRAND NAME	DOSAGE RANGE (mg)	DOSAGE FORMS AVAILABLE
Bendroflumethiazide	Naturetin	2.5–15	Tablets: 2.5, 5, and 10 mg
Benzthiazide	Exna, Hydrex, Proaqua	50–150	Tablets: 25 and 50 mg
Chlorothiazide	Diuril, Diachlor	1,000–2,000	Tablets: 250 and 500 mg Oral suspension: 250 mg/5 ml Injection: 500 mg/20 ml
Cyclothiazide	Anhydron	1–2	Tablets: 2 mg
Hydrochlorothiazide	Esidrix, HydroDiuril, Oretic, Hydromal	25–100	Tablets: 25, 50, and 100 mg
Hydroflumethiazide	Saluron, Diucardin	25–100	Tablets: 50 mg
Methyclothiazide	Enduron, Aquetensen	2.5–5	Tablets: 2.5 and 5 mg
Polythiazide	Renese	1–4	Tablets: 1, 2, and 4 mg
Trichlormethiazide	Naqua, Metahydrin, Aquazide, Diurese	1–4	Tablets: 2 and 4 mg

manifested by dizziness and weakness, particularly when therapy is being initiated.

Monitor the blood pressure daily in both the supine and erect positions.

Anticipate the development of postural hypotension and take measures to prevent an occurrence. Teach the patient to rise slowly from a supine or sitting position, and encourage him or her to sit or lie down if feeling "faint."

Side Effects to Report

Gastric Irritation, Nausea, Vomiting, Constipation

If gastric irritation occurs, administer with food or milk. If symptoms persist or increase in severity, report to the physician for evaluation.

Electrolyte Imbalance, Dehydration

The electrolytes most commonly altered are potassium (K^+), sodium (Na^+), and chloride (Cl^-). *Hypokalemia* is most likely to occur.

Many symptoms associated with altered fluid and electrolyte balance are subtle and interspersed with general symptoms of drug toxicity or the disease process itself.

Gather data relative to *changes* in the patient's mental status (i.e., alertness, orientation, confusion), muscle strength, muscle cramps, tremors, nausea, and general appearance.

Always check the electrolyte reports for early indications of electrolyte imbalance.

Keep accurate records of I/O, daily weights, and vital signs.

Hives, Pruritus, Rash

Report symptoms for further evaluation by the physician.

Pruritus may be relieved by adding baking soda to the bath water.

Hyperuricemia

This diuretic may inhibit the excretion of uric acid, resulting in hyperuricemia. Patients who have had previous attacks of gouty arthritis are particularly susceptible to additional attacks due to hyperuricemia.

Monitor the laboratory reports for early indications of hyperuricemia. Report to the physician, who then may add a uricosuric agent or allopurinol to the patient's medication regimen.

Hyperglycemia

Diabetic or prediabetic patients need to be monitored for the development of hyperglycemia, particularly during the early weeks of therapy.

Table 14.4
Thiazide-related Products

DIURETIC	BRAND NAME	DOSAGE RANGE (mg)	DOSAGE FORMS AVAILABLE
Chlorthalidone	Hygroton	50–200	Tablets: 25, 50, and 100 mg
Indapamide	Lozol	2.5–5	Tablets: 2.5 mg
Metolazone	Zaroxolyn, Diulo	2.5–10	Tablets: 2.5, 5, and 10 mg
Quinethazone	Hydromox	50–100	Tablets: 50 mg

Assess regularly for glycosuria and report if it occurs with any frequency.

Patients receiving oral hypoglycemia agents or insulin may require an adjustment in dosage.

Dosage and Administration

PO

Do not administer after midafternoon so that diuresis will not keep the patient awake at night.

Administer with food or milk to reduce gastric irritation.

Drug Interactions

Digitalis Glycosides

This diuretic may excrete excess potassium, leading to hypokalemia. If your patient is also receiving a digitalis glycoside, monitor closely for digitalis toxicity (anorexia, nausea, fatigue, blurred or colored vision, bradycardia, arrhythmias).

Corticosteroids (Prednisone, Others)

Corticosteroids may enhance the loss of potassium. Check potassium levels and monitor more closely for hypokalemia when these two agents are used concurrently.

Lithium

Thiazide diuretics may induce lithium toxicity. Monitor your patients for lithium toxicity manifested by nausea, anorexia, fine tremors, persistent vomiting, profuse diarrhea, hyperreflexia, lethargy, and weakness.

Indomethacin

Indomethacin inhibits the diuretic activity of this agent. The dose of thiazide may need to be increased, or indomethacin discontinued.

Maintain accurate I/O records and monitor for a decrease in diuretic activity.

Oral Hypoglycemic Agents, Insulin

Due to the hyperglycemic effects of the thiazide diuretics, dosages of insulin and oral hypoglycemic agents are frequently required.

Warfarin

Thiazide diuretics may antagonize the anticoagulant activity of warfarin. Monitor the prothrombin activity at regular intervals.

Potassium-Sparing Diuretics

Amiloride (am-il-or′eyd) *(Midamor)* (my-da′mor)

Amiloride is a relatively new potassium-sparing diuretic that also has weak antihypertensive activity. Its mechanism of action is unknown, but it acts at the distal renal tubule to retain potassium and excrete sodium, resulting in a mild diuresis. Amiloride is usually used in combination with other diuretics in patients with hypertension or congestive heart failure to help prevent hypokalemia that may result from other diuretics.

Side Effects

Side effects are usually quite mild and include anorexia, nausea, abdominal pain, flatulence, headache, and skin rash. Other side effects infrequently reported include muscle cramps, dizziness, constipation, fatiguability, and impotence.

Availability

PO—5 mg.

Dosage and Administration

Adult

PO—Initially 5 mg daily. Dosages may be increased in 5 mg increments up to 20 mg daily with close monitoring of electrolytes.

Administer with food.

Nursing Interventions

See also General Nursing Considerations for Patients Receiving Diuretic Therapy.

PATIENT CONCERNS: NURSING INTERVENTION/RATIONALE

Side Effects to Expect

Anorexia, Nausea, Vomiting, Flatulence

These side effects should be mild, particularly if the dose is administered with food. Persistent nausea and vomiting need to be evaluated for other causes, as well as for the development of electrolyte imbalance.

Headache

Monitor the blood pressure at regularly scheduled intervals since this agent is used for hypertension. Additional readings should be taken during headaches to determine if headaches are caused by the agents or by the hypertension.

Report persistence of headaches.

Side Effects to Report

Electrolyte Imbalance, Dehydration

The electrolytes most commonly altered are potassium (K^+), sodium (Na^+), and chloride (Cl^-). *Hyperkalemia* is most likely to occur. Report potassium levels above 5 mEq/liter.

Many symptoms associated with altered fluid and electrolyte balance are subtle and interspersed with general symptoms of drug toxicity or the disease process itself.

Gather data relative to *changes* in the patient's mental status (i.e., alertness, orientation, confusion), muscle strength, muscle cramps, tremors, nausea, and general appearance.

Always check the electrolyte reports for early indications of electrolyte imbalance.

Keep accurate records of I/O, daily weights, and vital signs.

Dosage and Administration

PO

Do not administer after midafternoon so that diuresis will not keep the patient awake at night.

Administer with food or milk to reduce gastric irritation.

Drug Interactions

Lithium

Amiloride may induce lithium toxicity. Monitor your patients for lithium toxicity manifested by nausea, anorexia, fine tremors, persistent vomiting, profuse diarrhea, hyperreflexia, lethargy, and weakness.

Potassium Supplements, Salt Substitutes

Amiloride inhibits potassium excretion. Do *not* administer with potassium supplements or use salt substitutes high in potassium because of the potentially dangerous effects of hyperkalemia.

Spironolactone (spy-ro-no-lak′tone)
(Aldactone) (al-dak′tone)

Spironolactone is a diuretic that is particularly useful in relieving edema and ascites that do not respond to the usual diuretics. It blocks the sodium-retaining and potassium-excreting properties of aldosterone, resulting in a loss of water with the increased sodium excretion. This drug may be given with thiazide diuretics to increase the effect of spironolactone and reduce the hypokalemia often induced by the thiazides.

Side Effects

Side effects are usually quite mild with spironolactone therapy but include drowsiness, lethargy, headache, cramping and diarrhea, and mental confusion.

Since the chemical structure of spironolactone is similar to that of certain hormones, an occasional male patient will report gynecomastia, reduced libido, and diminished erection, and females may complain of breast soreness and menstrual irregularities. These effects are quite reversible upon discontinuation of therapy.

Availability

PO—25 and 100 mg tablets.

Dosage and Administration

Adult

PO—Initially 50 to 100 mg daily. Maintenance dosage is usually 100 to 200 mg daily, but doses up to 400 mg may be prescribed.

Pediatric
PO—3.3 mg/kg/day. Readjust the dosage every 3 to 5 days.

Nursing Interventions

See also General Nursing Considerations for Patients Receiving Diuretic Therapy.

PATIENT CONCERNS: NURSING INTERVENTION/RATIONALE

Side Effects to Expect and Report
Mental Confusion

Perform a baseline assessment of the patient's alertness, drowsiness, lethargy, and orientation to time, date, and place before initiating drug therapy. Compare subsequent mental status and analyze on a regular basis.

Headache

Monitor the blood pressure at regularly scheduled intervals since this agent is used for hypertension. Additional readings should be taken during headaches to determine if headaches are caused by the agent or the hypertension. Report persistence of headaches.

Diarrhea

The onset of new symptoms since initiation of the drug therapy requires evaluation if persistent.

Electrolyte Imbalance, Dehydration

The electrolytes most commonly altered are potassium (K^+), sodium (Na^+), and chloride (Cl^-). *Hyperkalemia* is most likely to occur. Report potassium levels above 5 mEq/liter.
Many symptoms associated with altered fluid and electrolyte balance are subtle and interspersed with general symptoms of drug toxicity or the disease process itself.
Gather data relative to *changes* in the patient's mental status (i.e., alertness, orientation, confusion), muscle strength, muscle cramps, tremors, nausea, and general appearance.
Always check the electrolyte reports for early indications of electrolyte imbalance.

Keep accurate records of intake and output, daily weights and vital signs.

Dosage and Administration
PO

Do not administer after midafternoon so that diuresis will not keep the patient awake at night.
Administr with food or milk to reduce gastric irritation.

Drug Interactions

Potassium Supplements, Salt Substitutes

Spironolactone inhibits potassium excretion. Do *not* administer with potassium supplements or use salt substitutes high in potassium because of potentially dangerous effects from hyperkalemia.

Triamterene (try-am'ter-een)
(Dyrenium) (dy-reen'ee-um)

Triamterene is a very mild diuretic that acts by blocking the exchange of potassium for sodium in the distal tubule of the kidney. Potassium is retained, making it an effective agent to use in conjunction with the potassium-excreting diuretics such as the thiazides and furosemide.

Side Effects

Side effects of triamterene are generally quite mild. Those reported include dry mouth, leg cramps, photosensitivity, rash, nausea, vomiting, diarrhea, and weakness.

Availability

PO—50 to 100 mg capsules.

Dosage and Administration

Adult
PO—50 to 150 mg 2 times daily.

Nursing Interventions

See also General Nursing Considerations for Patients Receiving Diuretic Therapy.

PATIENT CONCERNS: NURSING INTERVENTION/RATIONALE

Side Effects to Expect and Report

Electrolyte Imbalance, Dehydration, Leg Cramps, Nausea, Vomiting, Weakness

The electrolytes most commonly altered are potassium (K^+), sodium (Na^+), and chloride (Cl^-). *Hyperkalemia* is most likely to occur. Report potassium levels above 5 mEq/liter.

Many symptoms associated with altered fluid and electrolyte balance are subtle and interspersed with general symptoms of drug toxicity or the disease process itself.

Gather data relative to *changes* in the patient's mental status (i.e., alertness, orientation, confusion), muscle strength, muscle cramps, tremors, nausea, and general appearance (drowsy, anxious, lethargic).

Always check the electrolyte reports for early indications of electrolyte imbalance.

Keep accurate records of I/O, daily weights, and vital signs.

Hives, Pruritus, Rash

Report symptoms for further evaluation by the physician.

Pruritus may be relieved by adding baking soda to the bath water.

Drug Interactions

Triamterene inhibits potassium excretion. Do *not* administer with potassium supplements or use salt substitutes high in potassium because of the potentially dangerous effects from hyperkalemia.

A Urinary Analgesic

Phenazopyridine hydrochloride (fen-ay-zo-peer'i-deen) *(Pyridium)* (py-rid'ee-um)

Phenazopyridine is an agent that, as it is excreted through the urinary tract, produces a local anesthetic effect on the mucosa of the ureters and bladder. It acts within about 30 minutes after oral administration and relieves burning, pain, urgency, and frequency associated with urinary tract infections. It also lessens bladder spasm, thus relieving the resulting urinary retention.

Phenazopyridine is also used for preoperative and postoperative surface analgesia in urologic surgical procedures and after diagnostic tests in which instrumentation was necessary. It is occasionally used to relieve the discomfort caused by the presence of an indwelling catheter.

Side Effects

Phenazopyridine produces a reddish-orange discoloration of the urine.

A yellowish tinge to the sclera or the skin may indicate accumulation caused by reduced renal function. The drug should be discontinued if this manifestation results.

Phenazopyridine is frequently used in combination with sulfonamides (Azo-Gantanol and Azo-Gantrisin). The same side effects apply, as well as those of the sulfonamides (see Index).

Availability

PO—100 and 200 mg tablets.

Dosage and Administration

Adult
PO—200 mg 3 times daily.
Pediatric (6 to 12 years of age)
PO—100 mg 3 times daily.

PATIENT CONCERNS: NURSING INTERVENTION/RATIONALE

Side Effects to Expect

Reddish-Orange Urine Discoloration

Be certain the patient understands that the color of the urine will become reddish-orange when this drug is used. There is no need for alarm.

Side Effects to Report

Yellow Sclera or Skin

The patient should report any yellowish tinge developing in the sclera (white portion) of the eye.

Drug Interactions

Urine Colorimetric Procedures

This medication will interfere with colorimetric diagnostic tests performed on urine. Consult your hospital laboratory for alternative measures.

Urinary Antimicrobial Agents

Urinary antimicrobial agents are substances that are excreted and concentrated in the urine in sufficient amounts to have an antiseptic effect on the urine and the urinary tract. Selection of the product to be used is based upon identification of the pathogens by the Gram stain or by urine culture in severe, recurrent, or chronic infections. Fluid intake should be encouraged so that there will be at least 2000 ml of urinary output daily. Treatment should be continued for at least a week after symptoms have subsided or the results of cultures have been negative.

The most common organisms found to infect the urinary tract are gram-negative bacilli. Of this group, *Escherichia coli* is responsible for the greatest number of infections. Four other groups of pathogens also found frequently in the urinary tract are *Aerobacter aerogenes*, *Klebsiella pneumoniae*, and organisms of the genera *Proteus* and *Pseudomonas*.

Cinoxacin, methenamine mandelate, nitrofurantoin, and nalidixic acid are used only for urinary tract infections. Other antibiotics that are also used to treat urinary infections are ampicillin, sulfisoxazole, co-trimoxazole, sulfamethazole, gentamicin, and carbenicillin. These agents are effective in a variety of tissue infections against many different microorganisms. Because of their use in multiple organ systems, they are discussed in detail (with nursing interventions) in Chapter 18, Antimicrobial Agents.

General Nursing Considerations for Patients Receiving Urinary Antimicrobial Therapy

See also General Nursing Considerations for Patients with Infectious Disease.

Patient Teaching Associated with Urinary Antimicrobial Therapy

POTENTIAL PATIENT NEEDS/PROBLEMS: NURSING INTERVENTION/RATIONALE

Communication and Responsibility

Encourage open communication concerning frustrations and anger as the patient attempts to adjust to the diagnosis and need for treatment.

The patient must be guided to gain insight into the condition in order to assume responsibility for the continuation of treatment. Keep reemphasizing those factors the patient can control to alter the progression of the disease, including maintenance of general health, nutritional needs, adequate rest and appropriate exercise, and continuation of prescribed medication therapy.

Prevention

Emphasize that permanent kidney damage and renal failure is a consequence of repeated urinary tract infections. *Prevention* is the key to avoiding this complication.

Adequate I/O, personal hygiene, completing all medications, and negative follow-up cultures are equally important.

Teach the female patient factors that may aid in preventing reinfection:

- Avoid nylon underwear (use cotton) and very tight, constricting clothing in the perineal area.
- Avoid frequent use of bubble bath.
- Avoid colored toilet paper, because the dye may cause irritations.
- Wash the perineal area immediately before and after sexual intercourse.
- Urinate immediately after intercourse.

Fluid Intake

All patients with urinary tract infections or calculi, or those patients undergoing urologic procedures need increased intake of fluids, especially water. Unless coexisting medical problems prohibit, have patients drink a minimum of eight 8-ounce glasses daily.

Perineal Irritation

If the patient complains of irritation or itching of the perineal area, request an order for protective or anesthetic ointments. Also consider the possibility of a secondary yeast infection, especially if the patient is taking antibiotics.

Expectations of Therapy

Discuss expectations of therapy with the patient: Pain and discomfort are usually relieved within 30 minutes after the administration of a urinary analgesic.

The symptoms of burning, frequency, urgency, and even incontinence improve steadily after antimicrobial therapy is initiated. Stress previously cited hygiene measures to prevent recurrence.

Changes in Expectations

Assess changes in expectations as therapy progresses and the patient gains understanding and skill in the management of the diagnosis. Recurrence of symptoms should be reported immediately.

Changes in Therapy through Cooperative Goal-Setting

Work mutually with the patient to encourage adherence to the prescribed treatment. When the patient feels that a change should be made in a treatment plan, encourage a discussion first with the physician.

Written Record

Enlist the patient's aid in developing and maintaining a written record (Table 14.2) of the monitoring parameters (i.e., burning, frequency or urgency of voiding, daily fluid intake, and temperature, if present) and response to prescribed therapies for discussion with the physician. Patients should be encouraged to take this record with them on follow-up visits.

Fostering Compliance

Discuss medication information and how it will benefit the patient's course of treatment. Seek cooperation and understanding of the following points, so that medication compliance may be enhanced:

1. Name
2. Dosage

3. Route and administration times
4. Anticipated therapeutic response
5. Side effects to expect
6. Side effects to report
7. What to do if a dosage is missed
8. When, how, or if to refill the medication prescription.

Difficulty in Comprehension

If it is evident that the patient and/or family does not understand all aspects of continuing therapy being prescribed (i.e., administration and monitoring of medications, need for increased fluid intake, follow-up appointments), consider the use of social service or visiting nurse agencies.

Associated Teaching

Give patients the following instructions:

Always inform the physician or dentist of any prescription or over-the-counter medication being taken. Over-the-counter medications should not be taken without first discussing them with your physician or pharmacist.

Always report side effects of rash, itching, or hives immediately. Nausea, vomiting, or diarrhea should also be reported for the physician's evaluation if it is a new symptom.

Take all of the medication as prescribed for the full course of treatment. Do not discontinue use when feeling improved; do not save for future use; do not give your medicine to another individual. Sudden discontinuation of certain medications may produce harmful effects.

Emphasize the importance of antibiotic therapy being continued until urine samples at follow-up visits have been negative for organisms.

Keep all medications out of the reach of children.

If pregnancy is suspected, consult an obstetrician as soon as possible about continuation of medication therapy.

At Discharge

Items to be sent home with the patient should:

1. Have written instructions for use.
2. Be labeled in a level of language and size of print appropriate for the patient.

3. If needed, include identification cards or bracelets.
4. Include list of additional supplies to be purchased after discharge.
5. Include a schedule of follow-up appointments.

Cinoxacin (sin-ox′ah-sin) (Cinobac) (sin-oh′bak)

Cinoxacin is an organic acid that is chemically related to nalidixic acid. Cinoxacin is effective in treating initial and recurrent urinary tract infections caused by *E. coli*, *Proteus mirabilis*, and other gram-negative microorganisms. It is not effective against *Pseudomonas* species, common pathogens in chronic urinary tract infections. Clinical studies indicate that cinoxacin may have milder side effects than nalidixic acid.

Side Effects

About 10% of patients will suffer reversible adverse effects from cinoxacin therapy. Most frequent are nausea (3%), vomiting, anorexia, diarrhea, and abdominal cramps (1%). Up to 3% of patients develop rash, perineal burning, urticaria, pruritus, or hives. Less than 2% of patients report headache and dizziness, and less than 1% report insomnia, photophobia, tingling sensations, and tinnitus.

Although it has not been reported, structural similarities with nalidixic acid indicate that hemolysis may occur in patients with glucose-6-phosphate dehydrogenase deficiency. Cinoxacin should be used with caution in these patients.

Although it has not been reported, structural similarities with nalidixic acid indicate that cinoxacin may produce false positive results with Clinitest. Clinistix or Tes-Tape may be used instead.

Availability

PO—250 and 500 mg capsules.

Dosage and Administration

Adult
PO—1 g daily in 2 to 4 divided doses for 7 to 14 days.
Pediatric
Not recommended for children under 12 years of age.

Nursing Interventions

See also General Nursing Considerations for Patients Receiving Urinary Antimicrobial Therapy.

See also General Nursing Considerations for Patients with Infectious Disease.

PATIENT CONCERNS: NURSING INTERVENTION/RATIONALE

Side Effects to Expect

Nausea, Vomiting, Anorexia, Abdominal Cramps

These side effects are usually mild and tend to resolve with continued therapy. Encourage the patient not to discontinue therapy without consulting his or her physician first.

Side Effects to Report

Perineal Burning, Urticaria, Pruritus, Hives

Burning with urination may be produced by the infection itself.

Notify the physician if any of these symptoms develop. Symptomatic relief may be obtained by the use of cornstarch or bicarbonate of soda to the bath water. The use of antihistamines or topical steroids is rarely required.

Headache, Tinnitus, Dizziness, Tingling Sensations, Photophobia

Report these symptoms for further evaluation.

Dosage and Administration

PO

Schedule medication administration to coincide with mealtime if gastrointestinal symptoms develop.

Drug Interactions

Probenecid

Probenecid may reduce urinary excretion of cinoxacin, thereby producing inadequate antimicrobial therapy and the possibility of developing resistant strains of microorganisms.

Clinitest

This drug may produce false-positive Clinitest results. Use Clinistix or Tes-Tape to measure urine glucose.

Methenamine mandelate (me-the'na-min man-del'ate)
(Mandelamine) (man-del'-ah-min)

Methenamine mandelate combines the action of methenamine and mandelic acid. Methenamine yields formaldehyde in the presence of an acidic urine. The formaldehyde released helps suppress the growth and multiplication of bacteria that may cause recurrent infection. Mandelic acid is present to help maintain the acidic urine. Ascorbic acid (vitamin C) is also frequently prescribed to help maintain the acidity of the urine.

Methenamine mandelate is used only in patients susceptible to chronic, recurrent urinary tract infections. It is not potent enough to be effective in patients suffering from a pre-existing infection. The infection should be treated with antibiotics until the urine is sterile; then methenamine is started to help prevent recurrence of the infection.

Side Effects

Side effects are rare, but when they do occur, the most common are nausea, vomiting, belching, skin rash, and pruritus.

Availability

PO—0.25, 0.5, and 1 g enteric-coated tablets; 0.25 and 0.5 g/5 ml suspension.

Dosage and Administration

Adult
PO—1 g 4 times daily after meals and at bedtime.

Nursing Interventions

See also General Nursing Considerations for Patients Receiving Urinary Antimicrobial Therapy.
See also General Nursing Considerations for Patients with Infectious Disease.

**PATIENT CONCERNS:
NURSING INTERVENTION/RATIONALE**

Side Effects to Expect

Nausea, Vomiting, Belching

These side effects are usually mild and tend to resolve with continued therapy. Encourage the patient not to

discontinue therapy without consulting his or her physician first.

Side Effects to Report

Hives, Pruritus, Rash

Report symptoms for further evaluation by the physician.
Pruritus may be relieved by adding baking soda to the bath water.

Bladder Irritation, Dysuria, Frequency

Notify the physician of these symptoms since they may indicate the presence of another urinary tract infection.

Dosage and Administration

pH Testing

Perform urine testing for pH at regular intervals. Report values above 5.5.

PO

Gastrointestinal symptoms may be minimized by administering with meals.
Do not crush the tablets! This will allow the formation of formaldehyde in the stomach, resulting in nausea and belching.

Drug Interactions

Acetazolamide, Sodium Bicarbonate

Acetazolamide and sodium bicarbonate produce an alkaline urine, preventing the conversion of methenamine to formaldehyde, thus inactivating the medication.

Sulfamethizole

Sulfamethizole may form an insoluble precipitate in acidic urine. Therefore, concurrent treatment with sulfamethizole and methenamine should be avoided.

Nalidixic acid (nal-ih-diks'ik)
(NegGram) (neg'gram)

Nalidixic acid may produce false-positive results with Clinitest. Clinistix or Tes-Tape may be used instead.

(NegGram), it has antibacterial activity against gram-negative bacteria. It may be used to treat initial and recurrent urinary tract infections caused by *E. coli*, *Proteus mirabilis*, and other gram-negative microorganisms. It is not effective against *Pseudomonas* species, common pathogens in chronic urinary tract infections.

Side Effects

The most common side effects of nalidixic acid include nausea and vomiting, drowsiness, headache, dizziness, and weakness.

Visual disturbances such as overbrightness of lights, changes in color perception, difficulty in focusing, and double vision may occur shortly after administration of each dose during the first few days of therapy.

Patients receiving nalidixic acid therapy should avoid undue exposure to sunlight since photosensitivity may occur.

Nalidixic acid may induce hemolysis in patients with glucose-6-phosphate dehydrogenase deficiency. Nalidixic acid should not be used in these patients.

Nalidixic acid may produce false-positive results with Clinitest. Clinistix or Tes-tape may be used instead.

Availability

PO—250 and 500 mg tablets; 250 mg/5 ml suspension.

Dosage and Administration

Adult
PO—1 g 4 times daily for 1 to 2 weeks. If therapy is to be prolonged for prophylaxis, administer 500 mg 4 times daily.

Pediatric
PO—55 mg/kg/24 hours in 4 divided doses. If therapy is to be prolonged for prophylaxis, administer 33 mg/kg/24 hours in 4 divided doses.

• *Do not* administer to infants under 3 months of age.

Nursing Interventions

See also General Nursing Considerations for Patients Receiving Urinary Antimicrobial Therapy.

See also General Nursing Considerations for Patients with Infectious Disease.

PATIENT CONCERNS: NURSING INTERVENTION/RATIONALE

Side Effects to Report

Nausea, Vomiting

These side effects are usually mild and tend to resolve with continued therapy. Encourage the patient not to discontinue therapy without first consulting the physician.

Visual Disturbances

During the first few days of therapy, difficulty focusing, double vision, and changes in brightness and colors may occur shortly after each dose is given. If these symptoms persist or occur later in therapy, notify the physician for further evaluation.

Photosensitivity

Patients should avoid exposure to direct sunlight and wear sunshades and long-sleeved garments outdoors while taking this medication. A severe burn requires medical attention.

Drowsiness, Headache, Dizziness, Weakness

These side effects are usually mild and tend to resolve with continued therapy. Encourage the patient not to discontinue therapy without consulting the physician first.

Dosage and Administration

PO

Administer with food or milk if gastrointestinal symptoms are evident.

Drug Interactions

Warfarin

This medication may enhance the anticoagulant effects of warfarin. Observe for the development of petechiae, ecchymoses, nosebleeds, bleeding gums, dark tarry stools, and bright red or coffee-ground emesis. Monitor the prothrombin time and reduce the dosage of warfarin if necessary.

Clinitest
This drug may produce false-positive Clinitest results. Use Clinistix or Tes-Tape to measure urine glucose.

Nitrofurantoin (ny-tro-fu-ran'to-in)
(Furadantin) (fur-ah-dan'tin),
(Macrodantin) (mak-ro-dan'tin)

Nitrofurantoin is an antibiotic that acts by interfering with several bacterial enzyme systems. It is active against many gram-positive and gram-negative organisms, such as *Streptococcus faecalis*, *E. coli*, and *Proteus* species. Nitrofurantoin is not active against *Pseudomonas aeruginosa* or *Serratia* species. This antibiotic is not effective against microorganisms in the blood or in tissues outside the urinary tract.

Side Effects

The most frequent side effects of nitrofurantoin are nausea, vomiting, and anorexia. This complication to therapy can be reduced by administration with food or milk.

Nitrofurantoin may tint the urine rust-brown to yellow.

Allergic reactions manifested by dyspnea, chills, fever, erythematous rash, and pruritus have been reported. Acute reactions usually develop within 8 hours in previously sensitized patients and within 7 to 10 days in patients who develop sensitivity during the course of therapy.

Nitrofurantoin may induce hemolysis in patients with glucose-6-phosphate dehydrogenase deficiency. Nitrofurantoin should not be used in these patients.

Nitrofurantoin may cause peripheral neuropathies, particularly in patients with renal impairment, anemia, diabetes, electrolyte imbalance, or vitamin B deficiency. Nitrofurantoin should be discontinued at the first sign of numbness or tingling in the extremities.

Availability

PO—25, 50, and 100 mg tablets and capsules; 25 mg per 5 ml suspension.
IV—180 mg in 20 ml vials.

Dosage and Administration

Note: Nitrofurantoin must be in the bladder in sufficient concentrations to be therapeutically effective. Nitrofurantoin therapy is *not* recommended for use in patients with a creatinine clearance of less than 40 ml/minute.

Adult
PO—50 to 100 mg 4 times daily for 10 to 14 days.
IV—Over 120 pounds: 180 mg every 12 hours, administered at a rate of 2 to 3 ml/minute. Replace intravenous therapy with oral administration as soon as possible.

Pediatric
Note: Do not administer to infants under 1 month of age.
PO—5 to 7 mg/kg/24 hours in four divided doses.
IV—See reconstitution instructions for adults. Under 120 pounds: 3 mg/kg every 12 hours at a rate of 2 to 3 ml per minute. Replace intravenous therapy with oral administration as soon as possible.

Nursing Interventions

See also General Nursing Considerations for Patients Receiving Urinary Antimicrobial Therapy.

See also General Nursing Considerations for Patients with Infectious Disease.

PATIENT CONCERNS: NURSING INTERVENTION/RATIONALE

Side Effects to Expect

Nausea, Vomiting, Anorexia

Administer with food or milk to reduce gastric irritation.

Urine Discoloration

Tell the patient that urine may be tinted rust-brown to yellow. This should be no cause for alarm.

Side Effects to Report

Dyspnea, Chills, Fever, Erythematous Rash, Pruritus

These symptoms are the early indications of an allergic reaction to nitrofurantoin.

Acute reactions usually occur within 8 hours in previously sensitized individuals, and within 7 to 10 days in patients who develop sensitivity during the course of therapy.

Discontinue the drug and notify the physician.

Peripheral Neuropathies

Discontinue the medication at the first sign of numbness or tingling in the extremities.

Second Infection

Report immediately the development of dysuria, pungent-smelling urine, or fever. These symptoms may be the early indication of a second infection due to an organism resistant to nitrofurantoin.

Dosage and Administration

PO

Administer with food or milk to reduce gastrointestinal side effects.

To maintain adequate urine concentrations, space the dosage at even intervals around the clock.

Suspension

Store in a dark amber container away from bright light.

Intravenous

Always read and follow the manufacturer's recommendations:

Reconstitution: Just before use, add 20 ml of dextrose 5% or sterile water to the vial and shake well. Each milliliter of this initial solution should be further diluted with an additional 25 ml of fluid. Therefore, 180 mg in 20 ml must be diluted to at least 500 ml of parenteral fluid for infusion.

- *Do not* dilute with solutions containing methyl- or propylparabens, phenol, or cresol as preservatives. These may cause nitrofurantoin to precipitate out of solution. Do not administer if a precipitate develops.

Drug Interactions

Clinitest

This drug may produce false-positive Clinitest results. Use Clinistix or Tes-Tape to measure urine glucose.

Antacids

Encourage the patient *not* to take products containing magnesium trisilicate (Escot Capsules, Gaviscon, Gelusil) concurrently with nitrofurantoin because the antacid may inhibit absorption of the nitrofurantoin.

Uricosuric Agents

Uricosuric agents act on the tubules of the kidneys to enhance the excretion of uric acid. Uric acid is a normal metabolite of cellular metabolism and is excreted by the kidneys under normal circumstances. For several reasons, however, uric acid can accumulate, resulting in acute attacks of gout, gouty arthritis, and deposits of urate tophi in joints. Hyperuricemia may be treated by inhibiting the production of uric acid with an agent known as allopurinol (see Index) or by enhancing the excretion of uric acid by the kidneys. Two agents effective in enhancing the excretion of uric acid are probenecid and sulfinpyrazone.

General Nursing Considerations for Patients Receiving Uricosuric Therapy

Gout requires prolonged medical management to prevent the long-term progression of debilitating joint disease and renal dysfunction. The nurse needs to carefully assess the individual initially for the presenting symptoms of the attack, and over a longer period for compliance with the therapeutic modalities prescribed. Baseline data need to be obtained so that symptoms, course of recovery, and degree of understanding and compliance with the management prescribed can be assessed in the future.

PATIENT CONCERNS: NURSING INTERVENTION/RATIONALE

Assessment of Current Gout Attack

Obtain data relative to the onset of this attack of gout.

Joint Involvement

Describe the specific location of involvement.

Pain

State the degree, location, intensity, duration, and radiation of joint pain being experienced.

Warmth, Color

Note the color and feel the warmth of affected areas.

Pain Relief

Is the pain relieved by hot or cold compresses? Or, have these proven intolerable?

Swelling

Inspect the affected areas for swelling.

Additional Symptoms

Ask about additional symptoms such as general malaise, headache, fatigue, fever, or anorexia.

Nutritional Compliance

In most cases, certain foods or alcoholic beverages may precipitate an attack. Ask for a food history, noting particularly whether the patient has eaten larger quantities of organ meats (liver, kidney), meat-based dishes (broth), seafood, or dried beans than usual.

Regimen Compliance

If previously treated for gout, obtain details of the prescribed treatment to assess for compliance.

Medication

Medications being taken.

Fluid Intake

The amount of fluid routinely ingested.

Diet

What type of diet had been prescribed? Ask the patient to describe his or her routine diet.

Patient Teaching Associated with Uricosuric Therapy

Communication and Responsibility

Encourage open communication concerning frustrations and anger as the patient attempts to adjust to the diagnosis and need for prolonged treatment. The patient must be guided to gain insight into the condition in order to assume responsibility for the continuation of treatment. Keep emphasizing those factors the patient can control to alter the disease process, including maintenance of general health, nutritional needs, adequate rest and appropriate exercise, and continuation of prescribed medication therapy.

NUTRITION

It is suggested, but not proven, that dietary alterations can relieve the symptoms of gout. Organ meats, meat-based dishes, seafood, and dried beans should be restricted from the diet until the desired uric acid level has been achieved.

Encourage the avoidance of specific foods or alcoholic beverages that may precipitate attacks.

MEDICATION

If the patient is taking uricosuric agents, maintaining the urine alkalinity can enhance uric acid excretion. The doctor may prescribe agents to increase urine alkalinity.

HYDRATION

Drink 8 to 12 8-ounce glasses of fluid daily while receiving uricosuric agents.

Expectations of Therapy

Discuss with the patient his or her expectations of therapy.

ACTIVITIES AND EXERCISE

Activities of daily living need to be resumed within the boundaries set by the patient and the physician.

During the acute attack, the patient may require bedrest.

PAIN RELIEF

Discuss the degree of joint pain relief with and without activity. Since effects on the joints are progressive, the degree of pain and associated activity will vary based on the individual's presenting symptoms and degree of joint involvement.

STRESS MANAGEMENT

Encourage the patient to openly express *feelings* with regard to this chronic illness. The adjustment to this situation involves working through great personal fears, frustrations, hostilities, and resentments associated with the loss of control within one's life.

Changes in Expectations

Assess changes in expectations as therapy progresses and the patient gains understanding and skill in the management of the diagnosis.

Changes in Therapy through Cooperative Goal-Setting

Work with the patient to encourage adherence to the prescribed treatment. When the patient feels that a change should be made in a treatment plan, encourage a discussion first with the physician.

WRITTEN RECORD

Enlist the patient's aid in developing and maintaining a written record (Table 14.5) of monitoring parameters (i.e., swelling, warmth, tenderness of particular joints, identification of foods that precipitate an attack, degree of pain relief, exercise tolerance) and response to prescribed therapies for discussion with the physician. Patients should be encouraged to take this record on follow-up visits.

FOSTERING COMPLIANCE

Throughout the hospitalization, discuss medication information and how it will benefit the course of treatment. Seek cooperation and understanding of the following points, so that medication compliance may be enhanced:

1. Name
2. Dosage
3. Route and administration times
4. Anticipated therapeutic response
5. Side effects to expect
6. Side effects to report
7. What to do if a dosage is missed
8. When, how, or if to refill the medication prescription.

DIFFICULTY IN COMPREHENSION

If it is evident that the patient and/or family does not understand all aspects of continuing therapy being prescribed (i.e., administration and monitoring of medications, diets, follow-up appointments), consider the use of social service or visiting nurse agencies.

ASSOCIATED TEACHING

Give the patients the following instructions:

Always inform the physician or dentist of any prescription or over-the-counter medication being taken. Over-the-counter medications should not be taken without first discussing them with a physician or pharmacist.

Always report side effects of rash, itching, or hives immediately. Nausea, vomiting, or diarrhea should also be reported for the physician's evaluation if it is a new symptom.

Take all of the medication as prescribed for the full course of treatment. Do not discontinue use when feeling improved; do not save for further use; do not give your medicine to another individual. Sudden discontinuation of certain medications may produce harmful effects.

Keep all medications out of the reach of children.

If pregnancy is suspected, consult an obstetrician as soon as possible about continuation of medication therapy.

At Discharge

Items to be sent home with the patient should:

1. Have written instructions for use.
2. Be labeled in a level of language and size of print appropriate for the patient.
3. If needed, include identification cards or bracelets.
4. Include a list of additional supplies to be purchased after discharge
5. Include a schedule of follow-up appointments.

Probenecid (pro-ben′eh-sid) ### *(Benemid)* (ben-′eh-mid)

Probenecid promotes renal excretion of a number of substances, including uric acid. It inhibits the reabsorption of urate in the kidney, which results in reduction of uric acid in the blood. Thus, probenecid is used to treat hyperuricemia and chronic gouty arthritis. It is not effective in acute attacks of gout and is not an analgesic.

Side Effects

The number of gouty attacks may increase during the first 6 to 12 months of treatment. Continue probenecid therapy without changing doses during these attacks. Treat the acute attack with colchicine or anti-inflammatory agents.

The most common adverse effects of probenecid therapy are gastrointestinal in nature. About 8% of patients will complain of anorexia, nausea, and vomiting. Use with caution in patients with a history of peptic ulcer disease.

About 5% of patients develop a hypersensitivity to probenecid, manifested by fever, pruritus, and rashes. If these symptoms develop, discontinue therapy.

A false-positive reaction for glucose in the urine may occur with Clinitest tablets, but not with Clinistix or Tes-Tape.

Availability

PO—500 mg tablets.

Dosage and Administration

Note: Do not start probenecid therapy during an acute attack of gout; wait 2 to 3 weeks.
Adult
PO—Initially 250 mg twice daily for 1 week, then 500 mg twice daily. The dosage may be increased by 500 mg every few weeks to a maximum of 2 to 3 g daily. Administer with food or milk to diminish gastric irritation.

- Maintain fluid intake at 2 to 3 liters daily.
- Do not administer to patients with a creatinine clearance of less than 40 ml/minute or a BUN greater than 40 mg/100 ml.
- Do not administer to patients with a history of blood dyscrasias or uric acid kidney stones.

Nursing Interventions

See also General Nursing Considerations for Patients Receiving Uricosuric Therapy.

**PATIENT CONCERNS:
NURSING INTERVENTION/RATIONALE**

Side Effects to Expect

Acute Gout Attacks

Patients should be told that the frequency of gout attacks may increase for the first few months of therapy.

The patient should continue therapy without changing the doses during the attacks.

Side Effects to Report

Nausea, Anorexia, Vomiting

Use with caution in patients with a history of peptic ulcer disease. Individuals who experience symptoms of ulcers, and are yet undiagnosed, should be encouraged to report gastrointestinal symptoms if they increase in intensity or frequency. Always report bright blood or "coffee-ground" vomitus or dark, tarry stools.

Hives, Pruritus, Rash

Therapy may have to be discontinued.

Dosage and Administration

Acute Attacks

Do not start therapy during an acute attack of gout; wait 2 to 3 weeks.

Gastric Irritation

Give oral medication with food or milk to diminish gastric irritation.

Fluid Intake

Maintain fluid intake at 8 to 12 8-ounce glasses daily.

Contraindication

Do not administer to patients with a history of blood dyscrasias or uric acid kidney stones.

Drug Interactions

Oral Hypoglycemic Agents

Monitor for hypoglycemia: headache, weakness, decreased coordination, general apprehension, diaphoresis, hunger, blurred or double vision.

The dosage of the hypoglycemic agent may need to be reduced. Notify the physician if any of the above symptoms appear.

Table 14.5

Example of a Written Record for Patients Receiving Medication for Gout

Medications	Color	To be taken

Name _____

Physician _____

Physician's phone _____

Next appt.* _____

Parameters		Day of discharge							Comments
Joint swelling	Location								
	Amount: Small, moderate, large								
Pain relief Poor ——— Improved ——— No pain 10 ——— 5 ——— 1									
Ability to perform exercise	No problem								
	Too painful								
	Produces discomfort								
Temperature of affected area	Red hot								
	Warm								
	Normal								
Color of joint	Red								
	White								
	Normal								
Sleep pattern	Cannot stand covers								
	Can sleep with covers								
Overall sleep evaluation: Poor ——— Okay ——— Good 10 ——— 5 ——— 1									
Fluid intake per day: Record # glasses per day									
List foods that generally cause an attack									

*Please bring this record with you to your next appointment.
Use the back of this sheet for additional information.

Dapsone, Indomethacin, Sulfinpyrazone, Rifampin, Sulfonamides, Naproxen, Penicillins, Cephalosporins, Methotrexate, and Clofibrate

Probenecid blocks the renal excretion of these agents. See individual drugs listed for side effects to report that may indicate development of toxicity.

Salicylates

Although an occasional aspirin will not interfere with the effectiveness of probenecid, regular use of aspirin or aspirin-containing products should be discouraged. If analgesia is required, suggest acetaminophen.

Antineoplastic agents

Probenecid is not recommended for increased uric acid levels caused by antineoplastic therapy because of the potential development of renal uric acid stones.

Clinitest

This drug may produce false-positive Clinitest results. Use Clinistix or Tes-Tape to measure urine glucose.

Sulfinpyrazone (sul-fin-py′rah-zone) (Anturane) (an′tu-rayn)

Sulfinpyrazone is a renal tubular blocking agent that inhibits the reabsorption of urate from the renal tubules, increasing the urinary excretion of uric acid and decreasing serum urate levels. It is used for long-term treatment of hyperuricemia associated with gout and gouty arthritis.

Side Effects

The number of gouty attacks may increase during the first 6 to 12 months of treatment. Continue sulfinpyrazone therapy without changing doses during these attacks. Treat the acute attack with colchicine or anti-inflammatory agents.

The most common adverse effects of sulfinpyrazone therapy are gastrointestinal in nature. Some patients will complain of anorexia, nausea, and vomiting. Use with caution in patients with a history of peptic ulcer disease.

About 3% of patients develop hypersensitivity to sulfinpyrazone, manifested by fever, pruritus, and rashes. If these symptoms develop, discontinue therapy. Patients who have developed hypersensitivities to oxyphenbutazone or phenylbutazone should not be placed on sulfinpyrazone therapy due to the possibility of cross-sensitivity.

Serious, potentially fatal blood dyscrasias including anemia, agranulocytosis, and thrombocytopenia have been associated with sulfinpyrazone therapy. Although the development of blood dyscrasias is quite rare, periodic differential blood counts are recommended.

Availability

PO—100 mg tablets, and 200 mg capsules.

Dosage and Administration

Note: Do not start sulfinpyrazone therapy during an acute attack of gout; wait 2 to 3 weeks.
Adult
PO—Initially 100 to 200 mg twice daily during the first week of therapy. The maintenance dose is usually 200 to 400 mg twice daily. Administer with food or milk to diminish gastric irritation.

- Maintain fluid intake at 2 to 3 liters daily.
- *Do not* administer to patients with a creatinine clearance of less than 40 ml/minute or a BUN greater than 40 mg/100 ml.
- *Do not* administer to patients with a history of blood dyscrasias or uric acid kidney stones.

Nursing Interventions

See also General Nursing Considerations for Patients Receiving Uricosuric Therapy.

PATIENT CONCERNS: NURSING INTERVENTION/RATIONALE

Side Effects to Expect

Acute Gout Attacks

Patients should be told that the frequency of gout attacks may increase for the first few months of therapy. The patient should continue therapy without changing the doses during the attacks.

Side Effects to Report

Nausea, Anorexia, Vomiting

Use with caution in patients with a history of peptic ulcer disease. Individuals who experience symptoms of ulcers, and are yet undiagnosed, should be encouraged to report gastrointestinal symptoms if they increase in intensity or frequency. Always report bright blood or "coffee-ground" vomitus or dark, tarry stools.

Hives, Pruritus, Rash

Therapy may have to be discontinued.

Dosage and Administration

Acute Attacks

Do not start therapy during an acute attack of gout; wait 2 to 3 weeks.

Gastric Irritation

Give oral medication with food or milk to diminish gastric irritation.

Fluid Intake

Maintain fluid intake at 8 to 12 8-ounce glasses daily.

Contraindications

Do not administer to patients with a creatinine clearance of less than 40 ml/minute or a BUN greater than 40 mg/100 ml.

Do not administer to patients with a history of blood dyscrasias or uric acid kidney stones.

Drug Interactions

Salicylates

Although an occasional aspirin will not interfere with the effectiveness of sulfinpyrazone, discourage regular use of aspirin or aspirin-containing products. If analgesia is required, suggest acetaminophen.

Antineoplastic Agents

Sulfinpyrazone is not recommended for increased uric acid levels caused by antineoplastic therapy because of the potential development of renal uric acid stones.

Warfarin

This medication may enhance the anticoagulant effects of warfarin. Observe for the development of petechiae, ecchymoses, nosebleeds, bleeding gums, dark tarry stools, and bright red or "coffee ground" emesis.

Monitor the prothrombin time and reduce the dosage of warfarin if necessary.

Drugs That Act on the Bladder

Oxybutynin chloride (ok-se-bu′ti-nin)
(Ditropan) (di′trow-pan)

Oxybutynin chloride is an antispasmodic agent that acts directly on the smooth muscle of the bladder to reduce the frequency of bladder contractions and delay the initial desire to void in patients with neurogenic bladder.

Oxybutynin should not be used in patients with glaucoma, myasthenia gravis, bowel disease such as ulcerative colitis, or obstructive uropathy such as prostatitis.

Side Effects

Side effects are usually dose-related and respond to a reduction in dosage. Routine side effects are dry mouth, decreased sweating, urinary hesitance and retention, blurred vision, tachycardia, palpitations, dilatation of the pupil, cycloplegia, drowsiness, insomnia, nausea, vomiting, constipation, and a bloated feeling. Allergic reactions have also been reported.

Availability

PO—5 mg tablets; 5 mg/5 ml syrup.

Dosage and Administration

Adult
PO—5 mg 2 or 3 times daily. Maximum dose is 20 mg daily.
Pediatric (over 5 years of age)
PO—5 mg twice daily. Maximum dose is 15 mg daily.

Nursing Interventions

See also General Nursing Considerations for Patients with Urinary System Disease.

PATIENT CONCERNS: NURSING INTERVENTION/RATIONALE

Side Effects to Expect

Dry Mouth, Urinary Hesitance, Retention

These side effects are usually dose-related and respond to a reduction in dose.

Relieve dry mouth by sucking on ice chips or hard candy or by chewing gum.

Constipation, Bloating

Encourage balanced nutrition and inclusion of fresh fruits and vegetables, for roughage, and an adequate fluid intake to help alleviate this complication. If this approach is unsuccessful, suggest a stool softener or bulk-forming supplement. Avoid laxatives.

Blurred Vision

Caution patients not to drive or operate power equipment until they have adjusted to this side effect.

Side Effects to Report

Above Symptoms

If any of the above symptoms intensifies, it should be reported to the physician for evaluation.

Drug Interactions

No clinically significant interactions have been reported.

Bethanechol chloride (be-tha′ne-kol) (Urecholine) (u-re-ko′leen)

Bethanechol is a parasympathetic nerve stimulant that causes contraction of the detrusor urinae muscle in the bladder, usually resulting in urination. It also may stimulate gastric motility, increase gastric tone, and restore impaired rhythmic peristalsis. Bethanechol is used in nonobstructive urinary retention, particularly in postoperative and postpartum patients.

Side Effects

Side effects are infrequent, but are usually extensions of the pharmacologic activity of parasympathetic stimulants. These include flushing of the skin, sweating, nausea, vomiting, headache, colicky pain, abdominal cramps, diarrhea, belching, and involuntary defecation.

Availability

PO—5, 10, 25, and 50 mg tablets.
SC—5 mg/ml in 1 ml vials.

Dosage and Administration

Adult
PO—10 to 50 mg 2 to 4 times daily. The maximum daily dose is 120 mg.
SC—2.5 to 5 mg.
   Note: If overdosage occurs, the pharmacologic actions of the drug can immediately be abolished by atropine.

Nursing Interventions

See also General Nursing Considerations for Patients with Urinary System Disease.

PATIENT CONCERNS: NURSING INTERVENTION/RATIONALE

Side Effects to Expect

Flushing of Skin, Headache

A pharmacologic property of the drug results in dilated blood vessels.

Side Effects to Report

Nausea, Vomiting, Sweating, Colicky Pain, Abdominal Cramps, Diarrhea, Belching, Involuntary Defecation

These effects are caused by a pharmacologic property of the drug. Consult the physician; a dosage adjustment may control these adverse effects.

Support the patient with diarrhea or involuntary defecation.

Dosage and Administration

SC

Have atropine sulfate available to counteract serious adverse effects.

Drug Interactions

Quinidine, Procainamide

Do not use concurrently with bethanechol. The pharmacologic properties of these agents counteract those of bethanechol.

Chapter 15

Drugs Affecting
the Endocrine System

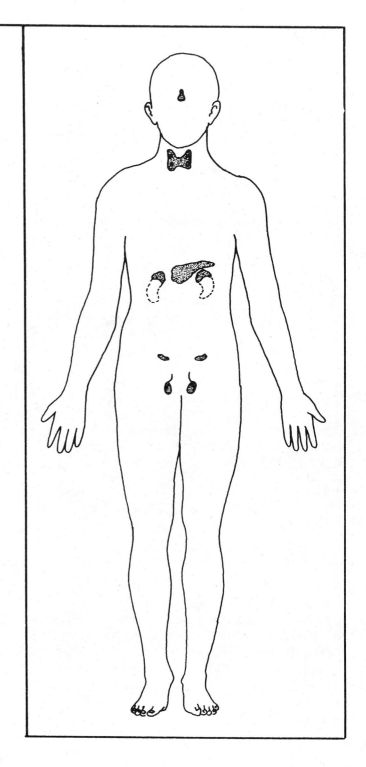

Objectives

After completing this chapter, the student should
be able to do the following:

1. Explain the major action and effects of drugs
   used to treat disorders of the endocrine system.
2. Identify baseline data the nurse should collect
   on a continuous basis for comparison and
   evaluation of drug effectiveness.
3. Identify important nursing assessments and
   interventions associated with the drug therapy
   and treatment of diseases associated with the
   endocrine system.
4. Identify health teaching essential for a
   successful treatment regimen.

Antidiabetic Agents

Diabetes Mellitus

Diabetes mellitus has traditionally been defined as a chronic, progressive disease manifested by abnormalities in carbohydrate, protein, and fat metabolism resulting from a lack of insulin. It has now been redefined as a group of diseases that have glucose intolerance (hyperglycemia) in common. The causes of these diseases are still unknown, but it is now recognized that different pathologic mechanisms are involved for different diseases.

Diabetes mellitus is appearing with increasing frequency in the United States as the number of older people in the population increases. In the U.S., approximately 4.5 million people are being treated for diabetes. Another 2 million have undiagnosed diabetes, and 5 million more will develop diabetes during their lives. Undiagnosed diabetic adults, with few or no symptoms, present a major challenge to the health profession. Because early symptoms of diabetes are minimal, the patient does not seek medical advice. Indications of the disease are discovered only at the time of routine physical examination. Those with a predisposition to developing diabetes include (1) people who have relatives with diabetes (they have two and one half times greater incidence of developing the disease), (2) obese people (85% of all diabetic patients are overweight), and (3) older people (4 out of 5 diabetics are over 45 years of age).

In 1979, the National Diabetes Data Group of the National Institutes of Health published a new classification system for diabetes that more accurately categorizes the various mechanisms associated with the diseases. The classification includes three clinical classes, characterized by either fasting hyperglycemia or abnormalities of glucose tolerance, and two statistical risk classes, with normal glucose tolerance, that are thought to be stages in the natural course of diabetes, see Table 15.1.

Type I, *insulin-dependent diabetes mellitus* (IDDM) is present in 5% to 10% of the diabetic population. It frequently occurs in juveniles, but it is now recognized that patients can become symptomatic for the first time at any age. The onset of this form of diabetes usually has a rapid progression of symptoms (a few days to a few weeks) characterized by polydipsia (increased thirst), polyphagia (increased appetite), polyuria (increased urination), increased frequency of infections, loss of weight and strength, irritability, and often ketoacidosis. There is no insulin secretion from the pancreas, and patients require administration of exogenous insulin. Insulin dosage adjustment is easily influenced by inconsistent patterns of physical activity and dietary irregularities.

Type II, *non-insulin-dependent diabetes mellitus* (NIDDM) represents about 90% of the diabetic population. It usually has a more insidious onset. The pancreas still maintains some capability to produce and secrete insulin. Consequently, symptoms are minimal or absent for a prolonged period. The patient may seek medical attention several years later only after symptoms of the disease are apparent. Patients may complain of weight gain or loss. Blurred vision may indicate diabetic retinopathy. Neuropathies may be first observed as numbness or tingling of the extremities (paresthesia), loss of sensation, orthostatic hypotension, impotence, and difficulty in controlling urination (neurogenic bladder). Nonhealing ulcers of the lower extremities may indicate chronic vascular disease. Fasting hyperglycemia can be controlled by diet in some patients, but other patients will require the use of supplemental insulin or oral hypoglycemia agents, such as tolbutamide or acetohexamide. Although the onset is usually after the fourth decade of life, NIDDM can occur in younger patients who do not require insulin for control.

The third subclass of diabetes mellitus includes additional types of diabetes that are a part of other diseases having features not generally associated with the diabetic state. Diseases that may have a diabetic component include pheochromocytoma, acromegaly, and Cushing syndrome. Other disorders included in this category are malnutrition, drugs and chemicals that induce hyperglycemia, defects in insulin receptors, and certain genetic syndromes.

The second clinical class, known as *gestational diabetes* (GDM) is reserved for women who show abnormal glucose tolerance during pregnancy. It does not include diabetic women who become pregnant. The majority of gestational diabetics will have a normal glucose

Table 15.1
National Diabetes Group Classification of Glucose Intolerance

CLASS	FORMER TERMINOLOGY
Clinical Classes	
Diabetes mellitus (DM)	
Type I: Insulin dependent (IDDM)	Juvenile diabetes, juvenile-onset diabetes, JOD, ketosis prone diabetes, brittle diabetes
Type II: Non-insulin-dependent (NIDDM)	Adult-onset diabetes, maturity-onset diabetes, ketosis resistant diabetes, stable diabetes, MOD
Nonobese NIDDM	
Obese NIDDM	
Other types associated with certain conditions and syndromes:	Secondary diabetes
1. Pancreatic disease	
2. Hormonal	
3. Drug or chemical induced	
4. Insulin receptor abnormalities	
5. Certain genetic syndromes	
6. Other types:	
Gestational diabetes (GDM)	Gestational diabetes
Impaired glucose tolerance (IGT)	Asymptomatic diabetes, chemical diabetes, borderline diabetes, latent diabetes
Nonobese IGT	
Obese IGT	
IGT associated with certain conditions and syndromes:	
1. Pancreatic disease	
2. Hormonal	
3. Drug or chemical induced	
4. Insulin receptor abnormalities	
5. Certain genetic syndromes	
Statistical Risk Classes	
Previous abnormality of glucose tolerance (PrevAGT)	Latent diabetes
Potential abnormality of glucose tolerance (PotAGT)	Prediabetes, potential diabetes

Modified from National Diabetes Data Group, *Diabetes* 28:1039–1057, Dec. 1979.

tolerance postpartum. Gestational diabetics must be reclassified after delivery into the category of diabetes mellitus, impaired glucose tolerance, or previous abnormality of glucose tolerance. Gestational diabetics have been put into a separate category because of the special clinical features of diabetes that develop during pregnancy and the complications associated with fetal involvement. These women are also at a higher risk of developing diabetes 5 to 10 years after pregnancy.

The third and last clinical class is for those patients found to have an *impaired glucose tolerance* (IGT). It is now thought that patients with IGT are at a higher risk for developing NIDDM or IDDM in the future. In many of these patients, however, the glucose tolerance returns to normal or persists in the intermediate range for years. Studies indicate that these patients have an increased susceptibility to atherosclerotic disease.

There are two groups of patients at risk for diabetes or impaired glucose tolerance—those with a previous abnormality and those with a potential abnormality of glucose tolerance. Therefore, the National Diabetes Data Group included two statistical risk classes in the new classification. The first risk class is for patients with a *previous abnormality of glucose tolerance* (PrevAGT). This class includes patients who now have a normal glucose tolerance but who have a history of previous diabetes mellitus or impaired glucose tolerance. Representatives of this class might be the gestational diabetic who has a normal glucose tolerance after delivery or an obese patient whose glucose tolerance has returned to normal because of diet control and weight loss. It is important to realize that PrevAGT patients are not diabetics and should not be labeled as such, but should be tested periodically for the development of diabetes.

The second statistical risk class is *potential abnormality of glucose tolerance* (PotAGT). This class is for patients who have never exhibited abnormal glucose tolerance but who are at an increased risk for developing abnormalities. Risk factors for the development of non-insulin-dependent diabetes include being the monozygotic twin of this type of diabetic, having a close relative (e.g., sibling, parent, or child) who is a non-insulin-dependent diabetic, and being obese. A person with islet cell antibodies, or who is a monozygotic twin of an insulin-dependent diabetic, or who is a sibling of an insulin-dependent diabetic has an increased probability of becoming an insulin-dependent diabetic.

Although the classification system of the National Diabetes Data Group was developed to facilitate clinical and epidemiologic investigation, the categorization of patients can also be helpful in determining general principles for therapy. Since a cure for diabetes mellitus is unknown at present, the minimal purpose of treatment is to prevent ketoacidosis, and symptoms resulting from hyperglycemia. The long-term objective of control of the disease must involve mechanisms to stop the progression of the complications of the disease. Major determinants involve a balanced diet, insulin or oral hypoglycemic therapy, routine exercise, and good hygiene. Patient education and reinforcement are extremely important to successful therapy. The intelligence and motivation of the diabetic patient, and an awareness of the potential complications, contribute significantly to the ultimate outcome of the disease and the quality of life the patient may lead.

Control of Diabetes Mellitus. Patients with diabetes can lead full and satisfying lives. However, unrestricted diets and activities are not possible. Dietary treatment of diabetes constitutes the basis for management of most patients, especially those with the Type II (NIDDM) form of the disease. With adequate weight reduction and dietary control, patients may not require the use of exogenous insulin or oral hypoglycemic drug therapy. Type I (IDDM) diabetics will always require exogenous insulin as well as dietary control because the pancreas has lost the capacity to produce and secrete insulin. The aims of dietary control are (1) the prevention of excessive postprandial hyperglycemia, (2) the prevention of hypoglycemia in those patients being treated with hypoglycemic agents or insulin, and (3) the achievement and maintenance of an ideal body weight. A return to normal weight is often accompanied by a reduction in hyperglycemia. The diet should also be adjusted to reduce elevated cholesterol and triglyceride levels in an attempt to retard the progression of atherosclerosis.

To help maintain adherence to dietary restrictions, the diet should be planned in relation to the patient's food preferences, economic status, occupation, and physical activity. Emphasis should be placed on what food the patient may have and what exchanges are acceptable. Food should be measured for balanced portions, and the patient should be cautioned not to omit meals or between meal and bedtime snacks.

All diabetic patients must receive adequate instruction on personal hygiene, especially regarding care of the feet, skin, and teeth. Infection is a common precipitating cause of ketosis and acidosis, and must be treated promptly.

Insulin is required to control Type I diabetes and for those patients whose diabetes cannot be controlled by diet, weight reduction, or oral hypoglycemic agents. Patients normally controlled with oral hypoglycemic agents will require insulin during situations of increased physiologic and psychologic stress, such as pregnancy, surgery, and infections. The dosage of insulin is usually adjusted according to the blood glucose levels and the degree of glucosuria. The patient should test the urine before each meal and at bedtime while the insulin is being regulated.

Another adjunct in the therapy of Type II diabetes is the use of oral hypoglycemic agents. They are recommended only in those patients who cannot be controlled by diet alone and who are not prone to develop ketosis, acidosis, and/or infections. Patients most likely to benefit from treatment are those who have developed diabetes after 40 years of age and who require less than 40 units of insulin per day.

General Nursing Considerations for Patients with Diabetes Mellitus

A major challenge in nursing is to teach the newly diagnosed diabetic patient all the necessary information to manage self-care and the disease process, and to prevent complications. The patient must be taught the entire therapeutic regimen—diet, activity level, urine or blood testing, the medication, self-injection techniques, prevention of complications, and the effective management of hypoglycemia or hyperglycemia. Many diabetics have difficulty understanding the critical balance among the dietary prescription, the prescribed medication, and the maintenance of general health. All are important to the control and effective management of the disease process.

PATIENT CONCERNS: NURSING INTERVENTION/RATIONALE

Management of Patients with Diabetes Mellitus

Nutritional Status

Diet is used alone or in combination with insulin or oral hypoglycemic agents to control diabetes mellitus. The diabetic patient, whether non-insulin-dependent or insulin dependent, must follow a prescribed diet to achieve optimal control of the disease.

NUTRITIONAL EVALUATION

The newly diagnosed diabetic requires a thorough nutritional evaluation. Information collected by the nurse or dietitian should include identification of the patient's average daily diet, the ability and willingness to prepare foods, food budget, and level of daily exercise.

People who are readmitted for treatment should be reevaluated for both nutritional knowledge and compliance with the prescribed dietary plan.

DIETARY PRESCRIPTION

The dietary prescription is based on providing the patient with the nutritional and energy requirements necessary to maintain an appropriate weight and lifestyle. Diabetics are encouraged to maintain a body weight slightly below an ideal weight based on height, gender, and frame size.

The diet for the obese diabetic, regardless of age, is calculated to achieve weight loss over the next several weeks to months. Once the optimal weight is attained, these patients are placed on a maintenance diet. (See a medical-surgical nursing text or a nutrition text for the details of dietary calculations and the specific foods contained on each of the exchange lists.)

Activity and Exercise

Maintenance of a normal lifestyle is to be encouraged. This includes exercise and activities the individual enjoys. The normal daily energy level is used in determining the dietary and medication requirements for the patient.

Just as it is important for the patient to maintain a diet, it is equally important to maintain a certain activity level. Patients who suddenly increase or decrease activity levels are susceptible to developing episodes of hyperglycemia or hypoglycemia. Both dietary and medication prescriptions may require adjustment if the patient does not plan to resume the previous exercise level.

Psychological Considerations

When first diagnosed, the patient may experience varying degrees of grief, anger, denial, or acceptance. Let the patient express these concerns and address those items that are considered to be of greatest importance first.

Foster the idea that the patient can control most aspects of diabetes by careful management of diet, medications, and activities. Having a sense of control is important to all people. Stress that learning to manage the disease process is the best means of preventing complications.

Medication

As stated in the introduction, insulin or oral hypoglycemic agent therapy may be required to control diabetes mellitus. No changes in therapy should be made without medical supervision.

HYPOGLYCEMIA

Hypoglycemia, or low blood sugar, can occur from too much insulin, insufficient food intake to cover the insulin given, imbalances caused by vomiting and diarrhea, and excessive exercise without additional carbohydrate intake.

Symptoms. Recognize and assess early symptoms of hypoglycemia: nervousness, tremors, headache, apprehension, sweating, and hunger. If uncorrected, hypoglycemia progresses to blurring of vision, lack of coordination, incoherence, coma, and death.

Treatment. If the patient is conscious and *able to swallow*, give 2 to 4 ounces of fruit juice with two teaspoons of sugar in it, or give a piece of candy such as Life-Savers or gum drops. (Chocolate contains fats which are utilized more slowly.) Repeat in 15 to 20 minutes if relief of symptoms is not evident.

If the patient is unconscious or *unable to swallow*, administer 20 to 50 ml of glucose 50%, IV. (Done only by a qualified individual.)

With any hypoglycemic reaction, notify the team leader, primary nurse, or head nurse, who will then contact the physician. The underlying cause of the hypoglycemia must be identified to prevent further occurrences.

HYPERGLYCEMIA

This condition (elevated blood sugar) occurs when the glucose available in the body cannot be transported into the cells for use, because of a lack of insulin necessary for the transport mechanism.

Symptoms. Symptoms of hyperglycemia are headache, nausea and vomiting, abdominal pain, dizziness, rapid pulse, rapid shallow respirations, and a fruity odor to the breath from acetone. If untreated, hyperglycemia may also cause coma and death.

Treatment. Treatment of hyperglycemia requires hospitalization, insulin, and close monitoring of the blood and urine glucose and ketones. Since hyperglycemia usually occurs due to another cause, the problem, often an infection, must also be identified and treated to control the hyperglycemia.

Prevention. The risk of hyperglycemia can be minimized by: taking the prescribed dose of insulin or oral hypoglycemic agent; maintenance of an accurate record of urine tests for glucose and ketones; adherence to the prescribed diet and exercise; and by reporting fevers, infection, or prolonged vomiting and/or diarrhea to the physician.

Complications Associated with Diabetes Mellitus

Peripheral Vascular Disease

The person with diabetes mellitus is more likely to suffer from peripheral vascular disease than the general population. Reduced blood supply to the extremities may result in intermittent claudication, numbness and tingling, and a greater likelihood of foot infections.

ASSESSMENT OF TISSUE OXYGENATION

Observe the color of each hand, finger, leg, and foot; report cyanosis or reddish-blue discolorations. Inspect the skin of the extremities for any signs of ulceration.

Temperature. Feel the temperature in each hand, finger, leg, and foot. Report paleness and coldness. Note that these symptoms will be increased if the limbs are elevated above the level of the heart.

Edema. Report edema, its extent, and whether relieved or unchanged when in a dependent position.

Peripheral Pulses. Record the pedal and radial pulses at least every four hours if circulatory impairment is found in that limb. Compare findings between each of the extremities. Report diminished or absent pulses immediately.

Limb Pain. Monitor pain in the patient carefully. Pain with exercise that is relieved by rest may be from claudication.

Care. Prevent ulcers, injury, and infection in the lower extremities with meticulous, regular care. See also General Nursing Considerations for Patients with Peripheral Vascular Disease in Chapter 10.

VISUAL ALTERATIONS

Visual changes are common in the patient with diabetes mellitus. These individuals frequently suffer from blurred vision associated with an elevated blood sugar. People known to be diabetic who complain to the nurse of intermittently blurred vision should be referred to their physician for a check of the blood sugar level. Once the hyperglycemia is controlled, the blurred vision usually clears.

Ask specific questions to elicit information on any visual problems that the patient may be experiencing. If visual impairment is present, plan for an appropriate degree of intervention. Special equipment is available for the visually impaired diabetic patient.

Blindness. In advanced stages of diabetes mellitus, the patient may suffer from changes (microangiopathies) in the small blood vessels of the eyes. Retinal hemorrhages, degeneration of retinal vascular tissue, cataracts, and eventual blindness may occur. The diabetic patient should have regular eye exams to allow early treatment of any apparent alterations.

RENAL DISEASE

Patients with diabetes may develop microangiopathies in the kidneys and are also more susceptible to urinary tract infections. Be alert for the development of proteinuria and elevations in serum creatinine and blood urea nitrogen levels. Report these to the physician.

INFECTION

Any type of infection can cause a significant loss of control of diabetes mellitus. Observe carefully for any signs of redness, tenderness, swelling, or drainage which occurs when there is any break in the skin. Patients should be taught to immediately report early signs of infection such as fever or sore throat.

During an infection, the dosage of insulin may require an adjustment to compensate for a change in metabolic rate, diet, and exercise.

NEUROPATHIES

A complication of diabetes mellitus is degeneration of nerves, usually in the extremities. Ask the patient to describe any sensations, such as numbness or tingling, being experienced in the extremities. Inspect the feet for blisters, ingrown toenails, or sores. Occasionally the patient will not be aware of these lesions due to the degeneration of nerves in the area.

Always test the water temperature before immersing a limb of a diabetic patient. Due to impaired sensation, the patient may be easily burned and unaware of it until later.

Neuropathies can also affect the autonomic nervous system. Patients with diabetes mellitus should always be closely assessed if nausea, diarrhea, constipation, or visual disturbances develop.

Discharge Planning

Prior to discharge, the patient must achieve a high degree of understanding of diabetes mellitus and its management. The patient and family members need to be included in the total educational program.

With the advent of shorter hospitalizations, it may be necessary to incorporate follow-up care by a visiting nurse association or a home health agency in the discharge planning.

The patient must understand the following:

- Recognition of the symptoms of hyperglycemia and hypoglycemia
- Dietary management and food preparation
- Urine or blood testing for glucose and ketones: time, recording, and interpretation of the results
- Injection technique and care of the equipment
- Medication preparation, dosage, frequency, storage, and refilling
- Appropriate hygiene and care of minor wounds

Provide psychological support and guidance for the patient and family. Give them every opportunity to ask questions concerning the patient's care. Reassess and reinforce the analysis of symptoms they should watch for and appropriate actions to take for complications that may develop.

Support to the family as they learn to cope with the integration of the diabetic's needs into the family, the job setting, or school.

Patient Teaching Associated with the Control of Diabetes Mellitus

Communication and Responsibility

Encourage open communication concerning frustrations and anger as the patient attempts to adjust to the diagnosis and the need for prolonged treatment. The patient must be guided to gain insight into the disorder in order to assume responsibility for the continuation of treatment. Keep emphasizing those factors the patient can control to alter progression of the disease, including maintenance of general health, nutritional needs, adequate rest and appropriate exercise, and continuation of the prescribed medication therapy.

SMOKING

Smoking causes vasoconstriction of blood vessels, aggravating microangiopathies associated with diabetes mellitus. Patients who smoke should be encouraged to quit.

NUTRITIONAL NEEDS

Explain the entire dietary prescription to the patient and family. Be certain to teach the dietary requirements of the patient to the person who will prepare the food.

Emphasize to the patient the importance of eating all of the prescribed foods at the proper times in order to cover the peak action of insulin or oral hypoglycemic therapy. Patients must understand how to properly substitute foods from the exchange lists to maintain a balance between nutritional requirements and insulin administration. Review with the patient the most common time when their particular drug regimen may cause hypoglycemia.

People who are readmitted for treatment should be reevaluated for both nutritional knowledge as well as for general understanding of all aspects of diabetic management. Never presume compliance or competence simply because the patient has long been diagnosed as a diabetic.

ACTIVITY AND EXERCISE

The prescribed diet and medication are carefully calculated to maintain the individual's lifestyle. Encourage the patient to report any major change in planned activity level so that appropriate adjustment can be made. Activities, such as changing from a sedentary job to one with physical labor, or starting to participate regularly in a strenuous sport, should be reported. The patient should also report discontinuation of a vigorous sport or a change to a more sedentary job.

PERSONAL HYGIENE

Explain the importance of maintaining personal hygiene. Encourage the patient to cleanse even a slight injury with soap and water and apply a topical antibiotic to the area. Instruct the patient not to use antiseptics that could cause skin irritations.

Teach patients to inspect their feet for developing callouses, blisters, sores, and ingrown toenails. Emphasize the importance of good foot care and properly fitting shoes to minimize complications.

Encourage the patient not to self-treat corns, callouses, or ingrown toenails. Products used for these problems may cause further damage, due to vasoconstriction, and are specifically contraindicated in patients with diabetes mellitus. (See also General Nursing Considerations for Patients with Peripheral Vascular Disease in Chapter 10.)

INFECTIONS

Encourage the patient to report immediately any signs of redness, tenderness, swelling, or draining which might occur where any break in the skin is located. Also report wounds that are slow in healing.

Avoid exposure to people known to have infections.

PSYCHOLOGICAL CONSIDERATIONS

Stress that learning to manage the entire disease process is the best means of preventing complications. Foster the idea that the individual can control many aspects of the disease by careful management of diet, medications, and activities.

Encourage individuals to return to as normal a lifestyle as possible. Help patients develop schedules that fit their pattern of life: are the patients late risers, early risers, work the midnight shift, or do they play a vigorous sport 3 or 4 times a week?

URINE GLUCOSE TESTING

Teach the patient to perform the urine test for glucose and ketones according to the methodology that will be used at home. Stress the need to follow the manufacturer's directions if products are changed at home. The patient must also notify the physician of the change in urine testing products.

The patient should test the urine for glucose at least four times daily during times of stress or infection. Report abnormalities to the physician, since additional doses of insulin may be required. (The usual times to test the urine are one half hour before meals and at bedtime.)

BLOOD GLUCOSE TESTS

Blood glucose tests may be required in patients who require small adjustments in daily insulin dosages. Teach the patient to perform the blood test according to the method that will be used at home.

Expectations of Therapy

Discuss the expectations of therapy (e.g., level of exercise, expectations for relief of symptoms, frequency of therapy use, degree of limitations, ability to maintain activities of daily living and/or work). If permanent visual impairment, atherosclerosis, or neuropathy are evident, discuss measures to control these factors.

Changes in Expectations

Assess changes in expectations as therapy progresses and the patient gains understanding and skill in the management of the diagnosis.

Role-play aspects of the patient's care with the patient or family (e.g., insulin preparation, urine tests, self-injection, control of hypoglycemic or hyperglycemic reactions). Have the participants practice by repeating the appropriate intervention for the presenting problem.

Changes in Therapy through Cooperative Goal-Setting

Work with the patient to encourage adherence to the prescribed treatment. When the patient feels that a change should be made in a treatment plan, encourage discussion with the physician.

WRITTEN RECORD

Enlist the patient's aid in developing and maintaining a written record of monitoring parameters (e.g., urine or blood glucose, insulin dosage, pertinent stress factors, exercise level, illnesses, or major changes in diet or other routine) for discussion with the physician. (See Table 15.2, example of written record.) Patients should be encouraged to take this record on follow-up visits.

FOSTERING COMPLIANCE

Throughout the hospitalization, discuss medication information and how it will benefit the course of treatment. Seek cooperation and understanding of the following points so that medication compliance may be enhanced:

1. Name: Be sure that the patient or family member is able to repeat the name of the type of insulin, and the onset, peak, and duration of the insulin or oral hypoglycemic agent prescribed. No change in insulin type, concentration, or brand should be made without medical supervision.

Table 15.2
Example of a Written Record for Patients Receiving Antidiabetic Agents

Medications	Color	To be taken

Name _____

Physician _____

Physician's phone _____

Next appt.* _____

Parameters		Day of discharge								Comments
Insulin/Oral agent Types: AM PM	Temperature / Weight									
	Site AM / Site PM									
	Units AM / Units PM									
Urine: (Use 2nd voided specimen) Sugar / Acetone	Before breakfast									
	Before lunch									
	Before supper									
	Bedtime									
Blood testing										
Diet	Eat all foods allowed									
	Unable to eat									
	Overate or indulged									
Lifestyle	Usual daily activities/exercise									
	Increased amount of exercise									
	Increased stress									
	Normal day-to-day stress									
Injuries or skin integrity	No visible changes in skin of feet									
	Cuts, bruises, open sores									
Hypoglycemia	Sweating, weak, shaky, hungry									
Hyperglycemia	Urinating frequently, poor appetite, ↑ thirst, weak, dizzy									

*Please bring this record with you to your next appointment.
Use the back of this sheet for additional information.

366

2. Dosage: Instruct the patient about the exact dosage of the prescription, and allow the patient to practice preparation and administration of insulin, as ordered.

3. Route and administration times (see Chapters 5, 6, and 7 on administration of medications): Be sure that the patient understands how to administer insulin or oral hypoglycemic agents. If the patient is on a sliding scale of insulin, based on urine or blood glucose values, be certain the patient understands the sliding scale and the amount of *regular* insulin prescribed.

4. Anticipated therapeutic responses: Diabetes is controlled within normal limits of the blood sugar level.

5. Side effects to expect: Fairly constant control of the diabetes with minimal side effects should be expected when the diet and prescription for insulin or oral hypoglycemia agents are followed.

6. Side effects to report: Occasional episodes of hypo- or hyperglycemia may occur if illness, stress, or infection is present, or if there is significant variation in diet or exercise. Frequent episodes should be reported to the physician for adjustment in therapy. (See above for treatment of hypo- or hyperglycemia.)

7. What to do if a dosage is missed: A diabetic patient cannot miss a dose of insulin and not develop hyperglycemia. A balanced diet, exercise level, and insulin dosage are crucial to the well-being of the diabetic patient.

8. When, how, or if to refill the medication prescription: Be sure that the patient understands how to refill prescriptions for insulin or oral hypoglycemic agents. When purchasing insulin, have the patient double-check the type and concentration (usually U-100) of insulin and the expiration date. The insulin should be stored in the refrigerator (not the freezer) prior to use. Once it is opened and being used, it can be stored at room temperature.

DIFFICULTY IN COMPREHENSION

If it is evident that the patient and/or family does not understand all aspects of the continuing therapy being prescribed (e.g., administration and monitoring of medications, exercises, diets, follow-up appointments) consider the use of social service or visiting nurse agencies.

ASSOCIATED TEACHING

Always inform the physician or dentist of any prescription or over-the-counter medication being taken.

Over-the-counter medications should not be taken without first discussing them with a physician or pharmacist. Medications such as aspirin and ascorbic acid can interfere with urine testing procedures. When necessary, ask the pharmacist for sugar-free products.

Always report side effects of rash, itching, or hives immediately. Diabetics just starting insulin therapy are more susceptible to allergic reactions at the site of injection. A change in source of insulin may be required.

Take all of the medication as prescribed for the full course of treatment. Do not discontinue use when feeling improved; do not save for future use; do not give your medicine to another individual. Sudden discontinuation of certain medications may produce harmful effects.

Keep all medications out of reach of children.

If pregnancy is suspected, consult an obstetrician as soon as possible about continuation of medication therapy and necessary adjustment during pregnancy.

At Discharge

Develop a list of specific equipment and supplies the patient will need when discharged. Keep in mind the cost of these supplies. Consider the following:

1. Syringes: Disposable syringes are convenient and presterilized, but are more expensive. (Be sure to tell the patient that disposable syringes are to be used once and then discarded.) Reusable syringes are less expensive, more easily read, and in some instances, paid for by insurance coverage.

2. Needles: Disposable needles are more convenient, but also more expensive. Stainless steel needles are easily resterilized and reused, but eventually become dull and must be discarded.

   Patients usually use a 26 or 27 gauge, ½ inch needle, but needles should be adjusted to the individual. An obese patient may require a 1 to 1½ inch needle length to properly inject the insulin.

3. Specialized Equipment: Magni-Guides are available for the visually impaired patient. This aid holds the vial of isulin, acts as a guide in withdrawing insulin, and has a magnifying glass to make reading the syringe scale easier. Special automatic insulin syringes are available for blind patients.

   Whenever possible, have the family purchase any reusable products the patient will be using. Vary teaching techniques to include the actual equipment the person will use at home.

4. Reusable Syringes and Needles: Teach proper sterilization techniques including the following:
Separate and clean the syringe parts and needles. Place in a strainer in a pan with sufficient water to completely cover all the equipment. Boil for 10 minutes and then remove from the water by lifting the strainer. Once cool, assemble the syringe parts. Store equipment immersed in 91% isopropyl alcohol in a syringe storage container, available at the pharmacy. If stored in this manner, allow to air dry before using with insulin.

If the patient is unable to boil the equipment (such as when traveling), wash all parts thoroughly and then completely immerse them in 91% isopropyl alcohol for 5 to 10 minutes. Allow to thoroughly air dry prior to using for insulin administration.

Items to be sent home with the patient should:

1. Have written instructions for use
2. Be labeled in language and size of print appropriate for the patient
3. If needed, include identification cards or bracelets
4. Include a list of additional supplies to be purchased after discharge (e.g., syringes, needles, alcohol, cotton balls, urine or blood glucose testing materials, insulin, dressings).
5. Include a schedule for follow-up appointments.

Insulins

Insulin is a hormone produced in the beta cells of the pancreas and is a key regulator of metabolism. Insulins from the pancreases of different animals have similar activity and thus may be used in human beings. Insulin is required for the entry of glucose into skeletal and heart muscle and fat. It also plays a significant role in protein and lipid metabolism. It is not required for glucose transport into the brain or liver tissue.

Insulin deficiency reduces the rate of transport of glucose into cells, producing hyperglycemia. Other metabolic reactions are also inhibited by the lack of insulin, resulting in the conversion of protein to glucose, hyperlipidemia, ketosis, and acidosis.

Insulin was discovered by Sir Frederick Banting, Charles Best, and John Macleod of Toronto, Canada, and was first made available to the public in 1922. Several preparations of insulin, isolated from beef and pork pancreas, are now commercially available.

Side Effects

Insulin overdose or decreased carbohydrate intake may result in hypoglycemia. If untreated, irreversible brain damage may occur. Hypoglycemia occurs most frequently when the administered insulin reaches its peak action (see Table 15.3). Hypoglycemia must be treated immediately. The following conditions may predispose a diabetic patient to a hypoglycemic (insulin) reaction: improper measurement of insulin dosage, excessive exercise, insufficient food intake, concurrent ingestion of hypoglycemic drugs and discontinuation of drugs (see Drug Interactions), or conditions (such as infection or stress) causing hyperglycemia.

Allergic reactions, manifested by itching, redness, and swelling at the site of injection are common occurrences in patients beginning insulin therapy. These reactions may be caused by modifying proteins in NPH or PZI insulin, the insulin itself, the alcohol used to cleanse the injection site or sterilize the syringe, the patient's injection technique, or the intermittent use of insulin. Spontaneous desensitization frequently occurs within a few weeks. Local irritation may be reduced by: changing to insulin without protein modifiers (the Lente series) or to insulins derived from another animal source; using unscented alcohol swabs or disposable syringes and needles; and checking the patient's injection technique. Acute rashes covering the whole body and anaphylactic symptoms are quite rare, but must be treated with antihistamines, epinephrine, and steroids.

Rotation of injection sites is important. Atrophy or hypertrophy of subcutaneous fat tissue may occur at the site of frequent insulin injections. The hypertrophic areas tend to be used more frequently by diabetic patients because the fat pad becomes anesthetized. In addition to the adverse cosmetic effects, the absorption rate of insulin from these sites becomes significantly prolonged and erratic. Loss of diabetic control may result, particularly in unstable, Type I diabetes.

Insulin resistance is an infrequent complication in the control of diabetic symptoms. Acute resistance may develop if the patient acquires an infection or experiences serious trauma, surgery, or emotional disturbances. This type of resistance subsides when the acute episode passes. Chronic insulin resistance may occur with the reinstitution of insulin therapy after a period of discontinuance. Resistance may be reduced by changing the animal sources of the insulin, using "purified" insulins, changing the use of glucocorticoids, or using specially prepared insulins with a slightly different chemical structure.

Availability

See Table 15.3.
In 1972, the American Diabetes Association recommended the elimination of production of U-40 and U-80 insulins. The U-80 insulins have been phased

Table 15.3
Commercially Available Forms of Insulin

TYPE OF INSULIN	MANU-FACTURER	STRENGTH (UNITS/ML)	SOURCE	IMPURITIES (PPM)	ONSET* (HR)	PEAK* (HR)	DURATION* (HR)	GLYCOSURIA†	HYPO-GLYCEMIA†
Fast-acting									
Insulin injection									
Actrapid	Novo	100	Pork	<10	0.5	2.5–5	8	Early AM[1]	Before lunch[3]
Insulin ("new")	Squibb	100	Pork	<25	0.5–1	3–6	6–8	Early AM[1]	Before lunch[3]
Insulin ("purified")	Squibb	40; 100	Pork	<10	0.5–1	3–6	6–8	Early AM[1]	Before lunch[3]
Regular Iletin I	Lilly	40, 100	Beef and pork	<25	0.5–1	3–6	6–8	Early AM[1]	Before lunch[3]
Regular Iletin II (Beef)	Lilly	100	Beef	<10	0.5–1	3–6	6–8	Early AM[1]	Before lunch[3]
Regular Iletin II (Pork)	Lilly	100; 500	Pork	<10	0.5–1	3–6	6–8	Early AM[1]	Before lunch[3]
Velosulin	Nordisk-USA	100	Pork	<10	0.5	1–3	8	Early AM[1]	Before lunch[3]
Prompt insulin zinc suspension									
Semilente Iletin I ("new")	Lilly	40; 100	Beef and pork	<25	0.5–1	4–6	12–16	Early AM[1]	Before lunch[3]
Semilente insulin	Squibb	100	Beef	<25	0.5–1	4–6	12–16	Early AM[1]	Before lunch[3]
Semitard	Novo	100	Pork	<10	1.5	5–10	16	Early AM[1]	Before lunch[3]
Intermediate-acting									
Isophane insulin suspension (NPH)									
Insulatard	Nordisk-USA	100	Pork	<10	1.5	4–12	24	Before lunch[2]	3 PM to supper[3]
Isophane insulin NPH ("purified")	Squibb	100	Beef	<10	1–1.5	8–12	24	Before lunch[2]	3 PM to supper[3]
NPH Iletin I	Lilly	40; 100	Beef and pork	<25	1–1.5	8–12	24	Before lunch[3]	3 PM to supper[3]
NPH Iletin II	Lilly	100	Beef or pork	<10	1–1.5	8–12	24	Before lunch[2]	3 PM to supper[3]
Protophane NPH	Novo	100	Pork	<10	1.5	4–12	24	Before lunch[2]	3 PM to supper[3]
Isophane insulin suspension and insulin injection									
Mixtard	Nordisk-USA	100	Pork	<10	0.5	4–8	24	Before lunch[2]	3 PM to supper[3]
Insulin zinc suspension									
Lentard	Nordisk-USA	100	Pork and beef	<10	2.5	7–15	24	Before lunch[2]	3 PM to supper[3]
Lente Iletin	Lilly	40; 100	Pork and beef	<25	1–1.5	8–12	24	Before lunch[2]	3 PM to supper[3]
Lente Iletin I	Lilly	100	Beef or pork	<25	1–1.5	8–12	24	Before lunch[2]	3 PM to supper[3]

(Table continues on p. 370.)

Table 15.3 (*continued*)

TYPE OF INSULIN	MANU-FACTURER	STRENGTH (UNITS/ML)	SOURCE	IMPURITIES (PPM)	ONSET* (HR)	PEAK* (HR)	DURATION* (HR)	GLYCOSURIA†	HYPO-GLYCEMIA†
Intermediate-acting (*continued*)									
Lente Iletin II	Lilly	100	Beef or pork	<10	1–1.5	8–12	24	Before lunch[2]	3 PM to supper[3]
Lente insulin	Squibb	40; 100	Beef	<10	1–1.5	8–12	24	Before lunch[2]	3 PM to supper[3]
Monotard	Novo	100	Pork	<10	2.5	7–15	22	Before lunch[2]	3 PM to supper[3]
Long-acting									
Protamine zinc insulin suspension									
Protamine zinc Iletin I	Lilly	40; 100	Beef and pork	<25	1–8	16–24	36+	Supper to bedtime[2]	2 AM to breakfast[3]
Protamine zinc Iletin II	Lilly	100	Beef or pork	<10	1–8	16–24	36+	Supper to bedtime[2]	2 AM to breakfast[3]
Protamine zinc insulin	Squibb	100	Beef and pork	<25	4–8	16–24	36+	Supper to bedtime[2]	2 AM to breakfast[3]
Extended insulin zinc suspension									
Ultralente Iletin I	Lilly	40; 100	Beef and pork	<25	4–8	16–18	36+	Supper to bedtime[2]	2 AM to breakfast[3]
Ultralente insulin	Squibb	100	Beef	<25	4–8	16–18	36+	Supper to bedtime[2]	2 AM to breakfast[3]
Ultratard	Novo	100	Beef	<10	4	10–30	36	Supper to bedtime[2]	2 AM to breakfast[3]

* The times listed are averages based on a newly diagnosed diabetic patient. Factors modifying these times include patient variation, site and route of administration and dosage.

† Most frequently occurs when insulin is administered at (1) bedtime the previous night, (2) before breakfast the previous day, (3) before breakfast the same day.

out and replaced by U-100 insulin. The U-40 concentration is still available for patients who require very small doses of insulin and for older Type I diabetics whose dosages are adjusted to it. Replacement with the U-100 form for all types of insulin will help reduce the chance of patient error in using multiple dosage forms and dually calibrated syringes. U-500 regular insulin (from pork) is also available for those patients with a resistance to insulin.

Over the past decade, significant progress has been made in improving the purity of insulin in an attempt to reduce allergenicity. Conventional insulins have always contained varying concentrations, greater than 10,000 parts per million (ppm), of proinsulin, glucagon, somatostatin, and other proteins from the pancreas. The FDA has named the more highly refined products, with less than 10 ppm of proinsulin, as "purified." All conventional insulins are now "cleaner," with less than

25 ppm of proinsulin content (see Table 15.3). Because purified insulins are more expensive and in limited supply, their use should be restricted to patients with specific indications, such as those using insulin for a short period of time (e.g., gestational diabetics, Type II diabetics undergoing surgery, nondiabetics receiving insulin as part of hyperalimentation solutions), patients with insulin resistance (using more than 100 to 200 units per day), patients with local cutaneous allergic reactions, patients with significant lipodystrophy, patients with renal transplants, and patients desensitized to pork insulin. The response is highly variable, but patients usually require less insulin.

Biosynthetic human insulin is now available for selected patients. Onset of action may be slightly more rapid than pork insulin and it is expected to have fewer allergic reactions associated with it than beef and pork insulins. The primary long-range advantage of human insulin is that a new source of insulin is now available to help meet a predicted worldwide shortage in the next decade.

All preparations of insulin (except biosynthetic insulin) are extracted from animal pancreas. The predominant sources are beef and pork, but sheep and fish may also be used. The extract is bioassayed, and the potencies are adjusted to provide concentrations of 40 units/ml (U-40), 100 units/ml (U-100), or 500 units/ml (U-500). Insulin can be modified by adding protein or protamine or by precipitating it in varying concentrations of zinc chloride. Depending on the amount of protamine used, and the type of crystals, insulin can be adjusted to have a short, intermediate, or long duration of action. See Table 15.3 for a comparison of commercially available forms of insulin.

Types of Insulin

- *Regular insulin* is used for its immediate onset of activity and short duration of action. It is the only form of insulin that is a clear solution (not a cloudy suspension). Also, it is the *only* dosage form of insulin that may be injected by *intravenous* as well as *subcutaneous* routes of administration. See Table 15.3 for the activity of the regular insulins, and Table 15.4 for mixing compatibility with other insulins.
- *Lente insulins* are derived from a manufacturing process that produces two physical forms, one crystalline and the other noncrystalline. The long-acting, crystalline form is marketed as *Ultralente*; the noncrystalline, fast acting compound is available as *Semilente*. The intermediate acting *Lente* insulin is a mixture containing approximately 30% noncrystalline Semilente and 70% crystalline Ultralente insulins.
- *Neutral protamine hagedorn (NPH) insulin* is an intermediate-acting insulin containing specific amounts of insulin and protamine. The activity of NPH is similar to that of a mixture of regular insulin and protamine zinc insulin (see Tables 15.3 and 15.4).
- *Protamine zinc insulin (PZI)* is modified by a manufacturing process to make it poorly soluble and slowly absorbed when injected subcutaneously. This process gives it a slow onset of action, but a long duration of activity (see Table 15.3).

Dosage and Administration

Maintenance Therapy for Newly Diagnosed Diabetic Patients. After ketoacidosis and hyperglycemia have been controlled and the patient can tolerate oral feedings, determine the total amount of regular insulin needed in 24 hours. The usual initial dose is 10 to 20

Table 15.4
Compatibility of Insulin Combinations

COMBINATION	RATIO	MIX BEFORE ADMINISTRATION
Regular + NPH	Any combination	2 to 3 months*
Regular + Lente	Any combination	2 to 3 months*
Regular + PZI†	1:1 = action like PZI alone	Immediately
	2:1 = action like NPH	Immediately
	3:1 = action like NPH + regular	Immediately
Lentes	Any combination	Stable indefinitely

* Must be used immediately to retain properties of regular insulin.

† PZI contains excess protamine that binds with regular insulin, prolonging the activity of regular insulin. Regular and PZI should not be mixed, but administered at separate sites at approximately the same time.

units of regular insulin, SC. Subsequent doses, administered one half hour before meals and at bedtime, are based on blood glucose and urine glucose levels. After control is established, the patient is converted to intermediate acting insulin, administered in doses that are 65% to 75% of the total dose of regular insulin required in 24 hours. Regular insulin is used as a supplement based on urine glucose levels. Adjustments in the intermediate acting insulin doses will be necessary. Divided doses (two-thirds in the morning, one-third in the evening) or combination therapy, using a mixture of insulins (see Table 15.4), may be required to maintain control, especially after the patient leaves the hospital and has changes in exercise and diet.

Maintenance Therapy for Known Diabetic Patients. Once ketoacidosis and hyperglycemia have been controlled and the patient can tolerate oral feedings, initiate maintenance therapy of one-half to two-thirds the previous dose of intermediate acting or combination insulin. Regular insulin is given as a supplement when indicated by blood sugar and urine glucose determinations. Adjust the maintenance dose of insulin until optimal control is achieved for the patient.

Note: "Control" of diabetic hyperglycemia is usually easier in the hospital than on an outpatient basis. Adjustments are almost always necessary after discharge due to changes in exercise and diet. Some physicians will allow patients to "spill," or exceed, a ¾% to 1% urine glucose while in the hospital so that after discharge a patient will spill a trace to ¼% as a result of changes in routine. Other physicians will stabilize a patient to a trace to ¼% urine glucose while in the hospital and drop the insulin dosage 5 units on discharge. There is less chance of a hypoglycemic reaction when using the second method, but regardless of the treatment program used, the discharged patient will have to be monitored frequently for medical and emotional adjustment to the new disease.

PATIENT CONCERNS: NURSING INTERVENTION/RATIONALE

Side Effects to Expect and Report

Hyperglycemia

Diabetic or prediabetic patients need to be monitored for the development of hyperglycemia, particularly during the early weeks of therapy.

Assess regularly for glycosuria and report if it occurs with any frequency.

Patients receiving insulin may require an adjustment in dosage.

Hypoglycemia

Monitor for the following signs of hypoglycemia: headache, nausea, weakness, hunger, lethargy, decreased coordination, general apprehension, sweating, blurred or double vision.

Hypoglycemia must be treated immediately. Mild symptoms may be controlled by the oral administration of a lump of sugar, orange juice, carbonated cola beverages, or candy. Severe symptoms may be relieved by the administration of intravenous glucose.

Notify the physician immediately if any of the above symptoms appear. The dosage of insulin may also have to be reduced.

Allergic Reactions

See Side Effects above. Notify the physician if allergic signs appear. Also check the patient's injection technique.

Lipodystrophies

Rotation of injection sites is important. Atrophy or hypertrophy of subcutaneous fat tissue may occur at the site of frequent insulin injections. The hypertrophic areas tend to be used more frequently by diabetic patients because the fat pad becomes anesthetized. In addition to the adverse cosmetic effects, the absorption rate of insulin from these sites becomes significantly prolonged and erratic. Loss of diabetic control may result, particularly in unstable Type I patients.

Administration

Mixing Insulins

See Chapter 6.

Administration Techniques

See Chapter 7.

Drug Interactions

Hyperglycemia

The following drugs may cause hyperglycemia (especially in prediabetic and diabetic patients); insulin dosages may require adjustment: acetazolamide, ethanol, corticosteroids, glucagon, dextrothyroxine, lithium, diuretics (thiazides, furosemide, bumetanide), oral contraceptives, diazoxide, phenothiazines, dobutamine, phenytoin, epinephrine, salicylates.

Diabetic or prediabetic patients need to be monitored for the development of hyperglycemia, particularly during the early weeks of therapy.

Assess regularly for glycosuria and report if it occurs with any frequency.

Hypoglycemia

The following drugs may cause hypoglycemia, thereby decreasing insulin requirements, in diabetic patients: acetaminophen, anabolic steroids (Dianabol, Durabolin), guanethidine, monoamine-oxidase inhibitors, propranolol, salicylates.

Monitor for the following signs of hypoglycemia: headache, nausea, weakness, hunger, lethargy, decreased coordination, general apprehension, sweating, blurred or double vision.

Notify the physician if any of the above symptoms appear.

Beta Adrenergic Blocking Agents

Beta adrenergic blocking agents (propranolol, timolol, nadolol, pindolol, others) may induce hypoglycemia, but may also mask many of the symptoms of hypoglycemia. Notify the physician if you suspect that any of the above symptoms appear intermittently.

Oral Hypoglycemic Agents

All of the oral hypoglycemic agents currently available are sulfonylureas. Sulfonylureas produce hypoglycemia by stimulating the release of insulin from the beta cells of the pancreas. They are of no value in the Type I diabetic, but are effective in Type II diabetic patients where the pancreas still has the capacity to secrete insulin. Sulfonylureas may be effective in the treatment of Type II diabetes mellitus that cannot be controlled by diet alone if the patient is not susceptible to developing ketosis, acidosis, or infections. Patients most likely to benefit from oral hypoglycemic treatment are those who develop signs of diabetes after age 40 and who require less than 40 units of insulin per day.

Side Effects

Patients receiving oral hypoglycemic therapy are as susceptible to hypoglycemia as diabetic patients on insulin therapy. Consequently, blood sugar levels and urine sugar levels must be monitored closely, especially in the early stages of therapy.

Side effects of sulfonylureas are infrequent and generally mild. The more common adverse reactions include allergic skin reactions and gastrointestinal symptoms of nausea, vomiting, anorexia, heartburn, and abdominal cramps. Blood dyscrasias, hepatotoxicity, and hypersensitivity reactions have rarely been reported.

Availability

See Table 15.5.

Dosage and Administration

See Table 15.5.

Individual dosage adjustment is essential for the successful use of oral hypoglycemic agents. A patient should be given a 1 month trial on maximum doses of the sulfonylurea being used before the patient can be considered a primary failure. If a patient represents a secondary failure (a patient initially controlled on oral agents), changing to an alternative sulfonylurea is occasionally successful in controlling blood sugar.

PATIENT CONCERNS: NURSING INTERVENTION/RATIONALE

Side Effects to Expect

Nausea, Vomiting, Anorexia, Abdominal Cramps

These side effects are usually mild and tend to resolve with continued therapy. Encourage the patient not to discontinue therapy without first consulting the physician.

Side Effects to Report

Hypoglycemia

Monitor for the following signs of hypoglycemia: headache, nausea, weakness, hunger, lethargy, decreased coordination, general apprehension, sweating, blurred or double vision.

Hypoglycemia must be treated immediately. Mild symptoms may be controlled by the oral administration of a lump of sugar, orange juice, carbonated cola beverages, or candy. Severe symptoms may be relieved by the administration of intravenous glucose.

Notify the physician immediately if any of the above symptoms appear. The dosage of oral hypoglycemic agents may also have to be reduced.

Hepatotoxicity

The symptoms of hepatotoxicity are: anorexia, nausea, vomiting, jaundice, hepatomegaly, splenomegaly,

---

Table 15.5
Oral Hypoglycemic Agents

GENERIC NAME	BRAND NAME	AVAILABILITY	INITIAL DOSAGE	DOSAGE RANGE	DURATION* (HOURS)
Acetohexamide	Dymelor	Tablets: 250, 500 mg	0.5 g daily	0.25–1.5 g daily	12–18
Chlorpropamide	Diabinese	Tablets: 100, 250 mg	100 mg daily	100–750 mg daily	24–72
Tolazamide	Tolinase	Tablets: 100, 250, 500 mg	100 mg daily	0.1–1 g daily	12–16
Tolbutamide	Orinase Sk-Tolbutamide	Tablets: 250, 500 mg	1 g 2 times daily	0.25–3 g daily	6–12

* The times listed are averages based on a newly diagnosed diabetic patient. Factors modifying these times include patient variation and dosage.

and abnormal liver function tests (elevated bilirubin, SGOT, SGPT, alkaline phosphatase, prothrombin time).

Blood Dyscrasias

Routine laboratory studies (RBC, WBC, and differential counts) should be scheduled. Stress the need to return for this laboratory work.

Monitor for the development of a sore throat, fever, purpura, jaundice, or excessive and progressively increasing weakness.

Dermatologic Reactions

Report a rash or pruritus immediately. Withhold additional doses pending approval by the physician.

Administration

PO

Adjust the dosage based on blood and urine sugar levels.

Drug Interactions

Hypoglycemia

The following drugs may enhance the hypoglycemic effects of the sulfonylureas: ethanol, methandrostenolone, chloramphenicol, warfarin, propranolol, salicylates, sulfisoxazole, guanethidine, oxytetracycline, monoamine-oxidase inhibitors, and phenylbutazone.

Monitor for the following signs of hypoglycemia: headache, nausea, weakness, hunger, lethargy, decreased coordination, general apprehension, sweating, blurred or double vision.

Notify the physician if any of the above symptoms appear.

Hyperglycemia

The following drugs, when used concurrently with the sulfonylureas, may decrease the therapeutic effects of the sulfonylureas: corticosteroids, phenothiazines, diuretics, oral contraceptives, thyroid replacement hormones, phenytoin, salicylates, diazoxide, and lithium carbonate.

Diabetic or prediabetic patients need to be monitored for the development of hyperglycemia, particularly during the early weeks of therapy.

Assess regularly for glycosuria and report if it occurs with any frequency.

Patients receiving insulin may require an adjustment in dosage.

Beta Adrenergic Blocking Agents

Beta adrenergic blocking agents (propranolol, timolol, nadolol, pindolol, others) may induce hypoglycemia, but may also mask many of the symptoms of hypoglycemia. Notify the physician if you suspect that any of the above symptoms appear intermittently.

Alcohol

Ingestion of alcoholic beverages during sulfonylurea therapy may infrequently result in an Antabuse-like reaction, manifested by facial flushing, pounding headache, feeling of breathlessness, and nausea.

In patients who develop an Antabuse-like reaction to alcohol, the use of alcohol and preparations containing alcohol (such as over-the-counter cough medications and mouthwashes) should be avoided during therapy and up to 5 days after discontinuation of sulfonylurea therapy.

Thyroid Hormones

The Thyroid Gland

The thyroid gland is a large, reddish, ductless gland in front of and on either side of the trachea, or windpipe. It consists of two lateral lobes and a connecting isthmus and is roughly butterfly shaped. It is enclosed in a covering of areolar tissue. The thyroid is made up of numerous closed follicles containing colloid matter, and is surrounded by a vascular network. This gland is one of the most richly vascularized tissues in the body.

As with other endocrine glands, thyroid gland function is regulated by the hypothalamus and the anterior pituitary gland. The hypothalamus secretes *thyrotropin releasing hormone* (TRH), which stimulates the anterior pituitary gland to release *thyroid stimulating hormone* (TSH). TSH stimulates the thyroid gland to release its hormones triiodothyronine (T_3) and thyroxine (T_4).

The thyroid hormones regulate general body metabolism. Imbalance in thyroid hormone production may also interfere with the following body functions: growth and maturation; carbohydrate, protein, and lipid metabolism; thermal regulation; cardiovascular function; lactation; and reproduction.

Two general classes of drugs used to treat thyroid disorders are (1) those used to replace thyroid hormones in patients whose thyroid glandular function is inadequate to meet metabolic requirements (hypothyroidism), and (2) antithyroid agents used to suppress synthesis of thyroid hormones (hyperthyroidism). Thyroid hormone replacements available are levothyroxine (T$_4$), liothyronine (T$_3$), liotrix, thyroglobulin, and thyroid, USP. Antithyroid agents to be discussed include iodides, propylthiouracil, and methimazole.

General Nursing Considerations for Patients Receiving Thyroid Therapy

---

PATIENT CONCERNS: NURSING INTERVENTION/RATIONALE

Hypothyroidism

Hypothyroidism is the result of inadequate thyroid hormone production. It may be caused by excessive use of antithyroid drugs used to treat hyperthyroidism, radiation exposure, surgery, acute viral thyroiditis, or chronic thyroiditis.

Myxedema

Myxedema is hypothyroidism that occurs during adult life. The onset of symptoms is usually quite mild and vague. Patients develop a sense of slowness in motion, speech, and mental processes. They often develop more lethargic, sedentary habits; have decreased appetites; are constipated; cannot tolerate cold; gain weight; become weak; and fatigue easily. The body temperature may be subnormal; the skin becomes dry, coarse and thickened; and the face appears puffy. Patients often have decreased blood pressure and heart rate, and develop anemia and high cholesterol levels. These patients have an increased susceptibility to infection and are very sensitive to small doses of sedative-hypnotics, anesthetics, and narcotics.

Cretinism

Congenital hypothyroidism occurs when a child is born without a thyroid gland or one that is hypoactive. The historical name of this disease is *cretinism*. Fortunately, this disorder is becoming rare because most states require diagnostic testing of the newborn for hypothyroidism.

In breast-fed infants symptoms are usually not recognized until the child is weaned. Over the next several weeks, the infant develops muscular hypotonia, dyspnea, decreased appetite, retarded growth, and skin and hair changes. The bottle-fed infant becomes a poor feeder, sleeps excessively, develops bradycardia, subnormal temperature, lethargy, inactivity, and constipation. If the hypothyroidism lasts for several months, permanent mental retardation may result.

Parents of infants who are diagnosed promptly need reassurance that the disease is treatable, but must also understand the need for lifelong treatment.

Parents of infants who were not diagnosed promptly require psychological support as well as direction in providing for additional needs of the infant. The nurse must demonstrate acceptance of the impaired child by caring for the infant in an accepting, caring manner. Emphasize to the parents the normal characteristics the child possesses and teach them how to maximize the learning potential of the infant.

Above all, LISTEN to the parents' concerns. Allow the parents to express their feelings, and respond in a nonjudgmental manner.

Diagnosis

Although the symptoms of hypothyroidism are fairly classical, the final diagnosis is usually not made until diagnostic tests have been completed. These tests include drawing serum levels of circulating T$_3$ and T$_4$ hormones. If the levels are low, the patient is considered to be hypothyroid. Further diagnostic testing is required to determine the cause of thyroid hypofunction.

Treatment of Hypothyroidism

Hypothyroidism can be treated quite successfully by replacement of thyroid hormones (see individual agents). After therapy is initiated, the dosage of thyroid hormone is adjusted until serum levels of the thyroid hormones are within the normal range.

Patient Teaching Associated with Thyroid Hormone Therapy

Communication and Responsibility

Encourage open communication concerning frustrations and anger as the patient attempts to adjust to the diagnosis and the need for prolonged treatment. The patient must be guided to gain insight into the disorder in order to assume responsibility for the continuation of the treatment. Keep emphasizing the factors the patient can control to alter progression of the disease, including the following:

NUTRITIONAL STATUS

A high-protein diet, low in calories and cholesterol, is usually prescribed. A weight reduction plan may also be required to reduce obesity.

CONSTIPATION

Since constipation is quite common among hypothyroid patients, encourage them to eat foods that supply roughage in the form of fresh fruits and vegetables, whole grains, and cereals.

People with constipation frequently drink too little water. Encourage patients to drink 8 to 10 8-ounce glasses of water each day.

Do not encourage elderly patients to use bran or bran products. Due to decreased muscle tone, bran can cause a fecal impaction.

ACTIVITY AND EXERCISE

Hypothyroid patients are often quite sedentary. With the support of the physician, begin the patient on an exercise plan to develop a pattern of daily activity. As symptoms improve, the patient will start feeling more willing to participate in the activities.

ENVIRONMENT

During the severe stages of the disease, control stressors and keep the patient warm. Explain to the family the need to provide a quiet, structured environment because the patient lacks the ability to respond to change and anxiety producing situations. It is important to inform the patient and family that the patient will return to the preillness level of capability when the thyroid levels return to normal.

Expectations of Therapy

Discuss the expectations of therapy (e.g., gradually increased level of exercise and activity, control of constipation, improved intellectual level, relief of depression, normal blood pressure and pulse, reduced weight, ability to maintain activities of daily living and/or work).

Changes in Expectations

Assess changes in expectations as therapy progresses and the patient gains understanding and skill in the management of the diagnosis.

Changes in Therapy through Cooperative Goal-Setting

Work with the patient to encourage adherence to the prescribed treatment. (It may be necessary to work initially with family members since the patient may be experiencing some degree of altered mental status and apathy.) When the patient feels that a change should be made in a treatment plan, encourage discussion first with the physician.

WRITTEN RECORD

Enlist the patient's (or family's) aid in developing and maintaining a written record of monitoring parameters. See Table 15.6 for a sample written record.

Prior to discharge, the nurse should start the recording process with the family and patient. Emphasize that the baseline data is a starting point, from which any deviations should be reported. The nurse should explain, in detail, how this data can assist the physician in managing the thyroid disorder. Patients should be encouraged to take this record on follow-up visits.

FOSTERING COMPLIANCE

Throughout the hospitalization, discuss medication information and how it will benefit the course of treatment. Seek cooperation and understanding of the following points so that medication compliance may be enhanced:

1. Name.
2. Dosage.
3. Route and administration times.
4. Anticipated therapeutic response: a gradual return to "normal" for the individual. Therapeutic response is usually noted after a short time on the medication. Reversal of symptoms should be complete within two to three months.
5. Side effects to expect.
6. Side effects to report (e.g., symptoms of hyperthyroidism). Notify the physician if the resting pulse rate is 100 or above and do not give the thyroid medication until specific directions are given.
7. What to do if a dosage is missed.
8. When, how, or if to refill the medication.

Table 15.6

Example of a Written Record for Patients Receiving Thyroid Medications

Medications	Color	To be taken

Name _____

Physician _____

Physician's phone _____

Next appt.* _____

Parameters	Day of discharge							Comments
Pulse								
Temperature								
Weight								
Desire to eat: Eat all the time Normal None 10 5 1								
Use this scale to rate tolerance of Heat / Cold Cannot tolerate Moderate toleration Normal 10 5 1								
Fatigue level: Tired all the time Normal Not tired; cannot stop 10 5 1								
Skin condition: Dry, leathery Oily Normal								
How I feel about life: Feel awful Getting better Feel good 10 5 1								
Tolerance for exercise: Difficulty breathing with exercise Normal Endless energy, no problem 10 5 1								

*Please bring this record with you to your next appointment.
Use the back of this sheet for additional information.

DIFFICULTY IN COMPREHENSION

If it is evident that the patient and/or family does not understand all aspects of the continuing therapy being prescribed (e.g., administration and monitoring of medications, exercises, diets, follow-up appointments for laboratory work, and monitoring by the physician), consider the use of social service or visiting nurse agencies.

ASSOCIATED TEACHING

Give the patient the following instructions:

Always inform the physician or dentist of any prescription or over-the-counter medication being taken. Over-the-counter medications should not be taken without first discussing them with a physician or pharmacist.

Always report side effects of rash, itching, or hives immediately. Nausea, vomiting, or diarrhea should also be reported for the physician's evaluation if it is a new symptom.

Take all of the medication as prescribed for the full course of treatment. Do not discontinue use when feeling improved; do not save for future use; do not give your medicine to another individual. Sudden discontinuation of certain medications may produce harmful effects.

Keep all medications out of reach of children.

If pregnancy is suspected, consult an obstetrician as soon as possible about continuation of medication therapy.

At Discharge

Items to be sent home with the patient should:

1. Have written instructions for use.
2. Be labeled in language and size of print appropriate for the patient.
3. If needed, include identification cards or bracelets.
4. Include a list of additional supplies that may need to be purchased after discharge.
5. Include a schedule for follow-up appointments.

Thyroid Replacement Hormones

Levothyroxine (le-vo-thy-rok'sen)
(Synthroid) (sin'throyd), *(Letter)*

Levothyroxine (T_4) is one of the two primary hormones secreted by the thyroid gland. It is partially metabolized to liothyronine (T_3), so that therapy with levothyroxine provides physiologic replacement of both hormones. It is now considered to be the drug of choice for hormone replacement in hypothyroidism.

Side Effects

Adverse effects of thyroid replacement preparations are dose related and may occur 1 to 3 weeks after changes in therapy have been initiated. Symptoms of adverse effects are tachycardia, anxiety, weight loss, abdominal cramping and diarrhea, cardiac palpitations, arrhythmias, angina pectoris, fever, and intolerance to heat.

Availability

PO—0.025, 0.05, 0.1, 0.125, 0.15, 0.175, 0.2, and 0.3 mg tablets.
INJ—100 µg/ml in 6 and 10 ml vials.

Dosage and Administration

Adult
PO—Therapy may be initiated in low doses of 0.025 mg daily. Dosages are gradually increased over the next few weeks to an average daily maintenance dose of 0.1 to 0.2 mg.

Nursing Interventions

See also General Nursing Considerations for Patients Receiving Thyroid Therapy.

**PATIENT CONCERNS:
NURSING INTERVENTION/RATIONALE**

Side Effects to Expect and Report

Signs of Hyperthyroidism

See Side Effects above. These signs are all indications of excessive thyroid replacement. Symptoms may require discontinuation of therapy. Patients may require up to a month without medication for toxic effects to fully dissipate.

Therapy must be restarted at lower dosages after symptoms have stopped.

Dosage and Administration

PO

The age of the patient, severity of hypothyroidism, and other concurrent medical conditions will determine the initial dosage and the interval of time necessary before increasing the dosage. Hypothyroid patients are quite sensitive to replacement of thyroid hormones. Monitor patients closely for adverse effects.

Drug Interactions

Warfarin

Patients with hypothyroidism require larger doses of anticoagulants. If thyroid replacement therapy is initiated while the patient is receiving warfarin therapy, the patient should have frequent prothrombin time determinations and should be counseled to observe closely for development of petechiae, ecchymoses, nosebleeds, bleeding gums, dark tarry stools, and bright red or "coffee-ground" emesis.

The dosage of warfarin may have to be reduced by one-third to one-half over the next 1 to 4 weeks.

Digitalis Glycosides

Patients with hypothyroidism require smaller doses of digitalis preparations. If thyroid replacement therapy is started while receiving digitalis glycosides, a gradual increase in the glycoside will be necessary to maintain adequate therapeutic activity.

Cholestyramine

To prevent binding of thyroid hormones by cholestyramine, administer at least 4 hours apart.

Hyperglycemia

Diabetic or prediabetic patients need to be monitored for the development of hyperglycemia, particularly during the early weeks of therapy.

Assess regularly for glycosuria and report if it occurs with any frequency.

Patients receiving oral hypoglycemic agents or insulin may require an adjustment in dosage.

Liothyronine (ly-o-thy'ro-neen)
(Cytomel) (sy'to-mel)

Liothyronine is a synthetic form of the natural thyroid hormone, triiodothyronine, T_3. Its onset of action is more rapid than levothyroxine's and it is occasionally used as a thyroid hormone replacement when prompt action is necessary. It is not recommended for patients with cardiovascular disease unless a rapid onset of activity is deemed essential.

Side Effects

See levothyroxine.

Availability

PO—5, 25, and 50 μg tablets.

Dosage and Administration

Adult
PO—The usual starting dose depends on the particular condition but is usually 25 μg daily. The usual maintenance dose is 25 to 75 μg daily.

Drug Interactions

See levothyroxine.

Nursing Interventions

See levothyroxine.

Liotrix (ly'o-triks)
(Euthroid) (you'throyd)
(Thyrolar) (thy'ro-lar)

This is a synthetic mixture of levothyroxine and liothyronine in a ratio of 4 to 1, respectively. A few endocrinologists prefer this combination because of the standardized content of the two hormones that results in consistent laboratory test results, more in agreement with the patient's clinical response. The two available commercial preparations of liotrix contain different amounts of each ingredient, so patients should not be changed from one preparation to the other unless differences in potency are considered.

Side Effects

See levothyroxine.

Availability

PO—Euthroid is available in 4 combination tablet strengths, and Thyrolar is available in 5 combination tablet strengths. See the manufacturer's literature for the strengths of each of the combination tablets.

Dosage and Administration

Adult
PO—Dosage range is 60 to 180 μg of levothyroxine and 15 to 45 μg of liothyronine, taken as one tablet daily, usually at breakfast.

Drug Interactions

See levothyroxine.

Nursing Interventions

See levothyroxine.

Thyroglobulin (thy-ro-glob'you-lin)
(Proloid) (pro'loyd)

Thyroglobulin is a protein obtained from a purified extract of hog thyroid. It contains thyroxine and tri-iodothyronine. It is effective in the treatment of inadequate thyroid hormone production. The potency of thyroglobulin is equal to that of thyroid, USP, but is twice as costly.

Side Effects

See levothyroxine.

Availability

PO—32, 65, 100, 130, and 200 mg tablets.

Dosage and Administration

Adult
PO—Dosage should be started in small amounts and increased gradually. Maintenance dose is 32 to 200 mg taken once daily, usually in the morning.

Drug Interactions

See levothyroxine.

Nursing Interventions

See levothyroxine.

Thyroid, USP

Thyroid, USP (desiccated thyroid) is derived from pig, beef, and sheep thyroid glands. Thyroid is the oldest thyroid hormone replacement available and the least expensive. Because of its lack of purity, uniformity, and stability, however, it is generally not the drug of choice for the initiation of thyroid replacement therapy.

Side Effects

See levothyroxine.

Availability

PO—16, 32, 65, 98, 130, 195, 260, and 325 mg tablets; 65, 130, and 195 mg enteric coated tablets.

Dosage and Administration

Adult
PO—Usual dosage range: 65 to 195 mg daily.

Drug Interactions

See levothyroxine.

Nursing Interventions

See levothyroxine.

Antithyroid Drugs

The synthesis of thyroid hormones and their maintenance in the bloodstream in sufficient amounts depend on sufficient iodine intake through food and water. Iodine is converted to iodide and stored in the thyroid gland before reaching the circulation.

Excessive formation of thyroid hormones and their escape into the circulatory system causes hyperthyroidism, also known as thyrotoxicosis, exophthalmic goiter, or Graves disease. Symptoms include increased metabolic rate, increased pulse rate (to perhaps 140 beats per minute), increased body temperature, restlessness, nervousness, anxiety, sweating, muscle weakness and tremors, and a complaint of feeling too warm. This condition is treated with antithyroid drugs or surgical removal of the thyroid gland.

An *antithyroid* drug is a chemical agent that interferes with the formation or release of the hormones produced by the thyroid gland.

General Nursing Considerations for Patients Receiving Antithyroid Therapy

PATIENT CONCERNS: NURSING INTERVENTION/RATIONALE

Hyperthyroidism

Hyperthyroidism is caused by excess production of thyroid hormones. Disorders that may cause hyperactivity of the thyroid gland are Graves disease, nodular goiter, thyroiditis, thyroid carcinoma, overdoses of thyroid hormones, and tumors of the pituitary gland.

The clinical manifestations of hyperthyroidism are rapid, bounding pulse (even during sleep); cardiac enlargement; palpitations; and arrhythmias. Patients are nervous and easily agitated. They develop tremors, a low grade fever, and weight loss, despite an increased appetite. Hyperactive reflexes and insomnia are also usually present. Patients are intolerant of heat; the skin is warm, flushed, and moist, with increased sweating; edema of the tissues around the eyeballs produces characteristic eye changes, including exophthalmos. Patients develop amenorrhea, dyspnea with minor exertion, hoarse, rapid speech, and have an increased susceptibility to infection.

Diagnosis

Elevated circulating thyroid hormone tests easily diagnose the hyperthyroidism. Further diagnostic studies are required to determine the cause of hyperthyroidism.

Treatment

Three types of treatment can be used to alter the hyperthyroid state: subtotal thyroidectomy, radioactive iodine, and/or antithyroid medications. Until treatment is under way, the patient requires nutritional and psychological support.

NUTRITIONAL STATUS

A high calorie diet (4,000 to 5,000 calories daily) with balanced nutrients may be required. Minimize stimulants such as tea, coffee, colas, and tobacco.

If the patient has diarrhea, avoid foods with a laxative effect (bran products, raw fruits and vegetables) if not tolerated.

Perform daily weights at the same time, in the same type of clothing on the same scale.

ACTIVITY AND EXERCISE

Promote rest and limit the extent of ambulation in order to prevent exhaustion. If an activity produces fatigue, discourage the patient from further exposures until the disease process responds to therapy.

PSYCHOLOGICAL ASPECTS

The hyperactivity caused by the disease requires the nurse to approach the patient calmly. Provide the family with an explanation of the patient's behavior.

Support the patient in working with the change in self-image. Assist with grooming and offer reassurance that treatment will allow a return to the preillness state.

ENVIRONMENT

Providing adequate rest is a nursing challenge because of the hyperactivity associated with the disease. Try to provide a cool room in a quiet area, and encourage the use of frequent back rubs, warm milk, and constructive methods to release nervous tension without overexerting the patient.

Patient Teaching Associated with Antithyroid Therapy

Communication and Responsibility

Encourage open communication concerning frustrations and anger as the patient attempts to adjust to the diagnosis and the need for prolonged treatment. The patient must be guided to gain insight into the disorder in order to assume responsibility for the continuation of the treatment. Keep emphasizing the factors the patient can control to alter progression of the disease, including maintenance of general health, nutritional needs, adequate rest, and continuation of the prescribed medication therapy as well as appropriate limitations on exercise.

Expectations of Therapy

Discuss with the patient the expectations of therapy (e.g., level of exercise, relief of dyspnea, reduction in tremors and irritability, return of energy without exhaustion, return of menses, ability to maintain activities of daily living and work).

Changes in Expectations

Assess changes in expectations as therapy progresses and the patient gains understanding and skill in the management of the diagnosis.

Changes in Therapy through Cooperative Goal-Setting

Work with the patient to encourage adherence to the prescribed treatment. When the patient feels that a change should be made in a treatment plan, encourage discussion first with the physician.

WRITTEN RECORD

Enlist the patient's aid in developing and maintaining a written record of monitoring parameters for discussion with the physician. See Table 15.7 for a sample written record. Patients should be encouraged to take this record on follow-up visits.

FOSTERING COMPLIANCE

Throughout the hospitalization, discuss medication information and how it will benefit the course of treatment. Seek cooperation and understanding of the following points so that medication compliance may be enhanced:

1. Name.
2. Dosage.
3. Route and administration times.
4. Anticipated therapeutic response.
5. Side effects to expect (e.g., headache, loss of taste).
6. Side effects to report (e.g., sore throat, fever, general malaise).
7. What to do if a dosage is missed.
8. When, how, or if to refill the medication.

DIFFICULTY IN COMPREHENSION

If it is evident that the patient and/or family does not understand all aspects of the continuing therapy being prescribed (e.g., administration and monitoring of medications, exercises, diets, follow-up appointments for laboratory work, and monitoring by the physician), consider use of social service or visiting nurse agencies.

ASSOCIATED TEACHING

Give the patient the following instructions:

Always inform the physician or dentist of any prescription or over-the-counter medication being taken. Over-the-counter medications should not be taken without first discussing them with a physician or pharmacist.

Always report side effects of rash, itching, or hives immediately. Nausea, vomiting, and diarrhea should also be reported for the physician's evaluation if it is a new symptom.

Take all of the medication as prescribed for the full course of treatment. Do not discontinue use when feeling improved; do not save for future use; do not give your medicine to another individual. Sudden discontinuation of certain medications may produce harmful effects.

Keep all medications out of reach of children.

If pregnancy is suspected, consult an obstetrician as soon as possible about continuation of medication therapy.

At Discharge

Items to be sent home with the patient should:

1. Have written instructions for use
2. Be labeled in language and size of print appropriate for the patient
3. If needed, include identification cards or bracelets
4. Include a list of additional supplies that may need to be purchased after discharge
5. Include a schedule for follow-up appointments

Radioactive Iodine (^{131}I)

Iodine-131 (^{131}I) is a radioactive isotope of iodine. When administered, it is absorbed into the thyroid gland in high concentrations. The liberated radioactivity destroys the hyperactive thyroid tissue, with essentially no damage to other tissues in the body.

Radioactive iodine is most commonly used for treating hyperthyroidism in the following individuals: older patients who are beyond the childbearing years, those with severe complicating diseases, those with recurrent hyperthyroidism after previous thyroid surgery, those who are poor surgical risks, and those who have unusually small thyroid glands.

Side Effects

Side effects include radioactive thyroiditis, which causes tenderness over the thyroid area and occurs during the first few days or few weeks after radioactive iodine therapy. Hyperthyroidism seldom recurs after therapy but it is possible, and can be especially dangerous in the patient with severe heart disease. Many patients who receive radioactive iodine develop hypothyroidism, which requres thyroid hormone replacement therapy.

Nursing Interventions

See also General Nursing Considerations for Patients Receiving Thyroid and Antithyroid Therapy.

Table 15.7

Example of a Written Record for Patients Receiving Antithyroid Medication

Medications	Color	To be taken

Name _____

Physician _____

Physician's phone _____

Next appt.* _____

Parameters	Day of discharge							Comments
Pulse								
Temperature								
Weight								
Desire to eat: Eat all the time Normal None ├──────┼──────┤ 10 5 1								
Use this scale to rate tolerance of Heat Cold Cannot tolerate Moderate toleration Normal ├──────┼──────┤ 10 5 1								
Fatigue level: Tired all the time Normal Not tired; cannot stop ├──────┼──────┤ 10 5 1								
Skin condition: Dry, leathery Oily Normal								
How I feel about life: Feel awful Getting better Feel good ├──────┼──────┤ 10 5 1								
Tolerance for exercise: Difficulty breathing with exercise Normal Endless energy, no problem ├──────┼──────┤ 10 5 1								

*Please bring this record with you to your next appointment.
Use the back of this sheet for additional information.

PATIENT CONCERNS: NURSING INTERVENTION/RATIONALE

Administration of Radioactive Iodine

Administration of radioactive iodine preparations seems simple: it is added to water and swallowed like a drink of water. It has no color or taste. The radiation, however, is quite dangerous.

- Minimize exposure as much as possible. Wear rubber gloves whenever administering radioactive iodine or disposing of the patient's excreta.
- If the radioactive iodine or the patient's excreta should spill, follow hospital policy. In general, collect the clothing, bedding, bedpan, urinal, and any other contaminated materials and place them in special containers for radioactive waste disposal.
- AVOID SPILLS! REPORT ANY ACCIDENTAL CONTAMINATION AT ONCE TO YOUR SUPERVISOR, HEAD NURSE, TEAM LEADER, OR INSTRUCTOR AND FOLLOW DIRECTIONS FOR HOSPITAL CONTAMINATION CLEAN-UP TECHNIQUE.
- Fill out an incident report.

Propylthiouracil (pro-pil-thy-o-you'rah-sil) *(PTU, Propacil)*

Propylthiouracil is an antithyroid agent that acts by blocking synthesis of T_3 and T_4 in the thyroid gland. Propylthiouracil does not destroy any T_3 or T_4 already produced, so there is usually a latent period of a few days to 2 weeks before symptoms improve once therapy is started. Propylthiouracil may be used for long-term treatment of hyperthyroidism or for short-term treatment prior to subtotal thyroidectomy.

Side Effects

The most common reaction (in 5% of all patients) that occurs with PTU is a urpuric, maculopapular skin eruption. Occasionally patients develop headaches, a loss of sense of taste, muscle and joint aches, and enlargement of the salivary glands and lymph nodes in the neck. Rarely, propylthiouracil may cause bone marrow suppression, hepatotoxicity, or nephrotoxicity.

Availability

PO—50 mg tablets.

Dosage and Administration

Adult
PO—Initially 100 to 150 mg every 6 to 8 hours. Dosage ranges up to 900 mg daily. The maintenance dose is 50 mg 2 or 3 times daily.

Nursing Interventions

See also General Nursing Considerations for Patients Receiving Thyroid and Antithyroid Therapy.

PATIENT CONCERNS: NURSING INTERVENTION/RATIONALE

Side Effects to Expect and Report

Purpuric, Maculopapular Rash

This skin eruption often occurs during the first 2 weeks of therapy and usually revolves spontaneously, without treatment. If pruritus becomes severe, a change to methimazole may be necessary. Cross-sensitivity is uncommon.

Headaches, Salivary and Lymph Node Enlargement, Loss of Taste

These side effects are usually mild and tend to resolve with continued therapy. Encourage the patient not to discontinue therapy without first consulting the physician.

Bone Marrow Suppression

Routine laboratory studies (RBC, WBC, and differential counts) should be scheduled. Stress returning for this laboratory work.

Monitor the patient for the development of a sore throat, fever, purpura, jaundice, or excessive, progressive weakness.

Hepatotoxicity

The symptoms of hepatotoxicity are: anorexia, nausea, vomiting, jaundice, hepatomegaly, splenomegaly, and abnormal liver function tests (e.g., elevated bilirubin, SGOT, SGPT, alkaline phosphatase, prothrombin time).

Nephrotoxicity

Monitor urinalyses and kidney function tests for abnormal results. Report increased BUN and creatinine, decreased urine output or decreased specific gravity (despite amount of fluid intake), casts or protein in the urine, frank blood or smoky-colored urine, or RBCs in excess of 0–3 on the urinalysis report.

Drug Interactions
Warfarin

Patients with hyperthyroidism require larger doses of anticoagulants. If antithyroid therapy is initiated while the patient is receiving warfarin therapy, the patient should have frequent prothrombin time determinations and should be counseled to observe closely for development of petechiae, ecchymoses, nosebleeds, bleeding gums, dark tarry stools, and bright red or "coffeeground" emesis.

The dosage of warfarin may have to be reduced over the next 1 to 4 weeks.

Digitalis Glycosides

Patients with hyperthyroidism require larger doses of digitalis preparations. If antithyroid replacement therapy is started while receiving digitalis glycosides, a gradual reduction in the glycoside will be necessary to prevent signs of toxicity. Monitor for the development of arrhythmias, bradycardia, increased fatigue, or nausea and vomiting.

Methimazole (meth-im'ah-zoal)
(Tapazole) (tap'ah-zoal)

Methimazole is another antithyroid agent similar in uses and side effects to propylthiouracil. It is effective for treatment of hyperthyroidism in preparation for subtotal thyroidectomy or radioactive iodine therapy.

Side Effects

See propylthiouracil.

Availability

PO—5 and 10 mg tablets

Dosage and Administration

Adult
PO—Initially 5 to 20 mg every 8 hours. Daily maintenance dosage is 5 to 15 mg.

Drug Interactions

See propylthiouracil.

Nursing Interventions

See propylthiouracil.

Corticosteroids

Corticosteroids are hormones secreted by the adrenal cortex of the adrenal gland. Corticosteroids are divided into two categories based on structure and biologic activity. The mineralocorticoids (desoxycorticosterone, aldosterone) are used to maintain fluid and electrolyte balance and to treat adrenal insufficiency caused by hypopituitarism or Addison disease. The glucocorticoids (cortisone, hydrocortisone, prednisone, others) are used to regulate carbohydrate, protein, and fat metabolism. Glucocorticoids have antiinflammatory and antiallergic activity and are prescribed for the relief of symptoms of rheumatoid arthritis, adrenal insufficiency, severe psoriasis, urticaria, chronic eczema, multiple myeloma, Hodgkin's disease, leukemias, and collagen diseases (Table 15.8).

General Nursing Considerations for Patients Receiving Corticosteroids

Minimum assessment data for patients receiving corticosteroids include baseline weights, blood pressure, and electrolyte studies. Monitoring of all aspects of intake, output, diet, electrolyte balance, and state of hydration are important to the long-term success of corticosteroid therapy.

PATIENT CONCERNS:
NURSING INTERVENTION/RATIONALE

Baseline Assessment
and Monitoring Parameters

Weight

Obtain the patient's weight on admission and use as a baseline in assessing therapy. Patients receiving corticosteroids have a tendency to accumulate fluid and gain weight, so the daily weights are an important tool in assessing ongoing therapy. Always perform daily weights

Table 15.8
*Corticosteroid Preparations**

GENERIC NAME	BRAND NAMES	DOSAGE FORMS
Betamethasone	Celestone, Valisone, Diprosone	Tablets, syrup, injection, cream, ointment, lotion, aerosol
Cortisone	Cortone	Tablets, injection
Desoxycorticosterone	Doca, Percorten	Injection
Dexamethasone	Decadron, Dexone, Hexadrol, Solurex, Dezone	Injection, cream, ointment, aerosol
Fludrocortisone	Florinef	Tablets
Fluocinolone	Fluonid, Synalar	Ointment, cream, solution
Flumethasone	Locorten	Cream
Fluprednisolone	Alphadrol	Tablets
Flurandrenolide	Cordran	Cream, ointment, tape, solution
Hydrocortisone (cortisol)	Cortef, Hydrocortone, Solu-Cortef, others	Tablets, suspension, injection, enema, gel, cream, ointment, lotion
Methylprednisolone	A-Methapred, Solu-Medrol, D-Med, Depo-Medrol	Tablets, injection, enema, ointment, cream, aerosol
Paramethasone	Haldrone	Tablets
Prednisolone	Hydeltrasol, Delta-Cortef, Sterane, others	Tablets, injection, cream, aerosol
Prednisone	Deltasone, Fernisone, Meticorten, Cortan, Orasone, Paracort, others	Tablets
Triamcinolone	Aristocort, Kenalog, Kenacort, Trilone, Amcort, others	Tablets, syrup, injection, ointment, cream, lotion, gel, aerosol

* For ophthalmic preparations, see Chapter 17.

1. Using the same scale
2. Using the same approximate weight of clothing
3. At the same time of day

Blood Pressure

Take a baseline blood pressure reading in both the supine and sitting positions. Since patients receiving corticosteroids accumulate fluid and gain weight, hypertension may develop. Periodic assessment of the blood pressure will be necessary.

Intake

Accurate I/O records should be kept during every shift, and totaled every 24 hours, for all patients receiving corticosteroid therapy. Measure and record *accurately* all fluids taken (oral, parenteral, rectal, and via tubes). Ice chips and foods, such as Jell-O, that turn to a liquid state need to be included. Irrigation solutions should be carefully measured, so that the difference between the amount instilled and that returned can be recorded as intake.

Remember to enlist the assistance of the patient, family, or other visitors in this process. Ask them to keep a record of how many glasses of water, glasses of juice, or cups of coffee were consumed. Then convert these to milliliters.

Output

Record all output from the mouth, urethra, rectum, wounds, and tubes (e.g., surgical drains, nasogastric tubes, indwelling catheters).

- Consistency, color, and quantity of liquid stools should be recorded.
- Urine output should include information on quantity, color, pH, odor, and specific gravity.
- All other secretions should be described by color, consistency, volume, and changes from previous collections, if possible.

Daily output is usually 1200 to 1500 cc, or 30 to 50 cc per hour. Always report urine output below this hourly rate. Keep the urinal or bedpan readily available.

Tell the patient and visitors not to "help" by dumping the bedpan or urinal, but rather, to use the call light and allow the hospital personnel to empty and record all output.

States of Hydration

DEHYDRATION

Assess, report, and record significant signs of dehydration in the patient. Observe for the following signs: poor skin turgor, sticky oral mucous membranes, a shrunken or deeply furrowed tongue, crusted lips, weight loss, deteriorating vital signs, soft or sunken eyeballs, weak pedal pulses, delayed capillary filling, excessive thirst, high urine specific gravity (or no urine output), and possible mental confusion.

SKIN TURGOR

Check skin turgor by gently pinching the skin together over the sternum, forehead, or on the forearm. In the well hydrated patient elasticity is present and the skin rapidly returns to a flat position. With dehydration, the skin remains pinched or peaked and returns very slowly to the flat, normal position.

ORAL MUCOUS MEMBRANES

When adequately hydrated, the membranes of the mouth feel smooth and glisten. With dehydration, they are sticky and appear dull.

LABORATORY CHANGES

The values of the hematocrit, hemoglobin, BUN, and electrolytes will appear to fluctuate, based on the state of hydration. When a patient is overhydrated, the values appear to drop due to "hemodilution." A dehydrated patient will show higher values due to *hemoconcentration.*

OVERHYDRATION

Increases in abdominal girth, weight gain, neck vein engorgement, and circumference of the medial malleolus are indications of overhydration.

- Measure the abdominal girth daily at the umbilical level;
- Measure the extremities bilaterally every day, approximately 5 cm above the medial malleolus;
- Weigh the patient daily using the same scale, at the same time, and in similar clothing.

Edema

Edema is excess fluid accumulation in the extracellular spaces.

PITTING EDEMA

Edema is considered to be *pitting* when an indentation remains in the tissue after pressure is exerted against a bony part such as the shin, ankle, or sacrum. The degree is usually recorded as 1+ (slight) to 4+ (deep).

Pale, cool, tight, shiny skin is another sign of edema.

Electrolyte Imbalance

Patients taking corticosteroids are particularly susceptible to the development of electrolyte imbalance. Physiologically, corticosteroids cause sodium retention (hypernatremia) and potassium excretion (hypokalemia).

Because the symptoms of most electrolyte imbalances are similar, the nurse should assess changes in the patient's mental status (e.g., alertness, orientation, confusion), muscle strength, muscle cramps, tremors, nausea, and general appearance.

SUSCEPTIBLE PATIENTS

Patients most likely to develop electrolyte disturbances are those who, in addition to receiving corticosteroids, have a history of renal or cardiac disease, hormonal disorders, massive trauma or burns, or are on diuretic therapy.

SERUM ELECTROLYTES

Monitor serum electrolyte tests and notify the physician of deviations from normal values.

HYPOKALEMIA

Serum potassium (K^+) levels below 3.5 mEq/liter should be reported.

Hypokalemia is especially likely to occur when a patient receiving corticosteroids develops vomiting, diarrhea, or heavy diuresis. All corticosteroids and diuretics, except the potassium sparing type, may cause hypokalemia.

HYPERKALEMIA

Serum potassium levels above 5.5 mEq/liter should be reported.

Hyperkalemia occurs most commonly when a patient is given excessive amounts of potassium supplements, either intravenously or orally. It may also occur as an adverse effect of potassium sparing diuretics.

HYPONATREMIA

Serum sodium (Na^+) below 135 mEq/liter should be reported.

HYPERNATREMIA

Serum sodium above 145 mEq/liter should be reported.

Remember the phrase "where the sodium goes, water goes." Corticosteroids cause retention of sodium by the kidneys, thus causing fluid retention. Hypernatremia can be aggravated when intravenous fluid intake exceeds output.

Behavioral Change

Patients receiving higher doses of corticosteroids are susceptible to psychotic behavioral changes. The most susceptible patients are those with a previous history of mental dysfunction. Perform a baseline assessment of the patient's ability to respond rationally to the environment and the diagnosis of the underlying disease. Make regularly scheduled mental status evaluations and compare the findings. Report the development of alterations.

Hyperglycemia

Corticosteroid therapy may induce hyperglycemia, particularly in prediabetic or diabetic patients. All patients need to be monitored for the development of hyperglycemia, particularly during the early weeks of therapy.

Assess regularly for glycosuria and report any frequent occurrences.

History of Ulcers

Patients receiving corticosteroid therapy develop a higher incidence of ulcer disease. Ask the patient about any previous treatment for an ulcer, heartburn, or stomach pain. Periodic testing of stools for occult blood may be ordered.

Patient Teaching Associated with Corticosteroid Therapy

Communication and Responsibility

Encourage open communication concerning frustrations and anger as the patient attempts to adjust to the diagnosis and the need for prolonged treatment. The patient must be guided to gain insight into the disorder in order to assume responsibility for the continuation of the treatment. Keep emphasizing the factors the patient can control to alter progression of the disease including maintenance of general health, nutritional needs, adequate rest and appropriate exercise, continuation of the prescribed medication therapy, and management of the underlying disease process for which the corticosteroids are being prescribed.

AVOID INFECTIONS

Advise the patient to avoid crowds or people known to have infections. Report even minor signs of an infection (e.g., general malaise, sore throat, or low-grade fever) to the physician.

NUTRITIONAL STATUS

Assist the patient to develop a specific schedule for spacing daily fluid intake and planning sodium restrictions, as prescribed by the physician.

If a high-potassium diet is prescribed, help the patient become familiar with foods that should be consumed.

If weight gain is a specific problem (not related to fluid accumulation), plan for calorie restrictions and spacing of daily intake.

Further dietary needs may include increases in vitamin D and calcium.

STRESS

Patients receiving high doses of corticosteroids do not tolerate stress very well. Patients should be instructed to notify the physician prior to exposure to additional stress, such as dental procedures. If a patient sustains an accidental injury or sudden emotional stress, the attending physician should be notified that the patient is receiving steroid therapy. An additional dose may be needed to support the patient through a stressful situation.

EXERCISE AND ACTIVITY

Encourage the patient to maintain the usual activities of daily living. Help the patient plan for appropriate alterations depending on the disease process and degree of impairment.

Encourage weight bearing to prevent calcium loss. Active and passive range of motion exercises maintain mobility and joint and muscle integrity.

Expectations of Therapy

Discuss the expectations of therapy with the patient. These drugs usually provide improvement of the symptoms for which the medication was prescribed. It must be remembered that the underlying disease process is not being cured through the use of these agents. Thus, for use with rheumatoid arthritis, the anticipated response would be improved mobility as a result of decreased joint pain and edema; for lesions of the skin, a reduction in inflammation; for adrenal insufficiency, gradual improvement of the presenting symptoms.

Changes in Expectations

Assess changes in expectations as therapy progresses and the patient gains understanding and skill in the management of the diagnosis. Although a patient may not be receiving corticosteroids any longer, the patient may require reinstitution of therapy during periods of stress, infection, surgery, or accidental injury.

Corticosteroids are usually reserved for treatment when all other therapies have been eliminated. Patients may have difficulty living with the side effects of corticosteroid therapy, but the alternative of the predrug symptoms offers little choice. It may be even more difficult for a patient to understand the need to decrease the dosage and allow incomplete symptom control because of adverse effects experienced.

Changes in Therapy through Cooperative Goal-Setting

Work with the patient to encourage adherence to the prescribed treatment. When the patient feels that a change should be made in a treatment plan, encourage discussion first with the physician.

WRITTEN RECORD

Enlist the patient's aid in developing and maintaining a written record of monitoring parameters (e.g., blood pressure, pulse, daily weight, degree of pain relief, exercise tolerance) (see Table 15.9) and response to prescribed therapies for discussion with the physician. Patients should be encouraged to take this record on follow-up visits.

FOSTERING COMPLIANCE

Throughout the hospitalization, discuss medication information and how it will benefit the course of treatment. Stress the need for regular and long-term treatment, if appropriate to the patient's disease. Seek the patient's cooperation and understanding of the following points so that medication compliance may be enhanced:

1. Name.
2. Dosage: The smallest possible dose is used to control the presenting symptoms for long-term therapy. NEVER stop taking the medication abruptly. A gradual withdrawal from the drug is required to prevent serious complications. The dosage must be regulated by the physician.
3. Route and administration times: Oral administration is usually done between 6 AM and 9 AM to minimize the suppressive activity on normal adrenal function. To minimize gastric irritation, administer with or after meals.

    Alternate-day therapy is sometimes used for long-term treatment.
4. Anticipated therapeutic response: Improvement in the presenting symptoms for which therapy has been prescribed.
5. Side effects to expect: See the discussion of glucocorticoids.
6. Side effects to report: Hyperglycemia, behavioral changes, signs of infection, exposure to stressful situations, or significant weight gain over a short period of time.
7. What to do if a dosage is missed: If one dose is missed, take it when remembered. If more than one is missed, consult your physician.
8. When, how, or if to refill the medication.

DIFFICULTY IN COMPREHENSION

If it is evident that the patient and/or family does not understand all aspects of the continuing therapy being prescribed (e.g., administration and monitoring of medications, exercises, diets, follow-up appointments) consider the use of social service or visiting nurse agencies.

ASSOCIATED TEACHING

Give patients the following instructions:

Always inform the physician or dentist of any prescription or over-the-counter medication being taken. Over-the-counter medications should not be taken without first discussing them with a physician or pharmacist.

Always report side effects of rash, itching, or hives immediately. Nausea, vomiting, or diarrhea should also be reported for the physician's evaluation if it is a new symptom.

Take all of the medication as prescribed for the full course of treatment. Do not discontinue use when feeling improved; do not save for future use; do not give your medicine to another individual. Sudden discontinuation of certain medications may produce harmful effects.

Keep all medications out of reach of children.

If pregnancy is suspected, consult an obstetrician as soon as possible about continuation of medication therapy.

Table 15.9
Example of a Written Record for Patients Receiving Corticosteroids

Medications	Color	To be taken

Name _____

Physician _____

Physician's phone _____

Next appt.* _____

Parameters		Day of discharge							Comments
Weight									
Blood pressure									
Pulse rate									
Notify doctor of sudden stress in life	Surgery, injury, trauma, death in family or of friend, events such as fights in family								
Pain relief? No relief 10 Improved 5 No pain 1									
Assessment of how I feel? Good 10 Improved 5 Bad 1									
Breast tenderness	None								
	Occasionally uncomfortable								
	Increasing								
Hair distribution	No changes seen								
	Hair growth increased: site ____								
Edema	Swelling noted (where)? ____								
	Time of day swelling occurs?								

*Please bring this record with you to your next appointment.
Use the back of this sheet for additional information.

At Discharge

Items to be sent home with the patient should:

1. Have written instructions for use.
2. Be labeled in language and size of print appropriate for the patient.
3. Include identification cards or bracelets that state the name of the doctor to contact in an emergency, as well as the drug name, dosage, and frequency of use.
4. Include a list of additional supplies to be purchased after discharge.
5. Include a schedule for follow-up appointments.

Mineralocorticoids

Desoxycorticosterone (DOCA)
(dez-ok′see-kort-ih-ko-stere-own)
(Percorten) (per-kort′en)

Desoxycorticosterone is a mineralocorticoid secreted by the adrenal glands. It affects fluid and electrolyte balance by acting on the distal renal tubules causing sodium and water retention, and potassium and hydrogen excretion. Desoxycorticosterone is used in combination with glucocorticoids to replace mineralocorticoid activity in patients who suffer from hypopituitarism or adrenocortical insufficiency (Addison disease), and for the treatment of salt losing adrenogenital syndrome.

Side Effects

Since desoxycorticosterone is a natural hormone, side effects are an extension of excessive use of desoxycorticosterone. Most side effects are associated with sodium accumulation and potassium depletion.

Availability

Injection—(Acetate) 5 mg/ml in 10 ml vials; (Pivalate) 25 mg/ml suspension in 4 ml vials.
Implant—(pellets) 125 mg.

Dosage and Administration

Adult
IM—Acetate (short-acting form) 2 to 5 mg daily. Inject into the upper outer quadrant of the gluteal region. Injection into the deltoid muscle should be avoided because of a high incidence of subcutaneous atrophy.

IM—Pivalate (long-acting form) 25 to 100 mg every 4 weeks.
Implant—Pellets are surgically implanted into the subcutaneous tissue every 8 to 12 months.

Drug Interactions

See Glucocorticoids.

Nursing Interventions

See General Nursing Considerations for Patients Receiving Corticosteroid Therapy.

Glucocorticoids

The major glucocorticoid of the adrenal cortex is cortisol. The hypothalamic pituitary axis regulates the secretion of cortisol by increasing or decreasing the output of *corticotropin releasing factor* (CRF) from the hypothalamus. CRF stimulates the release of *adrenocorticotropic hormone* (ACTH) from the pituitary gland. ACTH then stimulates the adrenal cortex to secrete cortisol. As serum levels of cortisol increase, the amount of CRF secreted by the hypothalamus is decreased, resulting in diminished secretion of cortisol from the adrenal cortex.

Glucocorticoids are most frequently prescribed for their antiinflammatory and antiallergic properties. They do not cure any disease, but rather relieve the symptoms of tissue inflammation. When used for the control of rheumatoid arthritis, relief of symptoms is noted within a few days. Joint and muscle stiffness, muscle tenderness and weakness, joint swelling, and soreness are all significantly reduced. When used for this purpose, it is important to assess the patient's predrug activity level. Relief of pain may lead to overuse of the diseased joints. Appetite, weight, and energy are increased, fever is reduced, and sedimentation rates are reduced, or return to normal. Anatomic changes and joint deformities that are already present remain unchanged. Symptoms usually return a short time after withdrawal of the glucocorticoids.

Glucocorticoids are also quite effective for relief of allergic manifestations, such as serum sickness, severe hay fever, status asthmaticus, and exfoliative dermatitis. In addition, they may be used for the treatment of shock and for *collagen* diseases, such as lupus erythematosus, dermatomyositis, and acute rheumatic fever.

Side Effects

Glucocorticoids are potent agents that produce many undesirable side effects as well as therapeutic benefits.

Unless immediate, life-threatening conditions exist, other therapeutic methods should be exhausted before corticosteroid therapy is initiated. Many of the side effects of the steroids are related to dosage and duration of therapy.

Possible side effects of the glucocorticoids include hyperglycemia, glycosuria, aggravation of diabetes mellitus symptoms, negative nitrogen balance, increase in white cell count, reduced resistance to infections, delay in wound healing, peptic ulcer formation, cataract formation, tendency for thrombosis and embolism, a rounded contour of the face, hirsutism, purplish or reddish striae of the skin, potassium depletion, retention of salt and water, and weight gain. Behavioral disturbances, ranging from nervousness and insomnia to manic-depressive (or schizophrenic) psychoses and suicidal tendencies, may develop, particularly with prolonged administration.

These drugs must be used with caution in patients with diabetes mellitus, congestive heart failure, hypertension, peptic ulcer, mental disturbance, and suspected infections.

Dosage and Administration

When therapeutic dosages are administered for a week or longer, one must assume that the internal production of corticosteroids is suppressed. Abrupt discontinuation of the glucocorticoids may result in adrenal insufficiency. Therapy should be withdrawn gradually. The time required to decrease glucocorticoids depends on the duration of treatment, the dosage amount, the mode of administration, and the glucocorticoid being used.

Nursing Interventions

See also General Nursing Considerations for Patients Receiving Corticosteroid Therapy

---

PATIENT CONCERNS: NURSING INTERVENTION/RATIONALE

Side Effects to Expect and Report

Electrolyte Imbalance, Fluid Accumulation

The electrolytes most commonly altered are potassium (K^+), sodium (Na^+), and chloride (Cl^-). Of these, *hypokalemia* is most likely to occur.

Many symptoms associated with altered fluid and electrolyte balance are subtle and interspersed with general symptoms of drug toxicity or the disease process itself.

Gather data relative to *changes* in the patient's mental status (e.g., alertness, orientation, confusion), muscle strength, muscle cramps, tremors, nausea, and general appearance (e.g., drowsy, anxious, lethargic).

Always check the electrolyte reports for early indications of electrolyte imbalance.

Keep accurate records of intake and output, daily weights, and vital signs.

Susceptibility to Infection

Always question the patient, *prior* to initiation of therapy, about any signs and symptoms that would indicate the presence of an infection. Corticosteroid therapy often masks symptoms of infection.

Monitor the patient closely for signs of infection such as sore throat, fever, malaise, nausea, or vomiting.

Encourage the patient to avoid exposure to infections.

Behavioral Changes

Psychotic behaviors are more likely to occur in patients with a previous history of mental instability.

Perform a baseline assessment of the patient's degree of alertness, orientation to name, place and time, and rationality of responses *prior* to initiating therapy. Make regularly scheduled mental status evaluations and compare the findings. Report the development of alterations.

Hyperglycemia

Diabetic or prediabetic patients need to be monitored for the development of hyperglycemia, particularly during the early weeks of therapy.

Assess regularly for glycosuria and report any frequent occurrences.

Patients receiving oral hypoglycemic agents or insulin may require an adjustment in dosage.

Peptic Ulcer Formation

Before initiating therapy, ask the patient about any previous treatment for an ulcer, heartburn, or stomach pain.

Periodic testing of stools for occult blood may be ordered. Antacids may also be recommended by the physician to minimize gastric symptoms.

Delayed Wound Healing

People who have recently had surgery require close monitoring of surgical sites for signs of dehisence.

Teach surgical patients to splint the wounds while coughing and breathing deeply.

Inspect surgical sites and report statements such as, "When I coughed, I felt something pop."

Visual Disturbances

Visual disturbances noted by patients receiving long-term therapy need to be reported. Glucosteroid therapy may produce cataracts.

Dosage and Administration

Abrupt Discontinuation

Patients who have received corticosteroids for at least one week must not abruptly discontinue therapy.

Symptoms of abrupt discontinuation include fever, malaise, fatigue, weakness, anorexia, nausea, orthostatic dizziness, hypotension, fainting, dyspnea, hypoglycemia, muscle and joint pain, and possible exacerbation of the disease process being treated.

Application

Topical corticosteroids are applied as directed by the manufacturer. Specific instructions regarding use of an occlusive dressing should be clarified.

Alternate Day Therapy

Alternate day therapy may be used to treat chronic conditions. Administration of corticosteroids is usually done between 6 AM and 9 AM to minimize suppression of normal adrenal function. Administer with meals to minimize gastric irritation.

Pediatric Patients

The correct dosage for a child is usually based on the disease being treated, rather than the weight of the patient. (Children may require monitoring of skeletal growth if prolonged therapy is required.)

Drug Interactions

Diuretics (Furosemide, Thiazides, Bumetanide, Others)

Corticosteroids may enhance the loss of potassium. Check potassium levels and monitor the patient more closely for hypokalemia when these two agents are used concurrently.

Many symptoms associated with altered fluid and electrolyte balance are subtle and interspersed with general symptoms of drug toxicity or the disease process itself.

Gather data relative to *changes* in the patient's mental status (e.g., alertness, orientation, confusion), muscle strength, muscle cramps, tremors, nausea, and general appearance (e.g., drowsy, anxious, lethargic).

Always check the electrolyte reports for early indications of electrolyte imbalance.

Keep accurate records of intake and output, daily weights, and vital signs.

Warfarin

This medication may enhance or decrease the anticoagulant effects of warfarin. Observe for the development of petechiae, ecchymoses, nosebleeds, bleeding gums, dark tarry stools, and bright red or "coffee-ground" emesis. Monitor the prothrombin time and adjust the dosage of warfarin if necessary.

The ulcerogenic potential of steroids requires close observation of patients taking anticoagulants to reduce the possiblity of hemorrhage.

Hyperglycemia

Diabetic or prediabetic patients need to be monitored for the development of hyperglycemia, particularly during the early weeks of therapy.

Assess regularly for glycosuria and report any frequent occurrences.

Patients receiving oral hypoglycemic agents or insulin may require an adjustment in dosage.

Gonadal Hormones

The Gonads

The *gonads* are the reproductive glands: the *testes* of the male and the *ovaries* of the female. In addition to producing sperm, the testes produce testosterone, the male sex hormone. Testosterone controls the development of the male sex organs and influences characteristics such as voice, hair distribution, and male body form. *Androgens* are other steroid hormones that produce masculinizing effects.

The *ovaries* produce estrogen and progesterone. These are hormones that stimulate maturation of the female sex organs. They influence breast development, voice quality, and the broader pelvis of the female body form. Menstruation is established because of the hormone production of the ovaries. *Estrogen* is responsible for most of these changes. *Progesterone* is thought to be concerned mainly with body changes that favor the implantation of the fertilized ovum, continuation of pregnancy, and preparation of the breasts for lactation.

General Nursing Considerations for Patients Receiving Gonadal Hormones

A complete physical examination is usually done as a part of the preliminary work-up prior to treatment of any disorders using gonadal hormones.

PATIENT CONCERNS: NURSING INTERVENTION/RATIONALE

Assessment

Purpose

Ask the patient to describe the current problems that initiated this visit. How long have the symptoms been present? Is this a recurrent problem? If so, how was it treated in the past?

Reproductive History

Have the patient describe the following, as appropriate:

- Age of menarche.
- Usual pattern of menses: duration, number of pads used, last menstrual period.
- Number of pregnancies, live births, miscarriages, abortions.
- Vaginal discharges, itching, infections, and how treated.
- Breast self-exam routine. (If not being performed regularly, explain the correct procedure.)
- Male patients should be asked whether testicular exams are performed. (If not being performed regularly, explain the correct procedure.)

History of Prior Illnesses

Any indication of hypertension, heart or liver disease, thromboembolic disorders, or cancers of the reproductive organs is of particular concern.

Medications, Smoking

Does the patient currently smoke, or is the patient taking any over-the-counter or prescription medication? Oral contraceptives?

Physical Examination

Record basic patient data: height, weight, and vital signs. Blood pressure readings are of particular concern so that recordings on future visits can be evaluated for any change.

Collect urine for urinalysis, and blood samples for hemoglobin, hematocrit, and other laboratory studies deemed appropriate by the physician. Generally, people with a family history of diabetes mellitus should be tested for hyperglycemia prior to starting gonadal hormone therapy.

The physical exam should include a breast examination and a pelvic examination including a Papanicolaou test.

Observe the distribution of body hair and the presence of scars.

Stress the need for periodic physical examinations while receiving gonadal hormones.

Patient Teaching Associated with Gonadal Hormone Therapy

Communication and Responsibility

Encourage open communication concerning frustrations and anger as the patient attempts to adjust to the diagnosis and the need for prolonged treatment. The patient must be guided to gain insight into the disorder and to assume responsibility for the continuation of the treatment. Keep emphasizing the factors the patient can control to alter progression of the disease including maintenance of general health, nutritional needs, adequate rest and appropriate exercise, and continuation of the prescribed medication therapy.

SMOKING

Explain the risks of continuing to smoke, especially when receiving estrogen or progestin therapy. (The incidence of fatal heart attacks is increased for women over 35 years of age.)

PHYSICAL EXAMINATION

Stress the need for regular periodic medical examinations and laboratory studies.

Expectations of Therapy

Discuss the expectations of therapy with the patient: (e.g., degree of pain relief, frequency of use of therapy, relief of menopausal symptoms, sexual maturation, regulation of menstrual cycle, sexual activity, maintenance of mobility and activities of daily living and/or work).

Changes in Expectations

Assess changes in expectations as therapy progresses and the patient gains understanding and skill in the management of the diagnosis.

Because there are a number of possible adverse effects, it is necessary to evaluate the effectiveness of the treatment prescribed in relation to the condition being treated and the severity of adverse effects being experienced.

Changes in Therapy through Cooperative Goal-Setting

Work with the patient to encourage adherence to the prescribed treatment. When the patient feels that a change should be made in a treatment plan, encourage discussion first with the physician.

WRITTEN RECORD

Enlist the patient's aid in developing and maintaining a written record of monitoring parameters (e.g., blood pressure, pulse, daily weight, degree of pain relief, menstrual cycle information, breakthrough bleeding, nausea, vomiting, cramps, breast tenderness, hirsutism, gynecomastia, masculinization, hoarseness, headaches, sexual stimulation) and responses to prescribed therapies for discussion with the physician. Patients should be encouraged to take this record on follow-up visits.

FOSTERING COMPLIANCE

Throughout the hospitalization, discuss medication information and how it will benefit the course of treatment. Seek the patient's cooperation and understanding of the following points so that medication compliance may be enhanced:

1. Name.
2. Dosage: The dosage will depend on the disease being treated and the agent being used.
3. Route and administration: Be certain the patient understands the route of administration and the times of administration in relation to the menstrual cycle.
4. Anticipated therapeutic response: See individual agents.
5. Side effects to expect: See individual agents.
6. Side effects to report: See individual agents.
7. What to do if a dosage is missed.
8. When, how, or if to refill the medication.

DIFFICULTY IN COMPREHENSION

If it is evident that the patient and/or family does not understand all aspects of the continuing therapy being prescribed (e.g., administration and monitoring of medications, exercises, diets, follow-up appointments) consider use of social service or visiting nurse agencies.

ASSOCIATED TEACHING

Give the patient the following instructions:

Always inform the physician or dentist of any prescription or over-the-counter medication being taken. Over-the-counter medications should not be taken without first discussing them with a physician or pharmacist.

Always report side effects of rash, itching, or hives immediately. Nausea, vomiting, or diarrhea should also be reported for the physician's evaluation if it is a new symptom.

Take all of the medication as prescribed for the full course of treatment. Do not discontinue use when feeling improved; do not save for future use; do not give your medicine to another individual. Sudden discontinuation of certain medications may produce harmful effects.

Keep all medications out of reach of children.

If pregnancy is suspected, consult an obstetrician as soon as possible about continuation of medication therapy.

At Discharge

Items to be sent home with the patient should:

1. Have written instructions for use.
2. Be labeled in language and size of print appropriate for the patient.
3. If needed, include identification cards or bracelets.
4. Include a list of additional supplies to be purchased after discharge (e.g., syringes, dressings).
5. Include a schedule of follow-up appointments.

Estrogens

The natural estrogenic hormone released from the ovaries is comprised of several closely related chemical compounds: *estradiol*, *estrone*, and *estriol*. The most potent is estradiol. It is metabolized to estrone, which is half as potent. Estrone is further metabolized to estriol, which is considerably less potent. Estrogens are responsible for the development of the sex organs during growth in the uterus, and maturation at puberty. They are also responsible for characteristics such as growth of hair, texture of skin, and distribution of body fat. Estrogens also affect the release of pituitary gonadotropins, cause capillary dilatation, fluid retention, protein metabolism, and inhibit ovulation and postpartum breast engorgement.

Estrogen products are used for relieving the hot flash symptoms of menopause; contraception; hormone replacement therapy after an oophorectomy; postpartum breast engorgement; in conjunction with appropriate diet, calcium, and physical therapy in the treatment of osteoporosis; and to slow the disease progress (and minimize discomfort) in patients with advanced prostatic cancer and certain types of breast cancer.

Side Effects

Estrogen-containing products all have somewhat similar adverse effects with similar dosages. Since estrogens affect so many body functions, there are many potential adverse effects associated with therapy. Each patient responds somewhat differently to various estrogenic products and dosages, based on the individual's body chemistry and duration of the therapy. Adverse effects associated with estrogen therapy, categorized by body system, are:

- Genitourinary: Breakthrough bleeding, changes in menstrual flow, dysmenorrhea, amenorrhea, infertility, and uterine growth changes.
- Gastrointestinal: Nausea, vomiting, abdominal cramps, bloating, jaundice, and colitis. There is a two- to threefold increase in risk of gallbladder disease in women receiving postmenopausal estrogens.
- Breast: Tenderness, enlargement and secretion.
- Cardiovascular: Hypertension, thrombophlebitis, pulmonary embolism, stroke, and myocardial infarction.
- Skin: Chloasma (pigmentary skin discoloration, usually yellowish brown patches or spots), loss of scalp hair, hirsutism, urticaria, localized dermatitis, erythema multiforme, and hemorrhagic eruption.

- Eyes: Intolerance to contact lenses.
- CNS: Headaches, migraine, dizziness, mental depression.
- Other: Changes in weight, hyperglycemia, edema, changes in libido, aggravation of porphyria.

The use of estrogens for long-term treatment of menopausal symptoms has been associated with a greater risk of endometrial cancer. The risk of endometrial cancer in estrogen users was 4.5 to 13.9 times greater than in nonusers and appears to depend on both duration of treatment and dose. When estrogens are used for the treatment of menopausal symptoms, the lowest dose that will control symptoms should be used, and medication should be discontinued as soon as possible. When prolonged treatment is required, the patient should be examined at least on a semiannual basis to determine the need for continued therapy. Cyclic administration of low doses of estrogen may carry less risk than continuous administration. There is no evidence that "natural" estrogens are more or less hazardous than synthetic estrogens in equivalent doses.

The use of estrogens during early pregnancy is contraindicated. Serious birth defects have been reported, and it has been found that the female offspring have an increased risk of developing vaginal or cervical cancer later in life.

Availability

See Table 15.10.

Dosage and Administration

See Table 15.10.

**PATIENT CONCERNS:
NURSING INTERVENTION/RATIONALE**

Side Effects to Expect

*Weight Gain, Edema, Breast
Tenderness, Nausea*

These symptoms tend to be mild and resolve with continued therapy. If they do not resolve, or become particularly bothersome, the patient should consult a physician.

Table 15.10

Estrogens

GENERIC NAME	BRAND NAME	AVAILABILITY	USES	DOSES
Chlorotrianisene	Tace	Capsules: 12, 25, 72 mg	Postpartum breast engorgement	PO: 12 mg 4 times daily for 7 days; or 50 mg every 6 hours for 6 doses; or 72 mg every 12 hours for 2 days Administer first dose within 8 hours after delivery
			Prostatic carcinoma	PO: 12–25 mg daily
			Menopause	PO: 12–25 mg daily cyclically*
			Atrophic vaginitis	PO: 12–25 mg daily cyclically*
			Female hypogonadism	PO: 12–25 mg daily for 21 days, followed by 5 days of progestin
Conjugated Estrogens	Premarin, Evestrone	Tablets: 0.3, 0.625, 1.25, 2.5 mg IV: 25 mg/5 ml vial Cream: 0.625 mg/g	Menopause	PO: 1.25 mg daily cyclically*
			Atrophic vaginitis	PO: 0.3–1.25 mg daily cyclically*
			Female hypogonadism	PO: 2.5–7 mg daily for 20 days, followed by 10 days off
			Ovarian failure or post-oophorectomy	PO: 1.25 mg daily cyclically*
			Osteoporosis	PO: 1.25 mg daily cyclically*
			Breast carcinoma	PO: 10 mg 3 times daily
			Prostatic carcinoma	PO: 1.25–2.5 mg 3 times daily
			Postpartum breast engorgement	PO: 3.75 mg every 4 hours for 5 doses; or 1.25 mg every 4 hours for 5 days
Diethylstilbestrol (DES)	Diethylstilbestrol	Tablets: 0.1, 0.25, 0.5, 1, 5 mg	Menopause, atrophic vaginitis	PO: 0.2–0.5 mg daily cyclically* Dosage range: up to 2 mg daily
		Vaginal suppositories: 0.1, 0.5 mg	Female hypogonadism, post-oophorectomy, ovarian failure	PO: 0.2–0.5 mg daily cyclically
			Prostatic carcinoma	PO: 1–3 mg daily
			Breast carcinoma	PO: 15 mg daily
			Postcoital contraception	PO: 25 mg 2 times daily for 5 days. Start within 24 hours, for emergency use only. Do not use routinely.
Esterified Estrogens	Estratab, Menest, Evex	Tablets: 0.3, 0.625, 1.25, 2.5 mg	Menopause, atrophic vaginitis	PO: 0.3–1.25 mg daily cyclically* Dosage range: 2.5–3.75 mg
			Female hypogonadism, post-oophorectomy, ovarian failure	PO: 2.5–7.5 mg daily cyclically
			Breast carcinoma	PO: 10 mg 3 times daily
			Prostatic carcinoma	PO: 1.25–2.5 mg 3 times daily
Estradiol	Estrace	Tablets: 1, 2 mg Injections: Cypionate in oil:	Menopause, atrophic vaginitis, hypogonadism,	PO: 1–2 mg daily cyclically* IM: Cypionate: 1–5 mg every 3–4 weeks

(*Table continues on p. 398.*)

Table 15.10 (*continued*)

GENERIC NAME	BRAND NAME	AVAILABILITY	USES	DOSES
Estradiol (*continued*)	Estrace (*continued*)	1, 5 mg/ml Valerate in oil: 10, 20, 40 mg/ml	post-oophorectomy, ovarian failure Postpartum breast engorgement Prostatic carcinoma Breast carcinoma	Valerate: 10–20 mg every 4 weeks IM: Valerate: 10–25 mg at end of first stage of labor PO: 1–2 mg 3 times daily IM: Valerate: 30 mg every 1–2 weeks PO: 10 mg 3 times daily
Estrone	Ogen, Estronol, Bestrone, Kestrone	Tablets: 0.625, 1.25, 2.5, 5 mg Injection: in oil: 2 mg/ml in water: 2, 5 mg/ml	Menopause, atrophic vaginitis Female hypogonadism, post-oophorectomy, ovarian failure Prostatic carcinoma	PO: 0.625–5 mg daily cyclically* IM: 0.1–0.5 mg 2–3 times weekly PO: 1.25–7.5 mg daily cyclically IM: 0.1–1 mg weekly Dosage range: 0.5–2 mg IM: 2–4 mg 2 or 3 times weekly
Ethinyl Estradiol	Estinyl, Feminone	Tablets: 0.02, 0.05, 0.5 mg	Menopause Female hypogonadism Breast carcinoma Prostatic carcinoma	PO: 0.02–0.05 mg daily cyclically* PO: 0.05 1–3 times daily for 2 weeks followed by 2 weeks of progesterone PO: 1 mg 3 times daily PO: 0.15–2 mg daily
Quinestrol	Estrovis	Tablets: 100 mcg	Menopause, hypogonadism, atrophic vaginitis, post-oophorectomy, ovarian failure	PO: Initially, 100 μg daily for 7 days; followed by 100 μg weekly starting 2 weeks after treatment starts

* Clinically = 3 weeks of daily estrogen followed by 1 week off.

Side Effects to Report

Hypertension, Hyperglycemia, Thrombophlebitis, Breakthrough Bleeding, Any Other Symptoms the Patient Recognizes as Being of Concern

These are all complications associated with estrogen therapy. It is extremely important that the patient is evaluated by the physician to consider alternative therapy.

Drug Interactions

Warfarin

This medication may diminish the anticoagulant effects of warfarin. Monitor the prothrombin time and increase the dosage of warfarin if necessary.

Phenytoin

Estrogens may inhibit the metabolism of phenytoin, resulting in phenytoin toxicity.

Monitor patients with concurrent therapy for signs of phenytoin toxicity: nystagmus, sedation, lethargy. Serum levels may be ordered, and a reduced dosage of phenytoin may be required.

Thyroid Hormones

Patients who have no thyroid function and who start on estrogen therapy may require an increase in thyroid hormone because estrogens reduce the level of circulating thyroid hormones. Do not adjust the thyroid dosage until the patient shows clinical signs of hypothyroidism.

Progestins

Progesterone, and its derivatives (the progestins), inhibit the secretion of pituitary gonadotropins, preventing maturation of ovarian follicles, and thus inhibit ovulation. Progestins are used primarily to treat secondary amenorrhea, breakthrough uterine bleeding, and endometriosis, but may also be used in combination with estrogens as contraceptives (see Oral Contraceptives in Chapter 19).

Side Effects

Side effects associated with administration of progestins are rare, but can include nausea, vomiting, diarrhea, breakthrough bleeding, oily scalp, acne, weight gain, edema, spotting, amenorrhea, headache, cholestatic jaundice, mental depression, and hirsutism.

The use of progestins in early pregnancy has been associated with birth defects. If pregnancy is suspected, the physician should be consulted immediately.

Availability

See Table 15.11.

PATIENT CONCERNS: NURSING INTERVENTION/RATIONALE

Side Effects to Expect

Weight Gain, Edema, Nausea, Vomiting, Diarrhea, Tiredness, Oily Scalp, Acne

These symptoms tend to the mild and resolve with continued therapy. If they do not resolve, or become particularly bothersome, have the patient consult the physician.

Side Effects to Report

Breakthrough Bleeding, Amenorrhea, Continuing Headache, Cholestatic Jaundice, Mental Depression

These are all complications associated with progestin therapy. It is extremely important that the patient is evaluated by the physician to consider alternatives in therapy.

Table 15.11
Progestins

GENERIC NAME	BRAND NAME	AVAILABILITY	USES	DOSES
Hydroxyprogesterone	Delalutin, Hydrosterone, Hylutin	Injection: 125, 250 mg/ml	Amenorrhea; Abnormal uterine bleeding	IM: 375 mg
			Uterine carcinoma	IM: 1 g weekly
Medroxyprogesterone	Provera, Amen, Curretab	Tablets: 2.5, 10 mg	Secondary amenorrhea Abnormal uterine bleeding	PO: 5–10 mg daily for 5–10 days
				PO: 5–10 mg daily for 5–10 days, beginning on the 16th or 21st day of the menstrual cycle
Norethindrone	Norlutin	Tablets: 5 mg	Amenorrhea, abnormal uterine bleeding	PO: 5–20 mg starting with the 5th and ending on the 25th day of the menstrual cycle
			Endometriosis	PO: 10 mg for 2 weeks; increase in increments of 5 mg/day every 2 weeks until 30 mg/day is reached
Norethindrone Acetate	Norlutate	Tablets: 5 mg	Amenorrhea, abnormal uterine bleeding	PO: 2.5–10 mg starting with the 5th and ending on the 25th day of the menstrual cycle
			Endometriosis	PO: 5 mg for 2 weeks; increase in increments of 2.5 mg/day every 2 weeks until 15 mg/day is reached
Norgestrel	Ovrette	Tablets: 0.075 mg	Oral contraceptive	PO: 1 tablet daily
Progesterone	Progelin	Injection: 25, 50, 100 mg/ml	Amenorrhea, functional uterine bleeding	IM: 5–10 mg for 6–8 consecutive days

Androgens

The dominant male sex hormone is *testosterone*. It is the primary natural androgen produced by the testicles. Androgens are responsible for the normal growth and development of male sex organs and for maintenance of secondary sex characteristics. These effects include the growth and maturation of the prostate, seminal vesicles. penis, and scrotum; the development of male hair distribution; laryngeal enlargement (Adam's apple); vocal chord thickening; alterations in body musculature, and fat distribution. Androgens are used to treat hypogonadism, eunuchism, androgen deficiency, prevention of postpartum pain, breast engorgement, and palliation of breast cancer in certain postmenopausal women.

Side Effects

Women receiving high doses of androgens may develop signs of masculinization manifested by a deepening of the voice, hirsutism, clitoral enlargement, acne, and menstrual irregularities.

In immobilized patients and patients with breast cancer, androgen therapy may cause hypercalcemia.

Androgens cause retention of sodium, potassium, and water. They may also cause gynecomastia and hepatotoxicity.

Androgens should generally not be used in prepubertal children because the drug may cause premature closure of the epiphyses, stopping bone growth.

Availability

See Table 15.12.

General Nursing Considerations for Patients Receiving Androgens

PATIENT CONCERNS: NURSING INTERVENTION/RATIONALE

Altered Self-Image/Self-Esteem

Assist female patients to manage the masculinizing effects caused by these agents.

Assist male patients to maintain self-esteem and provide stability by listening to the patient's concerns about difficulties with sexual maturation.

Activity and Exercise

Activity levels are based on the individual's tolerance and extent of disease pathology. Whenever possible, weight bearing should be encouraged to decrease calcium loss from the bones. In the absence of ambulation, provide for passive and active range of motion exercises.

Nutritional Status

Patients receiving androgens for breast carcinoma may be placed on a low calcium and high protein diet.

Table 15.12
Androgen

GENERIC NAME	BRAND NAME	AVAILABILITY	USES	DOSES
Short-acting				
Testosterone in water	Testosterone aqueous, Testaqua, Andro 100	IM: 25, 50, 100 mg/ml	Eunuchism, postpubertal cryptorchidism, impotence due to androgen deficiency	IM: 10–25 mg 2–3 times daily
			Postpartum breast engorgement	IM: 25–50 mg daily for 3–4 days
			Breast carcinoma	IM: 100 mg 3 times weekly
Testosterone in oil	Testosterone propionate, Testex	IM: 25, 50, 100 mg/ml	As above	As above
Long-acting				
Testosterone enanthate	Android–7, Testate, Delatestryl	IM: 100, 200 mg/ml	Eunuchism, androgen deficiency	IM: 200–400 mg every 4 weeks
			Oligospermia	IM: 100–200 mg every 4–6 weeks
Testosterone cypionate	Andro–cyp 100, Depotest, Duratest, Testa–C	IM: 50, 100, 200 mg/ml	As for testosterone enanthate	As for testosterone enanthate
Oral Products				
Methyltestosterone	Oreton Methyl, Testred, Virilon	Tablets: 10, 25 mg Capsules: 10 mg	Eunuchism	PO: 10–40 mg daily
			Cryptorchidism	PO: 30 mg daily
			Postpartum breast engorgement	PO: 80 mg daily for 3–5 days
			Breast carcinoma	PO: 200 mg daily
Fluoxymesterone	Holotestin, Ora–Testryl, Android-F	Tablets: 2, 5, 10 mg	Male hypogonadism Female:	PO: 2–10 mg daily
			breast carcinoma	PO: 15–30 mg daily
			postpartum breast engorgement	PO: 2.5 mg at onset of active labor; then 5–10 mg daily for 4–5 days

Many symptoms associated with altered fluid and electrolyte balance are subtle and interspersed with general symptoms of drug toxicity or the disease process itself.

Gather data relative to *changes* in the patient's mental status (e.g., alertness, orientation, confusion), muscle strength, muscle cramps, tremors, nausea, and general appearance (e.g., drowsy, anxious, lethargic).

Always check the electrolyte reports for early indications of electrolyte imbalance.

Keep accurate records of intake and output, daily weights, and vital signs.

Patients should report weight gains of more than 2 lbs per week. Diuretic therapy, with or without dietary reduction of salt, may be prescribed if edema is significant.

Masculinization

Females should be monitored for signs of masculinization (e.g., deepening of the voice, hoarseness, growth of facial hair, clitoral enlargement, and menstrual irregularities) during androgen therapy. The drug should usually be discontinued when mild masculinization is evident, since some adverse androgenic effects (such as voice changes) may not reverse with discontinuation of therapy. In consultation with her physician, the woman may decide that some masculinization is acceptable during treatment for carcinoma of the breast.

Males should be carefully monitored for the development of gynecomastia, priapism, or excessive sexual stimulation. These are indications of androgen overdose.

Hypercalcemia

Monitor patients for nausea, vomiting, constipation, poor muscle tone, and lethargy. These are indications of hypercalcemia, and are indications for discontinuation of androgen therapy.

Force fluids to minimize the possibility of renal calculi. Encourage the patient to drink 8 to 12 8-ounce glasses of water daily.

Perform weightbearing and active and passive exercises to the degree tolerated by the patient to minimize loss of calcium from bones.

Hepatotoxicity

The symptoms of hepatotoxicity are: anorexia, nausea, vomiting, jaundice, hepatomegaly, splenomegaly, and abnormal liver function tests (elevated bilirubin, SGOT, SGPT, alkaline phosphatase, prothrombin time).

Drug Interactions

Warfarin

Androgens may enhance the anticoagulant effects of warfarin. Observe for the development of petechiae, ecchymoses, nosebleeds, bleeding gums, dark tarry stools, and bright red or "coffee-ground" emesis. Monitor the prothrombin time and reduce the dosage of warfarin if necessary.

Oral Hypoglycemic Agents, Insulin

Monitor for hypoglycemia: headache weakness, decreased coordination, general apprehension, diaphoresis, hunger, blurred or double vision.

The dosage of the hypoglycemic agent or insulin may need to be reduced. Notify the physician if any of the above symptoms appear.

Corticosteroids

Concurrent use may increase the possiblity of electrolyte imbalance and fluid retention. See above for monitoring parameters.

Chapter 16

Drugs Affecting the Immune System

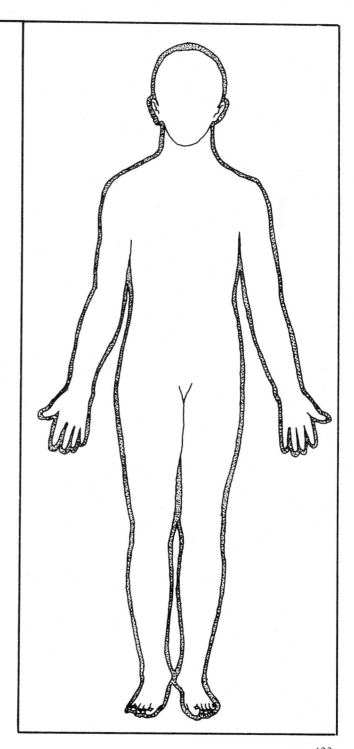

Objectives

After completing this chapter, the student should be able to do the following:

1. Explain the major actions and effects of drugs used to provide immunity.
2. Identify baseline data the nurse should collect on a continuous basis for comparison and evaluation of drug effectiveness.
3. Identify important nursing assessments and interventions associated with the drug therapy used in providing immunity.
4. Identify health teaching essential for a successful treatment regimen.

Immunity

Immunity is a state of resistance to disease. There are two kinds of immunity: natural and acquired. *Natural* immunity is endowed at birth and is retained for life. Microorganisms that live within a host organism such as a human being are harmless to that organism because it has natural defense mechanisms to ward off infection from the microorganism.

Acquired immunity may be *active* or *passive*. Active acquired immunity results when the host organism develops antibodies against the invading antigens, or microorganisms. Active immunity may be induced by artificial means, such as by injection of antigens. Examples of antigens include a suspension of living, inactivated organisms, such as the measles virus in measles vaccine, or a suspension of dead microorganisms, such as in typhoid vaccine. The antigen may be a toxin produced by a bacteria, such as the diphtheria toxin, or it may be an extract from the microorganism, such as the cell capsules of the influenza viruses used to make influenza vaccine.

Passive acquired immunity can be obtained in two ways: (1) an individual may be given the serum of an animal that has been actively immunized by injections with the specific microorganism that causes a particular disease, or (2) an individual may be given an injection of the serum of an immune person. This serum is rich in antibodies developed to protect the host against the specific disease antigen. *Passive* is used to describe this type of acquired immunity because the recipient's body plays no active part in the preparation of antibodies. The body does not produce antibodies to resist infection as it does in active immunity. As the blood is renewed, the acquired antibodies are lost, so the individual must be reimmunized periodically to maintain protection against that specific microorganism.

```
                  IMMUNITY
                     |
         +-----------+-----------+
      NATURAL              ACQUIRED
                         +----+----+
                      ACTIVE    PASSIVE
```

General Nursing Considerations for Patients Receiving Immunological Agents

Nurses need to remain current in their knowledge of the recommendations for administration of immunizations. Educating the public about the need for immunizations is a particular challenge since most young people who are now parents have not personally seen the crippling effects of the diseases that immunizations protect against.

In order to comply with immunization recommendations and to foster public health, several states have passed laws that require children to have certain immunizations before entering school. Exceptions are granted for medical reasons if approved by a physician. See Tables 16.1 to 16.3 for immunization schedules.

Many people wrongly believe that exposure to someone who has had the disease causes them to be immune to it, too. It should be stressed that exposure does *not* insure immunity.

A written record of all immunizations should be maintained. At the time of immunization, give the patient (or parents) (1) a record of the *exact* name, dosage, route of administration, and site of injection received (as appropriate to the medication type); (2) discharge instructions for the treatment of symptoms that may develop; and, (3) a schedule of additional immunizations that are needed. Suggest recording this information in the child's baby book or the family Bible.

PATIENT CONCERNS: NURSING INTERVENTION/RATIONALE

Screening before Administration of Immunologic Agents

History of Immunizations

Ask the patients if they have ever received any previous immunizations, and, if so, if they experienced any symptoms after the immunizations.

404

Table 16.1

Recommended Schedule for Active Immunization of Normal Infants and Children

RECOMMENDED AGE*	VACCINE†	COMMENTS
2 months	DTP-1‡, OPV-1§	Can be given earlier in areas of high endemicity
4 months	DTP-2, OPV-2	6-week to 2-month interval desired between OPV doses to avoid interference
6 months	DTP-3	An additional dose of OPV at this time is optional for use in areas with a high risk of polio exposure
15 months‖	MMR¶	
18 months‖	DTP-4, OPV-3	Completion of primary series
4–6 years**	DTP-5, OPV-4	Preferably at or before school entry
14–16 years	Td††	Repeat every 10 years throughout life

From Centers for Disease Control: *Morbid. Mortal. Week. Rep.* 32:2–16, Jan. 14, 1983.

* These recommended ages should not be construed as absolute; that is, 2 months can be 6–10 weeks, etc.

† For all products used, consult manufacturer's package enclosure for instructions for storage, handling, and administration. Immunobiologics prepared by different manufacturers may vary, and those of the same manufacturer may change from time to time. The package insert should be followed for a specific product.

‡ DTP—Diphtheria and tetanus toxoids and pertussis vaccine.

§ OPV—Oral, attenuated poliovirus vaccine contains poliovirus types 1, 2, and 3.

‖ Simultaneous administration of MMR, DTP, and OPV is appropriate for patients whose compliance with medical care recommendations cannot be assured.

¶ MMR—Live measles, mumps, and rubella viruses in a combined vaccine.

** Up to the seventh birthday.

†† Td—Adult tetanus toxoid and diphtheria toxoid in combination, which contains the same dose of tetanus toxoid as DTP or DT and a reduced dose of diphtheria toxoid.

History of Allergy

Take a thorough medication history BEFORE administering medications. People with a history of allergies, asthma, and chronic rhinitis are particularly susceptible to drug reactions.

Ask specifically about allergies. People with a history of allergy to eggs, feathers, aminoglycoside antibiotics, or horses may require intradermal skin testing before administration of the immunologic agent.

Infections

People with a current infection are generally not given immunizations because it is then difficult to determine whether the symptoms of the patient are due to the infection or are a reaction to the immunization.

Check the policy of your facility concerning the presence of "cold" symptoms; some institutions do give immunizations if symptoms are mild, while others postpone them entirely.

Immunosuppression

Do not administer live, attenuated virus vaccines to those with impaired immune systems. These patients are susceptible to infection from the virus.

People in direct contact with immunosuppressed patients should not receive oral polio vaccine. The live, attenuated virus is excreted from the immunized person's body and may infect the immunosuppressed patient.

Pregnancy

Always ask women of childbearing age if they are pregnant or likely to become pregnant within 3 months after immunization. Depending upon the immunologic agent, there is a risk of birth defects to the fetus.

Nursing Actions

Do not administer the medication if the person reports possible allergy, infection, pregnancy, or immunosuppression. Share all information obtained with the physician, who will decide whether to administer the medication.

When a definite drug allergy is identified, the patient's chart, unit Kardex, and identification bracelet should be carefully marked to alert all personnel to the specific agents the patient should *not* receive.

Table 16.2
*Recommended Immunization Schedule for Infants and Children up to Seventh Birthday Not Immunized at the Recommended Time in Early Infancy**

TIMING	VACCINE	COMMENTS
First visit	DTP-1,† OPV-1,‡ (If child is ≥ 15 months of age, MMR§)	DTP, OPV, and MMR can be administered simultaneously to children ≥ 15 months of age
2 months after first DTP, OPV		
2 months after second DTP	DTP-3	An additional dose of OPV at this time is optional for use in areas with a high risk of polio exposure
6–12 months after third DTP	DTP-4, OPV-3	
Preschool‖ (4–6 years)	DTP-5, OPV-4	Preferably at or before school entry
14–16 years	Td¶	Repeat every 10 years throughout life

From Centers for Disease Control: *Morbid. Mortal. Week. Rep.* 32:2–16, Jan. 14, 1983.

* If initiated in the first year of life, give DTP-1, 2, and 3, OPV-1 and 2 according to this schedule and give MMR when the child becomes 15 months old.

† DTP—Diphtheria and tetanus toxoids with pertussis vaccine. DTP may be used up to the seventh birthday.

‡ OPV—Oral, attenuated poliovirus vaccine contains poliovirus types 1, 2, and 3.

§ MMR—Live measles, mumps, and rubella viruses in a combined vaccine.

‖ The preschool dose is not necessary if the fourth dose of DTP and third dose of OPV are administered after the fourth birthday.

¶ Td—Adult tetanus toxoid and diphtheria toxoid in combination, which contains the same dose of tetanus toxoid as DTP or DT and a reduced dose of diphtheria toxoid.

Responding to Allergic Reactions

Observations

All patients should be watched closely for possible allergy for at least 20 to 30 minutes following the administration of an immunologic agent.

Emergency Cart

Know the location of the hospital emergency cart and the procedure for summoning it. In the event of suspected anaphylaxis, summon the physician and the emergency cart immediately.

Sites of Reactions

Although a serious reaction may occur with the first administration of a drug, repeated exposures to a previously sensitized substance can be fatal. Respond immediately to any signs of reaction:

- At the site of injection: swelling or redness, pain.
- Systemically: hives, nasal congestion and discharge, wheezing progressing to increasing dyspnea, pulmonary edema, tachycardia, hypotension, stridor, and sternal retractions.

Follow-Up

Following any reaction, the patient and family should be alerted to inform anyone treating them in the future that they are allergic to a specific drug.

Prevention of Disease Transmission

Needles and Syringes

Always use a separate needle and syringe, regardless of the expense, when administering injections of any type.

Disposal

Dispose of used needles and syringes in accordance with the hospital or clinic policy. Autoclaving to insure decontamination and sterilization is recommended to prevent disease transmission.

- Do not break or bend needles off used syringes, since you may puncture yourself. Place used disposable needles within the needle cap, and then place the capped needle in a rigid container which is specifically labeled for "contaminated" purposes.
- Syringes may go into this same container, or in a separate moisture-proof bag.
- These "contaminated" containers are then autoclaved or incinerated.

Hygiene

Thoroughly wash your hands between patients to prevent possible spread of disease.

PATIENT CONCERNS: NURSING INTERVENTION/RATIONALE

Communication and Responsibility

Encourage open communication concerning frustrations and anger as the patient attempts to adjust to the diagnosis and need for completion of treatment.

The patient must be guided to gain insight into the need for immunity and to assume responsibility for the continuation of treatment. Keep reemphasizing those factors the patient can control to alter the disease progression: maintenance of general health, nutritional needs, adequate rest and appropriate exercise, and continuation of prescribed immunizations to achieve immunity to the disease process, thereby preventing not only development of the disease but also complications that may arise from the disease and drug therapy.

Expectations of Therapy

Discuss expectations of therapy with the patient: prevention of the development of communicable disease for which immunization is being given. Assess changes in expectations as therapy progresses and the patient gains understanding of the need to complete all immunizations for effective prevention of disease.

Changes in Expectations

Assess changes in expectations as therapy progresses and the patient gains understanding of the immunization required.

Table 16.3
Recommended Immunization Schedule for Persons 7 Years of Age or Older

TIMING	VACCINE	COMMENTS
First visit	Td-1,* OPV-1,† and MMR‡	OPV not routinely administered to those ≥ 18 years of age
2 months after first Td, OPV	Td-2, OPV-2	
6–12 months after second Td, OPV	Td-3, OPV-3	OPV-3 may be given as soon as 6 weeks after OPV-2
10 years after Td-3	Td	Repeat every 10 years throughout life

From Centers for Disease Control: *Morbid. Mortal. Week. Rep.* 32:2–16, Jan. 14, 1983.

* Td—Tetanus and diphtheria toxoids (adult type) are used after the seventh birthday. The DTP doses given to children under 7 who remain incompletely immunized at age 7 or older should be counted as prior exposure to tetanus and diphtheria toxoids (for example, a child who previously received 2 doses of DTP needs only 1 dose of Td to complete a primary series).

† OPV—Oral, attenuated poliovirus vaccine contains poliovirus types 1, 2, and 3. When polio vaccine is to be given to individuals 18 years or older, IPV is preferred.

‡ MMR—Live measles, mumps, and rubella viruses in a combined vaccine. Persons born before 1957 can generally be considered immune to measles and mumps and need not be immunized. Rubella vaccine may be given to persons of any age, particularly to women of childbearing age. MMR may be used, since administration of vaccine to persons already immune is not deleterious.

Changes in Therapy through Cooperative Goal-Setting

Work with the patient to encourage adherence to the prescribed treatment. When the patient feels that a change should be made in a treatment plan, encourage a discussion first with the physician.

WRITTEN RECORD

Enlist the patient's aid in developing and maintaining a written record of monitoring parameters (Table 16.4) (i.e., rash, general malaise, arthralgias) and response to prescribed therapies for discussion with the physician. Patients should be encouraged to take this record with them on follow-up visits or to call the physician if symptoms become intense.

FOSTERING COMPLIANCE

Discuss medication information and how it will benefit the course of treatment. Seek cooperation and understanding of the following points so that medication compliance may be enhanced:

1. Name.
2. Dosage.
3. Route and administration times: Nurses need to foster maintenance of the administration schedule and the need to comply rigidly with appropriate storage of the immunologic agents.
4. Anticipated therapeutic response.
5. Side effects to expect: Most immunization clinics have routine orders for health teaching that state the usual symptoms to expect, such as pain, swelling, and tenderness at the injection site.

   The person may develop a subclinical case of the disease for which the vaccine was given. The person needs to understand what symptoms may develop and how to treat the fever, general malaise, or rash, should they occur. Check your institution's policies regarding routine orders.
6. Side effects to report: Always tells the patient to contact the physician or go to the nearest emergency room if these symptoms develop.
7. What to do if a dosage is missed.
8. When, how, or if to return for the next in a series of immunizations to become sufficiently immunized.

DIFFICULTY IN COMPREHENSION

If it is evident that the patient and/or family do not understand all aspects of continuing therapy being prescribed (i.e., need for follow-up appointments and completion of all required immunizations) consider the use of social service or visiting nurse agencies.

ASSOCIATED TEACHING

Always provide written information to the patient and family about the specific name of the agent that caused any reactions. Tell them always to inform all health workers (physicians, dentists, industrial nurses) of this reaction before receiving any treatment. Provide them with an allergy identification card and bracelet or necklace, if necessary.

Encourage the patient to report side effects of rash, itching, hives, or dyspnea immediately.

Always give the patient (1) a record of the *exact* name, dosage, route of administration and site of injection received (as appropriate to the medication type); (2) the discharge instructions for the treatment of symptoms that may develop; and, (3) a schedule of additional immunizations that are needed. Have the patient maintain a current record of all immunizations received.

If pregnancy is suspected, consult an obstetrician as soon as possible about continuation of medication therapy or series of immunizations.

Immune Serums

An immune serum is derived from the serum of a human being that has formed antibodies in the bloodstream against a specific disease. The immune serum is injected into the patient, whose specific antibodies that act on disease microorganisms provide passive acquired immunity.

Naturally produced human serums are obtained from the serum of patients who have recovered from a disease and still have the immune antibodies in their blood serum.

All of the immune serums listed in Table 16.5 are obtained from human plasma and contain gamma globulin. The plasma is pooled from blood donors from the general population or from donors who have been immunized against a specific disease.

Considerations for Use

These products are contraindicated in patients who are allergic to gamma globulin or who have produced antiimmunoglobulin A (IgA) antibodies.

Do not administer skin tests with these products. Local irritation from intradermal injection may easily be misinterpreted as a positive allergic response. True allergic reactions to human gamma globulin administered intramuscularly are extremely rare.

Table 16.4
Example of a Written Record for Patients Receiving Immune Agents (Vaccine or Immunization)

Medications	Color	To be taken

Name _____

Physician _____

Physician's phone _____

Next appt.* _____

Parameters		Day of injection									Comments
Temperature	8 AM / 12 N / 5 PM / Bed time										
Pulse											
Skin (rash)	Hivelike, fine red; itching present — (Yes or No)										
Joint discomfort	None										
	Aching										
	Painful										
Irritability	None										
	Mild										
	Unconsolable										
	Last ___ hr./ min.										
How I feel — Tired (10) 5 Okay (1)											
Dizziness	Faint when in upright position										
	Occasional										
	None										
Site of injection	Hot, swollen, and painful										
	Swollen, some discomfort										
	No problem										

*Please bring this record with you to your next appointment.
Use the back of this sheet for additional information.

Table 16.5
Immune Serums

GENERIC NAME	BRAND NAME	AVAILABILITY	COMMENTS
Hepatitis B immune globulin	H-BIG, HyperHep	IM: 1 and 5 ml vials	To be used after accidental exposure by "needle stick" or direct mucous membrane contact from blood, plasma, or serum containing hepatitis B antigen.
Immune globulin	Gamimune, Gammar	IV: 5% in 50 and 100 ml vials IM: 2 and 10 ml vials	Used for hepatitis A, hepatitis B, rubeola, rubella exposure. IV: Provides immediate antibody levels to provide protection for patients with immune deficiencies. IM: Requires 2–7 days for adequate antibody levels.
Lymphocyte immune globulin	Atgam	IM: 50 mg/ml in 5 ml ampules	Used in conjunction with other immunosuppressant therapy to prevent rejection of transplants.
Pertussis immune globulin	Hypertussis	1.25 ml vials	Used in infants for the prophylaxis and treatment of pertussis (whooping cough). Do not administer to patients over 7 years of age.
Rh₀ (D) immune globulin	RhoGAM, HypRho-D, Gamulin Rh	IM: 1:1000 dilution, single dose vials	Used in patients who are Rh negative who have been exposed to Rh positive blood. It prevents the formation of antibodies that may cause hemolysis if exposed to Rh positive blood again.
Tetanus immune globulin	Homo-tet, Hu-Tet, Hyper-Tet	IM: 250 unit vials and prefilled syringes	For patients exposed to tetanus who have not been immunized with tetanus toxoid.
Varicella-zoster immune globulin (VZIG)	Same	IM: 125 units in 2.5 ml vials	For use in immunodeficient children exposed to varicella-zoster (chicken pox).

After intramuscular injection, patients may have mild, localized tenderness and stiffness, which may persist for several hours after injection.

Although rare, allergic reactions, manifested by urticaria, angioedema, erythema, and low-grade fever, have been reported. Anaphylactic reaction, although even more rare, is more likely to develop in patients receiving intravenous immune globulin products who have received repeated infusions and who are highly allergic individuals. Epinephrine (1:1000) and other appropriate agents should be available to treat allergic reactions.

Availability

See Table 16.2 for available products.

Administration

See Table 16.5.
IM—Administer these agents intramuscularly (except Immune Globulin, Intravenous), preferably in the gluteal or deltoid region.

- Do not mix with any other product.

IV—Except for Immune Globulin, Intravenous (Gamimune), do not administer these products intravenously. A severe hypotensive reaction may result.

- Immune Globulin, Intravenous, may be diluted with dextrose 5% solution.

Nursing Interventions

See also General Nursing Considerations for Patients Receiving Immunologic Agents.

PATIENT CONCERNS: NURSING INTERVENTION/RATIONALE

Side Effects to Expect

Localized Tenderness

Inform patients that they may experience stiffness at the site of injection for several days.

Fever, Arthralgias, Generalized Aches and Pains

Monitor on a regular basis for the development of these symptoms. Be certain patients (or parents) know how to take a temperature.

Follow routine orders of the physician or clinic concerning the use of analgesics (usually acetaminophen; do not use aspirin or other antiinflammatory agents) for patient discomfort.

Side Effects to Report

Urticaria, Tachycardia, Hypotension

Allergic reactions need immediate treatment. Monitor patients for 20 to 30 minutes following administration. Have emergency supplies readily available.

Drug Interactions

Live Virus Vaccines

Antibodies in the immune globulin solutions may interfere with the immune response to live virus vaccination. Do not administer live virus vaccines for at least 3 months after the administration of immune globulin products.

Toxoids

A toxoid is a toxin that has been chemically modified to be nontoxic but still antigenic, thus inducing active, acquired immunity. The agent generally used for the detoxification of toxins is formaldehyde. Toxoids are available in the plain fluid form and as adsorbed and precipitated preparations. Aluminum hydroxide and aluminum phosphate are used to provide an adsorption surface for the adsorbed products, and alum is used for the precipitated products. The adsorbed and precipitated products are absorbed more slowly by the circulating and tissue fluids of the body and are excreted more slowly; thus, they provide immunizing levels longer than the plain fluid form of toxoid.

Considerations for Use

These products are contraindicated in patients who are allergic to any one of the individual toxoids. For example, if a patient is allergic to tetanus toxoid, do not administer diphtheria and tetanus toxoids, and pertussis vaccine (DPT). The patient may be immu-

nized, however, for diphtheria and pertussis by using individual immunologic products.

In general, do not use these products in patients with an acute infection or who are immunosuppressed. It is difficult to differentiate symptoms of disease from symptoms of reaction to the toxoid if the patient is ill. If a patient is immunosuppressed, it is unlikely that an adequate number of antibodies will be produced against the toxoid, thus leaving the patient unprotected.

Infants or children with cerebral damage, neurologic disorders, or a history of febrile convulsions should have their routine immunizations postponed until at least 1 year of age or, in the case of tetanus toxoid, administered first as a small dose to test the patient's tolerance to the toxoid.

Do not use toxoids as vaccines for treatment against active infection. Antitoxins or, preferably, specific immune globulins must be administered.

Localized reactions at the site of intramuscular injection are not uncommon. This reaction may be manifested by localized edema, itching, erythema, and induration, which will persist for several days. A nodule may be present at the site for several weeks.

Systemic allergic reactions are quite rare but are manifested by chills, fever, urticaria, generalized aches and pains, flushing, tachycardia, and hypotension. Epinephrine (1:1000) and other appropriate agents should be readily available to treat allergic reactions.

It is recommended that routine immunization schedules be postponed if an outbreak of poliomyelitis should occur. Complete the immunization schedule after the poliomyelitis infection is over.

Availability

See Table 16.6.

Administration

IM—Administer into the deltoid or midlateral muscles of the thigh. Do not inject the same muscle site more than once during the course of the routine immunization schedule.
SC, IV—*Do not* administer subcutaneously or intravenously.

Nursing Interventions

See also General Nursing Considerations for Patients Receiving Immunologic Agents.

Table 16.6
Toxoids

GENERIC NAME	BRAND NAME	AVAILABILITY	COMMENTS
Tetanus toxoid	Tetanus Toxoid, Fluid; Tetanus Toxoid, Adsorbed	SC: Fluid—0.5 ml syringes and vials, 7.5 ml vials IM: Adsorbed—0.5 ml syringes and vials, 5 ml vials	Tetanus Toxoid, Adsorbed, is recommended for all routine immunization and booster doses. Use is recommended for military personnel, farm and utility workers, firemen, and all other persons whose occupation may place them at risk for lacerations and abrasions. Do not administer if previous doses resulted in hypersensitivity or neurologic reactions.
Diphtheria toxoid	Diphtheria Toxoid Adsorbed (Pediatric)	IM: 5 ml vials	Recommended for use if a patient should not receive either Tetanus Toxoid or Pertussis Vaccine. Postpone immunization until age 2 if the infant has a history of seizure activity. Do not administer to children over 6 years of age.
Diphtheria and tetanus toxoids	Diphtheria and Tetanus Toxoids, Adsorbed, Pediatric and Adult Strengths	IM: 0.5 ml prefilled syringes, 5 ml vials	Administer the pediatric strength (TD) up to age 6. Administer the adult strength (Td) after age 6. Booster injections should be administered every 10 years. See comments above.
Diphtheria and tetanus toxoids, pertussis vaccine	Diphtheria, Tetanus, Pertussis Vaccine, Adsorbed-Connaught; Tri-Immunol; Ultrafined Triple Antigen	IM: 7.5 ml vials, 0.5 prefilled syringe	Recommended for routine immunizations in children between 2 months and 6 years of age. Children beyond the age of 7 years should not be immunized with pertussis vaccine. See comments above.

PATIENT CONCERNS: NURSING INTERVENTION/RATIONALE

Side Effects to Expect

Fever, Arthralgias, Generalized Aches and Pains

Monitor on a regular basis for the development of these symptoms. Be certain patients (or parents) know how to take a temperature.

Follow routine orders of the physician or clinic concerning the use of analgesics (usually acetaminophen; do not use aspirin or other antiinflammatory agents) for patient discomfort.

Side Effects to Report

Urticaria, Tachycardia, Hypotension

Allergic reactions need immediate treatment. Monitor patients for 20 to 30 minutes following administration. Have emergency supplies readily available.

Administration

IM

Administer intramuscularly using the correct length needle to ensure that the medication is being deposited into the muscle.

Since toxoids may be irritating to the tissues, 0.1 to 0.2 cc of air may be used to flush irritating medications from the needle into the muscle when being injected. (Check your institution's policy before administration.)

Drug Interactions

Chloramphenicol, Immunosuppressants

Chloramphenicol, corticosteroids, antimetabolites, and alkylating agents may inhibit production of antibodies against the toxoid. Discontinue chloramphenicol and immunosuppressant therapy before immunization.

Vaccines

Vaccines are suspensions of either live, attenuated or killed bacteria or viruses. They are administered as antigens to stimulate the production of antibodies by the host against the specific bacteria or virus. In contrast to short-term, passive immunity provided by immune serums and antitoxins, vaccines provide long-term, active immunity. Since vaccines must stimulate the production of antibodies, immunity is acquired over several days to weeks. Vaccines are administered prophylactically to prevent infection from specific organisms, whereas antitoxins and immune serums are administered after exposure to a specific organism for immediate protection. See Table 16.7.

Considerations for Use

Vaccines are contraindicated in patients who are allergic to the culture media (e.g., chick embryos), preservatives (e.g., thimerosal), or antibodies (e.g., neomycin) used in the manufacturing process.

Live, attenuated viruses should not be administered to patients with immune deficiencies or to those who are immunosuppressed. Replication of the virus may be enhanced in these patients.

Patients should not be immunized during a severe, febrile illness. It is difficult to differentiate symptoms of disease from symptoms of reaction to the vaccine if the patient is ill.

Live, attenuated virus vaccines should not be administered during pregnancy or to women who may become pregnant in the next 3 months. They have potential teratogenic effects on the developing fetus.

Do not use vaccines or toxoids for treatment against active infection. Antitoxins, or preferably, specific immune globulins must be administered.

Vaccinations are associated with a low risk of adverse effects, but reactions have been reported for all vaccines. These effects range from mild, local reactions to the very rare, severe systemic illness, such as anaphylaxis or paralysis. See Table 16.4 for precautions on individual vaccines.

Availability

See Table 16.7.

Administration

SC, IM—See individual manufacturer's recommendations.

Do not administer intravenously.

Storage at the correct temperature is imperative. *Do not* keep in the refrigerator door since this temperature is highly variable due to frequent opening. Place on the center shelf in the refrigerator, and periodically monitor the refrigerator temperature.

Nursing Interventions

See also General Nursing Considerations for Patients Receiving Immunologic Agents

---

PATIENT CONCERNS:
NURSING INTERVENTION/RATIONALE

Side Effects to Expect

Fever, Arthralgias, Generalized Aches and Pains

Monitor on a regular basis for the development of these symptoms. Be certain patients (or parents) know how to take a temperature.

Follow routine orders of the physician or clinic concerning the use of analgesics (usually acetaminophen; do not use aspirin or other antiinflammatory agents) for patient discomfort.

Side Effects to Report

Urticaria, Tachycardia, Hypotension

Allergic reactions need immediate treatment. Monitor patients for 20 to 30 minutes following administration. Have emergency supplies readily available.

Drug Interactions

Immunosuppressants

Corticosteroids, antimetabolites, and alkylating agents may inhibit production of antibodies against the vaccine. Discontinue immunosuppressant therapy before immunization.

Do not administer oral poliovirus vaccine to immunosuppressed children or to people who will come in contact with these children. The excreted virus can be transmitted to the immunosuppressed child.

Immune Serum Globulins

Antibodies in the immune globulin solutions may interfere with the immune response to live virus vaccines up to 3 months after administration of the globulin. It may be necessary to revaccinate persons who received immune globulins shortly after live virus vaccination.

Table 16.7

Vaccines

GENERIC NAME	BRAND NAME	AVAILABILITY	COMMENTS
Cholera vaccine	Cholera Vaccine	SC, IM: 1, 1.5, 20 ml vials	Killed virus; used primarily for immunity prior to traveling to an area of the world where cholera is still active. Only about 60% of patients injected gain immunity against cholera.
Influenza vaccine	Fluogen, Fluzone-Connaught	IM: 0.5, 5, 25 ml vials	Inactivated antigens of virus expected to be prevalent for the next year. Do not administer to patients allergic to eggs, chickens, and chick feathers. Recommended for patients over age 65 due to greater susceptibility and mortality from viral infections.
Measles (rubeola) vaccine	Attenuvax	SC: Single dose vials	Live, attenuated virus; administered to produce a mild measles infection. The mild infection then produces antibodies to prevent future, more serious measles infections.
Rubella vaccine	Meruvax II	SC: Single dose vials	Live, attenuated virus; administered to produce protection against german measles. Absolutely must not be administered to a female who might possibly become pregnant in the next 3 months. Vaccine contains Neomycin. Do not administer to patients allergic to aminoglycosides.
Measles, mumps, rubella vaccine	MMR II	SC: Single dose vials	Live, attenuated, viruses. Infants must be at least 15 months of age. Use with caution in children with a history of febrile convulsions, or cerebral injury. Defer vaccination for at least 3 months after blood transfusions. See also measles and mumps vaccines.
Mumps vaccine	Mumpsvax	SC: Single dose vials	Live, attenuated virus. Used for adult and pediatric immunizations against mumps. Mild fevers may occur within 30 days of immunization. Do not administer to patients allergic to aminoglycosides, eggs, chickens, or chick feathers. Discard reconstituted vial after 8 hours.
Pneumococcal vaccine, polyvalent	Pneumovax 23, Pnu-Immune 23	SC, IM: 1 and 5 dose vials	Cell capsules of 23 very prevalent or invasive pneumococcal bacteria that account for 85–90% of pneumococcal bacterial infections. Used in patients who have chronic illnesses who may be at greater risk for viral infections.
Poliovirus vaccine live, oral, trivalent (TOPV)	Orimune	PO: 0.5 ml doses	Live, attenuated viruses; stimulates natural infection without producing symptoms of the disease. Do not administer to immunosuppressed patients. Do not administer during febrile illness. Abolutely do not administer parenterally.
Rabies vaccine	Imovax WYVAC	IM: Single dose vials	Freeze-dried, suspension of inactivated rabies virus. Administered for patients who may be exposed to rabies, and for those who may have been exposed. If used post-exposure, an IM dose of rabies immune globulin (human) is also recommended. Soreness and swelling frequently occurs and mild febrile responses have been reported. Corticosteroids may interfere with immunity against rabies. Do not administer with rabies vaccine.

Antitoxins

Antitoxic serums are formed in the bodies of horses that have been injected with either diphtheria or tetanus toxin. The toxin acts as an antigen, stimulating the formation of antibodies against the toxin. Antitoxins are similar to immune serums in that they produce passive immunity.

Antitoxins are administered to treat a patient who has been exposed to either diphtheria or tetanus. The disadvantage of antitoxins is that there is a high in-cidence of hypersensitivity to horse blood, even though the products are highly purified. Tetanus immune globulin is recommended for the prevention and treatment of tetanus. The antitoxin should be used only if the immune globulin is not available. There is no immune globulin available for diphtheria.

Tests for sensitivity to horse serum should be made on patients before injection of antitoxins to prevent possibilities of hypersensitivity and anaphylactic shock. The antitoxin should be withheld if a reaction characterized by a red, swollen area develops around the site of the intradermal test injection.

Chapter 17

Drugs Affecting the Eye

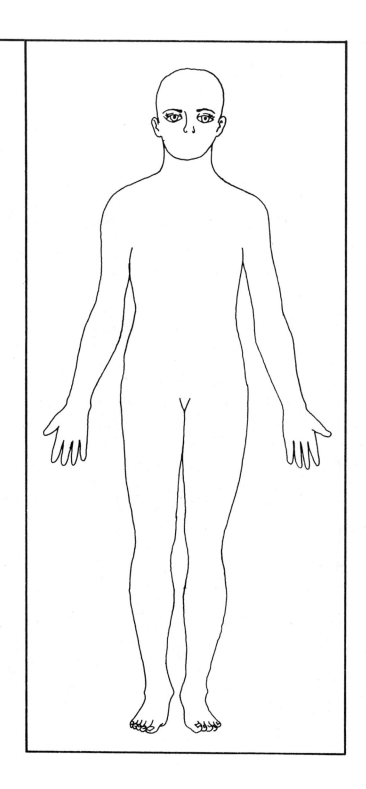

Objectives

After completing this chapter, the student should be able to do the following:

1. Explain the major actions and effects of drugs used to treat disorders of the eye.
2. Identify baseline data the nurse should collect on a continuous basis for comparison and evaluation of drug effectiveness.
3. Identify important nursing assessments and interventions associated with the drug therapy and treatment of diseases associated with the eye.
4. Identify health teaching essential for a successful treatment regimen.

The Eye

The eyeball has three coats or layers: the protective external, or corneoscleral, coat; the nutritive middle vascular layer, called the choroid; and the light-sensitive inner layer, or retina (Fig. 17.1).

The cornea, or outermost sheath of the anterior eyeball, is transparent to allow light to enter the eye. The cornea has no blood vessels but receives its nutrition from the aqueous humor and its oxygen supply by diffusion from the air and surrounding vascular structures. There is a thin layer of epithelial cells on the external surface of the cornea that is quite resistant to infection. An abraded cornea, however, is most susceptible to infection. The cornea has sensory fibers, and any damage to the corneal epithelium will cause pain. Seriously injured corneal tissue is replaced by scar tissue that is usually not transparent. The sclera, continuous with the cornea, is nontransparent and is the eye's white portion.

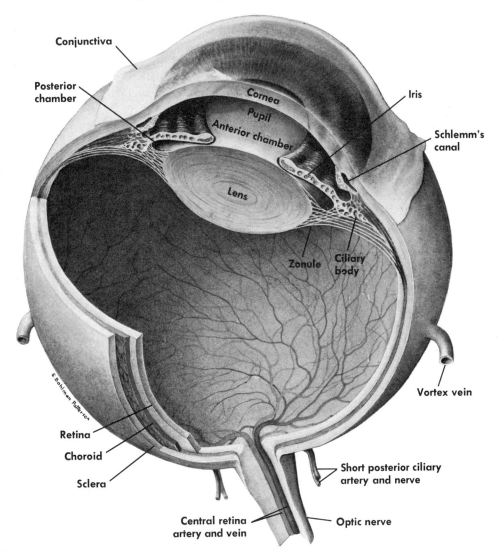

Fig. 17.1. *The human eye. (From Newell, F. W.: Ophthalmology, Principles and Concepts, ed. 4. The C.V. Mosby Co., St. Louis, 1978.)*

417

The iris is a diaphragm that surrounds the pupil and gives the eye its blue, green, hazel, brown, or gray color. The sphincter muscle within the iris encircles the pupil and is innervated by the parasympathetic nervous system. Contraction of the iris sphincter muscle causes the pupil to narrow; this is called *miosis*. The dilator muscle, which runs radially from the pupillary margin to the iris periphery, is sympathetically innervated. Contraction of the dilator muscle and relaxation of the sphincter muscle causes the pupil to dilate; this is called *mydriasis*.

Drugs that produce miosis (miotics) act similar to acetylcholine (cholinergic agents) at receptor sites in the sphincter muscle or interfere with cholinesterase activity (cholinesterase inhibitors), prolonging the activity of acetylcholine. Drugs that produce mydriasis (mydriatics) stimulate adrenergic receptors or inhibit the action of acetylcholine. Constriction of the pupil normally occurs with light or when the eye is focusing on nearby objects. Dilation of the pupil normally occurs in dim light or when the eye is focusing on distant objects.

The lens is a transparent, gelatinous mass of fibers encased in an elastic capsule situated behind the iris. Its function is to ensure that the image on the retina is in sharp focus. It does this by changing shape (accommodation). This occurs readily in youth, but with age the lens becomes more rigid and the ability to focus close objects is lost. The *near point*, or the closest point that can be seen clearly, recedes. With age, the lens may lose its transparency and become opaque, forming a cataract. Blindness can occur unless the cataract can be treated or surgically removed.

The lens has ligaments around its edge called zonular fibers that connect with the ciliary body. Tension on the zonular fibers helps to change the shape of the lens. In the unaccommodated eye, the ciliary muscle is relaxed and the zonular fibers are taut. For near vision, the ciliary muscle fibers contract, relaxing the pull on the ligaments and allowing the lens to increase in thickness. Accommodation depends on two factors: the ability of the lens to assume a more biconvex shape when tension on the ligaments is relaxed and ciliary muscle contraction. Paralysis of the ciliary muscle is termed *cycloplegia*. The ciliary muscle is innervated by parasympathetic nerve fibers.

The ciliary body secretes aqueous humor, which bathes and feeds the lens, posterior surface of the cornea, and iris. After it is formed, the fluid flows forward between the lens and the iris into the anterior chamber. It drains out of the eye through drainage channels located near the junction of the cornea and sclera into a meshwork that leads into the canal of Schlemm and into the venous system of the eye.

Eyelids, eyelashes, tears, and blinking all protect the eye. There are about 200 eyelashes for each eye. The eyelashes cause a blink reflex whenever a foreign body touches them, closing the lids for a fraction of a second to prevent the foreign body from entering the eye. Blinking, which is bilateral, occurs every few seconds during waking hours. It keeps the corneal surface free of mucus and spreads the lacrimal fluid evenly over the cornea. Tears are secreted by lacrimal glands and contain lysozyme, a mucolytic lubrication for lid movements. They wash away foreign agents and form a thin film over the cornea, providing it with a good optical surface. Tear fluid is lost by drainage into two small ducts (the lacrimal canaliculi) at the inner corners of the eyelids and by evaporation.

General Nursing Considerations for Patients with Disorders of the Eyes

The nurse has the important role of educating the public and promoting safety measures to protect the eyes from potential sources of injury. Health professionals can participate in this role during their daily contacts with people at work and in the community. The use of safety glasses in potentially hazardous situations, prevention of chemical burns from common household cleaning items or other agents at home or work, proper cleaning and wearing of contact lenses or glasses, and the selection of safe toys and play activities for children are examples of areas the nurse can teach the public about. These safety measures could significantly reduce the number of injuries that occur annually.

Nurses also play an important role in detection and implementation of the treatment process. The information the nurse assesses relative to eye disorders can be used as a baseline for subsequent response to the treatment plan. One of the greatest nursing challenges in the care of chronic eye disorders is to convince the patient of the need for long-term treatment and compliance with the therapeutic regimen.

POTENTIAL PATIENT NEEDS/PROBLEMS: NURSING INTERVENTION/RATIONALE

Indications of Disorders of the Eye

Observations by the Nurse

EYELIDS

Observe for complete closure of the eyelid. This is essential for protection of the cornea. All people with corneal anesthesia, fifth cranial nerve surgery, or who are unconscious must be protected from corneal damage.

Eye irrigations, the use of "artificial tears" such as methylcellulose, and closure of the eyes during anesthesia are practices used to insure protection.

Lid edema may be an indication of a systemic disease process or a tumor; report for further evaluation.

Exophthalmus (protusion of the eyeballs) should be evaluated and measures to protect the cornea instituted as part of the treatment plan.

PUPILS

Assess pupils for equality of size, roundness, and response to light. Always report irregular contour, unequal size, or decreased or unequal response to light.

EYELASHES

Inspect the eyes to be certain the eyelashes are not turned inward.

REDNESS, DRAINAGE

Persistent redness or discharge from the eyes should be evaluated. Emphasize for the patient that self-treatment with over-the-counter medications or eyewashes, or using another patient's eye medications, can be disastrous.

CROSSED EYES

Eyes that have recently shown signs of deviation from central gaze must be evaluated promptly.

NYSTAGMUS

Report nystagmus that always occurs in the same direction in response to eye movement in either direction.

HEMORRHAGE OR DRAINAGE

Drainage observed on the dressing should be reported immediately. Never remove the dressing to inspect the eyes unless given a specific order by the ophthalmologist.

Patient's Complaints

PAIN

Pain in the eye is not normal and should always be reported for immediate evaluation. Following ocular surgery, moderate discomfort may be expected; however, increasing pain is always a cause for immediate action. Notify the physician.

VISUAL ALTERATIONS

Complaints of "double vision," "halos" around lights, or the sudden occurrence of floating "spots" require physician evaluation.

Blurred vision, unrelated to eye medications, is not normal and all complaints of this should be followed up by examination.

Diagnostics Procedures

REFRACTION

Refraction is the part of an eye examination that determines whether a patient will benefit from wearing glasses. Anticholinergic agents are used to obtain the correct degree of dilation and paralysis of the ciliary muscles to allow examination of the interior of the eye.

INTRAOCULAR PRESSURE

Pressure within the eye is measured with a tonometer. Normal tonometer readings range between 12 and 22 mm Hg. Increased pressure may result in permanent damage to the eye tissue and the optic nerve.

Increased intraocular pressure is treated medically through the use of drugs to control rising pressure. If medications are ineffective, surgery may be required. Hourly tonometric readings may be required in some instances.

DYES

Dyes may be used to examine the cornea for abrasions or to identify viral infections. Since these solutions may become contaminated with use, it is imperative that new, sterile solutions be used.

Nursing Actions

VISUAL ACUITY

Patients with eye disorders should be carefully assessed for the degree of visual impairment. Provide for patient safety:

- Orient to new surroundings and leave furnishings in original place.
- Place the call light and other needed objects close to the patient.
- Assist with ambulation.
- Fix the food tray, cut up meat, if necessary, and pour liquids.
- Restrict the operation of tools or power equipment as appropriate to the degree of alteration present.

- Plan with the patient to call for assistance if needed for daily activities.
- If one eye is covered, place the patient in a room where the covered eye is away from the door so the patient can see who enters the room.

DISORIENTATION

The blind or those with both eyes patched may suffer from sensory deprivation that may result in disorientation:

- Always speak prior to touching a person with impaired vision.
- Check on the patient at frequent intervals; hold conversations and regularly orient him or her to date, time, and place.
- Try to arrange for a semiprivate room and a roommate who is alert, to provide stimulation.
- If the patient is agitated, contact the physician. It may be necessary to obtain an order to remove one eye patch.

INJURY

Provide for patient safety and prevent personal injury. Following surgery, caution the patient not to rub the eyes or try to touch under the dressings.

INFECTION

Always wash your hands before performing any procedure on the eye.

Use only sterile eye medications or dressings on the eyes.

Practice personal hygiene measures to prevent the introduction of an infection:

- Do not touch the eyes or rub them.
- Wipe one eye from the inner carthus outward; discard the tissue or cotton ball used; wash hands *before* proceeding to the second eye.
- When an infection is present, prevent cross-contamination. Always use a separate source of medication and droppers for each eye.
- Never touch the eyeball or face with the tip of the dropper or opening of the ointment container.
- When irrigating the eye, do not allow the solution to flow from one eye to the other.
- When inserting or removing contact lenses, wash your hands first, then follow the manufacturer's specific instructions regarding the cleansing and care of the lenses.
- Report any persistent redness or drainage from the eyes.

EMOTIONAL SUPPORT

Always let the patient know what limitations are being placed on him or her and the *reason* for the restrictions.

Give psychological support to the patient with an eye disorder. Fear of blindness may escalate anxiety and result in further tissue damage. Deal calmly with the patient's concerns. Let him or her vent anxieties.

ADMINISTRATION OF MEDICATIONS

See Administration of Eye Drops and Eye Ointments.

Patient Teaching Associated with Medications Used in the Eye

Communication and Responsibility

Encourage open communication concerning frustrations and anger as the patient attempts to adjust to the diagnosis and need for prolonged treatment. The patient must be guided to gain insight into the condition in order to assume responsibility for the continuation of treatment. Keep emphasizing those factors the patient can control to alter progression of the disease process, including maintenance of general health, nutritional needs, adequate rest and appropriate exercise, and continuation of prescribed medication therapy.

Expectations of Therapy

Discuss expectations of therapy with the patient (i.e., level of exercise, degree of pain relief, frequency of use of medications, relief of visual impairment, ability to maintain activities of daily living and work).

Changes in Expectations

Assess changes in expectations as therapy progresses and the patient gains understanding and skill in the management of the diagnosis.

Changes in Therapy through Cooperative Goal-Setting

Work with the patient to encourage adherence to the prescribed treatment. When the patient feels that a change should be made in a treatment plan, encourage discussion first with the physician.

WRITTEN RECORD

Enlist the patient's aid in developing and maintaining a written record of the monitoring parameters

(Table 17.1) (i.e., blood pressure and pulse with adrenergic agents, degree of visual disturbance, and progression of impairment) and response to prescribed therapies for discussion with the physician. Patients should be encouraged to take this record with them on follow-up visits.

FOSTERING COMPLIANCE

Throughout the hospitalization, discuss medication information and how it will benefit their course of treatment. Seek cooperation and understanding of the following points so that medication compliance may be enhanced:

1. Name
2. Dosage
3. Route and administration times: stress the need for maintaining the schedule
4. Anticipated therapeutic response particularly with glaucoma, control of intraocular pressure, and prevention of blindness
5. Side effects to expect
6. Side effects to report: see individual agents
7. What to do if a dosage is missed
8. When, how, or if to refill the medication prescription. Always keep an extra bottle of eye medication on hand. When refilling the prescriptions, always check the label on the new bottle to be sure the new supply is the same as the former bottle.

DIFFICULTY IN COMPREHENSION

If it is evident that the patient and/or family do not understand all aspects of continuing therapy being prescribed (i.e., administration and monitoring of medications, exercises, diets, follow-up appointments) consider the use of social service or visiting nurse agencies.

ASSOCIATED TEACHING

Give patients the following instructions:

Always inform the physician or dentist of any prescription or over-the-counter medication being taken. Over-the-counter medications should not be taken without first discussing them with your physician or pharmacist. This includes the use of eye washes.

Always report side effects of rash, itching, or hives immediately. Nausea, vomiting, or diarrhea should also be reported for the physician's evaluation if it is a new symptom.

Take all of the medication as prescribed for the full course of treatment. Do not discontinue use when feeling improved; do not save for future use; do not give your medicine to another individual. Sudden discontinuation of certain medications may produce harmful effects.

Keep all medications out of reach of children.

If pregnancy is suspected, consult an obstetrician as soon as possible about continuation of medication therapy.

At Discharge

Items to be sent home with the patient should:

1. Have written instructions for use
2. Be labeled in a level of language and size of print appropriate for the patient
3. If needed, include identification cards or bracelets
4. Include a list of additional supplies to be purchased after discharge (i.e., eye dressings, tissues, cotton balls, patches)
5. Include a schedule of follow-up appointments.

Glaucoma

Glaucoma is an eye disease characterized by abnormally elevated intraocular pressure, which may result from excessive production of the aqueous humor or from diminished ocular fluid outflow. Increased pressure, if persistent and sufficiently elevated, may lead to permanent blindness. There are three major types of glaucoma: primary, secondary, and congenital. Primary includes closed-angle or acute congestive glaucoma and open-angle, or chronic, simple glaucoma. These are diagnosed by the angle of the anterior chamber where aqueous humor reabsorption takes place. Open-angle glaucoma has an insidious onset, and its control demands long-term drug therapy. Drugs are also necessary for controlling the acute attack associated with closed-angle glaucoma. Secondary glaucoma may result from previous eye disease or may follow a cataract extraction and may require drug therapy for an indefinite period. Congential glaucoma requires surgical treatment.

Symptoms of chronic (open-angle) glaucoma include no symptoms in early stages, gradual loss of peripheral vision over a period of years, slow but persistent onset in older age groups, and persistent elevation of intraocular pressure, as determined by serial tonometric examinations and any other examinations the ophthamologist requires.

Cholinergic, anticholinesterase, adrenergic, and beta adrenergic blocking agents are used to treat glaucoma. The selection of the drug is determined to a great extent by the requirements of the individual patient.

Table 17.1

Example of a Written Record for Patients Receiving Eye Medications

Medications	Color	To be taken

Name _____

Physician _____

Physician's phone _____

Next appt.* _____

Parameters		Day of exam							Comments
Blood pressure									
Pain in eye (Right or Left)									
No pain in eyes									
Vision (clarity)	Blurred all the time								
	Occasionally hazy								
	Clear								
Side vision	Must turn head to see								
	Can see without turning head								
Vision since starting eye medication: No improvement Better Much better 10 5 1									
Headache	None								
	If yes, location								
	What were you doing when it started?								
Eye color Redness	Is redness improved by medication?								
Burning	Is burning improved by medication?								
Itching, rash	None								
	Sometimes associated with medication								
	Always occurs with medication								

*Please bring this record with you to your next appointment.
Use the back of this sheet for additional information.

422

Patient Teaching Associated with Glaucoma

ications are directed at decreasing the intraocular pressure through a variety of mechanisms (see individual medications).

PATIENT CONCERNS: NURSING INTERVENTION/RATIONALE

Communication and Responsibility

Encourage open communication concerning frustrations and anger as the patient attempts to adjust to the diagnosis and need for prolonged treatment. The patient must be guided to gain insight into the condition in order to assume responsibility for the continuation of treatment. Keep emphasizing those factors the patient can control to alter the disease process or progression, including the following:

Prevention

Persons with a family history of glaucoma should receive a yearly eye examination.

Prompt Diagnosis

Routine eye examination with tonometry as a part of a yearly physical should be encouraged, particularly in people over 40 years of age.

Patients experiencing alterations in peripheral vision, disturbance in ability to adjust to the dark, eye pain, or a general aching around the eyes should receive diagnostic evaluation as soon as possible.

Nutrition

General dietary intake of a well-balanced variety of nutrients, vitamins, and minerals is essential to good health.

Control

Once diagnosed, *constant control* for the remainder of one's life is essential to prevent blindness.

Medications

Adherence to the *specific* medication regimen prescribed for an individual must be stressed. Do not alter or omit medications; teach specific side effects to expect and how to manage these effects. All med-

Expectations of Therapy

Discuss expectations of therapy with the patient:

- With simple glaucoma, rigid compliance can control intraocular pressure and prevent further tissue damage. In some cases surgical intervention may be necessary.
- With closed-angle glaucoma, treatment with medications is tried first; surgical intervention is commonly required.

Activities and Exercise

To control intraocular pressure

- Avoid heavy lifting
- Avoid straining with defecation
- Avoid coughing
- Avoid bending and placing the head in a dependent position.

Pain Relief

With closed-angle glaucoma, the pain may be controlled with potent analgesics.

Nausea, Vomiting

Antiemetics to control nausea and vomiting and prevent further increases in intraocular pressure are essential. These symptoms are associated with closed-angle glaucoma.

Improved Vision

Degenerated tissue or damage to the optic nerve cannot be reversed. The main goal of therapy is to prevent further damage that may result in blindness.

Personal Safety

Provide for personal safety when visual acuity is diminished.

- Orient the patient to the surroundings.
- Assist in ambulation as appropriate to the degree of visual impairment.

• Do not allow the operation of equipment that might be dangerous to the visually impaired.

Changes in Expectations

Assess changes in expectations as therapy progresses and the patient gains understanding and skill in the management of the diagnosis.

Blurred Vision, Lacrimation, Redness

Many of the medications used cause temporary blurring of vision. With continued therapy this, as well as lacrimation and redness, subsides.

Changes in Therapy through Cooperative Goal-Setting

Work with the patient to encourage adherence to the prescribed treatment. When the patient feels that a change should be made in a treatment plan, encourage discussion first with the physician.

Written Record

Enlist the patient's aid in developing and maintaining a written record of the monitoring parameters: headache, blurred vision, pulse, and blood pressure. (Monitoring should correspond to the medications being taken.) Patients should be encouraged to take this record with them on follow-up visits.

Fostering Compliance

Throughout the patient's hospitalization, discuss medication information and how it will benefit the course of treatment. Seek cooperation and understanding of the following points so that medication compliance may be enhanced:

1. Name
2. Dosage
3. Route and time of administration: seek compliance and stress the need for adherence to the schedule to maintain the intraocular pressure at a stable level
4. Anticipated therapeutic response: control of intraocular pressure to prevent blindness
5. Side effects to expect: lacrimation and blurred vision

6. Side effects to report: decreasing vision, pain (see individual agents)
7. What to do if a dosage is missed
8. When, how, or if to refill the medication prescription. An extra bottle of medication should be kept on hand in case of contamination of the primary bottle.

   When refilling the prescription, always compare the new bottle with the information on the old prescription: name of drug, concentration or strength, directions, and expiration date.

Difficulty in Comprehension

If it is evident that the patient and/or family does not understand all aspects of continuing therapy being prescribed (i.e., administration and monitoring of medications, restrictions in exercises, need for follow-up appointments), consider the use of social service or visiting nurse agencies. Use of Ocusert may be appropriate depending on the patient's compliance.

Associated Teaching

Give patients the following instructions:

Always inform the physician or dentist of any prescription or over-the-counter medication being taken. Over-the-counter medications and eye washes should not be taken without first consulting with the physician or pharmacist.

Always report side effects of rash, itching, or hives immediately. Nausea, vomiting, or diarrhea should also be reported for the physician's evaluation if it is a new symptom.

Take all of the medication as prescribed for the full course of treatment. Do not discontinue use when feeling improved; do not save for future use; do not give your medicine to another individual. Sudden discontinuation of certain medications may produce harmful effects.

Keep all medications out of reach of children.

If pregnancy is suspected, consult an obstetrician as soon as possible about continuation of medication therapy.

At Discharge

Items to be sent home with the patient should:

1. Have written instructions for use.

2. Be labeled in a level of language and size of print appropriate for the patient.
3. If needed, include identification cards or bracelets
4. Include a list of additional supplies to be purchased after discharge (i.e., eye dressings, patches, cotton balls).
5. Include a schedule of follow-up appointments.

Cholinergic Agents

Cholinergic agents produce strong contractions of the iris (miosis) and ciliary body musculature (accommodation). These drugs lower the intraocular pressure in patients with glaucoma by widening the filtration angle, permitting outflow of aqueous humor. They may also be used to counter the effects of mydriatic and cycloplegic agents following surgery or ophthalmoscopic examination.

Advantages of cholinergic agents are that (1) they are effective in many cases of chronic glaucoma, (2) the side effects are less severe and less frequent than those of anticholinesterase agents, and (3) they give better control of intraocular pressure with fewer fluctuations in pressure.

Side Effects

A common side effect of cholinergic agents is difficulty in adjusting quickly to changes in light intensity. Reduced visual acuity may be most notable at night by older patients and in those patients developing lens opacities. Other common side effects are headaches in the suborbital or temporal region, conjunctival irritation and erythema, and induced myopia.

Rarely, a patient may develop signs of systemic toxicity, manifested by sweating, salivation, abdominal discomfort, diarrhea, bronchospasm, muscle tremors, hypotension, arrhythmias, and bradycardia. These symptoms are an indication of excessive administration. If accidental overdosage should occur during instillation, flush the affected eye with water or normal saline.

Availability

See Table 17.2.

Dosage and Administration

See individual agents.

Drug Interactions

No significant drug interactions have been reported.

Nursing Interventions

See also General Nursing Considerations for Patients with Disorders of the Eyes.

PATIENT CONCERNS: NURSING INTERVENTION/RATIONALE

Side Effects to Expect
Reduced Visual Acuity

The miosis induced by the cholinergic agents reduces visual acuity, particularly in areas of poor lighting. Advise patients to use caution while driving at night or performing hazardous tasks in poor light.

Blurred vision occurs particularly during the first 1 to 2 hours after instilling the medication.

Be sure to keep eye medications separate from other solutions.

The ability to read for long periods of time is decreased due to impairment of near-vision accommodation.

Provide for patient safety when visual impairment exists.

- In hospitals, orient to the hospital unit, furniture placement, and call light; place the bed in a low position.
- At home, do not move furniture or the individual's household or personal belongings.

Conjunctival Irritation, Erythema, Headache

These side effects are usually mild and tend to resolve with continued therapy. Encourage the patient not to discontinue therapy without first consulting the physician.

Pain, Discomfort

Because of pupillary constriction, an increase in pain or discomfort may occur, particularly in bright light. Stress the need for compliance and assure the patient that this will diminish with continued use.

Side Effects to Report
Systemic Side Effects

These side effects indicate overdosage or excessive administration. Report to the physician for dosage ad-

Table 17.2
Cholinergic Agents

GENERIC NAME	BRAND NAME	AVAILABILITY	DOSAGE	COMMENTS
Acetylcholine chloride, intraocular	Miochol Intraocular	1:100 solution	0.5–2 ml instilled into the eye during surgery	Used only during surgery to produce complete miosis within seconds. The duration of action is only a few minutes, so pilocarpine may be added to maintain miosis.
Carbachol, intraocular	Miostat Intraocular	0.01% solution	0.5 ml	Used only during surgery to produce complete miosis within 2–5 minutes.
Carbachol, topical	Isopto-Carbachol, Carbacel	0.75, 1.5, 2.25 and 3% solution	1–2 drops into eye 2–4 times daily	Miotic action lasts 4–8 hours. May be particularly useful in patients resistant to pilocarpine.
Pilocarpine	Isopto-Carpine, Pilocel, Pilocar, Akarpine, Almocarpine	0.25, 0.5, 1, 1.5, 2, 3, 4, 5, 6, 8, 10% solutions	1–2 drops up to 6 times daily. 0.5–4% solutions used most frequently.	Safest, most commonly used miotic for glaucoma. Also used to reverse mydriasis after eye examination. Onset is 15 minutes to 1 hour, and lasts for 2–3 hours.
Pilocarpine ocular therapeutic system	Ocusert Pilo-20 Ocusert Pilo-40	—	Inserted weekly, releases either 20 or 40 μg of pilocarpine per hour.	A small reservoir containing pilocarpine that is placed in a corner of the eye. Advantages: convenience, once-weekly dosing better continuous control of intraocular pressure less medication used, lower incidence of toxicity Disadvantages cost weekly insertions conjunctival irritation variable duration of action may fall out during sleep

justment. The adverse effects themselves usually do not need to be treated, since they will resolve by withholding cholinergic therapy.

Prevent systemic effects by carefully blocking the inner canthus for 1 to 2 minutes after instilling the medication to prevent absorption via the nasolacrimal duct.

During drug therapy, assess the blood pressure every shift and report significant changes from the baseline data.

Cholinesterase Inhibitors

Cholinesterase is an enzyme that destroys acetylcholine, the cholinergic neurotransmitter. The cholinesterase inhibitors prevent the metabolism of acetylcholine within the eye, causing increased cholinergic activity and resulting in decreased intraocular pressure and miosis. Thus, cholinesterase inhibitors are used in the treatment of glaucoma. Due to a higher incidence of side effects, however, they are reserved for patients who do not respond well to cholinergic agents.

Side Effects

A common side effect of anticholinesterase inhibitors is difficulty in adjusting quickly to changes in light intensity. Reduced visual acuity may be most notable at night by older patients and in those patients developing lens opacities.

Other common side effects are stinging, burning, headaches, conjunctival irritation and erythema, lid muscle twitching, brow-ache, and induced myopia with blurred vision.

Rarely, a patient may develop signs of systemic toxicity, manifested by sweating, salivation, vomiting, abdominal cramps, urinary incontinence, diarrhea, dyspnea, bronchospasm, muscle tremors, hypotension, arrhythmias, and bradycardia. These symptoms are an indication of excessive administration. If symptoms become severe, parenteral atropine should be administered. If accidental overdosage should occur during instillation, flush the affected eye with water or normal saline.

Availability

See Table 17.3.

Dosage and Administration

See individual agents.

Nursing Interventions

See also General Nursing Considerations for Patients for Disorders of the Eyes.

**PATIENT CONCERNS:
NURSING INVERVENTION/RATIONALE**

Side Effects to Expect

Reduced Visual Acuity

The miosis induced by the cholinesterase inhibitors reduces visual acuity, particularly in poorly lit areas. Advise patients to use caution while driving at night or performing hazardous tasks in poor light.

Conjunctival Irritation, Erythema, Headache, Lacrimation

These side effects are usually mild and tend to resolve with continued therapy. Encourage the patient not to discontinue therapy without first consulting the physician.

Table 17.3
Cholinesterase Inhibitors

GENERIC NAME	BRAND NAME	AVAILABILITY	DOSAGE	COMMENTS
Demecarium bromide	Humorsol	0.125, 0.25% solution	1–2 drops 1–2 times daily	Onset is within 1 hour; duration may be several days. Due to cumulative doses, use only the minimum dose necessary. Wipe excess solution away immediately.
Echothiophate iodide	Phospholine Iodide	0.03, 0.06, 0.125 0.25% solution	1 drop 1–2 times daily	Used most commonly in open-angle glaucoma. Onset occurs within 10–45 minutes, duration may be several days. After reconstitution, use within 1 month if stored at room temperature, 6 months if refrigerated. Tolerance may develop after prolonged use; a rest period will restore response.
Isoflurophate	Floropryl	0.025% ointment	¼ inch strip of ointment in conjunctiva every 8–72 hours.	When possible, apply at bedtime because of blurred vision. Due to cumulative doses, use only the minimum dose necessary.
Physostigmine	Eserine Isopto-Eserine	0.25% ointment 0.25, 0.5% solution	Ointment: small quantity up to 3 times daily. Solution: 2 drops up to 4 times daily.	May only be needed every other day. Do not use if solution turns pink to brown. Duration ranges 12–36 hours.

Side Effects to Report

Systemic Side Effects

These are an indication of overdosage or excessive administration. Report to the physician for treatment and dosage adjustment.

Drug Interactions

Carbamate and Organophosphate Insecticides and Pesticides

Gardeners, farmers, manufacturing employees, and others who are exposed to these pesticides and insecticides and who are receiving cholinesterase inhibitors should be warned of the added risk of systemic symptoms from absorption of these chemicals through the skin and respiratory tract. Respiratory masks and frequent washing and clothing changes are advisable.

Adrenergic Agents

Adrenergic agents have several uses in ophthalmology. Sympathomimetic agents cause pupil dilation, increased outflow of aqueous humor, vasoconstriction, relaxation of the ciliary muscle, and a decrease in the formation of aqueous humor. Adrenergic agents are used to treat open-angle glaucoma, to relieve congestion and hyperemia, and to produce mydriasis for ocular examinations.

Side Effects

The only common side effects are stinging, conjunctival irritation, and sensitivity to bright light. Pigmentary deposits in the conjunctiva, cornea, or lids may occur after prolonged use.

Systemic effect from ophthalmic instillation are uncommon and minimal. However, systemic absorption may occur via the lacrimal drainage system into the nasal pharyngeal passages. Systemic effects are manifested by palpitations, tachycardia, arrhythmias, hypertension, faintness, trembling, and sweating.

Use with caution in patients with hypertension, diabetes mellitus, hyperthyroidism, heart disease, arteriosclerosis, or long-standing bronchial asthma.

Availability

See Table 17.4.

Dosage and Administration

See individual agents.

Table 17.4
Adrenergic Agents

GENERIC NAME	BRAND NAME	AVAILABILITY	DOSAGE	COMMENTS
Epinephrine	Epifrin, Glaucon, Epitrate, Epinal, Eppy/N	0.25, 0.5, 1, 2% solutions	1–2 drops 1–2 times daily	Used to treat open-angle glaucoma, often in combination with cholinergic or beta-blocking agents. Duration of action is about 12 hours.
Dipivefrin hydrochloride	Propine	0.1%	1 drop every 12 hours	This drug has no activity itself, but is metabolized to epinephrine. It is used because it can penetrate the anterior chamber more readily than epinephrine, and is less irritating.
Hydroxyamphetamine hydrobromide	Paredrine	1% solution	1–2 drops	Used for pupillary dilation for diagnostic purposes. Duration is just a few hours.
Naphazoline hydrochloride	Vasoclear, Allerest, Naphcon, Albalon Liquifilm	0.012, 0.01, 0.1% solution	1–2 drops every 3–4 hours	Used as a topical vasoconstrictor.
Tetrahydrozoline hydrochloride	Murine Plus, Tetracon, Visine, Tetrasine	0.05% solution	1–2 drops 2 or 3 times daily	Used as a topical vasoconstrictor.

Nursing Interventions

See also General Nursing Considerations for Patients with Disorders of the Eyes.

PATIENT CONCERNS: NURSING INTERVENTION/RATIONALE

Side Effects to Expect

Sensitivity to Bright Lights

The mydriasis produced allows excessive amounts of light into the eyes, which causes the patient to squint. Use of sunglasses will help reduce the brightness. Caution the patient temporarily to avoid tasks that require visual acuity such as driving or operating power machinery.

Conjunctival Irritation, Lacrimation

These side effects are usually mild and tend to resolve with continued therapy. Encourage the patient not to discontinue therapy without first consulting the physician.

Side Effects to Report

Systemic Side Effects

These are indications of overdosage or excessive administration. Report to the physician for treatment and dosage adjustment.

Prevent systemic effects by carefully blocking the inner canthus for 1 to 2 minutes after instilling the medication to prevent absorption via the nasolacrimal duct.

Monitor the pulse rate and blood pressure and have the patient continue to do this at home; report significant changes from the baseline data.

Sweating, Trembling

Touch the patient and bedding to assess for diaphoresis (sweating), particularly when these agents are used in surgery where the patient is under sterile drapes, anesthetized, and unable to respond to verbal questioning.

Drug Interactions

Tricyclic Antidepressants

Tricyclic antidepressants (amitriptyline, imipramine, doxepin, others) may cause additive hypertensive effects. Monitor carefully for poor blood pressure control or a gradually increasing blood pressure.

Adrenergic Blocking Agent

Timolol maleate (tim'o-lol) (Timoptic) (tim-op'tik)

Timolol is a beta adrenergic blocking agent that reduces normal and elevated intraocular pressure. Unlike the anticholinergic agents, there is no blurred or dim vision or night blindness, because intraocular pressure is reduced with little or no effect on pupil size or visual acuity. Timolol is now used to reduce intraocular pressure in patients with chronic open-angle glaucoma, in aphakic patients with glaucoma, in certain cases of secondary glaucoma, and in ocular hypertension.

Side Effects

The only common side effects are stinging and conjunctival irritation.

Systemic effects from ophthalmic instillation are uncommon and minimal. Systemic effects are manifested by bradycardia, arrhythmias, hypotension, faintness, and bronchospasm.

Use with caution in patients with hypertension, diabetes mellitus, heart disease, arteriosclerosis, or long-standing bronchial asthma.

Availability

Ophthalmic—0.25 and 0.5% solution in 5, 10, and 15 ml dropper bottles.

Dosage and Administration

Initial therapy: 1 drop of 0.25% twice daily. Doses greater than 1 drop of 0.5% solution daily are rarely required.

Nursing Interventions

See also General Nursing Considerations for Patients with Disorders of the Eyes.

PATIENT CONCERNS: NURSING INTERVENTION/RATIONALE

Side Effects to Expect

Conjunctival Irritation, Lacrimation

These side effects are usually mild and tend to resolve with continued therapy. Encourage the patient not to discontinue therapy without first consulting the physician.

Side Effects to Report

Systemic Side Effects

These are an indication of overdosage or excessive administration. Report to the physician for treatment and dosage adjustment.

Record the blood pressure and pulse rate at specific intervals.

Drug Interactions

Beta Adrenergic Blocking Agents

Propranolol, atenolol, nadolol, pindolol, and metoprolol may enhance the systemic therapeutic and toxic effects of timolol.

Monitor for an increase in severity of side effects such as fatigue, hypotension and bradycardia.

Osmotic Agents

Osmotic agents are administered intravenously, orally, or topically to reduce intraocular pressure. These agents elevate the osmotic pressure of the plasma, causing fluid from the extravascular spaces to be drawn into the blood. The effect on the eye is reduction of volume of intraocular fluid, producing a decrease in intraocular pressure.

The osmotic agents are used to reduce intraocular pressure in patients with acute narrow-angle glaucoma, prior to iridectomy, and preoperatively and postoperatively in conditions such as congenital glaucoma, retinal detachment, cataract extraction, and keratoplasty, and in some secondary glaucomas.

Side Effects

Side effects include headache, nausea, vomiting, diarrhea, and thirst.

These agents should be used with caution in patients with cardiac, hepatic, or renal disease; the shift in body water may cause congestive heart failure or pulmonary edema.

In diabetic patients, the metabolism of the glycerin may cause hyperglycemia and glycosuria, so that diabetic patients should be observed for symptoms of acidosis.

Monitor vital signs, fluid and electrolyte balance, and urinary output of all patients.

Availability

See Table 17.5.

Dosage and Administration

See individual agents.

Nursing Interventions

See also General Nursing Considerations for Patients with Disorders of the Eyes.

PATIENT CONCERNS: NURSING INTERVENTION/RATIONALE

Side Effects to Report

Thirst, Nausea, Dehydration, Electrolyte Imbalance

The electrolytes most commonly altered are potassium (K^+), sodium (Na^+), and chloride (Cl^-).

Many symptoms associated with altered fluid and electrolyte balance are subtle and resemble general symptoms of drug toxicity or the disease process itself.

Gather data relative to *changes* in the patient's mental status (i.e., alertness, orientation, confusion), muscle strength, muscle cramps, tremors, nausea, and general appearance (drowsy, anxious, lethargic).

Always check the electrolyte reports for early indicators of electrolyte imbalance.

Keep accurate records of I/O, daily weights, and vital signs.

Headache

This is an indication of cerebral dehydration. It can be minimized by keeping the patient lying down.

Table 17.5
Osmotic Agents

GENERIC NAME	BRAND NAME	AVAILABILITY	DOSAGE	COMMENTS
Glycerin	Glyrol, Osmoglyn	50, 75% solutions	PO: 1–1.5 g/kg	An oral osmotic agent for reducing intraocular pressure. Administer 60–90 minutes prior to surgery. Use with caution in diabetic patients, monitor for hyperglycemia.
Isosorbide	Ismotic	100 g in 220 ml solution	PO: 1.5 g/kg (range— 1–3 g/kg) 2–4 times daily	An oral osmotic agent for reducing intraocular pressure. Onset of action is 30 minutes, duration is 5–6 hours. With repeated doses, monitor fluids and electrolytes. The solution will taste better if poured over cracked ice and sipped.
Mannitol	Osmitrol	5, 10, 15, 20, 25% solutions for infusions	IV: 1.5–2 g/kg as a 25% solution over 30 minutes	Used intravenously when oral methods are unacceptable. When used preoperatively, administer 60–90 minutes prior to surgery. Use an in-line filter since mannitol has a tendence to crystallize.
Urea	Ureaphil	40 g in 150 ml	IV: 1–1.5 g/kg	Administer as a 30% solution at an infusion rate not to exceed 4 ml/minute. Used when mannitol and oral methods are not available. Do not exceed 120 g daily. Use extreme caution against extravasation. Tissue necrosis may result. Do not infuse in veins of lower extremities due to the possibility of thrombus formation.

Circulatory Overload

These medications act on the blood volume as well by pulling fluid from the tissue spaces into the general circulation (blood). Assess the patient at regularly scheduled intervals for signs and symptoms of fluid overload, pulmonary edema, or congestive heart failure. Perform lung assessments; report the development of rales and increasing dyspnea, frothy sputum, or cough.

Dosage and Administration

Catheter

Be certain the patient has an indwelling catheter if these drugs are used during an operative procedure; check with the physician before scrubbing for the procedure.

IV

Assess the IV site at regular intervals for any signs of infiltration. Tissue necrosis may occur from infiltration into the surrounding tissue. If it occurs, stop the IV, report, then elevate the extremity and follow hospital protocol for extravasation.

Do not use veins in lower extremities for administration of these agents. This will minimize the occurrence of phlebitis and thrombosis.

Mannitol Crystals

Check the mannitol solution for crystals; *do not* administer if present. Follow directions in the literature accompanying the medication for a warm bath to dissolve the crystals and then cool the solution prior to administration.

Carbonic Anhydrase Inhibitors

Acetazolamide (ah-set-ah-zol'ah-myd)
(Diamox) (dy'ah-moks)

Dichlorphenamide (dy-klor-fen'ah-myd)
(Daranide) (dar'a-neyd)

Methazolamide (meth-ah-zol'ah-myd)
(Neptazane) (nep'tah-zain)

These three agents are inhibitors of the enzyme carbonic anhydrase. Inhibition of this enzyme results in a decrease in the production of aqueous humor, thus lowering intraocular pressure. These agents are used in conjunction with other treatment modalities to control intraocular pressure in both closed-angle and open-angle glaucoma.

Side Effects

Carbonic anhydrase inhibitors are sulfonamide derivatives and thus have the potential to cause adverse effects similar to those associated with sulfonamide antimicrobial therapy. These adverse effects, although rare, include dermatologic, hematologic, and neurologic reactions. For further discussion, see the sulfonamide section of Chapter 18.

Patients who are allergic to sulfonamides should not receive carbonic anhydrase inhibitors due to cross-sensitivity.

Side effects associated with carbonic anhydrase inhibitors are usually quite mild. They include gastric irritation, a numbness or tingling of the extremities, diuresis, and, occasionally, drowsiness and confusion.

Although infrequent, treatment with carbonic anhydrase inhibitors may lead to excessive diuresis with water dehydration and electrolyte imbalance.

Availability

Acetazolamide
PO—125, 250 mg tablets, 500 mg capsules.
IV—500 mg per vial.
Dichlorphenamide
PO—50 mg tablets.
Methazolamide
PO—50 mg tablets.

Dosage and Administration

Adult
PO—Acetazolamide: 250 mg to 1 g every 24 hours. Dichlorphenamide: 25 to 50 mg 1 to 3 times daily. Methazolamide: 50 to 100 mg, 2 or 3 times daily.

Nursing Interventions

See also General Nursing Considerations for Patients with Disorders of the Eyes.

PATIENT CONCERNS: NURSING INTERVENTION/RATIONALE

Side Effects to Report

Electrolyte Imbalance, Dehydration

The electrolytes most commonly altered are potassium (K^+), sodium (Na^+), and chloride (Cl^-). *Hypokalemia* is most likely to occur.

Many symptoms associated with altered fluid and electrolyte balance are subtle and resemble general symptoms of drug toxicity or the disease process itself.

Gather data relative to *changes* in the patient's mental status (i.e., alertness, orientation, confusion), muscle strength, muscle cramps, tremors, nausea, and general appearance (drowsy, anxious, lethargic).

Always check the electrolyte reports for early indications of electrolyte imbalance.

Keep accurate records of I/O, daily weight, and vital signs.

Dermatologic, Hematologic, Neurologic Reactions

See Sulfonamides in Chapter 18, Antimicrobial Agents.

Confusion

Perform a baseline assessment of the patient's degree of alertness and orientation to name, place, and time before initiating therapy. Make regularly scheduled subsequent mental status evaluations and compare findings. Report development of alterations.

Drowsiness

This side effect is usually mild and tends to resolve with continued therapy. Encourage the patient not to discontinue therapy without first consulting the physician.

Persons who are working around machinery, driving a car, pouring and giving medicines, or performing other duties in which they must remain mentally alert should not take these medications while working.

Dosage and Administration

Sulfonamides

Do not administer to patients allergic to sulfonamide antibiotics without prior physician approval. Observe closely for the development of hypersensitivity.

Gastric Irritation

If gastric irritation occurs, administer with food or milk. If symptoms persist or increase in severity, report for physician evaluation.

Drug Interactions

Quinidine

These diuretics may inhibit the excretion of quinidine. If your patient is also receiving quinidine, monitor closely for signs of quinidine toxicity (tinnitus, vertigo, headache, confusion, bradycardia, visual disturbances).

Digitalis Glycosides

Patients receiving these diuretics may excrete excess potassium, which leads to hypokalemia. If your patient is also receiving a digitalis glycoside, monitor closely for digitalis toxicity (anorexia, nausea, fatigue, blurred or colored vision, bradycardia, arrhythmias).

Corticosteroids (Prednisone, Others)

Corticosteroids may enhance the loss of potassium. Check potassium levels and monitor more closely for hypokalemia when these two agents are used concurrently.

Anticholinergic Agents

Anticholinergic agents cause the smooth muscle of the ciliary body and iris to relax, producing mydriasis (extreme dilation of the pupil) and cycloplegia (paralysis of the ciliary muscle). Ophthalmologists use these effects to examine the interior of the eye, to measure the proper strength of lenses for eyeglasses (refraction), and to rest the eye in inflammatory conditions of the uveal tract.

Side Effects

The pharmacologic effects of anticholinergic agents cause an increase in intraocular pressure. Use these agents with extreme caution in patients with a narrow anterior chamber angle, in infants, children, and the elderly, and in hypertensive, hyperthyroid, and diabetic patients. Discontinue therapy if signs of increased intraocular pressure or systemic effects develop.

The only common side effects seen with short-term use are stinging, conjunctival irritation, and sensitivity to bright light.

Prolonged use may result in systemic effects manifested by flushing and dryness of the skin, dry mouth, blurred vision, tachycardia, arrhythmias, urinary hesitancy and retention, vasodilation, and constipation.

Availability

See Table 17.6.

Dosage and Administration

See individual agents.

Nursing Interventions

See also General Nursing Considerations for Patients with Disorders of the Eyes.

PATIENT CONCERNS: NURSING INTERVENTION/RATIONALE

Side Effects to Expect

Sensitivity to Bright Lights

The mydriasis produced allows excessive light into the eyes, causing the patient to squint. Use of sunglasses will help reduce the brightness. Caution the patient to temporarily avoid tasks that require visual acuity such as driving or operating power machinery.

Conjunctival Irritation, Lacrimation

These side effects are usually mild and tend to resolve with continued therapy. Encourage the patient not to discontinue therapy without first consulting the physician.

Table 17.6
Anticholinergic Agents

GENERIC NAME	BRAND NAME	AVAILABILITY	DOSAGE	COMMENTS
Atropine sulfate	Isopto-Atropine, Atropisol	1% ointment, 0.5, 1, 2, 3%	Uveitis: 1–2 drops up to 3 times daily	Onset of mydriasis and cycloplegia is 30–40 minutes, duration is 7–12 days. Do not use in infants.
Cyclopentolate hydrochloride	Cyclogyl, AK-Pentolate	0.5, 1, 2% solutions	Refraction: 1 drop followed by another drop in 5–10 minutes	For mydriasis and cycloplegia necessary for diagnostic procedures. 1–2 drops of 1–2% pilocarpine allows full recovery within 3–6 hours. CNS disturbances of hallucinations, loss of orientation, restlessness, and incoherent speech have been reported in children.
Homatropine hydrobromide	Isopto-Homatropine Homatrocel	2 and 5% solutions	Uveitis: 1–2 drops every 3–4 hours	Onset of mydriasis and cycloplegia is 40–60 minutes; duration is 1–3 days.
Scopolamine hydrobromide	Isopto-Hyoscine	0.25% solution	Uveitis: 1–2 drops up to 3 times daily	Onset of mydriasis and cycloplegia is 20–30 minutes; duration is 3–7 days.
Tropicamide	Mydriacyl	0.5 and 1% solutions	Refraction: 1 or 2 drops, repeated in 5 minutes	Onset of mydriasis and cycloplegia is 20–40 minutes; duration is 6 hours. CNS disturbances of hallucinations, loss of orientation, restlessness, and incoherent speech have been reported in children.

Side Effects to Report

Systemic Side Effects

These are an indication of overdosage or excessive administration. Report to the physician for treatment and dosage adjustment. Children are particularly prone to develop systemic reactions.

Antiseptics

Silver Nitrate

Silver nitrate ophthalmic solution is used as an antiseptic agent, primarily as a prophylaxis against gonorrhea infection in the eyes of newborn infants (ophthalmia neonatorum).

Side Effects

A mild conjunctivitis manifested by localized erythema is reported in up to 20% of patients.

Availability

Ophthalmic—1% solution in wax ampules.

Dosage and Administration

Newborns. Immediately after delivery, instill 2 drops in each eye (see additional instructions below).

Nursing Interventions

See also General Nursing Considerations for Patients with Disorders of the Eyes.

PATIENT CONCERNS: NURSING INTERVENTION/RATIONALE

Side Effects to Expect

Conjunctivitis

This side effect is usually mild and tends to resolve within a day.

Dosage and Administration

Instillation

Immediately after delivery:

- Wash your hands before and after instillation.
- Using a separate gauze and sterile water for each eye, wash the unopened lids from the nose outward until free of all blood, mucus, or meconium.
- Separate the eyelids and instill 2 drops of 1% solution into the eye. Separate the lids far enough from the eyeball so that a pool of silver nitrate rests between the lids, on the eye.
- Allow the pool to remain for 30 seconds or longer.
- Do not irrigate the eyes with other solutions after the silver nitrate instillation.
- Take care not to get silver nitrate solution on skin or nails, since they will become discolored.

Anesthetics

Local anesthetics (Table 17.7) may be used in such ophthalmic procedures as removal of foreign objects, tonometry, gonioscopy, suture removal, and for short corneal and conjunctival procedures. Since the blink reflex is temporarily eliminated, it is wise to protect the eye with a patch after procedures are completed. Caution the patient not to rub the eyes; the patient could damage the eye and yet feel no pain.

Alpha chymotrypsin 1:5000 or 1:10,000 may be used during ocular surgery to dissolve zonular fibers that suspend the cataract in the eye.

Antibacterial Agents

Antibacterial agents (Table 17.8) are occasionally used in the treatment of superficial eye infections. Prolonged or frequent intermittent use of topical antibiotics should be avoided because of the possibility of hypersensitivity reactions and the development of resistant organisms, including fungi. If hypersensitivities

Table 17.7
Ophthalmic Anesthetics

GENERIC NAME	BRAND NAMES	AVAILABILITY
Cocaine hydrochloride	Various	1% to 4% solution
Proparacaine hydrochloride	Alcaine, Ophthetic, Ophthaine	0.5% solution
Tetracaine hydrochloride	Pontocaine Eye	0.5% solution, 0.5% ointment

or new infections appear during use, consult an ophthalmologist immediately. Refer to the Index for a discussion of these antibiotics.

Antifungal Agent

Natamycin (na-tah-my'sin)
(Natacyn) (na'tah-sin)

Natamycin is an antifungal agent effective against a variety of yeasts, including *Candida*, *Aspergillus*, and *Fusarium*. It is effective in the treatment of fungal blepharitis, conjunctivitis, and keratitis caused by susceptible organisms. If little or no improvement is noted after 7 to 10 days of treatment, resistance to the antifungal agent may have developed. Topical administration does not appear to result in systemic effects.

Side Effects

Side effects are quite mild, but include minor blurring of vision and increased sensitivity to light. If eye pain develops, discontinue use and contact an ophthalmologist immediately.

Availability

Ophthalmic—0.5% suspension.

Dosage and Administration

Fungal keratitis: 1 drop in the conjunctival sac at 1 or 2 hour intervals for the first 3 to 4 days. The dosage may then be reduced to 1 drop every 3 to 4 hours. Continue therapy for 14 to 21 days.

Nursing Interventions

See also General Nursing Considerations for Patients with Disorders of the Eyes.

PATIENT CONCERNS: NURSING INTERVENTION/RATIONALE

Side Effects to Expect

Sensitivity to Bright Lights

The slight mydriasis produced allows excessive amount of light into the eyes causing the patient to squint. Use of sunglasses will help reduce the brightness. Caution the patient to temporarily avoid tasks that require visual acuity such as driving or operating power machinery.

Table 17.8
Ophthalmic Antibiotics

ANTIBIOTIC	BRAND NAMES	AVAILABILITY
Bacitracin	Baciguent Ophthalmic	Ointment
Chloramphenicol	Chloromycetin Ophthalmic, Chloroptic, Econochlor, Ophthochlor	Drops, ointment
Chlortetracycline	Aureomycin Ophthalmic	Ointment
Erythromycin	Ilotycin Ophthalmic	Ointment
Gentamicin	Garamycin Ophthalmic	Drops, ointment
Polymyxin B	Polymyxin B Sulfate	Drops
Sulfacetamide	AK-Sulf, Sulf-10	Drops, ointment
Tetracycline	Achromycin Ophthalmic	Drops
Tobramycin	Tobrex Ophthalmic	Drops
Combinations		
Chloramphenicol/Polymyxin B	Chloromyxin Ophthalmic	Ointment
Neomycin/Polymyxin B	Statrol Ophthalmic	Ointment, drops
Neomycin/Polymyxin B/ Bacitracin	Mycitracin Ophthalmic, Neosporin Ophthalmic, Neotal	
Neomycin/Polymyxin B/ Gramicidin	Neosporin Ophthalmic	Drops

Blurred Vision, Lacrimation, Redness

Provide for patient safety during temporary visual impairment. Instruct the patient not to rub the eyes forcefully while tearing.

These side effects are usually mild and tend to resolve with continued therapy. Encourage the patient not to discontinue therapy without first consulting the physician.

Side Effects to Report

Eye Pain

If eye pain develops, discontinue use and consult an ophthalmologist immediately.

Therapeutic Effect

If, after several days on therapy the presenting symptoms are not improving or are gradually worsening, consult the physician treating the patient.

Antiviral Agents

Idoxuridine (i-doks-ur'i-deen)
(Dendrid) (den'drid) **(Stoxil)** (stok'sil)

Trifluridine (try-flur'i-deen)
(Viroptic) (vy-rhop'tik)

Idoxuridine and trifluridine are chemically related compounds used to treat herpes simplex keratitis. Idoxuridine is particularly effective against initial infections but is not very effective against deep infections or chronic, recurrent infections. Trifluridine is used to treat recurrent infections in those patients who are intolerant of or resistant to idoxuridine or vidarabine therapy; cross-sensitivity with these other agents has not been reported. Idoxuridine and trifluridine are not effective against bacteria, fungi, and *Chlamydia* infections.

Side Effects

Side effects are quite mild, since essentially no systemic absorption takes place. Patients may notice a mild, transient stinging, burning, and redness of the conjunctiva and sclera on instillation.

Other adverse effects that have rarely been reported include stromal edema, hypersensitivity reactions, and increased intraocular pressure.

Use of the ointment form (Stoxil) may cause temporary blurring of vision until the ointment is spread across the eyeball by the eyelid.

Availability

Ophthalmic—Idoxuridine: 0.1% solution and 0.5% ointment.
Trifluridine: 0.1% solution.

Dosage and Administration

Idoxuridine

Ophthalmic Solution: Initially 1 drop in each infected eye every hour during the day and every 2 hours after bedtime. After significant improvement, as shown by loss of staining with fluorescein, reduce the dose to 1 drop every 2 hours during the day and every 4 hours at night. Continue therapy for 3 to 5 days after healing appears to be complete to minimize recurrences.

Ophthalmic Ointment: Place a ribbon of ointment in the conjunctival sac of the infected eye 5 times daily, approximately every 4 hours, with the last dose at bedtime. Continue therapy for 3 to 5 days after healing appears to be complete to minimize recurrence.

Trifluridine

Ophthalmic Solution: Place 1 drop onto the cornea of the affected eye every 2 hours. Do not exceed 9 drops daily. Continue for 7 more days to prevent recurrence, using 1 drop every 4 hours (5 drops daily).

Note: For both agents, if significant improvement has not occurred in 7 to 14 days, other therapy should be considered. Do not exceed 21 days of continuous therapy due to potential ocular toxicity.

Nursing Interventions

See also General Nursing Considerations for Patients with Disorders of the Eye.

PATIENT CONCERNS: NURSING INTERVENTION/RATIONALE

Side Effects to Expect

Sensitivity to Bright Lights

The slight mydriasis produced allows excessive amounts of light into the eyes causing the patient to squint. Use of sunglasses will help reduce the brightness. Caution the patient to temporarily avoid tasks that require visual acuity such as driving or operating power machinery.

Visual Haze, Lacrimation, Redness, Burning

Provide for patient safety during temporary visual impairment. Instruct the patient not to rub the eyes forcefully while tearing.

These side effects are usually mild and tend to resolve with continued therapy. Encourage the patient not to discontinue therapy without first consulting the physician.

Dosage and Administration

Storage

Idoxuridine and trifluridine should be stored in the refrigerator. (Herplex Liquifilm does not require refrigeration.)

Drug Interactions

Boric Acid Solutions

Tell the patient not to use boric acid eye washes while using idoxuridine; local irritation may be enhanced.

Vidarabine (vy-dar′a-been)
(Vira-A) (vy′rah-ay)

Vidarabine is used topically as an ophthalmic ointment to treat keratitis and keratoconjunctivitis caused by herpes simplex virus types 1 and 2. Vidarabine does not show cross-sensitivity to idoxuridine or trifluridine and may be effective in treating recurrent keratitis that is resistant to idoxuridine and trifluridine. Vidarabine is not effective against infections caused by bacteria, fungi, or *Chlamydia*.

Side Effects

Minor side effects associated with the use of vidarabine ointment include temporary visual haze, burning, itching, redness, and lacrimation. Photophobia (sensitivity to bright light) occasionally occurs. Allergic reactions have rarely been reported.

Availability

Ophthalmic—3% ointment.

Dosage and Administration

Ophthalmic—Place a 1 cm ribbon of ointment inside the lower conjunctival sac of the infected eye 5 times daily at 3 hour intervals. Continue for an additional 5 to 7 days at a dosage of 1 cm twice daily after significant improvement has occurred to prevent recurrence of the infection.
IV—Not for ophthalmic use (see Index).

Nursing Interventions

See also General Nursing Considerations for Patients with Disorders of the Eyes.

**PATIENT CONCERNS:
NURSING INTERVENTION/RATIONALE**

Side Effects to Expect

Visual Haze, Lacrimation, Redness, Burning

Provide for patient safety during temporary visual impairment. Instruct the patient not to rub the eyes forcefully while tearing.

These side effects are usually mild and tend to resolve with continued therapy. Encourage the patient not to discontinue therapy without first consulting the physician.

Sensitivity to Bright Light

The slight mydriasis produced allows excessive light into the eyes, causing the patient to squint. Use of sunglasses will help reduce the brightness. Caution the patient to temporarily avoid tasks that require visual acuity such as driving or operating power machinery.

Side Effects to Report

Allergic Reactions

Discontinue therapy and consult an ophthalmologist immediately.

Corticosteroids

Corticosteroid therapy is indicated for allergic reactions of the eye and other acute, noninfectious inflammatory conditions of the conjunctiva, sclera, cornea, and anterior uveal tract (Table 17.9). Corti-

Table 17.9
Corticosteroids

GENERIC NAME	BRAND NAME	AVAILABILITY
Dexamethasone	Maxidex	Suspension
	AK-Dex	Ointment
Fluorometholone	FML Liquifilm	Suspension
Hydrocortisone	Hydrocortone	Ointment
Medrysone	HMS Liquifilm	Suspension
Prednisolone	Econopred Plus, Pred	Solution
	Mild, Inflamase,	Suspension
	Predulose, Metreton	

costeroid therapy must not be used in bacterial, fungal, or viral infections of the eye because corticosteroids decrease defense mechanisms and reduce resistance to pathologic organisms. This therapy should be used for a limited time only, and the eye should be checked frequently for an increase in intraocular pressure. Prolonged ocular steroid therapy may cause glaucoma and cataracts.

Other Ophthalmic Agents

Fluorescein Sodium

Fluorescein sodium is used in fitting hard contact lenses and as a diagnostic aid in identifying foreign bodies in the eye and abraded or ulcerated areas of the cornea. When sodium fluorescein is instilled in the eye, it stains the pathologic tissues green if observed under normal light, or bright yellow if viewed under cobalt blue light. Fluorescein sodium is available in 2% topical solution; 0.6, 1, and 9 mg strips for topical application; and 5, 10, and 25% solutions for injection into the aqueous humor. The strips have the advantage of being used once and then discarded. The solution carries the risk of bacterial contamination if used for several different patients. Product names include Fluorescite, Funduscein-25, Ful-Glo, and Fluor-I-Strip.

Artificial Tear Solutions

Artificial tear solutions are products made to mimic natural secretions of the eye. They provide lubrication for dry eyes. They may also be used as lubricants for artificial eyes. Most products contain variable concentrations of methylcellulose, polyvinyl alcohol, and polyethylene glycol. The dosage is 1 to 3 drops in each eye 3 to 4 times daily, as needed. Product names include Isopto Plain, Lacril, Tears Naturale, Nu-Tears, and Hypotears.

Ophthalmic Irrigants

These products are sterile solutions used for soothing and cleansing the eye, removing foreign bodies, in conjunction with hard contact lenses, or with fluorescein. Product names include Eye-Stream, Lavoptik Eye Wash, AK-Rinse, Collyrium, and Trisol.

Unit IV

Other Pharmacologic Agents

Chapter 18

Antimicrobial Agents

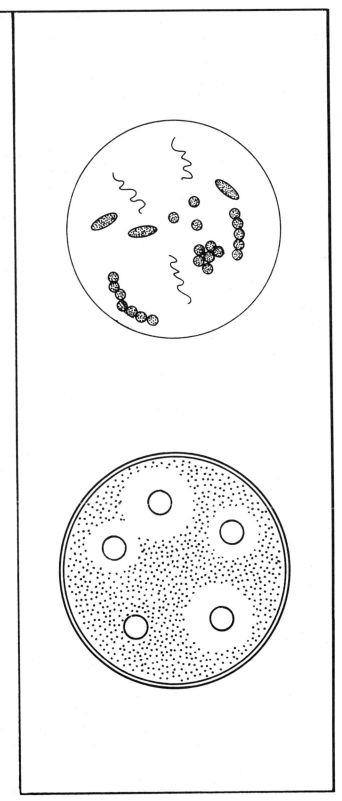

After completing this chapter, the student should be able to do the following:

1. Explain the major actions and effects of drugs used to treat infectious diseases.
2. Identify baseline data the nurse should collect on a continuous basis for comparison and evaluation of drug effectiveness.
3. Identify important nursing assessments and interventions associated with the drug therapy and treatment of infectious diseases.
4. Identify health teaching essential for a successful treatment regimen.

Introduction

Antimicrobial agents are chemicals that eliminate living microorganisms pathogenic to the patient. Antimicrobial agents may be of chemical origin, such as the sulfonamides, or may be derived from other living organisms. Those derived from other living microorganisms are called *antibiotics*; for example, penicillin was first derived from the mold *Penicillium notatum*. Most antibiotics used today are harvested from large colonies of microorganisms, purified, and chemically modified into semisynthetic antimicrobial agents. The chemical modification makes the antibiotic more effective against certain specific pathogenic organisms.

The selection of the antimicrobial agent must be based on the sensitivity of the pathogen and the possible toxicity to the patient. If at all possible, the infecting organisms should first be isolated and identified. Culture and sensitivity tests should be completed. The antimicrobial therapy is then started based on the sensitivity results and the clinical judgment of the physician.

Side Effects

Side effects common to all antimicrobial agents include: allergy, direct tissue damage, and superinfection.

Allergy. The severity of allergic reaction ranges from a mild rash to fatal anaphylaxis. Allergic reactions may develop within 30 minutes of administration (anaphylaxis, laryngeal edema, shock, dyspnea, or skin reactions) or may occur several days after discontinuance of therapy (skin rashes or fever). All patients must be questioned for previous allergic reactions, and allergy-prone patients must be observed closely. It is important not to label a patient "allergic" to a particular medication without adequate documentation. The medication that a patient claims he or she is allergic to may be a life-saving drug for him or her.

Direct Tissue Damage. All drugs have at least the potential to damage tissues of certain organs. Examples include kidney damage by the aminoglycosides and penicillins and liver damage by isoniazid. Fortunately, these adverse effects are rare. The physician will order certain laboratory tests during antimicrobial treatment

442

to help monitor the patient's therapy. Patients with preexisting disease, such as renal failure or hepatitis, will require lower doses to prevent toxicity.

Superinfection. Antimicrobial agents may induce overgrowth of resistant bacterial strains or fungal organisms. Superinfections occur most frequently with the use of broad spectrum antibiotics and with agents that diminish host resistance, such as corticosteroids and antineoplastic agents. Stomatitis, glossitis, itching and vulvovaginitis are often caused by candidal species of fungi. Viral infections may also develop, especially on the lips (cold sores) and oral mucosa (canker sores).

Common side effects of antimicrobial agents taken orally include nausea, vomiting, and diarrhea. These effects are often dose-related and result from changes in normal bacterial flora in the bowel, from irritation, and from superinfection. Symptoms resolve within a few days and rarely require discontinuation of therapy.

General Nursing Considerations for Patients with Infectious Diseases

Nurses need to consider the entire patient when administering and monitoring antimicrobial therapy. It is essential that the nurse be knowledgeable about the drugs themselves, including physiological parameters for monitoring expected therapeutic activity, as well as for potential adverse effects.

Basic principles of patient care should not be overlooked when treating a patient with infections:

1. Adequate rest with as little stress as possible. Rest also decreases metabolic needs and enhances the physiological repair process.
2. Nutritional management, including attention to hydration, proteins, fats, carbohydrates, minerals, and vitamins to support the body's needs during an inflammatory response.
3. Infection control, as mandated by hospital policy, regarding protective isolation to ensure that the infection is not spread to others.
4. Training the patient in personal hygiene measures, such as handwashing techniques, management of their excretions, and wound care.
5. Drug therapy specific to the type of microorganism causing the infection.

Principles of drug administration need to be followed for all pharmacologic agents administered. (Refer to Chapters 5–7 for a review of specific principles.) The patient may have coexisting medical or surgical diagnoses, be debilitated, or have a suppressed immune system so that an infectious process could be fatal. Routine monitoring of all individuals receiving antimicrobial therapy should include status of hydration, temperature, pulse, respirations, and blood pressure. Monitor at least every 4 hours and more frequently as the patient's clinical status warrants.

Nurses need to perform baseline assessments of their patients for the common side effects associated with each individual agent administered. Further routine assessments should be performed on a scheduled basis to detect and to prevent early indications of allergic reactions, tissue damage (nephrotoxicity, ototoxicity, hepatotoxicity), and superinfections.

The general nursing considerations presented in this section concerning allergic treatment apply to all drug therapy and patient monitoring. However, since antimicrobial therapy is ordered so frequently, it is appropriate to reemphasize them here.

PATIENT CONCERNS: NURSING INTERVENTION/RATIONALE

Allergy

Preventing Allergic Reactions

Take a thorough nursing history of any prior "allergic" problems that the patient has experienced.

Symptoms

Has the patient taken this medication before? If so, what symptoms (e.g., nausea, vomiting, diarrhea, rash, itching, or hives) developed when taking it that led him or her to state now that he or she is allergic? Ask the patient to describe the appearance of the rash, where it started, and the course of recovery.

Onset

How soon after starting the medication did the symptoms develop?

Other Medications

Was the patient also taking any over-the-counter medications (e.g., laxatives, antacids, cough or cold preparations, suntanning products, etc.)?

Other Allergies

Has the patient previously been allergic to dust, weeds, foods, or other environmental factors?

Asthma

Does the patient have a history of asthma or allergic rhinitis?

Susceptible Patients

People with a history of allergies, asthma, rhinitis, taking multiple drug preparations, or kidney or liver dysfunctions are particularly susceptible to drug reactions.

The elderly, because of physiological changes of aging, need close observations for therapeutic response or for toxicity to drugs administered.

Nursing Actions

Do not administer the medication if the person reports possible allergy; share all information obtained with the physician, who will decide whether to administer the drug.

If a definite drug allergy is identified, the patient's chart, unit Kardex, and an identification bracelet should be carefully marked to alert all personnel to the specific drugs the patient should not receive.

Responding to Allergic Reactions

All patients should be watched carefully for possible allergy for at least 20 to 30 minutes following administration of a medication.

EMERGENCY CART

Know the location of the hospital emergency cart and the procedure for summoning it. In the event of suspected anaphylaxis, summon the physician and the emergency cart immediately.

Sites of Reactions

Although a serious reaction may occur with the first administration of a drug, repeated exposures to a previously sensitized substance can be fatal. Respond immediately to any signs of reaction:

- At the site of injection: swelling or redness, pain.
- Systemically: hives, nasal congestion and discharge, wheezing progressing to dyspnea, pulmonary edema, stridor, and sternal retractions.

Monitoring

Monitor the patient's vital signs continuously. Report hypotension, increasing pulse, and respirations that become labored and shallow.

Follow-Up

Following any reaction, the patient and family should be alerted to inform anyone treating the patient in the future that he or she is allergic to a specific drug.

Preventing and Assessing Tissue Damage

Nephrotoxicity

Monitor urinalysis and kidney function tests for abnormal results. Report an increasing BUN and creatinine, decreasing urine output and/or decreasing specific gravity (despite amount of fluid intake), casts or protein in the urine, frank blood or smoky-colored urine, or RBCs in excess of 0–3 on the urinalysis report.

Many antimicrobial agents are potentially nephrotoxic (aminoglycosides, tetracyclines, cephalosporins). Concomitant therapy with diuretics enhances the likelihood of toxicity, particularly in the elderly or debilitated patient.

When renal function is impaired, most drug dosages must be decreased, or alternate drug therapy employed.

Ototoxicity

Damage to the eighth cranial nerve can occur from drug therapy, particularly from aminoglycosides. This may initially be manifested by dizziness, tinnitus, and progressive hearing loss.

Assess your patient for difficulty in walking unaided and assess the level of hearing daily. Intentionally speak to patients softly; note if they are aware that you said anything. Take particular notice of the individual patient who repeatedly says, "What did you say?" or those who start talking louder or progressively increase the volume on the television or radio.

Hepatotoxicity

Several drugs to be studied in this unit are potentially hepatotoxic (i.e., isoniazid, sulfonamides).

The liver is active in the metabolism of many drugs, and drug-induced hepatitis may occur. The actual liver damage may occur shortly after exposure to the pharmacologic agent or may not appear for several weeks after initial exposure. The symptoms of hepatotoxicity are anorexia, nausea, vomiting, jaundice, hepatomegaly, splenomegaly, and abnormal liver function tests (elevated bilirubin, SGOT, SGPT, alkaline phosphatase, prothrombin time).

Patients with preexisting hepatic disease such as cirrhosis or hepatitis will require lower doses of drugs metabolized by the liver.

Nausea, Vomiting, Diarrhea

Nausea, vomiting, and diarrhea are the "big three" adverse effects associated with antimicrobial drug therapy. When they occur, gather further data:

- Does the patient have a history of nausea, vomiting, or diarrhea before starting the drug therapy?
- How soon after starting the medication did the symptoms start?
- Since starting the medication, has the diet or water source changed in any way?
- Was the patient taking other drugs, either by prescription or over-the-counter, before the initiation of antibiotic therapy?
- How much fluid is the patient consuming when taking medications? Sometimes inadequate fluid intake may cause gastritis manifested by nausea. The physician may elect to give the antibiotic with food to decrease irritation even though absorption may be slightly decreased. When reporting any incidence of nausea and vomiting, all significant data should be collected and reported.
- For diarrhea, what was the pattern of elimination before drug therapy? Report diarrhea, and the character and frequency of stools as well as any abdominal pain promptly.

Superinfection

Superinfection may occur in patients receiving broad-spectrum antibiotic therapy, particularly in those who are immunosuppressed. Assess and report white patches in the mouth, cold sores, canker sores, vaginal itching or discharge, diarrhea, and recurrence of any fever. Cultures are taken, and additional antibiotics effective against the new organism are started.

Minimize exposure to people known to have an infection, and practice good personal hygiene measures.

Patient Teaching Associated with Antimicrobial Therapy

Communication and Responsibility

Encourage open communication concerning frustrations and anger as the patient attempts to adjust to the diagnosis and need for prolonged treatment. The patient must be guided to gain insight into the condition in order to assume responsibility for the continuation of treatment. Keep reemphasizing those factors the patient can control to alter the progression of the disease: maintenance of general health, nutritional needs, adequate rest and appropriate exercise, and continuation of prescribed medication therapy.

ADEQUATE REST

Rest decreases the metabolic needs of the body and enhances physiological repair.

NUTRITION

Adequate hydration, especially during fever, as well as intake of adequate nutrients to meet the energy needs is paramount so that the body will not break down its proteins and fats to meet energy requirements.

The dietary plan must be individualized to the patient's diagnosis and point of recovery.

PERSONAL HYGIENE

Teach thorough handwashing techniques to prevent the spread of infection. Protective isolation should be carried out in accordance with the hospital policies and procedures.

Tell the patient who has a wound infection not to touch the infected area.

For those patients with an upper respiratory infection, teaching proper handling and disposal of sputum tissues.

Expectations of Therapy

Discuss expectations of therapy with the patient: relief of burning and frequency of urination; relief of cough; end of drainage and healing of a wound; ability to maintain activities of daily living.

Changes in Expectations

Assess changes in expectations as therapy progresses and the patient gains understanding and skill in the management of the diagnosis.

Changes in Therapy through Cooperative Goal-Setting

Work with the patient to encourage adherence to the prescribed treatment. When the patient feels that a change should be made in a treatment plan, encourage the patient to discuss it first with the physician.

WRITTEN RECORD

Enlist the patient's aid in developing and maintaining a written record of his/her monitoring parameters (Table 18.1) (e.g., list presenting symptoms: cough with a large amount of phlegm, wound drainage; temperature; exercise tolerance) and response to prescribed therapies for discussion with the physician. Patients should be encouraged to take this record on follow-up visits.

FOSTERING COMPLIANCE

Throughout the patient's hospitalization, discuss medication information and how it will benefit the course of treatment. Seek cooperation and understanding of the following points, so that medication compliance may be enhanced:

1. Name
2. Dosage
3. Route and administration times
4. Anticipated therapeutic response
5. Side effects to expect
6. Side effects to report
7. What to do if a dosage is missed
8. When, how, or if to refill the medication prescription.

DIFFICULTY IN COMPREHENSION

If it is evident that the patient and/or family does not understand all aspects of continuing therapy being prescribed (i.e., administration and monitoring of medications, exercises, diets, follow-up appointments), consider the use of social service or visiting nurse agencies.

ASSOCIATED TEACHING

Give patients the following instructions:

Always inform the physician or dentist of any prescription or over-the-counter medication being taken.

Table 18.1
Example of a Written Record for Patients Receiving Antibiotics

Medications	Color	To be taken

Name _____

Physician _____

Physician's phone _____

Next appt.* _____

Parameters		Day of discharge								Comments
Temperature	on arising | 12 noon 5 PM | 9 PM									
Aspirin	Time; #tabs, e.g. 8am 2									
Acetaminophen	Time; #tabs, e.g. 12N 2									
Site of infection Scale + ++++ Small Severe	Redness									
	Pain									
	Drainage									
Cough and sputum Productive:	Color									
	Thickness									
	No cough									
Mouth and throat	Sore throat									
	No problem									
Dizziness	Walk unaided									
	Must use support									
	Walk with help									
Hearing	Had to ↑ volume of radio - TV									
	No difficulty									
Skin	Rash with itching									
	Rash - fine red									
	No itching									
	No rash									
Vaginal itching (Yes or No)										
Rectal itching (Yes or No)										

*Please bring this record with you to your next appointment.
Use the back of this sheet for additional information.

Over-the-counter medications should not be taken without first discussing them with a physician or pharmacist.

Always report side effects of rash, itching, or hives immediately. Nausea, vomiting, or diarrhea should also be reported for the physician's evaluation if it is a new symptom.

Take all of the medication as prescribed for the full course of treatment. Do not discontinue use when feeling improved; do not save for future use; do not give your medicine to another individual. Sudden discontinuation of certain medications may produce harmful effects.

Keep all medications out of reach of children.

If pregnancy is suspected, consult an obstetrician as soon as possible about continuation of medication therapy.

At Discharge

Items to be sent home with the patient should:

1. Have written instructions for use.
2. Be labeled in a level of language and size of print appropriate for the patient.
3. If needed, include identification cards or bracelets.
4. Include a list of additional supplies to be purchased after discharge (i.e., syringes, dressings).
5. Include a schedule for follow-up appointments.

Aminoglycosides

The aminoglycoside antibiotics are used primarily against gram-negative microorganisms that cause urinary tract infections, meningitis, wound infections, and life-threatening septicemias. They are a mainstay in the treatment of hospital-acquired gram-negative infections.

Side Effects

Two serious reactions may occur with the aminoglycosides: ototoxicity, manifested by dizziness, tinnitus, and deafness; and nephrotoxicity, manifested by protein and blood in the urine, particularly in patients receiving high doses, or medications for longer than 10 days. If any of these symptoms should occur, report it immediately. Continue to observe patients for ototoxicity after therapy has been discontinued. These adverse effects may appear several days later.

See Table 18.2 for aminoglycoside products available and dosage ranges.

Ampicillin, piperacillin, ticarcillin, mezlocillin, and azlocillin may rapidly inactivate aminoglycoside antibiotics. These agents should not be mixed together or administered at the same time at the same IV site.

Gentamicin and heparin are chemically incompatible. *Do not* mix together prior to infusion.

Nursing Interventions

See also General Nursing Considerations for Patients with Infectious Diseases.

PATIENT CONCERNS: NURSING INTERVENTION/RATIONALE

Side Effects to Report

Ototoxicity

Damage to the eighth cranial nerve can occur from aminoglycoside therapy. This may initially be manifested by dizziness, tinnitus, and progressive hearing loss.

Assess your patients for difficulty in walking unaided and assess their level of hearing daily. Intentionally speak softly; note if he or she is aware that you said anything. Take particular notice of the patient who repeatedly says, "What did you say?" or those who start talking louder or progressively increase the volume on the television or radio.

Nephrotoxicity

Monitor urinalysis and kidney function tests for abnormal results. Report an increasing BUN and creatine, decreasing urine output or decreasing specific gravity (despite amount of fluid intake), casts or protein in the urine, frank blood or smoky-colored urine, or RBCs in excess of 0–3 on the urinalysis report.

Dosage and Administration

Compatibilities

Do not mix other drugs in the same syringe or infuse together with other drugs. See Drug Interactions for incompatibilities.

Table 18.2
The Aminoglycosides

GENERIC NAME	BRAND NAME	AVAILABILITY	ADULT DOSAGE RANGE
Amikacin	Amikin	100 mg/2 ml vial 500 mg/2 ml vial 1 g/4 ml vial	IM, IV: 15 mg/kg/24 hr
Gentamicin	Garamycin	10, 40 mg/ml 60 mg/1.5 ml 80 mg/2 ml 100 mg/100 ml	IM, IV: Up to 240 mg/24 hr
Kanamycin	Kantrex, Klebcil	75,500 mg, 1 g vials	IM, IV: Up to 15 mg/kg/24 hr
Neomycin	Mycifradin	500 mg vial	IM: 15 mg/kg/24 hr
Netilmicin	Netromycin	10 mg/ml in 2 ml vials 25 mg/ml in 2 ml vials 100 mg/ml in 1.5 ml vials	IM, IV: 3–6.5 mg/kg/24 hr
Streptomycin	Streptomycin	400 and 500 mg/ml, 1 and 5 g vials	IM: 1–4 g/24 hr
Tobramycin	Nebcin	10 mg/ml in 2 ml vials 40 mg/ml in 1.2 g vials 40 mg/ml in 2 ml vials 60 mg/1.5 ml	IM, IV: Up to 5 mg/kg/24 hr

Laboratory

Check with the hospital laboratory regarding timing of aminoglycoside blood level tests.

After levels have been determined, assess whether results are normal or toxic.

Rate of Infusion

Consult with a pharmacist or see the individual package literature.

Drug Interactions

Nephrotoxic Potential

Cephalosporins and diuretics, when combined with aminoglycosides, may increase the nephrotoxic potential.

Monitor the urinalysis and kidney function tests for abnormal results.

Ototoxic Potential

Aminoglycosides, when combined with ethacrynic acid, bumetanide, and furosemide may increase ototoxicity. Therefore, nursing assessments for tinnitus, dizziness, and decreased hearing should be done regularly every shift.

Neuromuscular Blockade

Aminoglycoside antibiotics in combination with skeletal muscle relaxants may produce respiratory depression.

Check the anesthesia record in postoperative patients to see if skeletal muscle relaxants such as succinylcholine or pancuronium bromide were administered during surgery.

The nurse should monitor and assess the respiratory rate, depth of respirations, and chest movement; report apnea immediately. Since these effects may be seen for up to 48 hours after administration of skeletal muscle relaxants, continue monitoring respirations, pulse, and blood pressure beyond the usual postsurgical vital sign routine.

Heparin

Gentamicin and heparin are physically incompatible. *Do not* mix together before infusion.

Ampicillin, Piperacillin, Ticarcillin, Mezlocillin, Azlocillin

These penicillins rapidly inactivate aminoglycoside antibiotics. *Do not* mix together or administer together at the same IV site.

Cephalosporins

The cephalosporins are chemically related to the penicillins and have a similar mechanism of activity. The cephalosporins may be used as alternatives when patients are allergic to the penicillins, unless they are also allergic to the cephalosporins. The cephalosporins are used for certain pneumonias, urinary tract infections, abdominal infections, septicemias, and osteomyelitis.

Side Effects

Side effects of the cephalosporins are usually minor. The most common are nausea and diarrhea. Overgrowth of other organisms is manifested by oral thrush, genital and anal pruritus, genital candidiasis, vaginitis, and vaginal discharge.

Transient elevations of liver function tests (SGOT, SGPT, alkaline phosphatase) and renal function tests (BUN, serum creatinine) have been reported. Renal toxicity, as evidenced by proteinuria, hematuria, casts, decreased creatinine clearance, and decreased urine output, has also developed.

Hypoprothrombinemia, with and without bleeding, has been reported. These rare occurrences are most frequent in elderly, debilitated, or otherwise compromised patients with borderline vitamin K deficiency. Treatment with broad-spectrum antibiotics eliminates enough gastrointestinal flora to cause a further reduction in vitamin K synthesis. The hypoprothrombinemia is readily reversed by administration of vitamin K.

A false-positive reaction for glucose in the urine may occur with Clinitest tablets, but not with Tes-Tape or Diastix.

Phlebitis and thrombophlebitis are recurrent problems associated with intravenous administration of cephalosporins. Use small IV needles, large veins, and alternating infusion sites if possible to minimize irritation.

See Table 18.3 for products available and dosages.

Nursing Interventions

See also General Nursing Considerations for Patients with Infectious Diseases.

Table 18.3
The Cephalosporins

GENERIC NAME	BRAND NAME	AVAILABILITY	ADULT DOSAGE RANGE
Cefaclor	Ceclor	250, 500 mg capsules 125, 250 mg/5 ml suspension	PO: 250–500 every 8 hr; do not exceed 4 g/day
Cefadroxil	Duracef, Ultracef	500 mg capsules 1000 mg tablets 125, 250, 500 mg/5 ml suspension	PO: 1–2 g 1–2 times daily
Cefamandole	Mandol	500 mg, 1, 2 g vials	IM, IV: 0.5–1 g every 4–8 hr; do not exceed 12 g/24 hr
Cefazolin	Ancef, Kefzol	250, 500 mg, 1, 5, 10 g vials	IM, IV: 250 mg to 1.5 g every 6–8 hr
Cefoperazone	Cefobid	1, 2 g vials	IV: 1–3 g every 6–8 hr
Cefotaxime	Claforan	500 mg, 1, 2 g vials	IV: 1–2 g every 4–8 hr; do not exceed 12 g/day
Cefoxitin	Mefoxin	1, 2 g vials	IM, IV: 1–2 g every 6–8 hr; do not exceed 12 g/day
Ceftizoxime	Cefizox	1, 2 g vials	IV: 1–2 every 8–12 hr
Cefuroxime	Zinacef	750 mg, 1.5 g vials	IV: 750 mg to 1.5 g every 8 hr
Cephalexin	Keflex	250, 500 mg capsules 1000 mg tablets 100 mg/ml Peds suspension 125, 250 mg/5 ml suspension	PO: 250–1000 mg every 6 hr
Cephalothin	Keflin	1, 2, 4, 20 g vials	IM, IV: 500 mg to 2 g every 4–6 hr
Cephapirin	Cefadyl	500 mg, 1, 2, 4, 20 g vials	IM, IV: 500 mg to 1 g every 4–6 hr
Cephradine	Anspor, Velosef	250, 500 mg capsules 1000 mg tablets 125, 250 mg/5 ml suspension 1, 2, 4 g/vial	PO: 250–500 mg every 6 hr IM, IV: 500 mg to 1 g every 6 hr; do not exceed 8 g/day
Moxalactam	Moxam	1, 2 g vials	IV: 250 mg to 2 g 2–3 times daily; do not exceed 12 g daily

PATIENT CONCERNS: NURSING INTERVENTION/RATIONALE

Side Effects to Report

Diarrhea

Cephalosporins cause diarrhea by altering the bacterial flora of the gastrointestinal tract. The diarrhea is usually not severe enough to warrant discontinuing medication. Encourage the patient not to discontinue therapy without consulting the physician. When diarrhea persists, monitor the patient for signs of dehydration.

Superinfections

With cephalosporins, oral thrush, genital and anal pruritus, vaginitis and vaginal discharge may occur. Report promptly since these infections are resistant to the original antibiotic used.

Teach the importance of meticulous oral and perineal personal hygiene.

Abnormal Liver and Renal Function Tests

Monitor returning laboratory data and report abnormal findings to the physician.

Hypoprothrombinemia

Assess your patient for ecchymosis following minimal trauma, prolonged bleeding at an infusion site or from a surgical wound, or the development of petechiae, bleeding gums, or nosebleeds. Notify the physician of any of the signs of hypoprothrombinemia. The usual treatment is administration of vitamin K.

Thrombophlebitis

Carefully assess patients receiving IV cephalosporins for the development of thrombophlebitis.

Inspect the IV area frequently while providing care; inspect during dressing changes and at times the IV is changed to a new site. Always investigate pain at the IV site. Report redness, warmth, tenderness to touch, or edema in the affected part. If in lower extremities, dorsiflexion of the foot may cause pain in the calf area (Homan's sign). Compare findings in the affected limb with the unaffected limb.

Electrolyte Imbalance

If a patient develops hyperkalemia or hypernatremia, consider the electrolyte content of the antibiotics. Most of the cephalosporins have a high electrolyte content.

Drug Interactions

Nephrotoxic Potential

Patients receiving cephalosporins, aminoglycosides and diuretics concurrently should be assessed for signs of nephrotoxicity. Monitor urinalysis and kidney function tests for abnormal results. Report an increasing BUN and creatinine, decreasing urine output or decreasing specific gravity (despite amount of fluid intake), casts or protein in the urine, frank blood or smoky-colored urine, or RBCs in excess of 0–3 on the urinalysis report.

Probenecid

Patients receiving probenecid in combination with cephalosporins are more susceptible to toxicity due to the inhibition of excretion of the cephalosporins by probenecid. Monitor closely for adverse effects.

Alcohol

Avoid alcohol consumption during cefamandole, cefoperazone, moxalactam, and possibly ceftizoxime therapy. Patients will become flushed, tremulous, dyspneic, tachycardic, and hypotensive. Do not use over-the-counter preparations containing alcohol, such as mouthwash (Cepacol) or cough preparations, because of their alcohol content.

Penicillins

The penicillins were the first true antibiotics to be grown and used against pathogenic bacteria in human beings. They are still one of the most widely used classes of antibiotics today.

The penicillins act by interfering with the synthesis of bacterial cell walls. They are, therefore, most effective against bacteria that multiply rapidly. They do not hinder growth of human cells, because human cells have protective membranes but no cell wall.

The penicillins are used to treat middle ear infections (otitis media), pneumonia, meningitis, urinary tract infections, syphilis, gonorrhea, and as a prophylactic antibiotic for patients with rheumatic fever.

Side Effects

The most common side effects of orally administered penicillins are nausea, vomiting, epigastric distress, and diarrhea.

Adverse effects that may develop due to the use of large parenteral doses are: neurologic effects evidenced by hallucinations, hyperreflexia, seizures, and delirium;

electrolyte imbalances from sodium or potassium penicillin, ticarcillin, or carbenicillin manifested by cardiac arrhythmias, hyperreflexia, convulsions, and coma; and interstitial nephritis manifested by oliguria, proteinuria, hematuria, casts, azotemia, pyuria, fever and, rarely, a rash. All of these adverse effects are more common in elderly, debilitated patients with impaired renal function.

See Table 18.4 for products available and dosage ranges.

Nursing Interventions

See also General Nursing Considerations for Patients with Infectious Diseases.

**PATIENT CONCERNS:
NURSING INTERVENTION/RATIONALE**

Side Effects to Report

Diarrhea

Penicillins cause diarrhea by altering the bacterial flora of the gastrointestinal tract. The diarrhea is usually not severe enough to warrant discontinuation. Encourage the patient not to discontinue therapy without first consulting the physician. If diarrhea persists, monitor the patient for signs of dehydration.

Abnormal Liver and Renal Function Tests

Monitor returning laboratory data and report abnormal findings to the physician.

Thrombophlebitis

Carefully assess patients receiving IV penicillins for the development of thrombophlebitis.

Inspect the IV area frequently while providing care; inspect during dressing changes and at times the IV is changed to a new site. Always investigate pain at the IV site. Report redness, warmth, tenderness to touch, and edema in the affected part. If in lower extremities, dorsiflexion of the foot may cause pain in the calf area (Homan's sign). Compare the affected limb with the unaffected limb.

Electrolyte Imbalance

The electrolyte content of the antibiotics may cause hyperkalemia or hypernatremia, Most of the penicillins have a high electrolyte content.

Dosage and Administration

Compatibilities

Do not mix with other drugs in the same syringe or infuse together with other drugs. See Drug Interactions for incompatibilities.

Rate of Infusion

Consult with a pharmacist or see package literature.

Drug Interactions

Probenecid

Patients receiving probenecid in combination with penicillins are more susceptible to toxicity because probenecid inhibits excretion of the penicillins. Monitor closely for adverse effects.

This combination may be used to advantage in the treatment of gonorrhea and other infections where high levels are indicated.

Ampicillin and Allopurinol

When used concurrently, these two agents are associated with a high incidence of rash. Do not label the patient as allergic to penicillins until further skin-testing has verified that there is a true hypersensitivity to penicillins.

Antacids

Excessive use of antacids may diminish the absorption of oral penicillins.

Sulfonamides

The sulfonamides are not true antibiotics because they are not synthesized by microorganisms. However, they are highly effective antibacterial agents. Sulfonamides act by inhibiting bacterial biosynthesis of folic acid, which eventually results in bacterial cell death. Human cells do not synthesize folic acid so are not affected. Sulfonamides are used primarily to treat urinary tract infections and otitis media.

Side Effects

Due to an increasing frequency of organisms developing a resistance to sulfonamide therapy, and the

Table 18.4
The Penicillins

GENERIC NAME	BRAND NAME	AVAILABILITY	ADULT DOSAGE RANGE
Amoxicillin	Amoxil, Trimox, Larotid, Wymox, Polymox	125 mg chewable tablets 250 and 500 mg capsules 125 and 250 mg/5 ml suspension	PO: 250–500 mg/8 hr
Ampicillin	Amcill, Polycillin, Omnipen, Principen, Pensyn, Totacillin	0.125, 0.25, 0.5, 1, and 2 g vials 250 and 500 mg capsules 125, 250, 500 mg/5 ml suspension	IM, IV: 0.5 to 1 g/4–6 hr PO: 250–500 mg/6 hr
Azlocillin	Azlin	2, 3, 4 g vials	IV: 8–18 g/24 hr in 4–6 divided doses
Carbenicillin	Geopen, Pyopen	1, 2, 5, 10 g vials	IM: Do not exceed 2 g/ injection site IV: Up to 40 g/24 hr
Cloxacillin	Tegopen, Cloxapen	250 and 500 mg capsules 125 mg/5 ml suspension	PO: 250–500 mg/6 hr
Dicloxacillin	Dynapen, Pathocil, Veracillin	125, 250, and 500 mg capsules 62.5 mg/5 ml suspension	PO: 125–500 mg/6 hr
Methicillin	Celbenin, Staphcillin	1, 2, 4, 6 g vials	IM, IV: 1 g/4–6 hr
Mezlocillin	Mezlin	1, 2, 3, 4 g vials	IM, IV: Do not exceed 24 g/24 hr
Nafcillin	Nafcil, Unipen	0.5, 1, 2 g vials 250 and 500 mg tablets 250 mg/5 ml suspension	IM, IV: 0.5–1 g/4–6 hr PO: 250–500 mg/6 hr
Oxacillin	Bactocill, Prostaphlin	0.5, 1, 2, 4 g vials 250 and 500 mg capsules 250 mg/5 ml suspension	IM, IV: 0.5–1 g/4–6 hr PO: 250–500 mg/4–6 hr
Penicillin G, potassium or sodium	Pfizerpen, Pentids	Vials of 0.2, 0.5, 1, 5, and 10 million units Tablets of 1, 2, 2.5, 4, 5, and 800,000 units Suspension of 2, 2.5 and 400,000 units/5 ml	PO: 400,000 to 1.6 million units IM, IV: 600,000 to 30 million units daily
Penicillin V potassium	V-Cillin K, Betapen VK, Pen-Vee-K, Veetids	125, 250, and 500 mg tablets 125 and 250 mg/5 ml suspension	PO: 250–500 mg/6 hr
Piperacillin	Pipracil	2, 3, 4 g vials	IM, IV: 3–4 g every 4–6 hr, not to exceed 24 g/24 hr
Ticarcillin	Ticar	1, 3, and 6 g vials	IM: Do not exceed 2 g/ injection site IV: Up to 18 g/24 hr

unreliability of *in vitro* sulfonamide sensitivity tests, patients should be monitored closely for continued therapeutic response to treatment. This is particularly important in patients being treated for chronic and recurrent urinary tract infections.

Sulfonamides have many side effects, the most common of which are nausea and diarrhea. Rashes may represent more serious underlying disorders and should be reported immediately.

Patients receiving sulfonamides for more than 14 days should have routine red and white cell counts with differential completed periodically.

A false-positive reaction for glucose in the urine may occur with Clinitest tablets, but not with Tes-Tape or Diastix.

Patients should be encouraged to drink water several times daily while receiving sulfonamide therapy. Rarely, crystals form in the urinary tract if the patient becomes too dehydrated.

See Table 18.5 for products available and dosage ranges.

Nursing Interventions

See also General Nursing Considerations for Patients with Infectious Diseases.

PATIENT CONCERNS: NURSING INTERVENTION/RATIONALE

Side Effects to Report

Nausea, Vomiting, Anorexia, Diarrhea

These side effects are usually mild and tend to resolve with continued therapy. Encourage the patient not to discontinue therapy without first consulting the physician.

If the patient should become debilitated, contact the physician.

Dermatologic Reactions

Report a rash or pruritus immediately and withhold additional doses pending approval by the physician.

PHOTOSENSITIVITY

The patient should be cautioned to avoid exposure to sunlight and ultraviolet light. Suggest wearing long-sleeved clothing, a hat, and sunglasses when going to be exposed to sunlight. Discourage the use of artificial tanning lamps.

Hematologic Reactions

Routine laboratory studies (RBC, WBC, and differential counts) are scheduled for patients taking sulfonamides 14 days or longer. Stress returning for this laboratory work.

Monitor for the development of a sore throat, fever, purpura, jaundice or excessive, progressive weakness.

Neurologic Effects

Report the development of tinnitus, headache, dizziness, mental depression, drowsiness, or confusion.

Table 18.5

The Sulfonamides

GENERIC NAME	BRAND NAME	AVAILABILITY	ADULT DOSAGE RANGE
Sulfacytine	Renoquid	250 mg tablets	PO: Initial dose—500 mg, then 250 mg 4 times daily
Sulfadiazine	Microsulfon, Sulfadiazine	500 mg tablets	PO: Initial dose—2–4 g, then 4–8 g/24 hr in divided doses
Sulfamethizole	Thiosulfil, Proklar, Urifon	0.25, 0.5, 1 g tablets	PO: 0.5–1 g 3–4 times daily
Sulfamethoxazole	Gantanol, Urobak	0.5, 1 g tablets, 500 mg/5 ml suspension	PO: Initial dose—2 g, then 1 g/12 hr
Sulfasalazine	Azulfidine, S.A.S.-500	500 mg tablets, 250 mg/5 ml suspension	PO: Initial therapy—3–4 g daily in divided doses; maintenance dose is 2 g daily
Sulfisoxazole	Gantrisin, Sulfizin, SK-soxazole	500 mg tablets 500 mg/5 ml syrup 400 mg/ml vial	PO, IM, IV: Initial dose—2–4 g; maintenance dose is 4–8 g/24 hr divided into 3–6 doses
Sulfapyridine	Sulfapyridine	500 mg tablets	PO: Initial dose—500 mg 4 times daily, until controlled, then reduce to most effective dose
Triple Sulfas	Neotrizine Sulfaloid, Terfonyl	Tablets, suspension	PO: Initial dose—2–4g, followed by 2–4 g/24 hr divided into 3–6 hr doses
Co-trimoxazole	Bactrim, Septra	Tablets, suspension, infusion	PO: 2–4 tablets daily, depending on strength, disease being treated IV: 15–20 mg/kg/24 (based on trimethoprim) in 3–4 divided doses for up to 14 days
Erythromycin-sulfisoxazole	Pediazole	Suspension	PO: 2.5–10 ml every 6 hr depending on weight of patient

Dosage and Administration

Gastric Irritation

If gastric irritation occurs, administer with food or milk. If symptoms persist or increase in severity, report for physician's evaluation.

Fluid Intake

Adequate intake of 8 to 12 8-ounce glasses of fluid daily is encouraged to prevent crystal formation in the renal tubules. Report the development of hematuria immediately.

Drug Interactions

Oral Hypoglycemic Agents

Sulfonamides may displace sulfonylurea oral hypoglycemic agents (tolbutamide, acetohexamide, tolazamide, chlorpropamide) from protein-binding sites, resulting in hypoglycemia.

Monitor for hypoglycemia, headache, weakness, decreased coordination, general apprehension, diaphoresis, hunger, blurred or double vision.

The dosage of the hypoglycemic agent may need to be reduced. Notify the physician if any of the above symptoms appear.

Warfarin

This medication may enhance the anticoagulant effects of warfarin. Observe for the development of petechiae, ecchymoses, nosebleeds, bleeding gums, dark tarry stools, and bright red or "coffee-ground" emesis. Monitor the prothrombin time and reduce the dosage of warfarin if necessary.

Methotrexate

Sulfonamides may produce methotrexate toxicity when given simultaneously. Monitor patients on concurrent therapy for oral stomatitis and for signs of nephrotoxicity (oliguria, hematuria, proteinuria, casts, etc.).

Phenytoin

Sulfisoxazole may displace phenytoin from protein-binding sites, resulting in phenytoin toxicity.

Monitor patients on concurrent therapy for signs of phenytoin toxicity: nystagmus, sedation, lethargy (serum levels may be ordered). A reduced dosage of phenytoin may be required.

Tetracyclines

The tetracyclines are a class of antibiotics that are effective against both gram-negative and gram-positive bacteria. They act by inhibiting protein synthesis by bacterial cells. The tetracyclines are often used for patients allergic to the penicillins for the treatment of certain venereal diseases, urinary tract infections, upper respiratory tract infections, pneumonia, and meningitis. They are particularly effective against rickettsial and mycoplasmic infections.

Side Effects

The most common side effects of the tetracyclines are gastric upset, loss of appetite, vomiting, and diarrhea. Photosensitivity resulting in an exaggerated sunburn after short exposure has been reported.

Tetracyclines administered during the ages of tooth development (the last half of pregnancy through 8 years of age) may cause enamel hypoplasia and permanent staining of the teeth to a yellow, gray, or brown color. Tetracyclines are secreted in breast milk, so nursing mothers on tetracycline therapy are advised to feed their infants formula or cow's milk, as appropriate.

A false-positive reaction for glucose in the urine may occur between parenteral tetracycline and Clinitest tablets, but not between tetracycline and Tes-Tape or Diastix.

See Table 18.6 for products available and dosage ranges.

Nursing Interventions

See also General Nursing Considerations for Patients with Infectious Diseases.

PATIENT CONCERNS: NURSING INTERVENTION/RATIONALE

Side Effects to Report

Nausea, Vomiting, Anorexia, Abdominal Cramps, Diarrhea

These side effects are usually mild and tend to resolve with continued therapy. Encourage the patient not to discontinue therapy without first consulting the physician.

Table 18.6
The Tetracyclines

GENERIC NAME	BRAND NAME	AVAILABILITY	ADULT DOSAGE RANGE
Demeclocycline	Declomycin	150 mg capsules 150 and 300 mg tablets 75 mg/5 ml syrup	PO: 150 mg 4 times daily or 300 mg 2 times daily
Doxycycline	Vibramycin, Doxychel	100 and 200 mg vials 50 and 100 mg capsules 25 and 50 mg/5 ml syrup	IV: 100–200 mg 1 or 2 times daily PO: 200 mg on day 1, then 100 mg divided in 2 doses
Methacycline	Rondomycin	150 and 300 mg capsules 75 mg/5 ml syrup	PO: 150 mg 4 times daily or 300 mg 2 times daily
Minocycline	Minocin	100 mg vial 50 and 100 mg capsules 50 mg/5 ml syrup	PO, IV: 200 mg, followed by 100 mg/12 hr
Oxytetracycline	Terramycin, E.P. Mycin, Uri-Tet	100, 250, and 500 mg vials 125 and 250 mg capsules 125 mg/5 ml syrup	IM: 250 mg/24 hr or 100 mg/8 hr IV: 250–500 mg/12 hr; PO: 250–500 mg 4 times daily
Tetracycline	Achromycin, Tetracyn, Panmycin, Robitet, Sumycin	100, 250, and 500 mg vials 100, 250, and 500 mg capsules and tablets 125 mg/5 ml syrup	IM: 250–900 mg/24 hr IV: 250–500 mg/12 hr PO: 250–500 mg 4 times daily

Photosensitivity

The patient should be cautioned to avoid exposure to sunlight and ultraviolet light. Suggest wearing long-sleeved clothing, a hat, and sunglasses when going to be exposed to sunlight. Discourage the use of artificial tanning lamps. Notify the physician for the advisability of discontinuing therapy.

Dosage and Administration

PO

Emphasize taking medication 1 hour before or 2 hours after ingesting antacids, milk or dairy products, or products containing calcium, aluminum, magnesium, or iron (i.e., vitamins).

Drug Interactions

Warfarin

This medication may enhance the anticoagulant effects of warfarin. Observe for the development of petechiae, ecchymoses, nosebleeds, bleeding gums, dark tarry stools, and bright red or "coffee-ground" emesis. Monitor the prothrombin time and reduce the dosage of warfarin if necessary.

Methoxyflurane

If patients are receiving tetracycline and are scheduled for surgery, label the front of the chart "taking tetracycline." Fatal nephrotoxicity has been reported when methoxyflurane is administered to a person taking tetracycline.

Impaired Absorption

Iron, calcium-containing foods (milk and dairy products), calcium, aluminum, or magnesium preparations (antacids), and alkaline products (sodium bicarbonate) will decrease absorption of tetracycline. Administer all tetracycline products 1 hour before or 2 hours after ingesting these foods or products.

Exception: Food or milk does not interfere with the absorption of doxycycline.

Phenytoin, Carbamazepine

These agents reduce the half-life of doxycycline. Monitor patients for lack of clinical improvement from the infection.

Tooth Development

Do not administer tetracyclines to pregnant patients or to children under 8 years of age. The infant's or child's tooth enamel may be permanently stained (yellow, gray, or brown).

Lactation

Nursing mothers need to switch their babies to formula while on tetracyclines, since it is present in the breast milk.

Other Antibiotics

Chloramphenicol (klo-ram-fen'i-kol) *(Chloromycetin)* (klo-ro-my-se'tin)

Chloramphenicol is an antibiotic that acts by inhibiting bacterial protein synthesis. It is particularly effective in treating rickettsial infections, meningitis, and typhoid fever.

It must not be used in the treatment of trivial infections or when it is not indicated, such as in colds, influenza, throat infections, or as a prophylactic agent to prevent bacterial infection.

Side Effects

Serious and possibly fatal bone marrow suppression may occur after therapy is initiated with chloramphenicol. Early signs include sore throat, a feeling of fatigue, elevated temperature, and small petechial hemorrhages and bruises on the skin. If patients describe any of these symptoms, report them to your supervisor immediately.

Chloramphenicol may cause a false-positive urinary glucose reaction when Clinitest is used. Tes-Tape or Diastix may be used instead to test for the presence of glucose.

Gastrointestinal side effects include nausea, vomiting, diarrhea, glossitis, stomatitis, and an unpleasant taste in the mouth.

Availability

PO—250 and 500 mg capsules; 150 mg/5 ml suspension.
IV—100 mg/ml in 1 g vials.

Dosage and Administration

Adult

PO—50 to 100 mg/kg every 6 hours.
IM—Not recommended due to poor absorption and clinical response.
IV—As for PO administration. Reconstitute by adding 11 mg of sterile water for injection or dextrose 5% to 1 g of chloramphenicol to make a solution containing 100 mg/ml. Administer the calculated dose intravenously over a 1 minute period.

Pediatric

PO—Neonates: 25 mg/kg/24 hours in 4 equally divided doses. Infants over 2 weeks of age: 50 mg/kg/24 hours in 4 equally divided doses.
IM—Not recommended.
IV—As for PO dosages. Administer over 1 minute. Use only chloramphenicol sodium succinate intravenously in children.

Nursing Interventions

See also General Nursing Considerations for Patients with Infectious Diseases.

PATIENT CONCERNS: NURSING INTERVENTION/RATIONALE

Side Effects to Report

Hematologic

Routine laboratory studies (RBC, WBC, and differential counts) are scheduled for patients taking chloramphenicol 14 days or longer. Stress returning for this laboratory work.

Monitor for the development of a sore throat, fever, purpura, jaundice or excessive, progressive weakness.

Superinfections

Oral thrush, genital and anal pruritus, vaginitis, and vaginal discharge may occur. Report promptly, since these infections are resistant to the original antibiotic used.

Teach the importance of meticulous oral and perineal personal hygiene.

Drug Interactions

Warfarin

This medication may enhance the anticoagulant effects of warfarin. Observe for the development of petechiae, ecchymoses, nosebleeds, bleeding gums, dark tarry stools, and bright red or "coffee-ground" emesis. Monitor the prothrombin time and reduce the dosage of warfarin if necessary.

Oral Hypoglycemic Agents

Monitor for hypoglycemia: headache, weakness, decreased coordination, general apprehension, diaphoresis, hunger, blurred or double vision.

The dosage of the hypoglycemic agent may need to be reduced. Notify the physician if any of the above symptoms appear.

Phenytoin

Chloramphenicol inhibits the metabolism of phenytoin. Monitor patients with concurrent therapy for signs of phenytoin toxicity: nystagmus, sedation, lethargy. Serum levels may be ordered, and the dosage of phenytoin reduced.

Clindamycin (klin-dah-my'sin)
(Cleocin) (klee-o'sin)

Clindamycin is an antibiotic that acts by inhibiting protein synthesis. It is useful against infections caused by gram-negative aerobic organisms as well as a variety of gram-positive and gram-negative anaerobes.

Side Effects

Severe diarrhea may develop from the use of clindamycin. If diarrhea of more than five stools per day develops, notify the physician. The use of Lomotil, loperamide, or paregoric may prolong or worsen the condition. Large doses of Kaopectate may be effective in diminishing the diarrhea.

Patients may complain of a bitter taste since the medication is secreted in saliva.

Availability

PO—75 and 150 mg capsules, 75 mg/5 ml suspension.
IV—150 mg/ml in 2 and 4 ml ampules.

Dosage and Administration

Adult
PO—150 to 450 mg every 6 hours. *Do not* refrigerate the suspension. It is stable at room temperature for 14 days.
IM—600 to 2700 mg/24 hours. *Do not* exceed 600 mg per injection. Pain, induration, and sterile abscesses have been reported. Deep IM injection is recommended to help minimize this reaction.
IV—600 to 2700 mg/24 hours. Dilute to less than 6 mg/ml. Administer at a rate less than 30 mg/minute. Administration by IV push is not recommended.

Pediatric
PO—Suspension: 8 to 25 mg/kg/24 hours in 4 divided doses. Capsules: 8 to 20 mg/kg/24 hours in 4 divided doses. Capsules should be taken with a full glass of water to prevent esophageal irritation.
IM—15 to 40 mg/kg/24 hours in 4 divided doses.
IV—As for IM use. Dilute to less than 6 mg/ml and administer at a rate less than 30 mg/minute.

Nursing Interventions

See also General Nursing Considerations for Patients with Infectious Diseases.

PATIENT CONCERNS: NURSING INTERVENTION/RATIONALE

Side Effects to Report
Diarrhea

These side effects are usually mild and tend to resolve with continued therapy. Encourage the patient not to discontinue therapy without first consulting the physician.

Severe Diarrhea

Report diarrhea of five or more stools per day to the physician.

Blood or mucus in the stool should also be reported. *Warn patients not to treat diarrhea themselves when taking this drug.*

Dosage and Administration
PO

Do not refrigerate the suspension. It is stable at room temperature for 14 days.

IM

Deep IM injection is recommended to help minimize pain, indurations, and possible sterile abscess formation.

IV

It is not recommended that this drug be given by IV push. Dilute to less than 6 mg/ml and administer at a rate less than 30 mg/minute.

Drug Interactions

Impaired Absorption

Kaolin-pectin (Kaopectate) absorbs clindamycin. It is effective in stopping diarrhea that may occur with the administration of clindamycin.

Neuromuscular Blockade

Label charts of patients scheduled for surgery who are taking clindamycin. When combined with surgical muscle relaxants and/or aminoglycosides, neuromuscular blockade may result.

These combinations may potentiate respiratory depression. Check the anesthesia record of surgical patients. Monitor postoperative patients for a prolonged period for respiratory depression. This may occur 48 hours or more after the drug administration.

Theophylline Toxicity

Clindamycin, when given with theophylline, may result in theophylline toxicity. Observe for vomiting, dizziness, restlessness, and cardiac arrhythmias. The dosage of theophylline may need to be reduced.

Erythromycin

Therapeutic antagonism has been reported between clindamycin and erythromycin. Do not administer concurrently.

Erythromycin (e-rith-ro-my'sin)
(Erythrocin) (e-rith'ro-sin)

Erythromycin may be used as an alternative antibiotic for patients allergic to penicillin. It acts by inhibition of protein synthesis and is effective in treating respiratory tract infections, meningitis, syphilis, and gonorrhea, and may be used as prophylaxis against rheumatic fever.

Side Effects

The most common side effects of oral erythromycin products are epigastric distress, with possible nausea and vomiting.

Availability

PO—250, 333, and 500 mg enteric-coated tablets; 125, 200, 250, and 500 mg chewable tablets; 125, 250, 400, and 500 mg film-coated tablets; 250 mg enteric-coated pellets in capsules; 125, 200, 250, and 400 mg/5 mg suspension; 100 mg/ml and 100 mg/2.5 ml drops.
IV—250, 500, and 1000 mg vials for reconstitution.

Dosage and Administration

Adult
PO—250 mg 4 times daily for 10 to 14 days. Administer at least 1 hour before or 2 hours after meals.
IM—100 mg every 4 to 6 hours. Due to pain on injection and the possibility of sterile abscess formation, this route of administration is generally not recommended for multiple dose therapy.
IV—15 to 20 mg/kg/24 hours. Administer one-fourth of the total dose every 6 hours. Dilute the dosage in 100 to 250 mg of saline solution, or 5% dextrose and administer over 20 to 60 minutes. Thrombophlebitis after IV infusion is a relatively common side effect.
Pediatric
PO—30 to 50 mg/kg/24 hours in 4 divided doses. Doses of 60 to 100 mg/kg/24 hours may be necessary for severe infections.
IM—Not recommended in pediatric patients.
IV—15 to 20 mg/kg/24 hours in 3 divided doses.

Nursing Interventions

See also General Nursing Considerations for Patients with Infectious Diseases.

PATIENT CONCERNS: NURSING INTERVENTION/RATIONALE

Side Effects to Expect

Gastric Irritation

These side effects are usually mild and tend to resolve with continued therapy. Encourage the patient not to discontinue therapy without first consulting the physician.

Side Effects to Report

Thrombophlebitis

Carefully assess patients receiving IV erythromycin for the development of thrombophlebitis.
Inspect the IV area frequently while providing care; inspect during dressing changes and when the IV is changed to a new site. Always investigate pain at the

IV site. Report redness and edema in the affected part. If in lower extremities, dorsiflexion of the foot may cause pain in the calf area (Homan's sign). Compare the affected limb with the unaffected limb.

Dosage and Administration

PO

Administer at least 1 hour before or 2 hours after meals.

IM

Do not administer intramuscularly.

IV

Dilute the dosage in 100 to 250 mg of saline solution or 5% dextrose and administer over 20 to 60 minutes. Monitor for thrombophlebitis.

Drug Interactions

Theophylline Toxicity

Erythromycin, when given with theophylline, may result in theophylline toxicity. Observe for vomiting, dizziness, restlessness, and cardiac arrhythmias. The dosage of theophylline may need to be reduced.

Metronidazole (me-trow-nyd′a-zol)
(Flagyl) (fla′jil)

Metronidazole is a somewhat unusual medication in that it has antibacterial, trichamonicidal, and protozoacidal activity. Its mechanism of action is unknown. It is used to treat trichomoniasis, giardiasis, amebic dysentery, amebic liver abscess, and anaerobic bacterial infections.

Side Effects

The most common side effects are nausea, headache, anorexia, and occasionally vomiting, diarrhea, and abdominal cramping. An unpleasant metallic taste is also common. Thrombophlebitis occurs in about 6% of patients receiving parenteral therapy.

The most serious reactions are seizures and peripheral neuropathy. Patients receiving high doses, those with a history of seizure activity, and those with significant hepatic impairment may be at greater risk. Peripheral neuropathy, manifested as numbness of the extremities, has been reported after prolonged therapy. It appears to resolve after discontinuation of therapy, but this may take several weeks.

Overgrowth of oral and vaginal monilia may result in furry tongue, glossitis, vaginal itching and burning, and urethral irritation.

Metronidazole may impart a reddish-brown discoloration to the urine, especially when high doses are used.

Availability

PO—250 and 500 mg tablets.
IV—500 mg/vial.

Dosage and Administration

Adult
PO—Trichomoniasis
  1. Males and females: 250 mg 3 times daily for 7 days. Sexual partners must be treated concurrently to prevent reinfection.
  2. Single doses of 2 g, or 2 doses of 1 g each administered the same day appears to provide adequate treatment for trichomoniasis in both sexes.
Amebic dysentery: 750 mg 3 times daily for 5 to 10 days.
Amebic liver abscess: 500 to 750 mg 3 times daily for 5 to 10 days.
Giardiasis: 250 mg 2 to 3 times daily for 5 to 10 days.
Anaerobic bacterial infections
  1. Start with parenteral therapy initially.
  2. The usual *oral* dosage is 7.5 mg/kg every 6 hours. Do not exceed 4/24 hours. The usual duration is 7 to 10 days; infections of the bone and joint, lower respiratory tract and endocardium may require longer treatment.
IV—Anaerobic bacterial infections:
  1. Loading dose: 15 mg/kg infused over 1 hour.
  2. Maintenance dose: 7.5 mg/kg infused over 1 hour every 6 hours. Do not exceed 4 g/24 hours. Convert to oral dosages when clinical condition is stable.
  3. Dosage reduction is necessary in patients with hepatic impairment but not renal impairment.

Pediatric
PO—Trichomoniasis: 35 to 50 mg/kg/24 hours in 3 divided doses for 7 days.
  Amebiasis: 35 to 50 mg/kg/24 hours in 3 divided doses for 10 days.
  Giardiasis: 35 to 50 mg/kg/24 hours in 3 divided doses for 7 days.

Nursing Interventions

See also General Nursing Considerations for Patients with Infectious Diseases.

PATIENT CONCERNS: NURSING INTERVENTION/RATIONALE

Side Effects to Expect

Nausea, Vomiting, Anorexia, Abdominal Cramps

These side effects are usually mild and tend to resolve with continued therapy. Encourage the patient not to discontinue therapy without first consulting the physician.

Side Effects to Report

Seizures, Peripheral Neuropathy

Monitor patients for signs of numbness (paresthesia) in the extremities; report the extent and location. Teach safety measures to the patient experiencing neuropathy. Lack of sensation requires care in testing water temperature before immersing extremities and visual inspection for evidence of skin breakdown.

Assess the patient for development of seizures: nystagmus, muscle twitching, changes in effect.

Superinfections

With metronidazole, oral thrush, genital and anal pruritus, vaginitis and vaginal discharge may occur. Report promptly since these infections are resistant to the original antibiotic used.

Teach the importance of meticulous oral and perineal personal hygiene.

Thrombophlebitis

Carefully assess patients receiving IV metronidazole for the development of thrombophlebitis.

Inspect the IV area frequently while providing care; inspect during dressing changes, and when the IV is changed to a new site. Always investigate pain at the IV site. Report redness, warmth, tenderness to touch, and edema in the affected part. If in lower extremities, dorsiflexion of the foot may cause pain in the calf (Homan's sign). Compare the affected limb with the unaffected limb.

Drug Interactions

Alcohol

Use of alcohol and alcohol-containing preparations, such as over-the-counter cough medications, should be avoided during therapy and up to 48 hours after discontinuation of therapy.

Warfarin

This medication may enhance the anticoagulant effects of warfarin. Observe for the development of petechiae, ecchymoses, nosebleeds, bleeding gums, dark tarry stools, and bright red or "coffee-ground" emesis. Monitor the prothrombin time and reduce the dosage of warfarin if necessary.

Disulfiram

Combined use of disulfiram and metronidazole may result in mental confusion and psychoses. Concurrent therapy is not recommended.

Spectinomycin (spek-ti-no-my'sin) **(Trobicin)** (tro'bi-sin)

Spectinomycin is used specifically for the treatment of gonorrhea in both males and females. It has a particular advantage: most bacterial strains of gonorrhea respond to one administration of the recommended dosage. It is not effective in the treatment of syphilis.

Side Effects

Pain at the site of injection is a common side effect. Nausea, chills, urticaria, and fever are other side effects of single-dose therapy.

Dosage and Administration

Adult

IM—A 20-gauge needle is recommended. Injections should be made deep into the upper outer quadrant of the gluteal muscle. The usual dose for both males and females is 2 g. In geographic areas where penicillin-resistant gonorrhea is common, a dose of 4 g is recommended (2 g in each gluteal muscle).

Nursing Interventions

See also General Nursing Considerations for Patients with Infectious Diseases.

**PATIENT CONCERNS:
NURSING INTERVENTION/RATIONALE**

Dosage and Administration

IM

   Pain at the injection site is common. Give deeply in a large muscle mass. Devise a plan for rotation of injection sites if more than one injection is administered.

Anthelmintic Agents

The anthelmintic agents—mebendazole, piperazine citrate, pyrantel pamoate, pyrvinium pamoate, quinacrine hydrochloride, and thiabendazole—are the primary agents used in the treatment of intestinal worm infestations. They are discussed in greater detail elsewhere (see Index).

Fungal Infections

Fungal infections are becoming more common because modern antimicrobial and antineoplastic therapeutic agents are increasing the survival of the immunosuppressed host. Fungal infections can be subdivided into three categories:

1. Primary fungal pathogens that cause serious systemic infections in otherwise healthy persons.
2. Secondary fungal pathogens that produce fungal infections in the immunosuppressed patient.
3. Contagious, superficial fungal infections of the skin, hair, or nails.

Long-term therapy may be required to effectively manage the fungal infection. Stress the need for compliance for the full course of treatment and personal hygiene measures such as cleanliness and keeping infected skin surfaces dry.

*General Nursing Considerations for Patients
with Fungal Infections*

See General Nursing Considerations for Patients with Infectious Diseases.

Antifungal Agents

Amphotericin B (am-fo-tair′ih-sin)
(Fungizone) (fun-gi′zone)

Amphotericin B is a fungistatic agent that disrupts the cell membrane of fungal cells, resulting in a loss of cellular contents. Amphotericin B is used primarily for the treatment of systemic fungal infections and meningitis. It can also be used topically for candidal infections.

Side Effects

Side effects from topical preparations are usually quite minor. The cream may dry the skin. Both the lotion and the ointment may cause slight irritation, manifested by erythema, pruritus, or a burning sensation. Allergic dermatitis is quite rare.

Systemic side effects from intravenous use include headaches, chills, fever, malaise, muscle and joint pain, cramping, nausea, and vomiting. These adverse effects tend to be dose-related and may be minimized by slow infusion, reduction of dosage, and alternate-day administration. Antipyretics, antihistamines, and antiemetics may provide some symptomatic relief from the side effects.

Renal damage is a potential toxic effect of systemic amphotericin B therapy. Nephrotoxicity may be manifested by increases in excretion of uric acid, potassium, and magnesium, oliguria, granular casts in the urine, proteinuria, and increased BUN and serum creatinine levels. Report input and output, as well as a progressive decrease in daily urine volume or changes in visual characteristics.

Availability

Topical—3% cream, lotion, ointment.
IV—50 mg per vial.

Dosage and Administration

Adult
Topical—Apply liberally to candidal lesions 2 to 4 times daily. Any staining from cream or lotion preparations may be removed by soap and warm water, and any staining from amphotericin ointment may be removed by standard cleaning fluids.
IV—Initially 250 μg/kg over 6 hours. The daily dose is gradually increased as the patient develops tolerance. Dosage may range between 1 and 1.5 mg/kg on alternate days.

• Venous irritation may be diminished by the addition of 1200 to 1600 units of heparin and/or 10 to 15 mg of hydrocortisone or methylprednisolone to the infusion solution.

- Amphotericin B must be reconstituted with sterile water for injection without bacteriostatic agent.
- *Do not* use an in-line filter during infusion.
- The infusion must be protected from light during administration.
- The recommended infusion concentration is 1 mg/ 10 ml of dextrose 5% in water.

Nursing Interventions

See also General Nursing Considerations for Patients with Infectious Diseases.

PATIENT CONCERNS: NURSING INTERVENTION/RATIONALE

Side Effects to Expect

Topical Ointments/Lotions

Slight irritation may occur, causing erythema, pruritus, or burning sensations. If symptoms become severe, report for further evaluation by the physician.

Side Effects to Report

Nephrotoxicity

Monitor urinalysis and kidney function tests for abnormal results. Report an increasing BUN and creatinine, decreasing urine output or decreasing specific gravity (despite amount of fluid intake), casts or protein in the urine, frank blood or smoky-colored urine, or RBCs in excess of 0–3 on the urinalysis report.

Electrolyte Imbalance

The electrolytes most commonly altered are potassium (K^+) and magnesium (Mg^{++}). *Hypokalemia* is most likely to occur.

Many symptoms associated with altered fluid and electrolyte balance are subtle and resemble general symptoms of drug toxicity or the disease process itself.

Gather data relative to *changes* in the patient's mental status (i.e., alertness, orientation, confusion), muscle strength, muscle cramps, tremors, nausea, and general appearance (drowsy, anxious, lethargic).

Always check the electrolyte reports for early indications of electrolyte imbalance.

Keep accurate records of I/O, daily weights, and vital signs.

Malaise, Fever, Chills, Headache, Nausea, Vomiting

Check p.r.n. and standing orders for drugs (antihistamines, aspirin, antiemetics) that may alleviate these symptoms.

Thrombophlebitis

Carefully assess patients receiving IV amphotericin B for the development of thrombophlebitis.

Inspect the IV area frequently while providing care; inspect during dressing changes and when the IV is changed to a new site. Always investigate pain at the IV site. Report redness, warmth, tenderness to touch, and edema in the affected part. If in lower extremities, dorsiflexion of the foot may cause pain in the calf (Homan's sign). Compare the affected limb with the unaffected one.

Dosage and Administration

Staining

Staining on clothing caused by creams or lotion may be removed by soap and water; ointment stains require use of standard cleaning fluids.

IV

See above for reconstitution instructions.

Filters

Do not use an in-line filter during administration.

Light Protection

Cover the solution to protect it from light during administration.

Additives

Check for specific orders regarding the addition of heparin, hydrocortisone, or methylprednisone to diminish venous irritation.

Rate

Administer over 6 hours unless specifically ordered otherwise. Maintain close observation for thrombophlebitis.

Drugs Interactions

Corticosteroids (Prednisone, Others)

Corticosteroids may enhance the loss of potassium. Check potassium levels and monitor more closely for hypokalemia when these two agents are used concurrently.

Nephrotoxic Potential

Combining amphotericin B with other nephrotoxic agents such as aminoglycosides or diuretics should be done with extreme caution. Monitor closely for signs of nephrotoxicity.

Candicidin (kan-di-cyd′in)
(Vanobid) (van-o′bid)

Candicidin is a fungicidal agent used in the treatment of vaginal infections due to *Candida albicans* (monilia). It has an advantage in being approved for use during pregnancy.

Side Effects

Side effects are fairly rare with this product. A few patients may complain of irritation, and hypersensitivity sensitization has been reported.

Availability

Vaginal tablets—3 mg.
Vaginal ointment—75 g tubes.

Dosage and Administration

Intravaginal: One applicatorful of ointment or one vaginal tablet inserted high in the vagina 2 times daily, morning and at bedtime, for 14 days. During pregnancy, use the applicator only on recommendation from the physician. Digital insertion of tablets may be preferred.

Nursing Interventions

See also General Nursing Considerations for Patients with Infectious Diseases.

PATIENT CONCERNS: NURSING INTERVENTION/RATIONALE

Side Effects to Expect and Report

Irritation

This side effect is usually mild and tends to resolve with continued therapy. Encourage the patient not to discontinue therapy without first consulting her physician.

Dosage and Administration

Intravaginal

Give the patient the following instructions:

1. Wash the applicator in warm soapy water after each use, so that it does not become a vehicle for reinfection.
2. A pad may be used to protect clothing.
3. Refrain from sexual intercourse during therapy (or the male should wear a condom to avoid reinfection).
4. Contraception other than a diaphragm should be used when being treated with the vaginal ointment. Prolonged contact with petrolatum-based products may cause the diaphragm to deteriorate.

Drug Interactions

No clinically significant interactions have been reported.

Clotrimazole (klo-trim′ah-zole)
(Lotrimin) (lo′tri-min)

Clotrimazole is an antifungal agent that inhibits the growth of both dermatophytes and yeasts. It is effective in treating skin infections caused by species of fungi that burrow into superficial skin layers to cause athlete's foot and ringworm. It is also effective against *Candida albicans*, the yeastlike fungus that causes vulvovaginitis and inflammation of the corners of the mouth.

Side Effects

Adverse effects are rare with this medication, but if a patient should develop pruritus, urticaria, blistering, and erythema, the product should be discontinued. These signs are indications of hypersensitivity.

Availability

Vaginal tablets—100 mg.
Vaginal cream—1% in 45 and 90 g tubes.
Topical—1% cream, 1% lotion.

Dosage and Administration

Topical
Apply the cream or lotion to the affected areas and surrounding skin morning and evening and gently rub in. Relief of pruritus should be evident within 1 week.
Intravaginal
Insert one applicatorful of cream or one tablet high in the vagina 2 times daily, morning and at bedtime, for 7 days.

Nursing Interventions

See also General Nursing Considerations for Patients with Infectious Diseases.

**PATIENT CONCERNS:
NURSING INTERVENTION/RATIONALE**

Side Effects to Report

Pruritus, Itching, Blisters, Erythema

Withhold therapy until a physician has evaluated the patient.

Dosage and Administration

Topical

Response to therapy should be apparent within 7 days. Wash hands thoroughly before and immediately after application.

Intravaginal

Give the patient the following instructions:

1. Wash the applicator in warm soapy water after each use, so that it does not become a vehicle for reinfection.
2. A pad may be used to protect clothing.
3. Refrain from sexual intercourse during therapy (or the male should wear a condom to avoid reinfection).

4. Contraception other than a diaphragm should be used when the patient is being treated with the vaginal ointment. Prolonged contact with petrolatum-based products may cause the diaphragm to deteriorate.

Drug Interactions

No clinically significant drug interactions have been reported.

Flucytosine (flu-sy'toe-seen)
(Ancobon) (On-ko-bon')

Flucytosine is an antifungal agent. Its mechanism of action is unknown, but it is effective against susceptible candidal septicemia, endocarditis, urinary tract infections, cryptococcal meningitis, and pulmonary infections.

Side Effects

Nausea, vomiting, diarrhea, rash, anemia, leukopenia, thrombocytopenia, and elevation of hepatic enzymes, BUN, and creatinine have been reported. Other side effects include hallucinations, confusion, headache, sedation, and vertigo.

Availability

PO—250 and 500 mg capsules.

Dosage and Administration

Adult
PO—50 to 150 mg/kg/day divided into doses every 6 hours. Doses up to 250 mg/kg/day may be required in cryptococcal meningitis.

- Nausea may be reduced if the capsules are given a few at a time over 20 to 30 minutes.

Nursing Interventions

See also General Nursing Considerations for Patients with Infectious Diseases.

PATIENT CONCERNS: NURSING INTERVENTION/RATIONALE

Side Effects to Expect

Nausea, Vomiting, Diarrhea

These side effects are usually mild and tend to resolve with continued therapy. Encourage the patient not to discontinue therapy without first consulting the physician.

Side effects may be reduced by administering a few capsules at a time over 30 minutes.

Side Effects to Report

Hematologic, Rash

Monitor for the development of sore throat, fever, purpura, jaundice, or excessive, progressive weakness.

Nephrotoxicity

Monitor urinalysis and kidney function tests for abnormal results. Report an increasing BUN and creatinine, decreasing urine output or decreasing specific gravity (despite amount of fluid intake), casts or protein in the urine, frank blood or smoky-colored urine, or RBCs in excess of 0–3 on the urinalysis report.

Hepatotoxicity

The symptoms of hepatotoxicity are anorexia, nausea, vomiting, jaundice, hepatomegaly, splenomegaly, and abnormal liver function tests (elevated bilirubin, SGOT, SGPT, alkaline phosphatase, prothrombin time).

Drug Interactions

Amphotericin B

Flucytosine and amphotericin B display enhanced activity when used concurrently.

Griseofulvin (griz-ee-o-ful′vin)
(Fulvicin) (ful′vi-sin),
(Grifulvin) (gri-ful′vin)

Griseofulvin is a fungistatic agent used to treat ringworm of the scalp, body, nails, and feet. After griseofulvin is absorbed, it is incorporated into the keratin of the nails, skin, and hair in therapeutic amounts. The infecting fungus is not killed, but its growth into new cells is prevented. Once the cells are shed or removed, they are replaced by new cells free from the infection. Due to the slow growth of nails, treatment often requires several months.

Side Effects

Hypersensitivity reactions, manifested as skin rashes and urticaria, are relatively common adverse effects of griseofulvin. Other side effects include photosensitivity, oral thrush, nausea, vomiting, diarrhea, dizziness, and confusion.

During prolonged therapy, periodic laboratory tests should be completed to warn of changes in renal, hepatic, and hematopoietic function.

Availability

PO—125, 165, 250, 330, and 500 mg tablets and capsules; 125 mg/5 ml oral suspension.

Dosage and Administration

Adult
PO—Depending on the specific organism and the location of the infection, 500 mg to 4 g in single or divided doses daily.

- Absorption from the gastrointestinal tract may be increased by administering with a meal high in fat content.

Nursing Interventions

See also General Nursing Considerations for Patients with Infectious Diseases.

PATIENT CONCERNS: NURSING INTERVENTION/RATIONALE

Side Effects to Expect

Nausea, Vomiting, Anorexia, Abdominal Cramps

These side effects are usually mild and tend to resolve with continued therapy. Encourage the patient not to discontinue therapy without consulting his/her physician first.

Side Effects to Report

Urticaria, Rash, Pruritus

Report symptoms for further evaluation by the physician.

Pruritus may be relieved by adding baking soda to the bath water.

Confusion

Perform a baseline assessment of the patient's degree of alertness and orientation to name, place, and time *before* initiating therapy. Make regularly scheduled subsequent mental status evaluations and compare findings. Report development of alterations.

Dizziness

Provide for patient safety during episodes of dizziness; report for further evaluation.

Superinfections

With griseofulvin, oral thrush, genital and anal pruritus, vaginitis and vaginal discharge may occur. Report promptly since these infections are resistant to the original antibiotic used.

Teach the importance of meticulous oral and perineal personal hygiene.

Photosensitivity

The patient should be cautioned to avoid exposure to sunlight and ultraviolet light. Suggest wearing long-sleeved clothing, hat, and sunglasses when going to be exposed to sunlight. Discourage the use of artificial tanning lamps. Notify the physician for the advisability of discontinuing therapy.

Hematologic

Routine laboratory studies (RBC, WBC, and differential counts) are scheduled for patients taking griseofulvin 30 days or longer. Stress returning for this laboratory work.

Monitor for the development of a sore throat, fever, purpura, jaundice, or excessive, progressive weakness.

Nephrotoxicity

Monitor urinalysis and kidney function tests for abnormal results. Report an increasing BUN and creatinine, decreasing urine output or decreasing specific gravity (despite amount of fluid intake), casts or protein in the urine, frank blood or smoky-colored urine, or RBCs in excess of 0–3 on the urinalysis report.

Hepatotoxicity

The symptoms of hepatotoxicity are anorexia, nausea, vomiting, jaundice, hepatomegaly, splenomegaly, and abnormal liver function tests (elevated bilirubin, SGOT, SGPT, alkaline phosphatase, prothrombin time).

Dosage and Administration

PO

Administer with meals high in fat content to increase drug absorption. Stress that the drug may need to be given over a prolonged period to control the infection effectively.

Drug Interactions

Warfarin

This medication may diminish the anticoagulant effects of warfarin. Monitor the prothrombin time and increase the dosage of warfarin if necessary.

Barbiturates

The absorption of griseofulvin is impaired by combining it with barbiturates. If concurrent therapy cannot be avoided, administer the griseofulvin in divided doses 3 times daily.

Ketoconazole (key-toe-kon'a-zol) (Nizoral) (nis-o-ral')

Ketoconazole is an antifungal agent chemically related to miconazole. Both act by interfering with cell wall synthesis, causing leakage of cellular contents. Ketoconazole is used orally to treat candidiasis, chronic mucocutaneous candidiasis, oral thrush, candiduria, coccidioidomycosis, histoplasmosis, chromomycosis, and paracoccidioidomycosis.

Side Effects

Side effects are usually quite mild and resolve during continued therapy. Nausea and vomiting (3%) are usually controlled by administration just before or with a meal. Other side effects are pruritus (1.5%), abdominal pain (1.2%), rash, dizziness, constipation, diarrhea, fever, chills, and headache.

Gynecomastia has been reported in men, but tends to resolve during continued therapy.

Ketoconazole therapy has been associated with hepatotoxicity. Liver function tests are recommended before initiating therapy, and biweekly to monthly thereafter. Transient minor elevations in liver enzymes may occur during treatment; treatment should be discontinued if these elevations persist.

Availability

PO—200 mg tablets.

Dosage and Administration

Adults
PO—200 to 400 mg once daily. Absorption is improved when administered with food.
Pediatrics
PO—44 pounds or less: 50 mg once daily. 44 to 88 pounds: 100 mg once daily. More than 88 pounds: 200 mg once daily.

Nursing Interventions

See also General Nursing Considerations for Patients with Infectious Diseases.

**PATIENT CONCERNS:
NURSING INTERVENTION/RATIONALE**

Side Effects to Expect

Nausea, Vomiting

These side effects are usually mild and tend to resolve with continued therapy. Encourage the patient not to discontinue therapy without first consulting the physician. Administer with food or milk to reduce irritation.

Side Effects to Report

Hepatotoxicity

Liver function tests are recommended before initiating therapy, with follow-up tests biweekly to monthly.

The symptoms of hepatotoxicity are anorexia, nausea, vomiting, jaundice, hepatomegaly, splenomegaly, and abnormal liver function tests (elevated bilirubin, SGOT, SGPT, alkaline phosphatase, prothrombin time).

Pruritus, Rash

Report symptoms for further evaluation by the physician.
Pruritus may be relieved by adding baking soda to the bath water.

Dosage and Administration

PO

Administer with food to improve absorption.
Administer at least 2 hours before giving drugs that reduce stomach acidity.

Drug Interactions

Cimetidine, Dicyclomine, Antacids

Anticholinergic agents (dicyclomine, Donnatal, propantheline), antacids, and cimetidine diminish stomach acidity and decrease absorption of ketoconazole. Administer ketoconazole at least 2 hours before these medications.

Miconazole (my-kon-a-zol′) **(Monistat)** (mon-i′stat) **(Micatin)** (my-ka′tin)

Miconazole is an antifungal agent chemically related to ketoconazole. Both act by interfering with cell wall synthesis, causing cellular contents to leak. Topical miconazole is used to treat athlete's foot, jock itch, and vulvovaginitis. Parenteral miconazole is used to treat candidiasis, chronic mucocutaneous candidiasis, oral thrush, candiduria, coccidioidomycosis, histoplasmosis, chromomycosis, and paracoccidioidomycosis. Bladder irrigations may be used for fungal cystitis, and intrathecal injections may be used to treat fungal meningitis.

Side Effects

Topical use of miconazole is rarely associated with any adverse effects; however, if it causes irritation, burning, or erythema, discontinue use.

Avoid eye contact with any of the miconazole products. Wash eyes immediately if contact should occur.

Adverse effects associated with parenteral therapy include phlebitis (29%), pruritus (21%), nausea (18%), fever and chills (10%), rash (9%), and emesis (7%). Thrombocytopenia and transient drops in hematocrit and serum sodium values have also been reported. The incidence of nausea and vomiting can be reduced with the use of antihistaminic or antiemetic drugs given before infusion, or by reducing the dose, slowing the rate of infusion, and by avoiding administration after mealtime.

Availability

Topical—2% cream, lotion, or powder.
Vaginal suppositories—100 mg.
Vaginal cream—2%.
IV—10 mg/ml in 20 ml ampules.

Dosage and Administration

Adult

Topical—Gently rub the cream on the affected areas and surrounding skin, morning and evening. The lotion is recommended for use within skinfolds and is applied in a similar manner. Clinical improvement (relief from pruritus) should be evident within 7 days. If no improvement is noted within 4 weeks, reexamination and diagnosis should be considered.

Intravaginal—For treatment of candidiasis, insert one applicatorful intravaginally once daily at bedtime for 7 days.

IV—Coccidioidomycosis: 1800 to 3600 mg divided into 3 doses daily.

Cryptococcosis: 1200 to 2400 mg divided into 3 doses daily.

Candidiasis: 600 to 1800 mg divided into 3 doses daily.

Paracoccidioicomycosis: 200 to 1200 mg divided into 3 doses daily.

- Dilute all infusion solutions with at least 200 ml of 0.9% sodium chloride or dextrose 5% and administer over a period of 30 to 60 minutes.

Intrathecal—20 mg every 3 to 7 days as an adjunct to intravenous treatment of fungal meningitis. Administer undiluted by alternating lumbar, cervical, and cisternal punctures.

Bladder instillation—Instill 200 mg of miconazole in a diluted solution into the bladder. Frequency of administration is determined by the infecting microorganism.

Nursing Interventions

See also General Nursing Considerations for Patients with Infectious Diseases.

PATIENT CONCERNS: NURSING INTERVENTION/RATIONALE

Side Effects to Report with Topical Therapy

Irritation, Burning, Erythema

Withhold additional therapy until evaluated by the physician.

Eye Contact

Avoid contact with the eyes! Wash the eyes immediately with copious amounts of water.

Side Effects to Report with Parenteral Therapy

Phlebitis

Avoid IV infusion in the lower extremities and areas with varicosities. Use proper technique in starting the IV solution.

Always assess complaints of pain at the infusion site. If signs of inflammation accompany complaints, discontinue and restart elsewhere.

Pruritus, Rash, Fever, Chills

Report symptoms for further evaluation by the physician.

Pruritus may be relieved by adding baking soda to the bath water.

Nausea, Vomiting, Emesis

Nausea and vomiting can be reduced by:

- Use of antihistamines or antiemetic agents before infusion
- Reducing doses
- Slowing rate
- Avoiding administration after meals

Thrombocytopenia

Assess for signs of bleeding: petechiae, ecchymoses, nosebleeds, bleeding gums, dark tarry stools, bright red or "coffee-ground" emesis.

Dosage and Administration

Topical

Response to therapy should be apparent within 7 days. Wash hands thoroughly before and immediately after application.

Intravaginal

Give the following instructions:

1. Wash the applicator in warm soapy water after each use so that it does not become a vehicle for reinfection.
2. A pad may be used to protect clothing.
3. Refrain from sexual intercourse during therapy (or the male should wear a condom to avoid reinfection).
4. Contraception other than a diaphragm should be used when being treated with the vaginal ointment. Prolonged contact with petrolatum-based products may cause the diaphragm to deteriorate.

IV

Dilute all infusion solutions with a minimum of 200 ml of 0.9% sodium chloride or dextrose 5% and administer over a period of 30 to 60 minutes.

Give antihistamines or antiemetics before infusion; slow the rate if nausea and vomiting develop.

Bladder Instillation

Using aseptic technique, catheterize and infuse via an indwelling catheter. Clamp catheter for a specified period; open and drain, as ordered.

Drug Interactions

Warfarin

Parenteral miconazole may enhance the anticoagulant effects of warfarin. Observe for the development of petechiae, ecchymoses, nosebleeds, bleeding gums, dark tarry stools, and bright red or "coffee-ground" emesis. Monitor the prothrombin time and reduce the dosage of warfarin if necessary.

Nystatin (nys'tat-in)
(Mycostatin) (my-ko-staht'in)

Nystatin is an antifungal agent that acts by damaging the permeability of the fungal cell membrane. It is used in the treatment of candidal infections of the skin, mouth, vulvovaginal mucosa, and intestinal tract.

Side Effects

Side effects are quite uncommon with nystatin, although administration of the tablets and suspension may occasionally produce transient nausea, vomiting, and diarrhea.

Hypersensitivity to nystatin is quite rare; however, patients occasionally develop a contact dermatitis to the preservatives in the topical preparations.

Availability

Topical—Cream, ointment, powder, 100,000 units/g; lotion 100,000 units/ml.
PO—100,000 and 500,000 unit tablets; 100,000 units/ml suspension.
Vaginal tablets—100,000 units.

Dosage and Administration

Adult
PO—Gastrointestinal candidiasis: 500,000 to 1,000,000 units 3 three times daily.
Oral cavity: 400,00 to 600,000 units of suspension 4 times daily. The suspension should be retained in the mouth for several minutes before swallowing, if possible.
Vaginal—One tablet placed high in the vagina daily for 2 weeks. Even though symptomatic relief may appear within a few days, treatment should be continued for the full 2 weeks.
Topical—Apply to affected area 2 to 3 times daily. Continue treatment for 7 days after apparent cure. When treating topical candidal infections, the powder is recommended for moist lesions, for example, in skin folds or on the feet. The affected areas should be kept dry and exposed to air if possible. Concomitant therapy must include proper hygiene to prevent reinfection.
Pediatric:
PO—Infants: 200,000 units (2 ml) 4 times daily (1 ml in each side of the mouth). For premature and low-birth-weight infants, administer 100,000 units (1 ml) 4 times daily.
Children: As for adult doses.

Nursing Interventions

See also General Nursing Considerations for Patients with Infectious Diseases.

PATIENT CONCERNS: NURSING INTERVENTION/RATIONALE

Side Effects to Expect

Nausea, Vomiting, Diarrhea

These side effects are usually mild and tend to resolve with continued therapy. Encourage the patient not to discontinue therapy without first consulting the physician.

Hives, Pruritus, Rash

Report symptoms for further evaluation by the physician.

Pruritus may be relieved by adding baking soda to the bath water.

Dosage and Administration

PO

Have the patient retain the oral suspension in the mouth for several minutes before swallowing.

Intravaginal

Place one tablet high in the vagina daily for 14 days even if symptoms have improved.

Give the following instructions:

1. Wash the applicator in warm soapy water after each use so that it does not become a vehicle for reinfection.
2. A pad may be used to protect clothing.
3. Refrain from sexual intercourse during therapy (or the male should wear a condom to avoid reinfection).
4. Contraception other than a diaphragm should be used when the patient is being treated with the vaginal ointment. Prolonged contact with petrolatum-based products may cause the diaphragm to deteriorate.

Topical

Apply to infected area 2 to 3 times daily. Continue administration 7 days after apparent cure.

Powder is recommended for topical candidal infections where lesions are moist (skin folds or feet). Keep areas as dry as possible and open to air.

Teach hygiene measures to prevent reinfection. Wash hands thoroughly before and after application. Do not touch infected areas unnecessarily.

Drug Interactions

No clinically significant drug interactions have been reported.

Tuberculosis

Tuberculosis is an infectious disease caused by the bacteria *Mycobacterium tuberculosis*. This microorganism thrives in tissues with a relatively high oxygen content, so the infection is most commonly found in the lungs, kidneys, growing ends of bones, and the cerebral cortex. The organism is spread by airborne droplets from the cough or sneeze of a patient with pulmonary tuberculosis. It is not transmitted on objects such as dishes, clothing, or bedding. Family household contacts and those in institutions (hospitals, nursing homes, prisons) sharing an enclosed environment with a source case are at a major risk for infection.

Due to the long-term courses of therapy required to control tuberculosis, affected individuals need to be given particular encouragement to adhere to the treatment plan. The biggest nursing challenge in the treatment of tuberculosis is to sufficiently educate the patient to the need for prolonged drug therapy that may last up to 2 years.

General Nursing Considerations for Patients Receiving Antitubercular Therapy

See also General Nursing Considerations for Patients with Infectious Diseases.

Patient Teaching Associated with Antitubercular Therapy

PATIENT CONCERNS: NURSING INTERVENTION/RATIONALE

Communication and Responsibility

Encourage open communication concerning frustrations and anger as the patient attempts to adjust to the diagnosis and need for prolonged treatment. The patient must be guided to gain insight into the condition in order to assume responsibility for the continuation of treatment. Keep emphasizing those factors the patient can control to alter the disease process, including maintenance of general health, nutritional needs, adequate rest and appropriate exercise, and continuation of prescribed medication therapy.

Personal Hygiene

The patient must be taught to prevent the spread of infection to others by thorough handwashing and by covering the nose and mouth when sneezing or coughing.

The patient should also avoid other people with infections, children, and immunosuppressed or debilitated people.

Nutritional Status

Tuberculosis frequently occurs in patients with poor nutritional status. These individuals require a complete evaluation of their nutritional status, correction of deficiencies, and education about how to maintain a balanced diet.

Stress

Any person is going to be devastated by the news that he or she has an illness that prevents family socialization and employment, potentially for several months.

Encourage the patient to express feelings about this chronic illness. The adjustment to this situation involves working through great personal fears, frustrations, hostilities, and resentments associated with the loss of control within one's life.

Stress-producing factors within the family setting should be discussed and the individual should be allowed time to vent feelings in a nonthreatening, nonjudgmental atmosphere.

Professional psychological support and assistance from a social worker may be particularly appropriate.

Expectations of Therapy

Discuss expectations of therapy with the patient (i.e., time he or she will be unable to return to work, length of medication regimen, return to activities of daily living).

Changes in Expectations

Assess changes in expectations as therapy progresses and the patient gains understanding and skill in the management of the diagnosis.

Changes in Therapy through Cooperative Goal-Setting

Work with the patient to encourage adherence to the prescribed treatment. When the patient feels that a change should be made in a treatment plan, encourage discussion first with the physician.

Written Record

Enlist the patient's aid in developing and maintaining a written record of the monitoring parameters (Table 18.1) (i.e., weekly weights, amount and color of sputum, temperature, frequency of coughing, night sweats, tolerance to daily activities) and response to prescribed therapies for discussion with the physician. Patients should be encouraged to take this record on follow-up visits.

Fostering Compliance

Throughout the patient's hospitalization, discuss medication information and how it will benefit the course of treatment. Seek cooperation and understanding of the following points, so that medication compliance may be enhanced:

1. Name
2. Dosage
3. Route and administration times: give daily medications in one dose, usually on arising
4. Anticipated therapeutic response
5. Side effects to expect
6. Side effects to report
7. What to do if a dosage is missed
8. When, how, or if to refill the medication prescription.

Difficulty in Comprehension

If it is evident that the patient and/or family does not understand all aspects of continuing therapy being prescribed (i.e., administration and monitoring of medications, exercises, diets, follow-up appointments), consider the use of social service or visiting nurse agencies. Since this disease requires long-term therapy, it is not uncommon for these agencies to assume the responsibility for administering medications to noncompliant patients. If this approach is not successful, and the patient is still considered to be contagious, the person may require institutionalization.

Associated Teaching

Give patients the following instructions:

Always inform the physician or dentist of any prescription or over-the-counter medication being taken. Over-the-counter medications should not be taken without first discussing them with a physician or pharmacist.

Always report side effects of rash, itching, or hives immediately. Nausea, vomiting, or diarrhea should also be reported for the physician's evaluation if it is a new symptom.

Take all of the medication as prescribed for the full coursse of treatment. Do not discontinue use when feeling improved; do not save for future use; do not give your medicine to another individual. Sudden discontinuation of certain medications may produce harmful effects.

Keep all medications out of reach of children.

If pregnancy is suspected, consult an obstetrician as soon as possible about continuation of medication therapy.

At Discharge

Items to be sent home with the patient should:

1. Have written instructions for use.
2. Be labeled in a level of language and size of print appropriate for the patient.
3. If needed, include identification cards or bracelets.
4. Include a list of additional supplies to be purchased after discharge (i.e., syringes, dressings).
5. Include a schedule for follow-up appointments.

Antitubercular Agents

Ethambutol (e-tham'bu-tol)
(Myambutol) (my-am'bu-tol)

Ethambutol inhibits tuberculosis bacterial growth by altering cellular RNA synthesis and phosphate metabolism. Ethambutol must be used in combination with other antitubercular agents to prevent the development of resistant organisms.

Side Effects

General side effects that may occur with ethambutol therapy include dermatitis, pruritus, anorexia, nausea, vomiting, headache, dizziness, mental confusion, disorientation, and hallucinations.

Some patients receiving ethambutol develop blurred vision and green color blindness. These adverse effects disappear within a few weeks after therapy is discontinued.

Availability

PO—100 and 400 mg tablets.

Dosage and Administration

Adults
PO—Initial treatment: 15 mg/kg administered as a single dose every 24 hours.
Retreatment: 25 mg/kg as a single daily dose. After 60 days, reduce the dose to 15 mg/kg, and administer as a single dose every 24 hours.

Nursing Interventions

See also General Nursing Considerations for Patients with Infectious Diseases.

See also General Nursing Considerations for Patients Receiving Antitubercular Therapy.

**PATIENT CONCERNS:
NURSING INTERVENTION/RATIONALE**

Side Effects to Expect

Nausea, Vomiting, Anorexia, Abdominal Cramps

These side effects are usually mild and tend to resolve with continued therapy. Encourage the patient not to discontinue therapy without first consulting the physician.

Administer daily dose with food to minimize nausea and vomiting.

Side Effects to Report

Confusion, Hallucinations

Perform a baseline assessment of the patient's degree of alertness and orientation to name, place and time *before* initiating therapy. Make regularly scheduled subsequent mental status evaluations and compare findings. Report development of alterations. Provide for patient safety during episodes of altered behavior or periods of dizziness.

Blurred Vision, Red-Green Color Changes

Check for any visual alterations using a color vision chart before initiating therapy. Schedule subsequent evaluations on a regular basis. Report the development of visual disturbances for the physician's evaluation.

Dosage and Administration

PO

Administer once daily with food or milk to minimize gastric irritation.

The patient should be warned that omission or interrupted intake may result in drug resistance, reversal of clinical improvement, and increased susceptibility of family members and others to tuberculosis.

Drug Interactions

No clinically significant interactions have been reported.

Isoniazid (i-so-ny'ah-zid)
(INH), *(Hyzyd)* (hy'zid), *(Nydrazid)* (ny'dra-zid)

Isoniazid is used for the treatment of tuberculosis, but its mechanism of action is not known. It should be used in combination with other antitubucular agents for therapy of active disease.

Side Effects

Tingling and numbness of the hands and feet, nausea, vomiting, dizziness, and ataxia are relatively common side effects of isoniazid and are dose-related. Pyridoxine, 25 to 50 mg daily, is often recommended to reduce the incidence of these side effects.

Isoniazid may produce a false-positive reaction for urinary glucose with Clinitest tablets, but not with Tes-Tape or Diastix.

The incidence of hepatotoxicity increases with age. This reaction usually occurs within the first 3 months of therapy and is thought to be an allergic reaction. Early symptoms include fatigue, weakness, anorexia, and malaise.

Availability

PO—50, 100, and 300 mg tablets.
IM—100 mg/ml in 10 ml vials.

Dosage and Administration

Adult
PO—Treatment of active tuberculosis: 5 mg/kg to a maximum of 300 mg daily. Isoniazid should be used in conjunction with other effective antitubercular agents.
Prophylactic therapy: 300 mg daily in single or divided doses.
Concurrent administration of pyridoxine: 25 to 50 mg daily, recommended for prevention of peripheral neuropathies.
IM—As for PO administration.
Pediatric
PO—10 to 30 mg/kg/24 hours in single or divided doses. Infants and children tolerate larger doses than adults. Maximum dose is 500 mg daily.

Nursing Interventions

See also General Nursing Considerations for Patients with Infectious Diseases.

See also General Nursing Considerations for Patients Receiving Antitubercular Therapy.

**PATIENT CONCERNS:
NURSING INTERVENTION/RATIONALE**

Side Effects to Expect and Report

Tingling, Numbness

Concurrent use of pyridoxine will usually prevent the development of these common symptoms associated with this agent.

When paresthesias are present, the patient must be cautioned to inspect the extremities for any possible skin breakdown because of the diminished sensation.

Also caution patients not to immerse feet or hands in water without first testing the temperature.

Monitor patients with paresthesias for adequate nutrition.

Dizziness, Ataxia

Provide for patient safety and assistance in ambulation until either a dose adjustment or addition of pyridoxine provides symptomatic relief.

Hepatotoxicity

The incidence of hepatotoxicity increases with age and the consumption of alcohol.

The symptoms of hepatotoxicity are anorexia, nausea, vomiting, jaundice, hepatomegaly, splenomegaly, and abnormal liver function tests (elevated bilirubin, SGOT, SGPT, alkaline phosphatase, prothrombin time).

Dosage and Administration

PO

Administer on an empty stomach for maximum effectiveness. It is usually given as a single daily dose, but may be given in divided doses.

Pyridoxine is frequently given concurrently with isoniazid to diminish peripheral neuropathies, dizziness, and ataxia.

Drug Interactions

Disulfiram

Patients may experience changes in physical coordination and mental affect and behavior. Provide for patient safety and monitor the patient's mental status before and during therapy. If possible, avoid concomitant therapy.

Rifampin

Concurrent therapy may rarely result in hepatotoxicity. Patients on combined therapy should have liver function tests periodically.

Phenytoin

Isoniazid may inhibit the metabolism of phenytoin. Monitor patients receiving concurrent therapy for signs of phenytoin toxicity: nystagmus, sedation, lethargy. Serum levels may be ordered and the dosage of phenytoin reduced.

Clinitest

This drug may produce false-positive Clinitest results. Use Clinistix or Tes-Tape to measure urine glucose.

Rifampin (rif′am-pin) *(Rifadin)* (rif′ah-din)

Rifampin is used in combination with other agents against tuberculosis. It acts against enzymes within the bacterial cell that are required to produce DNA.

Side Effects

The more common adverse gastrointestinal effects are heartburn, anorexia, nausea, vomiting, cramps, gas, and diarrhea. Other side effects include headache, dizziness, mental confusion, visual disturbances, and generalized numbness.

Rifampin may tinge the urine, feces, saliva, sputum, sweat, and tears a red-orange color. No pathologic damage is caused by this color change, and it will disappear when the medication is discontinued.

Availability

PO—150 and 300 mg capsules.

Dosage and Administration

Adult
PO—600 mg once daily.
Pediatric
PO—10 to 20 mg/kg/24 hours with a maximum daily dose of 600 mg.

Nursing Interventions

See also General Nursing Considerations for Patients with Infectious Diseases.

See also General Nursing Considerations for Patients Receiving Antitubercular Therapy.

PATIENT CONCERNS: NURSING INTERVENTION/RATIONALE

Side Effects to Expect

Reddish-orange Secretions

Urine, feces, saliva, sputum, sweat, and tears may be tinged a reddish-orange color. The effect is harmless and will disappear after discontinuation of therapy.

Side Effects to Report

Nausea, Vomiting, Anorexia, Abdominal Cramps

These side effects are usually mild and tend to resolve with continued therapy. Encourage the patient not to discontinue therapy without first consulting the physician. Administer with food or milk to diminish irritation.

Dosage and Administration

PO

See note directly above. Patients should be warned that omission or interrupted intake may result in drug resistance, reversal of clinical improvement, and increased susceptibility of family members to tuberculosis.

Drug Interactions

Warfarin

This medication may diminish the anticoagulant effects of warfarin. Monitor the prothrombin time and increase the dosage of warfarin if necessary.

Isoniazid

Concurrent therapy may rarely result in hepatotoxicity. Patients on combined therapy should have liver function tests monitored periodically.

Quinidine, Diazepam

Rifampin stimulates the metabolism of these agents. Long-term combined therapy may require an increase in dosages for therapeutic effect.

Probenecid

Probenecid may reduce urinary excretion of rifampin. Monitor closely for rifampin toxicity.

Birth Control Pills

Rifampin interferes with the contraceptive activity of birth control pills. Counseling regarding alternate methods of birth control should be planned.

Viral Infections

Many viral infections are not treated with antiviral agents, but rather are treated symptomatically depending upon the causative virus. The basic assessments to be done by the nurse depend on the site of the infection, but would include monitoring patient hygiene and routine parameters, such as the vital signs. It is most important to assess the presenting symptoms.

General Nursing Considerations for Patients Receiving Antiviral Agents

See also General Nursing Considerations for Patients with Infectious Diseases.

Antiviral Agents

Acyclovir (a-sy′klo-veer)
(Zovirax) (zo-veer′ax)

Acyclovir is an antiviral agent that acts by inhibiting viral cell replication. It is used topically to treat initial infections of herpes genitalis and non-life-threatening cases of mucocutaneous herpes simplex virus infections in patients with suppressed immune systems. The intravenous form is used to treat initial and recurrent mucosal and cutaneous herpes simplex type 1 and 2 infections in immunosuppressed adults and children, and to treat severe initial clinical episodes of herpes genitalis who are not immunosuppressed.

Side Effects

Common adverse effects associated with topical application include pruritus, rash, and transient burning. Symptoms are mild and usually do not cause discontinuation of treatment.

Side effects that develop upon intravenous administration include phlebitis (14%), transient elevation in serum creatinine (4.7%), and rash or hives (4.7%). The adverse effects reported include diaphoresis, hematuria, hypotension, headache, and nausea. About 1% of patients have neurologic effects manifested by lethargy, obtundation, tremors, confusion, hallucinations, agitation, seizures, or coma.

Patients who are poorly hydrated, have reduced renal function, or who receive boluses of acyclovir are susceptible to renal tubular damage. This adverse effect is manifested by a rise in serum creatinine and blood urea nitrogen (BUN), hematuria, and a decrease in renal creatinine clearance.

Availability

Topical—5% ointment.
IV—500 mg per vial in 10 ml vials.

Dosage and Administration

Adult

Topical—Apply to each lesion every 3 hours, 6 times daily for 7 days. A finger cot or rubber gloves should be used to avoid the spread of virus to other tissues and persons.

- *Do not* apply to the eyes. It is not an ophthalmic ointment.

IV—*Note:* Bolus or rapid intravenous infusions may result in renal tubular damage.

- Acyclovir is reconstituted with 10 ml of preservative-free sterile water for injection to provide a solution concentration of 50 mg/ml. The solution is stable for 12 hours. This solution should be further diluted by a glucose and electrolyte intravenous fluid to a concentration of 1 to 7 mg/ml prior to administration (stable for 24 hours). Infuse over at least 1 hour to well-hydrated patients. Observe for phlebitis at the infusion site.
- Dose for patients with normal function: 5 mg/kg every 8 hours for 5 to 7 days.

Pediatric

Topical—As for adult patients.
IV—Patients over 12 years of age: 250 mg/m^2 every 8 hours for 7 days, at a constant infusion rate over 1 hour.

Nursing Interventions

See also General Nursing Considerations for Patients with Infectious Diseases.

PATIENT CONCERNS: NURSING INTERVENTION/RATIONALE

Side Effects to Expect

Pruritus, Rash, Burning

Report symptoms for further evaluation by the physician.
Pruritus may be relieved by adding baking soda to the bath water.

Side Effects to Report

Intravenous Therapy

PHLEBITIS

Avoid IV infusion in the lower extremities and areas with varicosities. Use proper technique in starting the IV solution.

Carefully assess at regularly scheduled intervals for signs of developing phlebitis. Inspect for redness, warmth, tenderness to touch, edema, or pain.

Rash, Hives

Assess, describe, and chart the location and extent of these presenting symptoms. Report for further evaluation.

Diaphoresis

Diaphoresis can be serious if the patient is not well hydrated. Assess hydration state, monitor electrolytes, and provide for nursing interventions (i.e., clean, dry linens, adequate fluid intake).

Nephrotoxicity

Monitor urinalysis and kidney function tests for abnormal results. Report an increasing BUN and creatinine, decreasing urine output or decreasing specific gravity (despite amount of fluid intake), casts or protein in the urine, frank blood or smoky-colored urine, or RBCs in excess of 0–3 on the urinalysis report.

Hypotension

Record the blood pressure in both a supine and sitting position before and during the administration of this drug. Caution the patient to rise slowly from a supine and sitting position.

Confusion

Perform a baseline assessment of the patient's degree of alertness and orientation to name, place, and time *before* initiating therapy. Make regularly scheduled subsequent mental status evaluations and compare findings. Report development of alterations.

Dosage and Administration

Topical

Apply the ointment using a finger cot or latex gloves to avoid spread to other tissues and persons.
Use meticulous handwashing technique before and after applying the ointment. DO NOT apply to the eyes; it is not an ophthalmic ointment.

IV

See above for instructions on reconstitution.
Bolus or rapid infusion may result in renal damage. Infuse over at least 1 hour to a well-hydrated patient.

Drug Interactions

Probenecid

Probenecid may reduce urinary excretion of acyclovir. Monitor closely for signs of toxicity from acyclovir.

Amantadine hydrochloride (ah-man'tah-deen) *(Symmetrel)* (sim'eh-trel)

Amantadine is an antiviral agent that has specific activity against the influenza A virus. Its primary use now, however, is as an anti-Parkinson's disease agent. It does not treat the underlying disease, but reduces its clinical manifestations. It is described in greater detail elsewhere (see Index).

Idoxuridine (eye-doks-yur'ih-deen) *(Stoxil)* (stok-sil')

Idoxuridine is an antiviral agent used to treat viral infections of the eye. It is discussed in greater detail elsewhere (see Index).

Trifluridine (tir-flur'ih-deen) *(Viroptic)* (vi-rop'tik)

Trifluridine is an antiviral agent used to treat viral infections of the eye. It is discussed in greater detail elsewhere (see Index).

Vidarabine (vi-dar'a-been) *(Vira-A)* (vi'ra ay)

Vidarabine is an antiviral agent that acts by inhibiting viral cell replication. It is used intravenously in the treatment of encephalitis caused by herpes simplex virus and topically as an ophthalmic ointment to treat keratitis and keratoconjunctivitis caused by herpes simplex virus types 1 and 2. Vidarabine does not show cross-sensitivity to idoxuridine and may be effective in treating recurrent keratitis that is resistant to idoxuridine.

Side Effects

Minor side effects associated with the use of vidarabine ointment include temporary visual haze, burning, itching, redness, and tearing. Photophobia—sensitivity to bright light—occasionally occurs, but can be minimized by wearing sunglasses. Allergic reactions have rarely been reported.

The most common side effects from intravenous vidarabine are nausea, vomiting, diarrhea, anorexia, and weight loss. These reactions begin on the second or third day of therapy and resolve in another 1 to 4 days. Hallucinations, psychosis, confusion, tremor, and dizziness may be dose-related and are reversed after discontinuation of therapy.

Intravenous vidarabine should be used with caution in patients with impaired liver or kidney function and in patients susceptible to fluid overload or cerebral edema.

Availability

Topical—3% ophthalmic ointment.
IV—200 mg/ml in 5 ml vials.

Dosage and Administration

Adult
Ophthalmic—Place a 1 cm ribbon of ointment inside the lower conjunctival sac of the infected eye, 5 times daily at 3 hour intervals. Continue for an additional 5 to 7 days at a dosage of 1 cm twice daily after reepithelialization has occurred to prevent recurrence of the infection.
IV—15 mg/kg daily for 10 days. Administer for 12 to 24 hours using an in-line filter (0.45 micron or smaller). Make sure that vidarabine is completely dissolved. It requires 2.2 ml of fluid to dissolve 1 mg of vidarabine (1 liter dissolves 450 mg at 77°F). Dissolution may be facilitated by prewarming the IV infusion fluid to 95–105°F. Dilute just prior to administration and use within 48 hours. *Do not* refrigerate the solution. Administer with any parenteral fluid, except blood, protein, and lipid products (hyperalimentation fluids).

Nursing Interventions

See also General Nursing Considerations for Patients with Infectious Diseases.

**PATIENT CONCERNS:
NURSING INTERVENTION/RATIONALE**

Side Effects to Expect and Report

Ophthalmic Ointment

VISUAL HAZE, TEARING, REDNESS, BURNING

Provide for patient safety during temporary visual impairment. Instruct the patient not to rub the eyes forcefully when tearing.

These side effects are usually mild and tend to resolve with continued therapy. Encourage the patient not to discontinue therapy without first consulting the physician.

PHOTOPHOBIA

Wearing sunglasses minimizes this effect.

Intravenous Therapy

NAUSEA, VOMITING, ANOREXIA

These symptoms usually resolve in 1 to 4 days. Perform daily weights; monitor fluid loss carefully.

CONFUSION

Perform a baseline assessment of the patient's degree of alertness and orientation to name, place, and time *before* initiating therapy. Make regularly scheduled subsequent mental status evaluations and compare findings. Report development of alterations so that dosage adjustments may be made.

NEPHROTOXICITY

Monitor urinalysis and kidney function tests for abnormal results. Report an increasing BUN and creatinine, decreasing urine output or decreasing specific gravity (despite amount of fluid intake), casts or protein in the urine, frank blood or smoky-colored urine, or RBCs in excess of 0–3 on the urinalysis report.

HEPATOTOXICITY

The symptoms of hepatotoxicity are anorexia, nausea, vomiting, jaundice, hepatomegaly, splenomegaly, and abnormal liver function tests (elevated bilirubin, SGOT, SGPT, alkaline phosphatase, prothrombin time).

BLOOD DYSCRASIAS

Monitor the WBC, RBC, and platelet counts. Report decreasing numbers. Monitor for the development of a sore throat, fever, purpura, or excessive progressive weakness.

Dosage and Administration

Ophthalmic

Use meticulous handwashing before and after application of eye ointment. *Do not* contaminate the tip of the applicator by touching the eye.

IV

See IV reconstitution instructions above.
Be certain it is completely dissolved prior to administration.
Administer with any parenteral solution, except blood, protein, and lipid products (hyperalimentation solutions).

Drug Interactions

Allopurinol

In question at the time of this writing is the possibility that the metabolism of vidarabine may be inhibited by allopurinol. Monitor for an increased frequency of toxic effects, if the two agents are used concurrently.

Urinary Antimicrobial Agents

The urinary antiinfective agents, including cinoxacin, methenamine mandelate, nalidixic acid, nitrofurantoin, and phenazopyridine, are mainstays in urinary antimicrobial therapy. They are discussed in greater detail in Chapter 14, Drugs Affecting the Urinary System.

Chapter 19

Obstetric and Gynecologic Agents

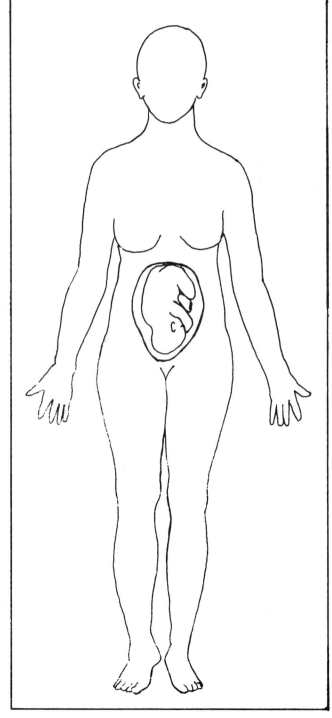

Objectives

After completing this chapter, the student should be able to do the following:

1. Explain the major action and effects of drugs used in obstetrics.
2. Identify baseline data the nurse should collect on a continuous basis for comparison and evaluation of drug effectiveness.
3. Identify important nursing assessments and interventions associated with the drug therapy associated with obstetrics.
4. Identify health teaching essential for a successful treatment regimen.

General Nursing Considerations
for Obstetrical Patients

See also Drugs Affecting the Endocrine System, Analgesics and Sedatives, and Diuretics.

PATIENT CONCERNS:
NURSING INTERVENTION/RATIONALE

Assessment of the Pregnant Woman

Prenatal Visit

CLIENT HISTORY

Obtain basic historical information about the woman and family concerning diseases, surgeries, and deaths.

MENSTRUAL HISTORY

Gather data about menstrual pattern (i.e., age of initial onset, duration and frequency of monthly periods, date of last full menstrual cycle, any bleeding since the last full menstrual period).

CONTRACEPTIVE USE

Gather data about contraceptive use (i.e., use of condoms, foam, diaphragm, sponge, the "pill," IUDs).

OBSTETRICAL HISTORY

Ask the woman the number of previous live births, stillbirths, "miscarriages," or induced abortions. If any of the deliveries were premature, obtain additional information about the infant's age of gestation, survival of the child, any suspected causes, and infections.

Ask if RhoGAM was given for Rh factor incompatibility.

Current Information

MEDICATIONS

Ask the woman if she takes any medications regularly. Include over-the-counter medications.

If she is not currently taking any medications, ask whether any have been taken over the past 6 months. Determine which have been prescribed and for what purpose.

ALCOHOL OR STREET DRUGS

Determine use of alcohol or street drugs of any kind, including what, how much, and how frequently.

HEALTH PROBLEMS

Ask the patient if she has ever been treated for:

- Kidney or bladder problems
- High blood pressure, heart disease, or rheumatic fever
- Hypothyroidism or hyperthyroidism
- Diabetes mellitus ("high blood sugar" or "sugar in the urine")
- Allergies to any foods, drugs, or environmental substances

If the woman answers "yes" to any of these questions, gather more information about what physician made the diagnosis, when the disorder occurred, and how it was treated.

EATING AND ELIMINATION

What are the woman's favorite foods, how often does the patient eat, and what has the patient eaten in the last 3 days?

What is the patient's elimination pattern? How often does the patient have bowel movements; what is the stool consistency and color; is there ever any bleeding; and are laxatives ever needed? If so, how often?

SOCIAL HISTORY

Capitalize on the individual's strengths:

Determine how the woman feels about this pregnancy (e.g., excited; nervous; baby is unwanted).

Who makes up her support group: husband, boyfriend, friends, family?

Ask the woman about her employment status and what type of work she performs.

Determine the woman's level of education and general interest in learning more about effective management of the pregnancy.

Also find out about woman's economic status. Will referral to social services agencies be necessary?

Physical Examination

Assist the individual to undress and prepare for examination.

URINE SPECIMEN

Have the individual void and save the specimen. (Give instructions on how to obtain a clean-catch specimen.)

HEIGHT AND WEIGHT

Weigh the woman and measure the current height.

BLOOD PRESSURE

Try to give the individual time to become more comfortable with the interviewer before taking the initial blood pressure reading. If elevated, recheck in about 10 minutes or when she appears to be more relaxed.

Ask again if any prior treatment has been given for high blood pressure. If so, inquire about the onset, treatment, and degree of control achieved.

PULSE

Count the pulse for 1 full minute. Report irregularities in rate, rhythm, or volume. On subsequent visits, anticipate an increase in rate of approximately 10 beats per minute during the course of the pregnancy.

RESPIRATIONS

Record the rate of respirations. As the pregnancy progresses, observe for hyperventilation and thoracic breathing.

TEMPERATURE

Record the temperature. Tell the client to report any elevations to the physician immediately for further evaluation. If temperature currently is elevated, ask about any signs of infection or exposure to persons with a known infection or communicable disease.

PELVIC EXAM

Assist the patient to prepare for the pelvic examination. Gather supplies for the physician and assist appropriately. A Papanicolaou (Pap) smear is usually performed as part of the examination. Mark specimens

appropriately, noting name, date, age, any hormone therapy, and date of last menstrual period.

BLOOD STUDIES

Blood samples for CBC, hemoglobin, hematocrit, rubella titer, Rh factor, and, occasionally, a VDRL, may be ordered drawn at this initial visit.

Schedule of Follow-up Visits

Explain that at each follow-up visit, the following will be done: weighing and necessary dietary teaching; measuring blood pressure, pulse, and respirations; examination of the abdomen with measurement of fundal height and fetal heart sounds. Any problems or concerns will be discussed. Hemoglobin and hematocrit may be periodically rechecked.

The pregnant woman who does not experience complications is usually examined once monthly for the first 6 months, every 2 weeks in the seventh and eighth months, and weekly during the last month of pregnancy. Vaginal exams are usually performed on the initial visit and are not repeated until 2 to 3 weeks prior to the estimated date of confinement (EDC) or "due date," at which time the cervical status, degree of engagement, and fetal presentation are evaluated.

Weight Gain

A weight gain of 2 to 4 pounds during the first trimester, 11 pounds during the second trimester, and 11 pounds during the third trimester is usual.

Stress the need to report a weight gain of 2 or more pounds in any 1 week for further evaluation.

Assessment of Pregnant Patients at Risk

Bleeding Disorders

Miscarriage and abortion are major causes of bleeding during the first and second trimesters of pregnancy. Bleeding during the third trimester may be due to placenta previa or abruptio placenta.

BLEEDING PATTERN

It is important to take a careful history of the onset and advancement of the bleeding symptoms. Gather specific information about the onset, duration, amount (number of pads used), color and any clots or tissue seen.

PAIN

Ask the patient to describe any pain being experienced. Has the patient had any backache or pelvic cramping, sharp abdominal pain, faintness, or pain in the shoulder area?

VITAL SIGNS

Whenever bleeding is present, the vital signs should be taken and compared to previous baseline data on the patient's records. Continue to monitor the vital signs at regular intervals to detect the development of shock: restlessness, perspiration, pallor, clammy skin, dyspnea, tachycardia, and blood pressure changes. Record the fetal heart rate at regular intervals.

LABORATORY STUDIES

When bleeding is present, blood studies for hemoglobin, hematocrit, WBCs, human chorionic gonadotropin (HCG) titer, and type and cross-match for blood may be ordered.

OTHER PROCEDURES

Other diagnostic procedures such as culdoscopy, sonography, laparoscopy, fetoscopy, and pregnancy tests may be performed.

ACTIVITY LEVEL

Bedrest and sedation are usually prescribed. Uterine relaxants such as ritodrine may also be required.

TERMINATION OF PREGNANCY

If bleeding occurs near the EDC, the infant may be delivered by cesarean birth.

If it appears that an incomplete abortion (miscarriage) has occurred, the woman may be hospitalized for observation, possible D&C (dilatation and curettage), and fluid replacement.

If a pregnancy is to be terminated (aborted), the following methods may be used:

- Before 12 weeks gestation: Suction curettage or dilatation and evacuation (D&E).
- 12 to 20 weeks gestation: Intraamniotic instillation of hypertonic saline (20% solution) or prostaglandin adminstered intraamniotically, intramuscularly, or by vaginal suppository.
- Intrauterine fetal death after 20 weeks of gestation: Prostaglandin suppositories with or without oxytocin augmentation.

Rh Factor. An Rh-negative mother may receive RhoGAM within 72 hours of the termination of pregnancy.

Rubella Vaccine. If the patient's rubella titer is low, an appropriate time for inoculation is immediately after pregnancy.

Patient Instructions. Persons having an abortion procedure should be instructed concerning personal care:

- Do not use tampons for one to two weeks; use pads.
- Do not douche.
- Report bleeding that is heavier than a normal "period" that persists for more than 24 hours.
- Do not engage in sexual intercourse for at least the first week following the abortion.
- Take temperature twice daily (noon and bedtime) for a few days, and report any elevations above 100°F.
- Stress the need for keeping the follow-up visit with the physician.
- Review contraceptive methods if necessary.

Psychologic Aspects. Encourage the persons involved in the loss of an infant to talk about their feelings of loss, grief, sadness, or anger. Listen and allow them to vent feelings. Give answers (if known) regarding future pregnancies. Refer for other counseling as appropriate. Anticipate that depression may develop over the next few weeks and may need treatment.

Pre-eclampsia and Eclampsia

Pre-eclampsia and eclampsia are now called *pregnancy-induced hypertension* (PIH). The term *toxemia of pregnancy* is no longer used because there is no evidence that a "toxin" produces the hypertension, edema, and proteinuria characteristic of the disease.

Pre-eclampsia is seen most often in the last 10 weeks of gestation, during labor, and in the first 12 to 48 hours after delivery. The etiology is unknown and the only cure for pre-eclampsia is termination of the pregnancy. Eclampsia is present when the mother develops seizures and coma in addition to the hypertension, edema, and proteinuria.

PIH occurs in 5 to 7% of all pregnancies. Women predisposed to the disease are those of lower socioeconomic status, teenagers with first pregnancies, and those with a history of chronic hypertension, diabetes mellitus, hydatidiform mole, renal disease, or multiple pregnancy (twins or triplets). Approximately one-third of women who have had PIH will develop it in a subsequent pregnancy.

Pre-eclamptic patients may be treated conservatively at home by limiting daily activity and instruction to eat adequate proteins in the form of lean meat, fish, poultry, and eggs. If the patient develops significant hypertension, edema, weight gain, and proteinuria, she may require hospitalization for more adequate control of the symptoms and to prevent the development of seizures.

HISTORY AND PHYSICAL

Carefully assess the patient for a history of predisposing disease or social factors.

VITAL SIGNS

Assess vital signs (temperature, blood pressure, pulse, and respirations) and compare to baseline readings. ALWAYS report sudden development of hypertension. (An elevation of systolic pressure 30 mm Hg or more above prior readings; or systolic blood pressure of 140 mm Hg or more; or a diastolic pressure of 90 mm Hg or more.)

EDEMA

All patients hospitalized for pre-eclampsia or eclampsia should be monitored for intake and output.

Daily hydration is maintained via oral or intravenous routes. Generally, 1000 ml plus the amount of urine output over the past 24 hours is allowed for intake.

Carefully assess for edema of any body parts (i.e., fingers, hands, face, legs, ankles).

Monitor daily weights and instruct the patient to report a weight gain of 2 lbs or more in any 1 week.

Salt intake is generally maintained at a normal level, although heavy use should be discouraged.

LABORATORY DATA

Urine. Always use a clean-catch specimen since vaginal discharge or the presence of RBCs may cause a positive test for proteinuria. An indwelling catheter may be necessary in severe cases both to monitor the amount of urine output and to obtain specimens for testing. Test the protein content and specific gravity hourly. Report steadily decreasing hourly output, or output < 30 ml/hr.

Electrolytes. Assess regularly and report abnormal findings.

Clotting Studies. Assess for possible thrombocytopenia.

BUN. The blood urea nitrogen is usually not elevated unless the patient has renal disease.

Uric Acid. Report increasing serum uric acid levels. There is a fairly good correlation with the severity of the pre-eclampsia–eclampsia. (Keep in mind that thiazide diuretics cause an increase in uric acid levels.)

Hematocrit. The hematocrit rises as the patient loses water from the intravascular space to the extravascular space or the patient becomes dehydrated due to inadequate hydration.

Serum Estriols, L/S Ratio. These laboratory tests give an indication of fetal maturity.

SEIZURES

Increased drowsiness, hyperreflexia, visual disturbances, and development of severe pain are indications of a worsening condition. Report these symptoms IMMEDIATELY.

If the patient does develop seizures, give supportive care, provide a nonstimulating environment, and have oxygen, suction, and a padded tongue blade available.

Record the respiratory and heart rates, degree of cyanosis, and duration of the seizure.

Continuously monitor fetal heart rate and movements.

Be alert for the start of labor or signs of other complications such as pulmonary edema, disseminated intravascular coagulation, congestive heart failure, abruptio placenta, or cerebral hemorrhage.

DRUG TREATMENT

Sedatives. A sedative, such as diazepam or phenobarbital, is sometimes given to encourage quiet rest.

Antihypertensives. The vasodilator hydralazine is generally used to control blood pressure. It may be administered orally or intravenously, depending upon the severity of the condition. If given IV, monitor the maternal and fetal heart rates, and the mother's blood pressure every 2 to 3 minutes after the initial dose, and every 10 to 15 minutes thereafter. The diastolic pressure is usually maintained at 90 to 100 mm Hg.

Anticonvulsants. Magnesium sulfate ($MgSO_4$) is the treatment of choice for seizure activity (see Index).

Premature Labor

Premature labor is labor that occurs before the end of the 37th week of gestation, resulting in the birth of an infant usually weighing less than 2500 g.

The overall incidence of prematurity in the United States is 9 to 10%; the incidence in blacks is 18 to 19%. Prematurity is responsible for almost two-thirds of infant deaths.

CAUSES

Among the causes of premature labor are premature rupture of membranes, maternal factors such as diabetes, pre-eclampsia–eclampsia, uterine anomalies, multiple pregnancies, fetal or uterine infection, and renal and cardiovascular diseases. In approximately two-thirds of cases, no specific cause can be identified.

STOPPING PRETERM LABOR

Early labor may be an indication of obstetrical complications such as infection, fetal death, hemorrhage, or severe pre-eclampsia–eclampsia. Close assessment by the physician is necessary before it is deemed appropriate to stop labor.

Non-Drug Treatment. If it is decided to stop labor, the patient should first be on bedrest, well-hydrated, and possibly sedated to relieve anxiety. These measures alone will stop labor in many patients.

Drug Treatment. If labor does not stop spontaneously, drugs such as ritodrine, terbutaline, or magnesium sulfate may be used to stop uterine contractions. Isoxsuprine and ethanol have been used in the recent past, but have generally been replaced by more effective agents such as ritodrine (see Index).

Glucocorticoids. Glucocorticoids, usually betamethasone, may be administered IM to the mother to accelerate fetal lung maturation and prevent hyaline membrane disease. It is used in cases where it is anticipated that premature labor should be stopped for only 36 to 48 hours, such as with premature rupture of the membranes.

Normal Labor and Delivery

History

Upon admission to the hospital, obtain the following information:

- Name and age
- Obstetrical history: gravida, para, abortions, fetal deaths, birth weight of previous children, complications during previous deliveries
- Estimated due date, estimated gestational age, and first day of last menstrual period (LMP)

- Prenatal care: type and amount, any significant problems
- Prenatal education: type and extent of childbirth preparation
- Plan for infant feeding
- Status of membranes: intact, ruptured, time ruptured, amount and color of fluid that escaped.
- Status of labor: time of onset of contractions, frequency, duration and intensity of contractions, how patient is coping with contractions
- Time of last meal

Physical Examination

Assess for:

- Height and weight
- Vital signs (temperature, blood pressure, pulse, and respirations)
- Presence of edema
- State of hydration
- Size and contour of abdomen and fundus
- Frequency of contractions
- Fetal heart rate
- Vaginal examination: cervical dilatation and effacement, status of membranes, and presentation and position of fetus.

Laboratory Tests

URINALYSIS

Obtain a clean-catch urine specimen and test for glucose and protein. Send to the lab for microscopic examination.

BLOOD

Obtain a blood specimen for CBC, hemoglobin, hematocrit, serology tests, and maternal blood type.

Other Admission Routines

PERINEAL PREP

The physician may order the perineal and pubic area to be shaved, to aid in postpartum repair of the perineum.

ENEMA

The physician may order this to empty the lower bowel, thus reducing the possibility of contamination during delivery.

Activity and Exercise

During the early stages of labor, some women may ambulate. Check the institutional rules.

Basic Needs

During labor, provide pain relief, comfortable positioning, back rubs, pelvic rocking, effleurage, and support for the coach and woman when necessary. Encourage rest between contractions throughout labor.

VOIDING

Encourage women in labor to void at least every 2 hours. Check for bladder distension.

NUTRITIONAL STATUS

Maintain adequate hydration by giving ice chips or clear liquids. Check the status of hydration as labor progresses by observing the mucous membranes, dryness of lips, and skin turgor.

Do not give solid foods unless specifically approved by the physician.

LEG CRAMPS AND MUSCLE SPASMS

Encourage leg extension and dorsiflexion of the foot to relieve spasms and cramping.

SWEATING

Keep a sponge available for wiping and cooling the face.

DRY MOUTH

Provide ice chips, mouthwash, or glycerine swabs, and help the mother brush her teeth if she desires.

PRIVACY

During the early phases of labor, provide the mother and coach as much privacy as possible. Give correct information when asked, and inform the couple of any procedures to be done.

Ongoing Monitoring

As labor progresses, continue to monitor the maternal and fetal vital signs and the frequency, duration, and intensity of uterine contractions.

Report contractions with a duration of 90 seconds or more, and those not followed by complete uterine relaxation. Report abnormal patterns on the fetal monitor such as decreased variability, late decelerations, and variable decelerations.

Continue to assist the coach when necessary.

As vaginal discharge increases, wash the perineum with warm water and dry the area. Change the bedsheets, pad, and gown when necessary.

After Delivery

Record:

- The time of delivery and position of the infant
- The type of episiotomy and type of suture used in repair, if appropriate
- Any anesthetic or analgesic used during repair
- Time of placental delivery
- Any complications such as additional bleeding or neonatal distress.

Medications

Administer and record oxytocic and lactation suppressants, if ordered.

Assessments

The vital signs should be checked every 15 minutes during the first hour or until the woman is stable, then every 30 minutes for the next 2 hours.

Inspect the perineum and note any abnormal swelling or bruising.

Check the fundal height and firmness every 15 minutes for 1 hour, then every 30 minutes for the next 4 hours.

Describe the amount of lochia, the color and the presence of any clots every 15 minutes for 1 hour; every 30 minutes for 4 hours; hourly for the next 12 hours.

Continue to monitor the state of hydration and elimination.

Support the physiological and psychological needs of the mother and father. Allow them to spend as much time with the infant as possible.

Postpartum Care

Postpartum is the time between delivery and return of the reproductive organs to prepregnancy status.

Rh Factor

An Rh-negative mother may receive *RhoGAM* within 72 hours of the completion of the pregnancy.

Rubella Vaccine

If the mother's rubella titer is low, an appropriate time for inoculation is immediately after pregnancy.

Assessments

FUNDUS

Continue to assess the fundal height and position until the woman is discharged.

LOCHIA

The lochia progresses from blood red to a more watery or pinkish color. Always report lochia that appears fresh after the discharge has been dark or diminished.

BREASTFEEDING

On delivery, the breasts secrete a thin yellow fluid called colostrum. Within 3 to 4 days, breast milk becomes available. This may produce some discomfort for the mothers as the breasts become congested. She may need to use a breast pump to prevent engorgement.

The quantity of breast milk varies among mothers. The diet, fluid intake, and level of anxiety all effect lactation. Oxytocin nasal spray may be necessary to help encourage milk letdown.

Remind the woman that breastfeeding is not a form of contraception. Alternative methods of contraception should be used if the patient does not desire to become pregnant immediately.

Mothers not desiring to breastfeed can be given lactation suppressants to inhibit milk secretion (see Index).

Prior to Discharge

Review methods of contraception if necessary.

Follow-Up Exam

The mother usually returns for a thorough exam at the physician's office 6 to 8 weeks after delivery.

Patient Teaching Associated with Pregnancy

Communication and Responsibility

Encourage open communication with the expectant family. They must be guided to gain insight into the pregnancy in order to assume responsibility for the continuation of care. Keep emphasizing those things the family can do to optimize the chances for a healthy baby, including maintenance of general health, nutritional needs, adequate rest and appropriate exercise, and continuation of prescribed medication therapy.

Expectations of Therapy

Discuss the expectations of therapy.

ADEQUATE REST, RELAXATION

Assist the individual to plan for adequate rest periods throughout the day to prevent fatigue, irritability, and overexhaustion.

Talk with the individual about planning rest periods during lunch breaks at work, when preschoolers are napping, or when the husband is home to care for children. A short period of relaxation in a reclining chair or just with the feet up may be beneficial when there is no time for sleep during the day.

Advise the patient to avoid long periods of standing in one place and to perform some daily activities while sitting.

ACTIVITY AND EXERCISE

Generally the woman can continue to perform common activities of daily living.

New attempts at strenuous exercise (e.g., jogging, aerobics) should not be started during pregnancy. Daily walks in the fresh air are encouraged.

Any changes in activity level should be discussed with the physician BEFORE starting.

Encourage good posture and participation in prenatal classes where exercises to strengthen the abdominal muscles and to relax the pelvic floor muscles are taught.

The woman should avoid lifting heavy objects or conditions that might cause physical harm, especially as the pregnancy progresses and the individual's balance may be affected.

EMPLOYMENT

Advice about continued employment should be based on the type of job, working conditions, amount of lifting, standing, or exposure to toxic substances, and the individual's state of health.

GENERAL PERSONAL HYGIENE

Encourage maintenance of general hygiene through daily tub baths or showers. Tub baths near the end of pregnancy may be discouraged because of the danger of slipping and falling while getting in and out of the tub. Tub baths should not be taken once the membranes have ruptured.

Encourage the use of plain soap and water to cleanse the genital area and prevent odors. The woman should *not* use deodorant sprays because of possible irritation. Tell the pregnant woman that an increase in vaginal discharge is common. Discharge that is yellowish or greenish, foul-smelling, or causes irritation and itching should be reported for further evaluation.

CLOTHING

Encourage the mother to dress in nonconstricting clothing.

As the pregnancy progresses, the mother may be more comfortable with a maternity girdle to support the abdomen. Encourage the mother to wear a well-fitting brassiere to provide proper support for the breasts. She should avoid restrictive circular garters which may impede circulation.

Encourage low-heeled, well-fitting shoes that provide good support. Properly fitting shoes can prevent lower back fatigue as well as tired feet.

ORAL HYGIENE

Encourage the mother-to-be to have a thorough dental exam at the beginning of the pregnancy. She should tell the dentist she is pregnant at the time of the examination.

Encourage thorough daily brushing, flossing, and use of an appropriate mouthwash.

SEXUAL ACTIVITY

Refer to an obstetrical text for discussion of alterations in sexuality during pregnancy. The wide range of feelings, needs, and intervention deserve more consideration than can be presented in this text.

SMOKING AND ALCOHOL

The mother-to-be should be encouraged to abstain from smoking or drinking during pregnancy. A vast amount of data now points out that smoking or drinking is potentially dangerous to the fetus. An increased incidence of neonatal mortality, low birth weight, and prematurity has been reported.

NUTRITIONAL NEEDS

Balanced nutrition is always to be encouraged, but is especially important throughout the course of the pregnancy. The Recommended Daily Allowances vary based on the individual's age, weight at the time of pregnancy, and daily activity level. At all times allowances must be made to maintain the nutritional needs of the mother and fetus. Refer to a nutrition text for specific recommendations.

Encourage limiting the caffeine content of the diet during pregnancy. Limit the consumption of coffee, tea, cola beverages, and cocoa. Tell the mother-to-be to check the labels for specific caffeine content since many soft drinks contain a significant quantity of caffeine.

BOWEL HABITS

Assess the individual's usual pattern of elimination and anticipate its continuance until later in pregnancy. Pressure on the lower bowel from the presenting part of the fetus may cause constipation and hemorrhoids. Stool softeners or a mild laxative may be prescribed if problems persist.

Encourage the consumption of fresh fruits, vegetables, whole grain and bran products, along with an adequate intake of six to eight 8-ounce glasses of fluid daily.

DOUCHING

Discourage any type of douching unless specifically prescribed for the individual by the physician.

Be certain when douching is prescribed that the patient is given simple, explicit instructions.

HEARTBURN

Tell the woman to avoid highly spiced foods and any foods that she knows have caused heartburn in the past. (See Chapter 13.)

Changes in Expectations

Assess changes in expectations as pregnancy progresses. Teach the woman how to deal with discomforts such as development of a backache, leg cramps, hemorrhoids, and edema.

Changes in Therapy through Cooperative Goal-Setting

Work with the mother-to-be to encourage adherence to the regimen. When she feels that a change should be made in a treatment plan, encourage discussion with the physician.

WRITTEN RECORD

Enlist the mother's aid in developing and maintaining a written record of monitoring parameters (Tables 19.1, 19.2) (i.e., blood pressure, pulse, daily weights, presence and relief of discomfort, exercise tolerance, fetal movement) and response to prescribed therapies for discussion with the physician. The woman should be encouraged to take this record on follow-up visits.

The woman should always report immediately loss of fluid vaginally, dizziness, double or blurred vision, severe headache, abdominal pain or persistent vomiting, fever, edema of the face, fingers, legs, or feet, and weight gain in excess of 2 lbs per week.

FOSTERING COMPLIANCE

Throughout the pregnancy, discuss medication information and how it will benefit the course of treatment. Seek cooperation and understanding of the following points so that medication compliance may be enhanced:

1. Name
2. Dosage
3. Route and administration times
4. Anticipated therapeutic response
5. Side effects to expect
6. Side effects to report
7. What to do if a dosage is missed
8. When, how, or if to refill the medication prescription.

DIFFICULTY IN COMPREHENSION

If it is evident that the patient and/or family does not understand all aspects of continuing therapy being prescribed (i.e., administration and monitoring of medications, exercises, diets, follow-up appointments) consider the use of social service or visiting nurse agencies.

ASSOCIATED TEACHING

Give the following instructions:

Always inform the physician or dentist of any prescription or over-the-counter medication being taken. Over-the-counter medications should not be taken without discussing them first with the physician or pharmacist.

Always report side effects of rash, itching, or hives immediately. Nausea, vomiting, or diarrhea should also be reported for the physician's evaluation if it is a new symptom.

Take all of the medication as prescribed for the full course of treatment. Do not discontinue use when feeling improved; do not save for future use; do not give your medicine to another individual. Sudden discontinuation of certain medications may produce harmful effects.

Keep all medications out of reach of children.

At Discharge

Items to be sent home with the pregnant woman should:

1. Have written instructions for use.
2. Be labeled in a level of language and size of print appropriate for the patient.
3. If needed, include identification cards or bracelets.
4. Include a list of additional supplies to be purchased after discharge (i.e., syringes, pads, dressings).
5. Include a schedule for follow-up appointments.

Uterine Stimulants

Dinoprostone (die'no-prahs-tone) (Prostaglandin E-2) (Prostin E-2)

Dinoprostone, or prostaglandin E-2, is a uterine and gastrointestinal smooth muscle stimulant. When used during pregnancy, it increases the frequency and strength of uterine contraction and produces cervical softening and dilatation. Dinoprostone is used to expel uterine contents in cases of intrauterine fetal death, benign hydatidiform mole, missed spontaneous miscarriage, and second trimester abortion. Occasionally, oxytocin and dinoprostone are used together to shorten the duration of time required to expel uterine contents.

Side Effects

The most frequently observed gastrointestinal side effects are nausea, vomiting, and diarrhea.

Temperature elevations about 38°C (100.6°F) occur within 15 to 45 minutes and continue for up to 6 hours in 50 to 70% of patients.

Headache, chills, and shivering occur in about 10% of patients receiving dinoprostone. Transient hypotension with a drop in diastolic pressure of 20 mm Hg, dizziness, flushing, and arrhythmias have all been reported.

Fragments of uterine contents are frequently left in the uterus after evacuation. Patients should be manually examined to prevent the development of fever, infection, and hemorrhage.

Table 19.1
Example of a Written Record for Patients Receiving Prenatal Care

Medications	Color	To be taken

Name _____

Physician _____

Physician's phone _____

Next appt.* _____

Parameters		Day of exam							Comments
Weight									
Blood pressure									
Pulse									
Pain	Cramps?								
	Backache?								
	Abdominal pain?								
Bleeding	With cramps?								
	# pads used per day								
	Describe color (bright or dark red)								
Edema	Morning								
	Evening								
	Other								
	Location: Hands, feet, ankles?								
Fatigue All day — After exercise — Normal 10 5 1									
Exercise Poor toleration — Moderate toleration — Normal 10 5 1									
Fetal movement	Normal?								
	None?								
Bowel movements Constipated — Normal — Diarrhea 10 5 1									

*Please bring this record with you to your next appointment.
Use the back of this sheet for additional information.

Table 19.2

Example of a Written Record for Patients Receiving Postpartum Care

Medications	Color	To be taken

Name _____

Physician _____

Physician's phone _____

Next appt.* _____

Parameters		Day of discharge							Comments
Weight									
Blood pressure	AM/PM								
Pulse	AM/PM								
Lochia	# pads/day?								
	Color of vaginal discharge								
Cramps Frequent 10 Moderate 5 None 1									
Breast tenderness	↑ discomfort								
	↓ discomfort								
	No problem								
Nipple condition	Sore								
	Cracking								
	No problem								
Sexual activity	Persistently painful								
	Uncomfortable								
	Normal								
Bowel movements	Constipation								
	Normal								

*Please bring this record with you to your next appointment.
Use the back of this sheet for additional information.

Availability

Vaginal suppository—20 mg.

Dosage and Administration

Adult

Intravaginal—Insert 1 suppository high into the posterior vaginal fornix. Patients should remain supine for at least 10 minutes after each insertion. Suppositories should be inserted every 2 to 5 hours, depending on uterine activity and tolerance to side effects.

PATIENT CONCERNS: NURSING INTERVENTION/RATIONALE

Side Effects to Expect

Nausea, Vomiting, Diarrhea

Premedication with an antiemetic such as prochlorpromazine and an antidiarrheal agent (loperamide or diphenoxylate) will reduce, but usually not completely eliminate, these adverse effects.

Fever

Sponge baths with water or alcohol and maintaining fluid intake may provide symptomatic relief.

Aspirin does not inhibit dinoprostone-induced fever.

Patients should be observed for clinical indications of intrauterine infection. Monitor temperature and vital signs every ½ hour.

Side Effects to Report

Orthostatic Hypotension

Although infrequent and generally mild, dinoprostone may cause some degree of orthostatic hypotension manifested by dizziness, flushing, and weakness, particularly when therapy is initiated.

Monitor the blood pressure in both the supine and standing positions.

Anticipate the development of postural hypotension and take measures to prevent its occurrence. For ambulatory patients, teach the patient to rise slowly from a supine or sitting position, and encourage her to sit or

lie down if feeling faint. Report rapidly falling blood pressure, as well as bradycardia, paleness, or other alterations in vital signs.

Drug Interactions

No clinically significant interactions have been reported.

Ergonovine maleate (er-go-no′veen mal-ee-ate)
(Ergotrate Maleate) (er′go-trayt)

Methylergonovine maleate (meth-il-er-go-no′veen mal-ee-ate)
(Methergine) (meth′er-jin)

Ergonovine and methylergonovine are structurally similar ergot derivatives that share similar actions. Both drugs directly stimulate contractions of the uterus. Small doses produce uterine contractions with normal resting muscle tone; intermediate doses cause more forceful and prolonged contractions with an elevated resting muscle tone; and large doses cause severe, prolonged contractions. Due to this sudden, intense uterine activity, which is dangerous to the fetus, these agents cannot be used for induction of labor. However, since these agents produce more sustained contractions than oxytocin, small doses of ergonovine and methylergonovine are used in postpartum patients to control bleeding and maintain uterine firmness.

Side Effects

The most common side effects are nausea and vomiting, and these are fairly infrequent. Other rare side effects reported include hypertension, dizziness, dyspnea, tinnitus, headache, and palpitations. Patients may also complain of abdominal cramping.

Availability

PO—0.2 mg tablets.
INJ—0.2 mg/ml in 1 ml ampules.

Dosage and Administration

Note: Use with extreme caution in patients with hypertension, pre-eclampsia, heart disease, venoatrial shunts, mitral valve stenosis, sepsis, or hepatic or renal impairment.

Adult

PO—0.2 mg every 6 to 8 hours after delivery for a maximum of 1 week.
IM—0.2 mg every 2 to 4 hours, to a maximum of 5 doses.

**PATIENT CONCERNS:
NURSING INTERVENTION/RATIONALE**

Side Effects to Expect

Nausea, Vomiting

These side effects are usually mild and tend to resolve with continued therapy. Encourage the patient not to discontinue therapy without first consulting the physician.

Abdominal Cramping

This is normally an indication of therapeutic activity, but, if severe, reduction or discontinuation of dosage may be necessary.

Side Effects to Report

Hypertension

Certain patients, especially those who are eclamptic or previously hypertensive, may be particularly sensitive to the hypertensive effects of these agents. These patients have a higher incidence of developing generalized headaches, severe arrhythmias, and strokes. Monitor the patient's blood pressure and pulse rate and rhythm. Report immediately if the patient complains of headache or palpitations.

Drug Interactions

Inhibition of Prolactin

Do not use ergonovine in patients who wish to breastfeed. Methylergonovine may be used as an alternative, since it will not inhibit stimulation of milk production by prolactin.

Caudal or Spinal Anesthesia

Hypertension and headaches may develop in patients who have received caudal or spinal anesthesia followed by a dose of either methylergonovine or ergonovine. Monitor the patient's blood pressure and heart rate and rhythm.

Oxytocin (ok-se-to'sin) *(Pitocin)* (pih-to'sin)

Oxytocin is a hormone produced in the hypothalamus and stored in the pituitary gland. When released, it stimulates the smooth muscle of the uterus, blood vessels, and the mammary glands. When administered during the third trimester of pregnancy, active labor may be initiated.

Oxytocin is the current drug of choice for inducing labor at term and for augmenting uterine contractions during the first and second stages of labor. Oxytocin is routinely administered immediately postpartum to control uterine atony and postpartum hemorrhage. Oxytocin may also be administered intranasally to promote milk letdown and to treat breast engorgement during lactation.

Side Effects

Side effects that may occur include nausea, vomiting, hypotension, tachycardia, and arrhythmias.

Oxytocin has some minor antidiuretic activity. When administered in large doses or over prolonged periods with electrolyte-free solutions, water intoxication may occur.

Overdosage of oxytocin may cause hyperstimulation of the uterus, resulting in severe contractions with possible abruptio placentae, cervical lacerations, impaired uterine blood flow, and fetal trauma.

Availability

IV—10 units/ml in 1 and 10 ml vials and 1 ml disposable syringes.
Nasal Spray—40 units/ml in 2 and 5 ml squeeze bottles.

Dosage and Administration

Induction of Labor
IV—Initial rate: 1 to 2 mU/minute. It is strongly recommended that an infusion pump be used to help control the rate of oxytocin infusion. Most pregnancies close to term will respond well to 2 to 10 mU/minute. Rarely will a patient require more than 20 mU/minute. Those patients at 32 to 36 weeks of gestation often require 20 to 30 mU/min or more to develop a laborlike contraction pattern. Rates of infusion should not be altered more frequently than every 20 to 30 minutes. It is frequently necessary to reduce or discontinue the infusion as spontaneous uterine activity develops and labor progresses.
Augmentation of Labor
IV—Occasionally a labor that started spontaneously may not progress satisfactorily. Labor may be augmented by oxytocin infusions at rates of 0.5 to 2 mU/minute.

Postpartum Hemorrhage

IM—10 units given after delivery of the placenta.
IV—10 to 40 units may be added to 100 ml of fluid and electrolyte solution and run at a rate necessary to control uterine atony.

Milk Letdown

Intranasal spray—1 spray or 3 drops may be instilled into 1 or both nostrils 2 to 3 minutes before nursing or pumping of the breasts.

PATIENT CONCERNS: NURSING INTERVENTION/RATIONALE

Side Effects to Expect

Uterine Contractions

Oxytocin infusions should be monitored by both a tocometer (measures uterine contractions) and a fetal heart monitor.

Maintain an ongoing record of the frequency, duration, and intensity of uterine contractions. Duration of contractions over 90 seconds requires the flow rate of the oxytocin to be slowed or discontinued.

Nausea, Vomiting

Although infrequent, these side effects may occur. Reduction in dosage may control symptoms.

Side Effects to Report

Fetal Distress

Fetal heart rate should be monitored continuously, but especially closely during uterine contractions. (Normal fetal heart rate = 120 to 160 beats per minute.) Indications of fetal distress may be manifested by tachycardia (>160 bpm) followed by bradycardia (<120 bpm). As the degree of distress progresses, bradycardia occurs more frequently and lasts longer than 15 seconds after contractions.

If the infant develops sudden distress, reduce the oxytocin infusion to the slowest possible rate according to hospital policy, turn the mother to the left lateral position, administer oxygen by nasal cannula or face mask, and call the physician immediately.

Hypertension, Hypotension

Check the mother's blood pressure and pulse rate at least every 30 minutes while infusing oxytocin. Report trends upward or downward, since oxytocin may cause hyper- or hypotension.

Water Intoxication

Oxytocin can alter fluid balance by stimulating antidiuretic hormone, causing the body to accumulate water. This is particularly more likely to occur if oxytocin is administered with electrolyte solutions.

Symptoms of water intoxication include drowsiness, listlessness, headache, confusion, anuria, edema, and, in extreme cases, seizures.

Dehydration

Since mothers are routinely placed NPO during labor, an occasional patient may develop dehydration even though an IV is running. Monitor urine output, dry crusted lips, and requests for water. Report to the physician and request ice chips and additional IV fluids if appropriate.

Postpartum Hemorrhage

Hemorrhage may be caused by uterine atony, retained fragments of placenta, or lacerations of the vaginal tract. Less frequent causes include defective blood clotting mechanisms, uterine eversion, and uterine infections.

Oxytocin is routinely administered after delivery of the placenta to cause the uterus to contract and to decrease blood loss.

Always check the height of the fundus of the uterus (usually at umbilical level) every 5 minutes following delivery; massage if necessary to maintain firmness. Report if not firm or the height is rising. (This may be an indication of urinary retention or a uterus filling with blood.)

Check the vaginal flow rate on each perineal pad at least every ½ hour.

Check and record the mother's vital signs as ordered by the physician, or every 15 minutes until stable; every 30 minutes for 2 hours; then every hour until definitely stable. Report unstable vital signs immediately.

Administration

Starting the Infusion

Oxytocin administered IV should be added to the solution after the IV is shown to be patent and running.

Rate

Careful monitoring of the prescribed rate of infusion is imperative. Should the IV line suddenly open, the resulting severe contractions could be extremely dangerous to the mother.

Infusion Pump

A constant infusion pump is recommended for control of the rate of administration. Keep in mind that a pump can still fail; continue to monitor the number of drops per minute from the drip chamber.

Drug Interactions

Anesthetics

Monitor the blood pressure and heart rate and rhythm closely. Report significant changes in the blood pressure or pulse.

For those patients receiving a local anesthetic containing epinephrine, report any complaints of sweating, fever, chest pain, palpitations, or severe "throbbing" headache immediately.

Uterine Relaxants

Hydroxyprogesterone (hi-drox′ee-pro-jest′er-own) *(Delalutin)* (del-ah′ lew-tin)

Hydroxyprogesterone inhibits the secretion of the pituitary hormones—luteinizing hormone (LH) and follicle-stimulating hormone (FSH)—and inhibits uterine contractions in the pregnant uterus. It is used in obstetrics to prevent habitual miscarriage. It is not effective once premature labor has started, but it may possibly be effective if administered periodically after the twentieth week of pregnancy.

Side Effects

There are essentially no side effects associated with hydroxyprogesterone therapy. The most common side effect is pain at the injection site. Rarely, hydroxyprogesterone may induce fluid retention. There is a slightly increased incidence of blood clot formation and thrombophlebitis.

Availability

Injection—125 mg/ml in 10 ml vials; 250 mg/ml in 5 ml vials.

Dosage and Administration

Note: Do not administer during the first 4 months of pregnancy. Teratogenicity may result.

Adult

IM—250 mg once weekly injected deeply into the upper outer quadrant of the gluteal muscle.

PATIENT CONCERNS: NURSING INTERVENTION/RATIONALE

Side Effects to Report

Fluid Retention

Weigh patients on a regular basis and monitor for an increase in blood pressure or edema.

Thrombophlebitis

Patients should be encouraged to report any symptoms of pain in the calves or chest, sudden shortness of breath, coughing of blood, severe headache, dizziness, faintness, or changes in vision as soon as possible.

Administration

IM

Administer by deep injection into the upper, outer quadrant of the gluteal muscle.

Drug Interactions

No clinically significant interactions have been reported.

Ritodrine hydrochloride (rih′toh-dreen) *(Yutopar)* (u′toh-par)

Terbutaline sulfate (ter-bew′tal-een) *(Bricanyl)* (brih-can′il)

Ritodrine and terbutaline are beta adrenergic receptor stimulants, acting predominantly on the beta-2 receptors, but, especially in higher dosages, the beta-1 receptors as well. Stimulation of the beta-2 receptors produces relaxation of the uterine, bronchial, and vascular smooth muscle. Beta-1 receptor stimulation causes an increased heart rate.

Because of selective relaxant properties on the uterus, causing a reduction in the intensity and frequency of uterine contractions, these agents are used in cases of premature labor where it has been determined that there is no underlying pathology that would indicate that pregnancy should be allowed to progress to termination.

Side Effects

Unfortunately, the receptors that are stimulated by beta receptor agents to cause relaxation of the smooth muscle of the uterus are found in other tissues as well as the reproductive system. They are found in the muscles of the heart, blood vessels, bronchopulmonary tree, gastrointestinal, urinary, and central nervous systems. They also help regulate fat and carbohydrate metabolism. For this reason, we can expect to see many side effects from these agents, particularly if used too frequently or in higher doses than recommended.

The most common side effects are dose related. These include maternal and fetal tachycardia, averaging 130 and 164 beats per minute, respectively; tremor, nervousness, heart palpitations, and dizziness. Maternal systolic blood pressure increases to a range of 96 to 162 mm Hg, while diastolic pressures drop to a range of 0 to 76 mg Hg. Other side effects that may occur less frequently include nausea, vomiting, headache, restlessness, drowsiness, sweating, and tinnitus.

Ritodrine and terbutaline routinely increase serum glucose and insulin levels, though these tend to return to normal within 48 to 72 hours with continued infusion. Diabetic patients should be monitored closely.

Serum potassium levels may drop during IV administration. Urinary losses generally do not increase; much of the losses are actually due to intracellular redistribution, which will return to the blood after discontinuation of therapy.

Patients known to have hypertension, hyperthyroidism, diabetes mellitus, or cardiac disease with arrhythmias may be particularly sensitive to adverse reactions and must be observed closely.

Neonatal adverse effects are infrequent, but hyperglycemia, hypoglycemia, hypocalcemia, hypotension, and paralytic ileus have been reported.

Availability

Ritodrine
PO—10 mg tablets.
Injection—10 mg/ml in 5 ml ampules.

Terbutaline
PO—2.5 and 5 mg tablets.
Injection—1 mg/ml in 1 ml ampules.

Dosage and Administration

See Tables 19.3 to 19.6.

PATIENT CONCERNS: INTERVENTION/RATIONALE

Side Effects to Report

Tachycardia, Palpitations

Since most symptoms are dose-related, alterations should be reported to the physician. Monitor the mother's and infant's heart rates and rhythms at regular intervals throughout therapy. Report heart rates significantly higher than baseline values.

Always report palpitations and suspected arrhythmias.

Table 19.3
Guidelines for Use of Ritodrine ind Premature Labor

1. Initiate a control IV of dextrose 5%, Ringer's lactate, or saline solution and administer 400 to 500 ml in 15 to 20 minutes before the initiation of the medication. Then decrease to 100 to 125 ml/hr.
2. Make a ritodrine infusion solution using Table 19-4. The usual concentration is 3 ampules in 500 ml of parenteral solution, but weaker or stronger concentrations may be used depending on the patient's fluid requirements.
3. Have the patient recline in the left lateral position.
4. The usual initial dosage is 50 to 100 μg/minute. Increase by 50 μg/minute every 10 minutes until labor is inhibited or side effects prevent further increases in dosage. The effective dose is usually 150 to 350 μg/minute. Frequent monitoring of maternal uterine contractions, heart rate, and blood pressure and fetal heart rate is mandatory, with dosage individually titrated according to response.
5. Fluid input and output, breath sounds, and blood glucose and serum electrolyte levels must be monitored periodically to prevent fluid overload, hyperglycemia, or hypokalemia.
6. The IV infusion is maintained for 8 to 12 hours after cessation of uterine contractions.
7. Start oral ritodrine tablets 30 to 60 minutes before discontinuation of IV therapy. The initial doses are 10 mg every 2 hours for the first 24 hours, then 10 to 20 mg every 4 to 6 hours, depending on uterine activity and side effects.
8. Recurrence of premature labor may be treated starting the guidelines over again. Labor may be arrested on lower IV dosages, depending on the patient's compliance with the oral medication regimen.

Table 19.4
*Ritodrine Solution Concentrations and Rates**

5 ml amps/500 ml†		1	2	3	4	5
mg/500 ml		50	100	150	200	250
μg/ml		100	200	300	400	500
μgtts/min	ml/min	μg/min	μg/min	μg/min	μg/min	μg/min
5	0.08	8	16	24	32	40
10	0.16	16	32	48	64	80
15	0.25	25	50	75	100	125
20	0.33	33	66	99	132	165
25	0.41	41	82	123	164	205
30	0.5	50	100	150	200	250
35	0.58	58	116	174	232	290
40	0.66	66	132	198	264	330
45	0.75	75	150	225	300	375
50	0.83	83	166	249	332	415
55	0.91	91	182	273	364	455
60	1.00	100	200	300	400	500

* Using a microdrip administration set—60 gtts/ml.

† Dilute in 500 ml of 0.9% sodium chloride, dextrose 5%, 10% dextran 40 in 0.9% sodium chloride, 10% fructose, Ringer's solution, or Hartmann's solution.

Usual initial dose is 50 to 100 μg/min. Increase by 50 μm/min every 10 min until desired result is attained. The effective dose usually lies between 150 and 350 μg/min. Frequent monitoring of maternal uterine contractions, heart rate, and blood pressure and of fetal heart rate is mandatory, with dosage individually titrated according to response.

(From Clayton, B. D., *Pharmacology in Nursing*, 3rd ed. St. Louis, C. V. Mosby Co., 1984.)

Tremors

Tell the patient to notify the physician if tremors develop after starting any of these medications. A dosage adjustment may be necessary.

Nervousness, Anxiety, Restlessness, Headache

Perform a baseline assessment of the patient's mental status (degree of anxiety, nervousness, alertness); compare at regular intervals to the findings obtained. Report escalation of tension.

Nausea, Vomiting

Monitor all aspects of the development of these symptoms.

Administer the oral medication with food and a full glass of water or milk. Report if the symptoms are not relieved.

Dizziness

Provide for patient safety during episodes of dizziness; report for further evaluation.

Baseline Studies

Obtain baseline laboratory data (serum glucose, chloride, sodium, hematocrit and carbon dioxide) BEFORE initiation of therapy. Monitoring should continue for alterations in baseline data. Report any changes immediately for physician evaluation.

HYPERGLYCEMIA

Diabetic or prediabetic patients need to be monitored for the development of hyperglycemia, particularly during the early days of therapy.

Assess regularly for glycosuria and report if it occurs with frequency.

Insulin requirements may double in these patients during ritodrine or terbutaline therapy.

ELECTROLYTE IMBALANCE

The electrolyte most commonly altered is potassium (K^+). *Hypokalemia* is most likely to occur.

Many symptoms associated with altered fluid and electrolyte balance are subtle.

Gather data relative to *changes* in the patient's mental status (i.e., alertness, orientation, confusion), muscle

Table 19.5

*Guidelines for Use of Terbutaline with Premature Labor**

1. Initiate a control IV of dextrose 5%, Ringer's lactate, or saline solution and administer 400 to 500 ml in 15 to 20 minutes before initiation of the medication. Then decrease to 100 to 125 ml/hr.
2. Add 20 mg of terbutaline to 1000 ml of dextrose 5%.
3. Place the patient in a left lateral, horizontal position with a blood pressure cuff in position.
4. Administer a loading dose of 250 μg IV over 1 to 2 minutes. Monitor very closely for hypotension.
5. Start the infusion at a rate of 10 μg IV (30 ml/hr) using Table 19.6.
6. Increase the infusion rate by 3.5 μg/minute (10 ml/hr) every 10 minutes until labor has stopped or a maximum dose of 26 μg/minute (80 ml/hr) has been attained.
7. Maintain the effective dose for 1 hr or more, then begin decreasing the rate by 2 μg/min (6 ml/hr) every 30 minutes until the lowest effective dose is reached. Maintain the total IV fluid intake at 125 ml/hr.
8. When the lowest effective IV dose is reached, begin PO terbutaline, 2.5 mg every 4 hours.
9. If labor has stopped, discontinue the IV infusion 24 hr after PO administration was initiated if the uterus is not irritable.
10. Continue the PO regimen (2.5 mg every 4 hr or 5 mg every 8 hr) until 36 weeks gestation.
11. If labor begins again, restart the IV infusion as above.

* NOTE: Terbutaline is not approved by the FDA for use in premature labor. It may be used, however, in emergency situations when the physician judges that it is in the best interests of the patient and infant.

When terbutaline is used for premature labor, a sometimes significant drop in blood pressure (due to vasodilatory effects) can be observed at the time of the loading dose and when the infusion is started. Blood pressure and pulse monitoring should be done before and every 5 minutes after the loading dose has been administered and the infusion started, until the patient is stable. Use continuous fetal monitoring. If the maternal pulse exceeds 120 beats/minute and does not decrease with an increase in fluids or when the patient is rolled on her left side, or if there is any evidence of a decrease in uterine perfusion, discontinue the infusion.

strength, muscle cramps, tremors, nausea, and general appearance (drowsy, anxious, lethargic).

Always check the electrolyte reports for early indications of electrolyte imbalance.

Keep accurate records of I/O, daily weights, and vital signs.

The Neonate

Neonatal adverse effects are infrequent, but hyperglycemia, followed by hypoglycemia, and hypocalcemia, hypotension, and paralytic ileus have been reported. Monitor these newborns closely over the next several hours. Make sure that the infant's sleep after birth is not masking these conditions.

Administration

IV Rate

Use of an infusion pump is absolutely essential to the safe delivery of these agents.

PO

Administer with food or milk to reduce gastric irritation.

Drug Interactions

Drugs That Enhance Toxic Effects

Tricyclic antidepressants (imipramine, amitriptyline, nortriptyline, doxepine, others), monoamine oxidase inhibitors (tranylcypromine, isocarboxazid, parglyine) and other sympathomimetic agents (metaproterenol, isoproterenol, others).

Monitor for increases in severity of drug effects such as nervousness, tachycardia, tremors, and arrhythmias.

Drugs That Reduce Therapeutic Effects

Beta adrenergic blocking agents (propranolol, timolol, nadolol, pindolol, others).

Corticosteroids

Concurrent use may rarely result in pulmonary edema. There is a higher incidence in patients with multiple pregnancy, occult cardiac disease, and fluid overload. Persistent tachycardia may be a sign of impending pulmonary edema. Observe patient closely, monitoring fluid input and output, breath sounds, and heart rate, as well as the patient's anxiety level and state of well-being.

Antihypertensive Agents

Sympathomimetic agents may reduce the therapeutic effects of antihypertensive agents. Monitor blood pressure for an indication of loss of antihypertensive control.

Table 19.6

*Terbutaline Infusion Rate**

ml/hr	15	20	30	40	50	60	70	80	90
μg/min	5	6.6	10	13	16	20	23	26	30

* Administer 20 mg/1000 ml or 20 μg/ml.
(From Clayton, B. D., *Pharmacolog̈ty in Nursing*, 3rd ed. St. Louis, C. V. Mosby Co., 1984.)

Anesthetics

Concurrent use with general anesthetics may result in additional hypotensive effects. Monitor the blood pressure and heart rate and rhythm regularly.

Lactation Suppressants

Chlorotrianisene (klo-ro-try-an′e-seen)
(Tace) (tase)

Chlorotrianisene is a long-acting, synthetic estrogen used in obstetrics to inhibit lactation and reduce the frequency of postpartum breast engorgement in patients who do not wish to breastfeed. It acts by inhibiting the action of prolactin, a pituitary hormone that is necessary for milk production.

Side Effects

Side effects associated with short-term estrogen therapy are usually quite minimal. The most common side effect is nausea. There is a slightly increased incidence of blood clot formation and thrombophlebitis. Patients should be encouraged to report any symptoms of pain in the calves or chest, sudden shortness of breath, coughing of blood, severe headache, dizziness, faintness, or changes in vision as soon as possible.

Availability

PO—12, 25, and 72 mg capsules.

Dosage and Administration

Adult
PO—Postpartum breast engorgement: 12 mg 4 times daily for 7 days, 50 mg every 6 hours for 6 doses, or 72 mg every 12 hours for 2 days. The first dose must be given within 8 hours after delivery.

PATIENT CONCERNS: NURSING INTERVENTION/RATIONALE

Side Effects to Expect

Nausea

Although infrequent, a few patients do experience nausea.

Side Effects to Report

Thrombophlebitis

Although this is a rare occurrence, patients should report any pain in the calves or chest, sudden shortness of breath, coughing of blood, severe headache, dizziness, faintness, or changes in vision as soon as possible.

Drug Interactions

Reduced Therapeutic Response

The following agents may counteract the prolactin-inhibiting effects of chlorotrianisene: carbidopa, ethanol, haloperidol, methyldopa, metoclopramide, phenothiazines, reserpine, and thiothixene.

Testosterone enanthate (tes-tos′ter-own en-an′thate) and estradiol valerate (es-tra-dy′ol val′er-ate) (Deladumone OB) (deh-la-due-mone′ oh-bee)

Deladumone OB is a long-acting combination estrogen-androgen product used in obstetrics to inhibit lactation and postpartum breast engorgement in patients who do not wish to breastfeed. Both estrogens and androgens may inhibit the secretion of prolactin, a pituitary hormone that stimulates milk production.

Side Effects

There are essentially no side effects associated with a single injection of Deladumone OB other than pain at the site of injection. There is a slightly higher incidence of blood clot formation and thrombophlebitis.

Availability

IM—2 ml prefilled syringe containing 360 mg testosterone enanthate and 16 mg of estradiol valerate.

Dosage and Administration

Adult
IM—2 ml of Deladumone OB is administered just before the second stage of labor (complete cervical dilation and effacement) by deep injection into the upper, outer quandrant of the gluteal muscle.

PATIENT CONCERNS: NURSING INTERVENTION/RATIONALE

Side Effects to Report

Thrombophlebitis

Patients should be encouraged to report any symptoms of pain in the calves or chest, sudden shortness of breath, coughing of blood, severe headache, dizziness, faintness, or changes in vision as soon as possible.

Administration

IM

Administer by deep injection into the upper, outer quadrant of the gluteal muscle.

Drug Interactions

Decreased Therapeutic Response

Carbidopa, ethanol, haloperidol, methyldopa, metoclopramide, phenothiazines, reserpine, and thiothixene. These drugs stimulate elevated prolactin levels, increasing milk production.

Oral Contraceptives

The oral (hormonal) contraceptives (birth control pills, BCPs) were first available in 1960. They now represent one of the most common forms of artificial birth control in use in the United States. It is estimated that approximately one-third of all women between 18 and 44 years of age use oral contraceptives.

There are two types of oral contraceptives in general use: (1) the combination pill, which is taken for 21 days of the menstrual cycle and contains both an estrogen and a progestin (see Fig. 19.1) and (2) the "mini-pill," which is taken every day and contains only a progestin (see Fig. 19.2 and Table 19.7).

Estrogens and progestins, to some extent, induce contraception by inhibiting ovulation. The estrogens block pituitary release of follicle-stimulating hormone (FSH), preventing the ovary from developing a follicle from which the ovum is released. Progestins inhibit pituitary release of luteinizing hormone (LH), the hormone responsible for release of the ovum from the follicle. Other mechanisms play a contributory role in preventing conception. Estrogens and progestins alter (1) cervical mucus by making it thick and viscous,

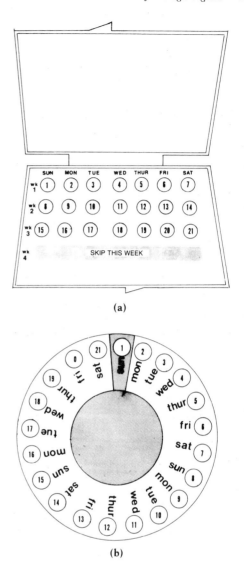

Fig. 19.1 *21-day packages (a and b). With either style package, take oral contraceptive pills for 21 days, wait one week, and start a new package on the next Sunday.*

inhibiting sperm migration, (2) mobility of uterine and oviduct muscle, reducing transport of both sperm and ovum, and (3) the endometrium, impairing implantation of the fertilized ovum.

The mini-pills or progestin-only pills represent a relatively new direction in oral contraceptive therapy. Many of the adverse effects of combination-type contraceptives are due to the estrogen component of the tablet. For those women particularly susceptible to adverse effects of estrogen therapy, the mini-pill provides an alternative. Women who might prefer the mini-pill are those with a history of migraine headaches, hypertension, mental depression, weight gain and breast tenderness, and those who want to breastfeed postpartum. The mini-pill is not without its disadvantages,

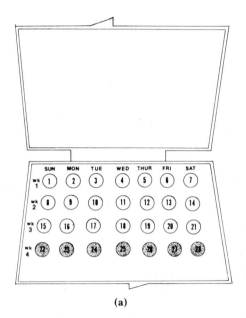

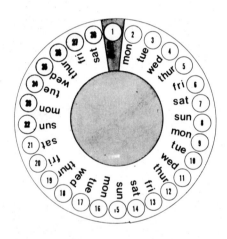

Fig. 19.2 *28-day packages (a and b). Take one pill daily; start a new package on the day after finishing the last package.*

however. Between 30 and 40% of women on the mini-pill continue to ovulate. Birth control is maintained by progestin activity on cervical mucus, uterine and fallopian transport, and implantation. There is a slightly higher incidence of both uterine and tubal pregancy. Dysmenorrhea, manifested by irregular periods, infrequent periods, and spotting between periods, is common among women taking the mini-pill.

Side Effects

Twenty-five years of clinical experience with literally millions of women have shown that birth control pills are not as "safe" as indicated by earlier studies. However use of oral contraceptives must be considered in light of the potential risks and complications stemming from pregnancy. There are minor adverse effects, major adverse effects, and contraindications to use of oral contraceptive therapy.

About 40% of women using oral contraceptives will suffer some side effects. Hormones such as estrogens and progestins have many other actions that affect nearly every organ system within the body. The most common side effects are related to the dose of estrogen and progestin in each product. Nausea, headaches, weight gain, spotting, depression, fatigue, chloasma, yeast infection, vaginal itching or discharge, and changes in libido are common side effects.

Disease states that may be aggravated by continued use of oral contraceptives are hypertension, gallbladder disease, diabetes mellitus, severe varicose veins, seizure disorders, oligomenorrhea or amenorrhea, and rheumatic heart disease.

The list of absolute contraindications to the use of oral contraceptives is somewhat variable depending on the clinician and the particular case history of each woman. However, women with any of the following conditons should strongly consider other forms of contraception: a history of thromboembolic disease, stroke, malignancy of breast or the reproductive system, renal or liver disease, severe mental depression, suspected pregnancy, and repeated contraceptive failure.

Availability

See Table 19.7.

Dosage and Administration

The estrogenic component of the combination-type pills is responsible for most of the adverse effects associated with therapy. The FDA has recommended that therapy be initiated with a product containing a low dose of estrogen. Side effects must be reviewed in relation to individual case histories, but many physicians initiate therapy with Norinyl 1 + 50 or Ortho Novum 1/50. Therapy, and therefore products, may be adjusted based on the incidence of side effects.

Patient Instructions

See Patient Concerns: Nursing Intervention/Rationale

Table 19.7
Oral Contraceptives

| | PROGESTIN | | | | | | ESTROGEN | | |
BRAND NAME	NORETHINDRONE (mg)	NORETHINDRONE ACETATE (mg)	NORGESTREL (mg)	ETHYNODIOL DIACETATE (mg)	NORETHYNODREL (mg)	LEVONORGESTREL (µg)	ETHINYL ESTRADIOL (µg)	MESTRANOL (µg)	OTHER
COMBINATION-TYPE*									
Brevicon (21,28)†	0.50						35.00		
Demulen (21,28)				1.00			50.00		
Enovid 5 mg (20)					5.00			75.00	
Enovid E (20,21)					2.50			100.00	
Loestrin 1/20 (21,28)		1.00					20.00		
Loestrin 1.5/ 3.0 (28)		1.50					30.00		
Logynon (See Trinordiol)‡									
Lo/Oural (21)			0.30				30.00		
Modicon (21,28)	0.50						35.00		
Norinyl 1 + 35 (21,28)	1.00						35.00		
Norinyl 1 + 50 (21,28)	1.00							50.00	
Norinyl 1 + 80 (21,28)	1.00							80.00	
Norinyl 2 mg (21)	2.00							100.00	
Norlestrin 1/ 50 (21,28)		1.00					50.00		Ferrous fumarate 75mg
Norlestrin Fe 1/50 (28)		1.00					50.00		
Norlestrin 2.5/ 50 (21)		2.50					50.00		
Norlestrin Fe 2.5/50 (28)		2.50					50.00		Ferrous fumarate 75 mg
Ortho-Novum 1/35 (21,28)	1.00						35.00	50.00	
Ortho-Novum 1/50	1.00							80.00	
Ortho-Novum 1/80 (21,28)	1.00							100.00	
Ortho-Novum 2 (21)	2.00						35.00		
Ortho-Novum 10/11 (21,28)	10 tabs–0.5						35.00		
	11 tabs–1.0						35.00		
Ortho-Novum 7/7/7 (21)‡	7 tabs–0.5						35.00		
	7 tabs–0.75						35.00		
	7 tabs–1.0							35.00	

(*Table continues on p. 502.*)

Table 19.7 (continued)

| BRAND NAME | PROGESTIN | | | | | | ESTROGEN | | |
	NORETHINDRONE (mg)	NORETHINDRONE ACETATE (mg)	NORGESTREL (mg)	ETHYNODIOL DIACETATE (mg)	NORETHYNODREL (mg)	LEVONORGESTREL (µg)	ETHINYL ESTRADIOL (µg)	MESTRANOL (µg)	OTHER
Ovcon-35 (28)	0.40							50.00	
Ovcon-50 (28)	1.00						50.00		
Ovral (21,28)			0.50					100.00	
Ovulen (20,21,28)				1.00			35.00		
Tri-Norinyl (21)‡	7 tabs–0.5						35.00		
	7 tabs–1.0						35.00		
	7 tabs–0.5					7 tabs–50	30.00		
Trinordiol (21)‡						7 tabs–75	40.00		
						7 tabs–125	30.00		
PROGESTIN ONLY‡									
Micronor (35)	0.35								
Nor-OD (42)	0.35								
Ovrette (28)			0.075						

* Products contain 20 or 21 hormone tablets/package.

† 21 hormone tablets/package plus 7 inert tablets.

‡ Products contain 20 or 21 hormone tablets/package.

§ Products contain all active hormone tablets.

PATIENT CONCERNS: NURSING INTERVENTION/RATIONALE

Side Effects to Expect

Nausea, Weight Gain, Spotting, Changed Menstrual Flow, Missed Periods, Depression, Mood Changes, Chloasma, Headaches

These are the most common side effects of hormonal contraceptive therapy. If these symptoms are not resolved after 3 months of therapy, the woman should return to the physician for reevaluation and a possible change in prescription.

Side Effects to Report

Vaginal Discharge, Breakthrough Bleeding, Yeast Infection

These symptoms represent the development of secondary disorders. Examination, a change in oral contraceptive, and possible treatment with other medications may be necessary.

Blurred Vision, Severe Headaches, Dizziness, Leg Pain, Chest Pain, Shortness of Breath, Acute Abdominal Pain

Report as soon as possible. These side effects are usually of minor consequence, but they may be early indications of very serious adverse effects.

Administration

Before Initiating Therapy

The patient should have a complete physical examination that includes blood pressure, pelvic and breast examination, Papanicolaou (Pap) smear, urinalysis, and hemoglobin or hematocrit.

Instructions for Using Combination Oral Contraceptives

When to start the pill: Start the first pill on the first Sunday after your period begins. Take one pill daily, at the same time daily, until the pack is gone. If using a 21-day pack, wait 1 week and restart on the next

Sunday. If using a 28-day pack, start a new pack the day after finishing the last pack. Use another form of birth control (condoms, foam) during this first month. You may not be fully protected by the pill during the first month.

MISSED PILLS

If you miss 1 pill, take it as soon as you remember it; take the next pill at the regularly scheduled time. If you miss 2 pills, take 2 pills as soon as you remember and 2 the next day. Spotting may occur when 2 pills are missed. Use another form of birth control (condoms, foam) until you finish this pack of pills. If you miss *3 or more*, start using another form of birth control immediately. Start a new pack of pills on the next Sunday even if you are menstruating. Discard your old packs of pills. Use other forms of birth control through the next month after missing 3 or more pills.

MISSED PILLS AND SKIPPED PERIODS

Return to your physician for a pregnancy test.

SKIPPING ONE PERIOD BUT NOT MISSING A PILL

It is not uncommon for a woman to occasionally miss a period when on the pill. Start the next pack on the appropriate Sunday.

SPOTTING FOR TWO OR MORE CYCLES

See your physician.

PERIODIC EXAMINATIONS

A yearly examination should include tests for blood pressure, pelvic examination, urinalysis, breast examination, and Papanicolaou smear.

DISCONTINUING THE PILL FOR CONCEPTION

Because of a possibility of birth defects, discontinue the pill 3 months before attempting pregnancy. Use other methods of contraception for these 3 months.

DURATION OF ORAL CONTRACEPTIVE THERAPY

Many physicians prefer to have their patients discontinue the pill for 3 out of every 28 months. This allows the body to return to a normal cycle. Be sure to use other forms of contraception during this time. Long-term use (3 or more years) must be determined on an individual basis.

SIDE EFFECTS TO BE REPORTED AS SOON AS POSSIBLE

Severe headaches, dizziness, blurred vision, leg pain, shortness of breath, chest pain, and acute abdominal pain. Although these side effects are usually of minor consequence, absence of serious adverse effects must be confirmed.

NOTE

When being seen by a physician or a dentist for other reasons, be sure to mention that you are currently taking oral contraceptives.

Instructions for Using the Mini-Pill

Starting the mini-pill: start on the first day of menstruation. Take 1 tablet daily, every day, regardless of when your next period is. Tablets should be taken at about the same time every day.

MISSED PILLS

If you miss 1 pill, take it as soon as you remember, and take your next pill at the regularly scheduled time. Use another form of birth control until your next period.

If you miss 2 pills, take 1 of the missed pills immediately and take your regularly scheduled pill that day on time. The next day, take the regularly scheduled pill as well as the other missed pill. Use another method of birth control until your next period.

MISSED PERIODS

Some women note changes in the time as well as duration of their periods while using mini-pills. These changes are to be expected. If menses occurs every 28 to 30 days, ovulation may still be occurring. For maximal safety, use alternate forms of contraception on days 10 through 18. If irregular bleeding occurs every 25 to 45 days, ovulation is probably not occurring on a regular basis. You may feel more comfortable if you use other forms of contraception with the mini-pill or discuss switching to an estrogen-containing (combination) contraceptive.

If you have taken all tablets correctly, but do not have a period for over 60 days, speak to your physician concerning a pregnancy test.

NOTE

Report sudden, severe abdominal pain, with or without nausea and vomiting, to your physician immediately. There is a higher incidence of ectopic pregnancy with the mini-pill, since it does not inhibit ovulation in all women.

SIDE EFFECTS TO BE REPORTED AS SOON AS POSSIBLE

Severe headaches, dizziness, blurred vision, leg pain, shortness of breath, chest pain, and acute abdominal pain. Although these side effects are usually of minor consequence, absence of serious adverse effects must be confirmed.

DURATION OF ORAL CONTRACEPTIVE THERAPY

Many physicians prefer to have their patients discontinue the pill for 3 out of every 18 months. This allows the body to return to a normal cycle. Be sure to use other forms of contraception during this time. Long-term use (3 or more years) must be determined on an individual basis.

DISCONTINUING THE PILL FOR CONCEPTION

Because of a possibility of birth defects, discontinue the pill 3 months before attempting pregnancy. Use other methods of contraception for these 3 months.

Drug Interactions

Warfarin

This medication may diminish the anticoagulant effects of warfarin. Monitor the prothrombin time and increase the dosage of warfarin if necessary.

Phenytoin

Monitor patients with concurrent therapy for signs of phenytoin toxicity: nystagmus, sedation, lethargy. Serum levels may be ordered, and a reduced dosage of phenytoin may be required.

Thyroid Hormones

Patients who have no thyroid function and who start on estrogen therapy may require an increase in thyroid hormone because the estrogens reduce the level of circulating thyroid hormones. The thyroid dosage is not adjusted until the patient shows clinical signs of hypothyroidism.

Phenobarbital

Phenobarbital may enhance the metabolism of estrogens to the extent that there is inadequate contraceptive protection. Changing to an oral contraceptive with a higher estrogen content or using another form of contraception (foam, condoms) is recommended.

Ampicillin, Isoniazid, Rifampin

The use of another form of contraception (foam, condoms) is recommended.

Benzodiazepines

Oral contraceptives appear to have a variable effect on the metabolism of benzodiazepines. Those that have reduced metabolism with an increase in therapeutic response are alprazolam, chlorazepate, chlordiazepoxide, diazepam, flurazepam, halazepam, and prazepam. Benzodiazepines that have enhanced metabolism and reduced therapeutic activity when taken with oral contraceptives are lorazepam, oxazepam, and temazepam. Adjust the dosage of benzodiazepine accordingly.

Phenytoin, Primidone, Carbamazepine

The efficacy of the oral contraceptive may be impaired. Breakthrough bleeding may be an indication of this interaction. Adjustment in dosage of oral contraceptive and the use of alternate methods of contraception (foam, condoms) should be considered.

Other Agents

Clomiphene citrate (klom′ih-feen si′trayt) (Clomid) (klo′mid)

Clomiphene is a chemical compound that is structurally similar to natural estrogens. When administered, it binds to estrogen-receptor sites, reducing the number sites available for circulating estrogens. The receptors send back false signals to the hypothalamus and pituitary gland, indicating a lack of circulating estrogens. The hypothalamus responds by increasing the secretion of hypothalamic releasing factor. This stimulates the pituitary gland to release luteinizing hormone (LH) and follicle stimulating hormone (FSH), which in turn stimulate the ovaries to release ova for potential fertilization. Thus, clomiphene is used to induce ovulation in women who were not ovulating due to reduced circulating estrogen levels. Studies indicate that pregnancy occurs in 25 to 30% of patients treated. Multiple pregnancies may occur in 5 to 10% of patients treated.

Side Effects

Side effects of clomiphene therapy tend to be quite mild and are generally dose related. Common side effects include flushing, resembling menopausal hot flashes, and abdominal symptoms, resembling cyclic ovarian pain (mittelschmerz) and premenstrual symptoms. Nausea, vomiting, diarrhea, light-headedness and dizziness, and constipation have been reported less often.

Visual disturbances such as blurred or double vision, irritation from bright lights (photophobia) and "seeing spots before the eyes" may occur, particularly with higher doses.

Availability

PO—50 mg tablets.

Dosage and Administration

Note: It is mandatory that patients have a complete physical examination to rule out other pathologic causes for lack of ovulation before the initiation of clomiphene therapy.

Patients must be informed of the possibility of multiple pregnancy and the importance of timing sexual intercourse at the time of ovulation, usually 6 to 10 days after the last day of treatment.

Clomiphene should not be administered if pregnancy is suspected. Basal temperatures should be followed for the month following therapy. If the body temperature follows a biphasic distribution (peaks twice within a few days), and is not followed by menses, the next course of clomiphene therapy should not be scheduled until pregnancy tests have been completed.

Adult

PO—50 mg daily for 5 days. Start therapy at any time if there has been no recent bleeding. If spontaneous bleeding occurs before therapy, start on or about the fifth day for 5 days.

If ovulation does not occur after the first course, give a second course of 100 mg/day for 5 days. Start this course no earlier than 30 days after the previous course.

A third course may be administered at 100 mg/day for 5 days, but most patients who respond will have done so in the first 2 courses. Reevaluation of the patient is necessary.

PATIENT CONCERNS: NURSING INTERVENTION/RATIONALE

Side Effects to Expect

Nausea, Vomiting, Diarrhea, Constipation, Abdominal Cramps

These side effects are usually mild and tend to resolve with continued therapy. Encourage the patient not to discontinue therapy without first consulting physician.

Side Effects to Report

Severe Abdominal Cramps

Patients should be informed to report significant abdominal or pelvic pain and bloating that develops during therapy.

Visual Disturbances

Patients developing visual blurring, spots, or double vision should report for an eye examination. The drug is usually discontinued, and visual disturbances pass within a few days to weeks following discontinuation.

Caution the patient to temporarily avoid tasks that require visual acuity such as driving or operating power machinery.

Dizziness

Provide for patient safety during episodes of dizziness; report for further evaluation.

Administration

Possible Pregnancy

Clomiphene should not be administered if pregnancy is suspected. Instruct the patient on how to take and record basal temperatures, and how to report a biphasic temperature distribution.

Timing of Intercourse

The timing of intercourse is important to the success of therapy. Make sure the patient understands the importance of having intercourse during the time of ovulation, usually 6 to 10 days after the last dose of medication.

Drug Interactions

No clinically significant drug interactions have been reported.

Magnesium Sulfate

Magnesium is an ion normally found in the blood in concentrations of 1.8 to 3 mEq/liter. When administered parenterally in doses sufficient to produce levels above 4 mEq/liter, the drug may depress the central nervous system and block peripheral nerve transmission, producing anticonvulsant effects and smooth muscle relaxation. It is used primarily in obstetrics for the control of seizure activity associated with pre-eclampsia or eclampsia. It may also be used to inhibit premature labor in patients who cannot tolerate ritodrine. When used as an anticonvulsant, blood levels should be maintained at 4 to 7.5 mEq/liter.

Side Effects

Patients maintained at a magnesium serum level between 3 and 5 mEq/liter rarely show any side effects from hypermagnesemia. At levels about 5 to 7.5 mEq/liter, patients start showing increasing signs of toxicity that correlate fairly well to serum levels. Early signs of maternal toxicity are complaints of "feeling hot all over" and "being thirsty all the time," flushed skin color, and sweating. Patients may then become hypotensive, have depressed patellar, radial, and biceps reflexes, and have flaccid muscles. Later signs of hypermagnesemia are CNS depression shown first by anxiety, then confusion, lethargy, and drowsiness. If serum levels continue to increase, cardiac depression and respiratory paralysis may result. Magnesium sulfate should be administered with extreme caution to patients with impaired renal function and those patients whose urine output is less than 100 ml over the past 4 hours.

Overdosage may be treated with artificial respirations and the administration of calcium gluconate.

Availability

Injection—10, 12.5, and 50% solutions.

Dosage and Administration

Anticonvulsant
IM—Loading dose: 10 g of 50% solution (20 ml) is divided into two doses of 5 g each (10 ml) and is injected by deep intramuscular injection into each buttock. (1% lidocaine or procaine may be added to each syringe to reduce the pain on injection.) The IM loading dose is usually administered at the same time as 4 g are administered intravenously (see below). Maintenance dose: 4 to 5 g of 50% solution (10 ml) IM every 4 hours in alternate buttocks.
IV—Loading dose: 4 g of magnesium sulfate is added to 250 ml of 5% dextrose in water and infused slowly at a rate of 10 ml/minute. (The IV loading dose is usually administered at the same time as a 10 g IM loading dose.) Maintenance dose: 1 to 2 g/hr by continuous infusion.

Note: Deep tendon reflexes, intake and output, vital signs, and orientation to the environment must be monitored on a regular, ongoing basis.

PATIENT CONCERNS:
NURSING INTERVENTION/RATIONALE

Side Effects to Report
Deep Tendon Reflexes

The presence or absence of patellar reflex (knee jerk reflex), biceps reflex, or radial reflex are primary monitoring parameters for magnesium sulfate therapy.

The patellar reflex should be monitored hourly if the patient is receiving a continuous IV infusion, or before every dose if being administered intermittently IM or IV. If the reflex is absent, further dosages should be withheld until it returns. If the patellar reflex cannot be used due to epidural anesthesia, the biceps or radial reflex may be used.

Intake and Output

Magnesium toxicity is more likely to occur in patients with reduced renal output. Report urine outputs of less than 30 ml/hr or less than 100 ml over a 4 hour period. Observe the color and measure the specific gravity.

Note any other fluid and electrolyte loss such as vaginal bleeding, diarrhea or vomiting.

Vital Signs

Vital signs (blood pressure and heart rate and rhythm) should be measured every 15 to 30 minutes when a patient is receiving a continuous IV infusion. Take vital signs before and after each administration for those patients receiving intermittent therapy.

The respiratory rate should be at least 16 breaths per minute before the administration of further doses of magnesium sulfate.

Do not administer additional doses if there is a reduced respiratory rate, drop in blood pressure, fetal heart rate or other signs of fetal distress.

Confusion

Perform a baseline assessment of the patient's degree of alertness and orientation to name, place, and time BEFORE initiating therapy. Make regularly scheduled mental status evaluations to assure that the patient is oriented.

Overdose

The antidote for magnesium intoxication (shown by respiratory depression and heart block) is calcium gluconate. A 10% solution of calcium gluconate should be kept at the patient's bedside ready for use. The dosage is 5 to 10 mEq (10 to 20 ml) IV over a 3 minute period.

Administer CPR until the patient responds appropriately.

Administration

IM

Intramuscular injection is very painful. Avoid if possible, or administer in conjunction with a local anesthetic.

IV

It is absolutely essential that an infusion pump be used to help control the infusion of the loading dose and continuous drip.

Drug Interactions

CNS Depressants

CNS depressants, including barbiturates analgesics, general anesthetics, tranquilizers and alcohol will potentiate the CNS depressant effects of magnesium sulfate.

Periodically check the patient's orientation to make sure the patient is not suffering from magnesium toxicity.

Neuromuscular Blockade

Concurrent use of neuromuscular blocking agents and magnesium sulfate will further depress muscular activity. Monitor the patient closely for depressed reflexes and respiration.

Chapter 20

Antineoplastic Drugs

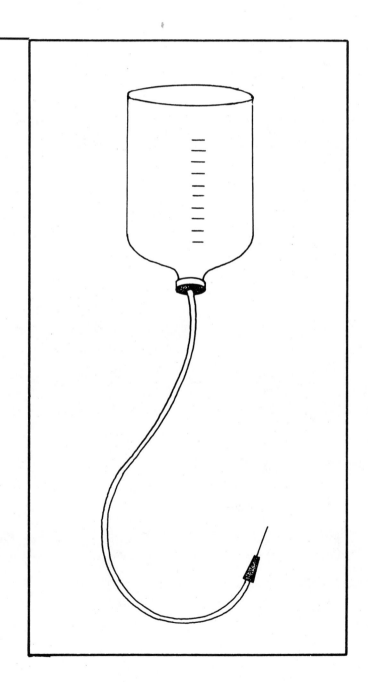

Objectives

After completing this chapter, the student should be able to do the following:

1. Identify baseline data the nurse should collect on a continuous basis for comparison and evaluation of drug effectiveness.
2. Identify important nursing assessments and interventions associated with the drug therapy and treatment of cancer.
3. Identify health teaching essential for a successful treatment regimen.

Cancer

Cancer is a disorder of cellular growth. It is a collection of abnormal cells that grow more rapidly than do normal cells, lose the ability to perform specialized functions, invade surrounding tissues, and develop growths in other tissues (metastases).

Cancer is a leading cause of death in the United States. Unfortunately, the number of persons dying from malignant disease increases each year. Early diagnosis and treatment is still one of the most important factors in providing a more optimistic prognosis for those patients stricken with the many forms of neoplastic disease.

Treatment of cancer often requires a combination of surgery, radiation, and chemotherapy. Recent advances in understanding the causes of cancer, cellular and molecular biology, and tumor immunology have enhanced the role that antineoplastic agents may play in therapy.

General Nursing Considerations for Patients Receiving Antineoplastic Agents

Adaptation to the Diagnosis. No other disease seems to evoke fear and anxiety equal to the impact that the diagnosis of cancer has on the patient and family. When the diagnostic workup is completed and revealed to the patient and family, a period of adjustment is needed. Initially the response is often one of shock and disbelief. Each member of the patient's support group, as well as the patient himself, has to learn to deal with the diagnosis and establish a personal perspective of its meaning. In addition, some patients must also adjust to an altered body image, for example, due to the loss of a breast or the creation of a colostomy, while simultaneously experiencing a sense of loss of control of their life, their future, and their family unit.

As the days pass, the patient starts to focus on the details of the disease and the prognosis. The patient ultimately views the future in light of the extent of disease involvement that has already occurred. Many patients search for the meaning of their illness and intellectualize the process. Other patients sink into self-blame with thoughts such as "Why didn't I do a breast exam every month?" Some individuals may be-come passive and withdrawn, while others make a commitment to control the disease.

The Family Unit. Members of the family unit require careful assessment for the nurse to plan their involvement in the patient's care. Within any family group there are a number of rules, often unspoken, that form the basis of the unit's values. During an illness such as cancer, the roles that specific individuals play in the family may be changed. The person with cancer may be so emotionally overwhelmed or incapacitated by the diagnosis that another member of the family may have to temporarily or permanently assume his role. In some families, the adjustment to different persons in new roles may be quite difficult and require time for transition. During this transition, the patient often develops feelings of guilt and frustration in forcing these changes upon the family.

Various patterns of bonding within a family or support group often occur during an illness. Some of the involved parties may experience closeness while others become "outsiders" waiting for acceptance and a chance to be involved. The nurse must be aware of these relationships and make provisions for the needs of all persons affected. Since relationships are an ever-changing process, the nurse must plan for periodic reevaluation of the family unit and shifts within it during the course of the patient's treatment.

When working with the patient's support group, it is important to remember that not all units function effectively, although they may have been operating for some time. Working within the boundaries that exist, rather than trying to change these relationships, may be essential to maintaining communication with the group. Occasionally the nurse will identify a member of the support group who subconsciously wants the patient to remain a dependent, and who therefore does not encourage compliance with the treatment plan or help the patient function at an optimal level.

Remember that not everyone is capable of becoming actively involved in the patient's care. Some members want to be active participants, while others are not emotionally capable of tolerating it. The inability to participate may produce guilt, which should not be overlooked when planning and intervening in the care.

Incorporation of the family unit should be carefully evaluated so that the degree of participation is individualized to the needs of all parties concerned. Many times the family needs as much, or more, support as the patient.

Trust and Positivism. The health team must foster a trusting relationship with the patient. Develop a genuine concern for the patient; take time to be an active *listener*, not a talker. Work with the patient's needs and concerns, then try tactfully to find out what threats the patient perceives from this illness. Answer questions and concerns; take action on even trivial matters so that the patient believes in you and responds with trust. The trust the patient has in the nurse, the physician, and others managing care can have a very significant influence on the response to therapy. Foster hope for the "control" of the disease, for the prolongation of a functional life, and for the effective management of any difficulties that might be encountered.

Provide Alternatives. Give the patient appropriate choices that allow involvement in the decisions to be made concerning selection of care. Encourage the patient to maintain the best health possible within the boundaries of the illness. Include the patient in selection of diet, planning activities, scheduling rest periods, and personal care. Stress what the patient *can* do, not what he or she cannot do.

Limit the amount of information given to the facts that are significant at this point in the plan of care and to the degree of symptoms present. Emphasize the prevention of complications through maintenance of nutrition and hydration, commitment to hygiene, avoidance of exposure to persons with infection, and safety measures to prevent accidental personal injury.

The Treatment Plan. The treatment plan for the patient is developed by the physician and is based on the specific type of cancer cells (malignancy), the location, and the extent of tissue or organ involvement. The nurse should be knowledgeable of the primary site, any metastases the patient has and the symptoms the individual is experiencing before initiation of therapy.

Carefully assess all current symptoms the patient is exhibiting so that subsequent data may be compared to these findings for analysis of the therapeutic effectiveness of the agents being used or the detection of adverse effects.

PATIENT CONCERNS: NURSING INTERVENTION/RATIONALE

Assessment of the Patient

Type of Cancer

Read the patient's chart to determine the type of cancer, location, and extent of involvement.

Perform an initial assessment of the patient and of the current symptoms based on the site of the cancer and degree of tissue or organ involvement.

Ascertain the extent of the patient's knowledge and understanding of the diagnosis. Check the physician's progress notes as well.

Emotional Status

Patients often exhibit varying degrees of anxiety or depression as a response to this type of diagnosis.

Tactfully obtain information from the individual regarding fears, feelings, and concerns.

THE PATIENT'S VIEWPOINT

Try to gain a perspective of the illness from the patient's viewpoint, and how the patient perceives that the cancer will affect the family and close friends. Assist the individual in expressing feelings. Spend time with the patient. Sometimes not much will be said; be patient and understanding.

COPING MECHANISMS

Ask the patient how he or she normally copes with very stressful situations (i.e., talking it out, yelling, throwing things, ignoring the situation, drinking, etc.).

Who is the patient's confidant? Involve this individual, if possible, in meeting the patient's care needs.

VERBAL AND NONVERBAL MESSAGES

Identify both the verbal and nonverbal messages conveyed. Take note of the patient's general appearance, tone of voice, inflections, and gestures used. Try to pick up on subtle clues and confirm their meaning with the patient.

Evaluate the psychological issues that the patient is perceiving—loss of control, self-esteem, body part; guilt.

NURSING PLANS

Plan for nursing intervention based on the alterations that are significant to the patient's behavior, mood, and physical needs.

Pain

Cancer patients experience varying degrees of pain. Carefully assess the severity, location, duration, and any activities that increase or decrease the pain.

Pain relief is generally achieved by starting with the weakest medication that provides relief. It is gradually increased as needed. Medications are changed to more potent forms as the need is identified.

Nutritional Status

Elicit data from the patient about normal eating patterns, food likes and dislikes, and elimination pattern. This information will serve as a baseline for future comparisons.

WEIGHT

Has there been a weight loss or gain in the past year?

EATING PATTERN

Ask the patient to describe the diet over the past 24 hours. Evaluate the data for types of foods from each of the four food groups, the quantity eaten, and the amount of time spent in eating. Ask if the eating pattern has changed over recent months and to what does the patient attribute any changes identified.

Ask whether certain foods cause bloating, indigestion, or diarrhea, and how much seasoning and spices are put on foods.

FLUID INTAKE

Ask the patient to describe fluid intake: how much water, coffee, teas, soft drinks, fruit juice, and alcoholic beverages.

Personal Hygiene

ORAL HYGIENE AND DENTAL CARE

What is the status of the patient's teeth? When was a dentist last seen? Is any dental work currently in progress?

If the patient wears dentures, do they fit well or have there been recent problems in use? How does the patient care for the dentures?

Do not use glycerin and lemon swabs routinely used in hospitals for oral hygiene. (See Patient Teaching for specific recommendations.)

BOWEL HABITS

Ask the patient to describe a pattern of normal elimination (number of stools per day, color, and consistency).

Administration of Chemotherapy

Goal of Treatment

Controlling the cancer cell growth is the primary goal of treatment.

Patient Dosage

The dosage and frequency of administration is calculated by the physician. Finding the therapeutic dose that is not too toxic to the patient is done by calculation of the patient's body surface area and body weight as well as by monitoring laboratory tests and the patient's symptomatic response.

Accurate Drug Identification

Read the physician's order and check the drug name exactly. These drugs are extremely potent and the wrong drug or dose could be fatal to the patient.

Accurate Identification of Administration Route

Chemotherapeutic drugs must be administered by specific routes for optimal effect. It is important to use the specified route.

Look for the details of administration (i.e., IV drip, bolus, diluted or undiluted, mixed in a specific solution, or added to a preexisting IV) and whether other medications should also be administered at the same time. (Review Chapters 5–7 on administration of medications.)

Mixing the Medication

Chemotherapeutic agents that require reconstitution prior to use should *always* be mixed under a laminar vertical flow hood to protect yourself and those around you. Chemotherapeutic agents are potentially carcinogenic.

Personnel preparing these drugs should do so wearing gloves and safety glasses to prevent exposure to these agents. If accidental spill should occur, wash the area with copious amounts of water.

Preparation of the agent should be done immediately prior to administration. Always follow specific instructions from the manufacturer regarding the amount and type of diluent used and stability prior to administration.

IV Administration

See also Chapter 6, on intravenous administration of medications for details of vein selection and venipuncture, and for complications of IV medication administration.

Before administering antineoplastic agents intravenously, check the venipuncture patency by giving 5 to 10 ml of normal saline through the needle before giving the agent. After administering the agent, again flush with 5 to 10 ml of saline.

Maintain a constant vigil for extravasation. Stop infusing the drug if the patient complains of burning or stinging. Watch for localized swelling and redness at the injection site. Know the hospital protocol for treatment of an infiltration and have equipment and drugs readily available for use.

Oral Administration

Give the drug and dosage exactly as prescribed; usually, all the medication is given at one time, but there may be exceptions.

If vomiting occurs shortly after administration, report to the physician for directions.

Maintain accurate records of the drugs on the medication flow sheet. The flow record should also contain pertinent laboratory data such as WBC, RBC, and platelet counts. With this information, the most appropriate dosing schedule can be established.

When the patient is administering the medications, all aspects of the scheduling, dosage, side effects to expect, and those to report must be carefully taught.

Adverse Effects Associated with Chemotherapy

Unfortunately, most chemotherapeutic agents are not very specific in the types of cells destroyed. Many normal cells in addition to abnormal cells are destroyed, thus causing many side effects.

Nausea, Vomiting

Nausea and vomiting occur with most antineoplastic treatments. Try not to suggest their occurrence to the patient: do not have the emesis basin out. Administer antiemetics or sedatives as ordered. Chart the degree of effectiveness achieved when antiemetics are given. Report poor control to the physician. Changing the antiemetic medication ordered or the route of administration may improve control.

Hydration

Monitor the patient's state of hydration. Check skin turgor, mucous membranes, softness of the eyeballs, etc. Electrolyte reports require vigilant observation; report abnormal findings to the physician. Fluid replacement via intravenous administration or total parenteral nutrition may be appropriate in some circumstances.

Positioning

Hospitalized patients may be sedated. Position the patient on his side to prevent aspiration.

Changes in Bowel Patterns

Depending on the treatment, the patient may develop diarrhea or constipation.

DIARRHEA

Record the color, frequency, and consistency. Include watery stools in the output record. Check for occult blood. Provide for adequate hydration and administer any drugs ordered to relieve the symptoms.

Check the anal area for irritation, provide for hygiene measures and protect from excoriation with products such as A & D Ointment or zinc oxide ointment.

Encourage adequate fluid intake and dietary alterations such as use of boiled milk and low roughage foods to control diarrhea.

Request an order for antidiarrheal drugs such as Kaopectate or Lomotil and administer appropriately.

Total parenteral nutrition may be necessary if symptoms persist.

CONSTIPATION

Compare this symptom with the patient's usual pattern of elimination. Many persons do not normally defecate daily.

Perform daily assessment of bowel sounds when the patient is hospitalized.

When a patient is constipated, the physician usually orders stool softeners or laxatives, fluids, and a diet that enhances normal defecation. Observe carefully for signs of an impaction (i.e., the urge to defecate without results, or oozing of a highly colored, watery solution from the rectum). Always report any abdominal pain or absence of bowel sounds.

Oral Stomatitis

Stomatitis, manifested by erythema, ulcerations, or white patchy membranes, can be very uncomfortable and may interfere with the patient's nutrition.

Teach the patient meticulous oral hygiene with an anesthetic mouthwash, soft-bristled toothbrush, and a bland, nonirritating diet. Do not wait until problems develop to start the care.

Inspect the mouth daily for any signs of bleeding gums or infection. White glistening areas, white patches, or yellow areas which are usually surrounded by a red halo should be reported immediately for treatment. Antifungal mouthwashes may be initiated if fungal infections are present. If the patient wears dentures, check the fit periodically throughout the course of therapy. Encourage leaving the dentures out at least 8 to 10 hours daily to decrease potential irritating effects.

It may be necessary during periods of marked decrease in platelets (under 20,000/mm^3) to stop brushing the teeth entirely. Perform oral hygiene care every 2 hours, in addition to just before and after meals.

Use of commercial mouthwashes may increase dryness in the oral cavity. These products contain alcohol that may dry and irritate the mucous membranes.

Alopecia

Depending upon the type of medication required, patchy hair loss may develop in various parts of the body. When administering certain agents, a scalp tourniquet may be applied before treatment and left in place for 10 to 15 minutes to reduce this effect. Check the hospital procedure manual.

Neurotoxicity

Ask the patient about any changes in sensation or the development of tremors or incoordination. Observe the patient's gait and check tendon reflexes.

Musculoskeletal Complaints

All complaints of pain over a bony area, muscle weakness, and myalgia require follow-up. Check the calcium level in the laboratory reports at regular intervals and report deviations. Check x-ray reports for any indication of bone metastases. Notify the physician of any complaints that would possibly indicate a fracture. Keep the patient in bed until an examination is completed to rule out a fracture.

Bone Marrow Depression

Monitor laboratory reports for leukopenia (WBC < 1,000/mm^3); for thrombocytopenia (platelet count < 20,000/mm^3) or for erythropenia (reduced RBCs). Some patients will require transfusions of white cells, platelets, or RBCs.

Infection

Prevent infection by use of measures appropriate to the degree of suppression (i.e., reverse isolation, avoidance of persons with known infections). Use meticulous personal hygiene and report the earliest signs of infection.

Activity and Exercise

Adjust the individual's activity level to the degree of impairment, laboratory alterations, and coordination, gait, or level of strength.

Introduce appropriate measures to conserve the patient's energy and need for oxygen to the tissues. Provide frequent rest periods. Assist with ambulating, if necessary.

It may be necessary to limit the number, frequency, and length of visitors' stays.

Maintain active and passive range-of-motion exercises; introduce measures to prevent foot drop or contractures.

Thrombocytopenia

Provide for patient safety and avoid unnecessary trauma:

- Use an electric razor; avoid taking repeated blood pressure readings or using the same extremity for measurement.
- Give parenteral medications only when absolutely necessary. Apply direct pressure to the site for an

extended period of time and be certain local bleeding is controlled. Use the smallest gauge needle possible.

- Avoid enemas or rectal temperature because of the danger of damage to the mucosa and bleeding.
- Test all bowel movements for occult blood.
- Inspect the patient's skin daily for petechiae, ecchymoses, or areas of skin breakdown.
- Follow a specific turning schedule and give thorough skin care. Do not overexpose to the sun.

Patient Teaching Associated with Cancer Chemotherapy

Communication and Responsibility

Encourage open communication concerning frustrations and anger as the patient attempts to adjust to the diagnosis and need for prolonged treatment. The patient must be guided to gain insight into the disorder in order to assume responsibility for the continuation of the treatment. Keep emphasizing those factors the patient can control to alter the progression of the disease:

STRESS MANAGEMENT

Some of the stressors observed in the patient coming for chemotherapy may be a belief in the effectiveness treatment or a lack of faith in its outcomes. Trust in the care-givers and the plan of treatment are of immense importance.

The patient's perspective of the illness and its effect on her or himself, the family, and their ability to maintain the activities of daily living need to be discussed. Encourage the individual to express feelings about this illness and its impact on lifestyle.

Control. Provide the patient with appropriate choices during care and chemotherapy to make sure he or she does not feel totally dominated by the disease or by the care-givers.

The degree of control will vary with each patient's situation. For example, allow choices in the scheduling of the times of chemotherapy and laboratory studies; try to adjust these so that the person can maintain a work schedule.

Take *time* to explain the procedures. Be calm, supportive, genuine, and warm.

Listen to the patient's concerns; take action to try to resolve appropriate problems, no matter how trivial. Let the patient know that personal *needs* are important.

Encourage the patient to maintain as normal a lifestyle as possible. Stress what the patient *can* do, not what he or she cannot do.

Loss. Let the patient talk about the loss of a body part, loss of the ability to be a provider, or loss of the ability to receive or convey intimacy.

If the person is unable to provide for personal care, this too may be expressed in various ways (e.g., frustration, anger, yelling, despondency).

Intimacy. Care-givers often do not consider the individual's ability to give or accept intimacy. Remember tact and diplomacy to avoid invading the person's privacy.

Involve appropriate members of the support group in the care of the patient to the degree the situation warrants.

Anxiety. Provide the patient with information about the plan of care and treatment. Do not overwhelm patients with too much too fast, or information that is not needed.

Teach relaxation techniques and personal comfort measures, such as a warm bath to relieve stress.

Referral for biofeedback or other relaxation techniques, such as visual imagery, may be appropriate.

Stress produced within the family may be significant. Deal with these problems if possible; refer for professional counseling if necessary.

Support Groups. Support groups such as *Make Today Count* may be quite helpful. These groups provide the patient and family members with role models who are effectively coping with similar problems.

NUTRITIONAL STATUS

Patient teaching must be individualized to the presenting problems, to the patient's experience, and to the nutritional history information. The major goal is to maintain the individual's weight and intake of foods to meet nutritional needs.

Weight Loss, Anorexia, Altered Taste. Encourage the patient to eat favorite dishes and frequent, small servings of high-protein, bland foods if having difficulty with nausea. If nutritional supplements are needed, serve them attractively.

Encourage the patient to try washing the mouth with saline or sodium bicarbonate mouthwash immediately before eating. This will sometimes relieve the "bad taste" the individual is experiencing.

Nausea and Vomiting. Persons experiencing nausea and vomiting from chemotherapy require special efforts to maintain nutritional needs.

Coke syrup, soda crackers, non-citrus juice, tepid tea, popsicles, or iced beverages may relieve nausea. Experiment with food temperatures—sometimes warm fluid such as broth works well.

The time the individual eats may need to be changed to the evening or late at night. Do not try to feed the patient who is experiencing nausea or vomiting episodes.

Administer antiemetics as prescribed by the physician. Report the effectiveness of response to the physician. Since antiemetics produce a sedative effect, provide for patient safety. Suggest having a family member or friend drive the patient home if having outpatient therapy. Have the patient report nausea and vomiting that lasts longer than 24 hours.

Some patients experience anticipatory nausea and vomiting before receiving each dose of medication. Relaxation techniques and visual imagery are being used effectively to manage these responses.

Fluid Intake. Unless contraindicated by co-existing medical conditions, encourage the patient to maintain a fluid intake of 8 to 12 8-ounce glasses of fluid daily to prevent dehydration.

ORAL HYGIENE

Before starting chemotherapy, any needed dental care should be completed. Have the patient discuss the condition with the physician and dentist.

Patient Education. Teach the patient to practice oral hygiene measures: Inspect the mouth daily for signs of bleeding gums or areas of yellow or white patches with red halos. If found, they should be reported to the physician for evaluation and treatment.

Equipment. Use a soft-bristled toothbrush or water cleanser (on a low setting) to prevent tissue damage.

Frequency. Measures of oral hygiene should be completed after meals and every 2 hours thereafter for adequate care.

Mouthwashes. Recommend that the patient not use commercially prepared mouthwashes. These products contain alcohol, which may cause further drying of the mouth and irritate rather than relieve the problem.

Use one tablespoonful of salt or hydrogen peroxide in 8 ounces of water; or ½ teaspoonful of baking soda in 8 ounces of water.

Oral Dryness. Dryness can be relieved by chewing gum and sucking on ice chips or popsicles. Dry lips can be coated with cocoa butter, KY Jelly, petroleum jelly, or lip balm.

Artificial saliva is available (Moi-Stir, Ora-lub, or Salivart).

Pain in the Oral Area. For painful oral lesions, try using the following:

- Xylocaine Viscous 2% before meals to relieve pain. Care must be taken to make sure the patient is not burned by the food, since the entire mouth and throat are anesthetized.
- Milk of magnesia can be used to rinse the mouth and coat the mucous membranes.
- Kaopectate stirred in water may be used as a mouthwash to coat painful oral lesions.
- Mycostatin tablets may be used as lozenges to reduce candidal oral infections.

Food Irritants. Oral irritation and stomatitis may be aggravated by salty foods, raw vegetables, some spices, alcohol, vinegar, tomatoes, and citrus fruits.

Poor Denture Fit. Denture fit should be carefully checked and poor fit discussed with the physician and dentist. Remove the dentures at night to reduce irritation to gum tissue.

DIARRHEA

Provide adequate hydration during periods of diarrhea.

Dietary alterations to maintain low residue content should be encouraged in small frequent servings: milk, tender meat, fish, fowl, strained meat-based broth or soup, vegetable puree, ripe bananas, fruit juice, gelatin desserts, puddings, or custard.

During severe symptoms, clear liquids, broth, and clear fruit juices may be tolerated.

Prolonged diarrhea may require more vigorous treatment in a hospital setting. Always report increasing numbers of stools or a lack of response to antidiarrheal therapy.

Encourage the patient to report any black or dark, tarry stools or abdominal pain.

Personal Hygiene. Teach the patient to cleanse the perianal area thoroughly and to apply protective ointment as needed. Stress that the patient must cleanse hands after this procedure.

CONSTIPATION

Instruct the patient about appropriate foods to eat and the need for adequate fluid intake. Foods containing bulk, whole-grain breads or cereal, and stewed prunes may be helpful.

Instruct the patient about the use of any laxative or stool softener that has been prescribed.

Expectations of Therapy

ACTIVITIES AND EXERCISE

Maintain the individual's activities of daily living at the highest level consistent with symptoms. The level will vary throughout the course of therapy. Most patients are concerned with being able to continue as much of a normal lifestyle as possible.

- When therapy is first initiated, an increase in fatigue may be experienced for the first 2 to 4 weeks.
- Encourage frequent rest periods to avoid becoming unnecessarily overtired.
- Involve family members in planning assistance with activities, based on the degree of impairment present. Provide for patient safety at all times.

ENVIRONMENT

Tell the patient to avoid crowds or persons with known infections. Report even the slightest sign of an infection so that vigorous treatment may be started immediately. Teach meticulous personal hygiene measures, especially the importance of handwashing.

BLEEDING

Tell the patient to report bleeding gums, dark tarry stools, nosebleeds, bruises, or developing red spots (petechiae). Prevent accidental injury. Suggest the use of a safety or electric razor, not a standard razor.

Tell the patient not to use aspirin or aspirin-containing products.

Have female patients report menstrual flow that is excessive, bright red in color, or that lasts for a prolonged period of time.

PAIN

One of the greatest fears of cancer patients is pain. If this concern is expressed, reassure the patient that pain can be effectively controlled. Additional information is available on pain management under the section on Analgesics (see Index).

ALOPECIA

Hair loss may be expected with chemotherapy. Suggest the use of scarves, wigs, or turbans and ask the individual for suggestions.

During treatment, do not use hot curling irons or hair dryers. Avoid brushing, and comb gently. Shampoo less frequently and use a protein-based shampoo.

Tell the patient that hair loss may be evident for several weeks after administration of the chemotherapy. Regrowth usually starts within 8 weeks.

SKIN DISORDERS

Rashes and itching may occur with chemotherapy. Suggest the use of products such as Alpha Keri or Calamine lotion, or baking soda baths, and avoiding overexposure to the sun.

SEXUAL ACTIVITY

The patient should resume sexual activities as soon as possible after hospitalization. Patients need to be told to use birth control during and for 1 to 2 years following treatment with chemotherapy or radiation. (Many chemotherapeutic agents cause sterility or possible teratogenicity.)

Changes in Expectations

Assess changes in expectations as therapy progresses and the patient gains understanding and skill in the management of the diagnosis.

Deal with the patient's concerns and questions prior to initiating specific teaching regarding medications or other needs. Determine what symptoms the patient is experiencing and how the patient expects they will be altered.

Changes in Therapy through Cooperative Goal-Setting

Work with the patient to encourage adherence to the prescribed treatment. When the patient feels that a change should be made in a treatment plan, encourage discussion first with the physician.

WRITTEN RECORD

Enlist the patient's aid in developing and maintaining a written record of monitoring parameters (Table 20.1) (i.e., fatigue level, weight gain or loss, nausea, vomiting, diarrhea, constipation, pain relief) and response to prescribed therapies for discussion with the physician. Patients should be encouraged to take this record on follow-up visits.

This record will need modification throughout the course of treatment. It should be based on the symptoms exhibited by the patient. The ultimate aim should be to evaluate the therapeutic response achieved when a change in therapy is prescribed.

Table 20.1

Example of a Written Record for Patients Receiving Antineoplastic Agents

Medications	Color	To be taken

Name _____

Physician _____

Physician's phone _____

Next appt.* _____

Parameters		Day of discharge								Comments
Temperature	AM / PM	/	/	/	/	/	/	/	/	
Pain level Severe 10 Moderate 5 None 1	8 AM									
	Noon									
	6 PM									
	Night									
Fatigue level Sleeps all day 10 Tired 5 Normal 1										
Fear and anxiety Anxious 10 5 Calm 1										
Nausea: Degree of relief Good 10 Moderate 5 Poor 1	Time of day									
Appetite Good 10 Normal 5 Poor 1										
Oral hygiene Normal 10 Moderate pain 5 Severe pain 1										
Bleeding (Yes or No)	Nosebleeds									
	Bruising									
Bowel movements	Color: brown, tarry									
	Diarrhea: Number of stools									
	Normal									

*Please bring this record with you to your next appointment.
Use the back of this sheet for additional information.

517

FOSTERING COMPLIANCE

Throughout the course of treatment, discuss medication information and how it will benefit the treatment. Seek cooperation and understanding of the following points so that medication compliance may be enhanced:

1. Name.
2. Dosage.
3. Route and administration times: Teaching must be adapted to the approach being recommended.
4. Anticipated therapeutic response: General improvement in the patient's overall symptoms and mental response (i.e., decreased pain, increased appetite, and ability to maintain activities of daily living).
5. Side effects to expect: Always research the particular drug your patient is receiving and be able to tell the patient what symptoms are expected. Common side effects include nausea and vomiting, diarrhea or constipation, oral stomatitis, increased fatigue, bleeding complications, alopecia, dyspnea, and peripheral neuropathy.

    Laboratory work to assess the degree of liver and kidney function and bone marrow depression is usually done to monitor the ability of the body to metabolize the antineoplastic agents.

    The nurse should explain the need for regular laboratory studies as a part of the method of evaluating the success of the agents administered. Any alterations from the normal values are reported to the physician for evaluation and modification of treatment.
6. Side effects to report: Always report signs of infection, abdominal pain, inability to defecate, bleeding, or increasing pain that is not controlled by the analgesic currently prescribed. Individualize the reporting of symptoms to the patient's disease state and the medications being used in the treatment plan.
7. What to do if a dosage is missed.
8. When, how, or if to refill the medication prescription.

DIFFICULTY IN COMPREHENSION

If it is evident that the patient and/or family does not understand all aspects of continuing therapy being prescribed (i.e., administration and monitoring of medications, exercises, diets, follow-up appointments) consider the use of social service or visiting nurse agencies.

ASSOCIATED TEACHING

Whenever possible, discuss the need for dental work with the physician and the advisability of having it completed prior to the initiation of chemotherapy.

Always inform the physician or dentist of any prescription or over-the-counter medication or chemotherapy being taken.

Over-the-counter medications should not be taken without first discussing them with a physician or pharmacist.

Always report side effects of rash, itching, or hives immediately. Nausea, vomiting, or diarrhea should also be reported for the physician's evaluation if it is a new symptom.

Take all of the medication as prescribed for the full course of treatment. Do not discontinue use when feeling improved; do not save for future use; do not give your medicine to another individual. Sudden discontinuation of certain medications may produce harmful effects.

Keep all medications out of reach of children.

If pregnancy is suspected, consult an obstetrician as soon as possible about continuation of medication therapy.

At Discharge

Items to be sent home with the patient should:

1. Have written instructions for use.
2. Be labeled in a level of language and size of print appropriate for the patient.
3. If needed, include identification cards or bracelets.
4. Include a list of additional supplies to be purchased after discharge (e.g., for oral hygiene measures: soft-bristled toothbrush, mouthwash substitutes).
5. Include a schedule for follow-up appointments.

Chemotherapeutic Agents

Chemotherapeutic agents currently used are classified as (1) alkylating agents, (2) antimetabolites, (3) natural products (plant alkaloids, antibiotics, other synthetic agents), and (4) hormones. The mechanisms by which these agents cause cell death have not yet been fully determined. See Table 20.2 for a list of drug names, dosages, uses, and adverse effects associated with therapy.

Table 20.2
Cancer Chemotherapeutic Agents

DRUG	USUAL DOSAGE	TOXICITY ACUTE	TOXICITY DELAYED	MAJOR INDICATIONS
Alkylating agents				
Busulfan (Myleran)	2–8 mg/day for 2–3 weeks PO; stop for recovery; then maintenance	None	Bone marrow depression	Chronic granulocytic leukemia
Carmustine (BCNU)	As single agent: 100–200 mg/m^2 IV; over 1–2 hr infusion every 6–8 weeks In combination: 30–60 mg/m^2 IV Use gloves, since solution may cause skin discoloration	Nausea and vomiting; pain along vein of infusion	Granulocyte and platelet suppression Hepatic and renal toxicity	Brain, colon, breast, lung, Hodgkin's disease, lymphosarcoma, myeloma, malignant melanoma
Chlorambucil (Leukeran)	Start 0.1–0.2 mg/kg/day PO; adjust for maintenance	None	Bone marrow depression (anemia, leukopenia, and thrombocytopenia) can be severe with excessive dosage	Chronic lymphocytic leukemia, Hodgkin's disease, non-Hodgkin's lymphoma, trophoblastic neoplasms
Cyclophosphamide (Cytoxan)	40 mg/kg IV in single or in 2–8 daily doses or 2–4 mg/kg/day PO for 10 days; adjust for maintenance	Nausea and vomiting	Bone marrow depression, alopecia, cystitis	Hodgkin's disease and other lymphomas, multiple myeloma, lymphocytic leukemia, many solid cancers
Lomustine (CCNU)	130 mg/m^2 PO once every 6 weeks	Severe nausea and vomiting; anorexia	Thrombocytopenia, leukopenia, alopecia, confusion, lethargy, ataxia	Brain, colon, Hodgkin's disease, lymphosarcoma, malignant melanoma
Mechlorethamine (nitrogen mustard; HN$_2$, Mustargen)	0.4 mg/kg IV in single or divided doses	Nausea and vomiting	Moderate depression of peripheral blood count	Hodgkin's disease and other lymphomas, bronchogenic carcinoma
Melphalan (1-phenylalanine mustard; Alkeran)	0.25 mg/kg/day for 4 days PO; 2–4 mg/day as maintenance or 0.1–0.15 mg/kg/day for 2–3 weeks	None	Bone marrow depression	Multiple myeloma, malignant melanoma, ovarian carcinoma, testicular seminoma
Thiotepa (triethylenethio-phosphoramide)	0.2 mg/kg IV for 5 days	None	Bone marrow depression	Hodgkin's disease, bronchogenic and breast carcinomas
Antimetabolites				
Cytarabine hydrochloride (arabinosyl cytosine; Cytosar)	2–3 mg/kg/day IV until response or toxicity or 1–3 mg/kg IV over 24 hr for up to 10 days	Nausea and vomiting	Bone marrow depression megaloblastosis	Acute leukemia
Fluorouracil (5-FU, FU)	12.5 mg/kg/day IV for 3–5 days or 15 mg/kg/week for 6 weeks	Nausea	Oral and gastrointestinal ulceration, stomatitis and diarrhea, bone marrow depression	Breast, large bowel, and ovarian carcinoma
Mercaptopurine (6-MP, Purinethol)	2.5 mg/kg/day PO	Occasional nausea and vomiting, usually well tolerated	Bone marrow depression, occasional hepatic damage	Acute lymphocytic and granulocytic leukemia, chronic granulocytic leukemia

(*Table continues on p. 520.*)

Table 20.2 (*continued*)

| DRUG | USUAL DOSAGE | TOXICITY | | MAJOR INDICATIONS |
		ACUTE	DELAYED	
Methotrexate (amethopterin; MTX)	2.5–5.0 mg/day PO; 0.4 mg/kg rapid IV daily 4–5 days (not over 25 mg) or 0.4 mg/kg rapid IV twice/week	Occasional diarrhea, hepatic necrosis	Oral and gastrointestinal ulceration, bone marrow depression (anemia, leukopenia, thrombocytopenia), cirrhosis	Acute lymphocytic leukemia, choriocarcinoma, carcinoma of cervix and head and neck area, mycosis fungoides, solid cancers
Thioguanine (6-TG)	2 mg/kg/day PO	Occasional nausea and vomiting, usually well tolerated	Bone marrow depression	Acute leukemia
Plant alkaloids				
Vinblastine sulfate (Velban)	0.1–0.2 mg/kg/week IV or every 2 weeks	Nausea and vomiting, local irritant	Alopecia, stomatitis, bone marrow depression, loss of reflexes	Hodgkin's disease and other lymphomas, solid cancers
Vincristine sulfate (Oncovin)	0.01–0.03 mg/kg/week IV	Local irritant	Areflexia, peripheral neuritis, paralytic ileus, mild bone marrow depression	Acute lymphcytic leukemia, Hodgkin's disease and other lymphomas, solid cancers
Antibiotics				
Bleomycin (Blenoxane)	10–15 mg/m^2 once or twice a week, IV or IM to total dose 300–400 mg	Nausea and vomiting, fever, very toxic	Edema of hands, pulmonary fibrosis, stomatitis, alopecia	Hodgkin's disease, non-Hodgkin's lymphoma, squamous cell carcinoma of head and neck, testicular carcinoma
Dactinomycin (actinomycin D; Cosmegen)	0.015–0.05 mg/kg/week (1–2.5 mg) for 3–5 weeks IV; wait for marrow recovery (3–4 weeks), then repeat course	Nausea and vomiting, local irritant	Stomatitis, oral ulcers, diarrhea, alopecia, mental depression, bone marrow depression	Testicular carcinoma, Wilms' tumor, rhabdomyosarcoma, Ewing's and osteogenic sarcoma, and other solid tumors
Doxorubicin (Adriamycin)	60–90 mg/m^2 IV, single dose or over 3 days; repeat every 3 weeks up to total dose 500 mg/m^2	Nausea, red urine (not hematuria)	Bone marrow depression, cardiotoxicity, alopecia, stomatitis	Soft tissue, osteogenic and miscellaneous sarcomas, Hodgkin's disease, non-Hodgkin's lymphoma, bronchogenic and breast carcinoma, thyroid cancer
Mithramycin (Mithracin)	0.025–0.050 mg/kg every 2 days for up to 8 doses, IV	Nausea and vomiting, hepatotoxicity	Bone marrow depression (thrombocytopenia), hypocalcemia	Testicular carcinoma, trophoblastic neoplasms
Mitomycin C (Mutamycin)	0.05 mg/kg/day IV for 5 days	Nausea and vomiting "flulike syndrome"	Bone marrow depression, skin toxicity; pulmonary, renal, CNS effects	Squamous cell carcinoma of head and neck, lungs, and cervix; adenocarcinoma of the stomach, pancreas, colon, rectum; adenocarcinoma and duct cell carcinoma of the breast

Table 20.2 (continued)

DRUG	USUAL DOSAGE	TOXICITY ACUTE	TOXICITY DELAYED	MAJOR INDICATIONS
Streptozocin (Zanosar)	As single agent: 1.0–1.5 mg/m^2/week for 6 consecutive weeks with 4 weeks observation In combination: 400–500 mg/m^2 for 4–5 consecutive days with 6 weeks observation	Hypoglycemia, severe nausea and vomiting	Moderate but transient renal and hepatic toxicity, hypoglycemia, mild anemia, leukopenia	Pancreatic islet cell tumors
Other synthetic agents				
Dacarbazine (DTIC-Dome; DIC)	4.5 mg/kg/day IV for 10 days; repeated every 28 days	Nausea and vomiting "flulike syndrome"	Bone marrow depression (rare)	Metastatic malignant melanoma
Hydroxyurea (Hydrea)	80 mg/kg PO single dose every 3 days or 20–30 mg/kg/day PO	Mild nausea and vomiting	Bone marrow depression	Chronic granulocytic leukemia
Mitotane (Lysodren)	6–15 mg/kg/day PO	Nausea and vomiting	Dermatitis, diarrhea, mental depression	Adrenal cortical carcinoma
Procarbazine hydrochloride (Methyl hydrazine; ibenzmethylzin; Matulane)	Start 1–2 mg/kg/day PO; increase over 1 week to 3 mg/kg; maintain for 3 weeks, then reduce to 2 mg/kg/day until toxicity	Nausea and vomiting	Bone marrow depression, CNS depression	Hodgkin's disease, non-Hodgkin's lymphoma, bronchogenic carcinoma
Tamoxifen (Nolvadex)	20–40 mg daily in two divided doses	Nausea, vomiting, hot flashes	Increased bone and tumor pain, thrombocytopenia, leukopenia, edema, hypercalcemia	Breast cancer (estrogen sensitive)
Hormones				
Diethylstilbestrol (DES)	15 mg/day PO (1 mg in prostate cancer)	None	Fluid retention, hypercalcemia, feminization, uterine bleeding; if during pregnancy, may cause vaginal carcinoma in offspring	Breast and prostate carcinomas
Dromostanolone propionate (Drolban)	100 mg 3 times a week IM	None	Fluid retention, masculinization, hypercalcemia	Breast carcinoma
Ethinyl estradiol	3 mg/day PO	None	Fluid retention, hypercalcemia, feminization, uterine bleeding	Breast and prostate carcinomas
Fluoxymesterone	10–20 mg/day PO	None	Fluid retention, masculinization, cholestatic jaundice	Breast carcinoma
Hydroxyprogesterone caproate	1 g IM twice a week	None	None	Endometrial carcinoma
Medroxyprogesterone acetate	100–200 mg/day PO; 200-600 mg twice a week	None	None	Endometrial carcinoma, renal cell, breast cancer
Prednisone	10–100 mg/day PO	None	Hyperadrenocorticism	Acute and chronic lymphocytic leukemia, Hodgkin's disease, non-Hodgkin's lymphomas

(Table continues on p. 522.)

Table 20.2 (continued)

| DRUG | USUAL DOSAGE | TOXICITY | | MAJOR INDICATIONS |
		ACUTE	DELAYED	
Testolactone (Teslac)	100 mg 3 times a week IM	None	Fluid retention, masculinization	Breast carcinoma
Testosterone enanthate	600–1200 mg/week IM	None	Fluid retention, masculinization	Breast carcinoma
Testosterone propionate	50–100 mg, IM 3 times a week	None	Fluid retention, masculinization	Breast carcinoma

Modified from Carter, S. K., and Kershner, L. M.: *Pharmacy Times* 41(8):56, 1975.

Chapter 21

Miscellaneous Agents

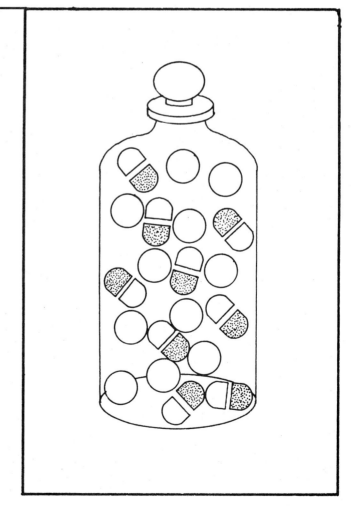

Objectives

After completing this chapter, the student should be able to do the following:

1. Identify baseline data the nurse should collect on a continuous basis for comparison and evaluation of drug effectiveness.
2. Identify important nursing assessments and interventions associated with the drug therapy.
3. Identify health teaching essential for a successful treatment regimen.

Patient Teaching Associated with Medication Therapy

PATIENT CONCERNS: NURSING INTERVENTION/RATIONALE

Communication and Responsibility

Encourage open communication concerning frustrations and anger as the patient attempts to adjust to the diagnosis and need for prolonged treatment. The patient must be guided to gain insight into the condition in order to assume the responsibility for the continuation of treatment. Keep emphasizing those factors the patient can control to alter the progression of the disease, including maintenance of general health, nutritional needs, adequate rest and appropriate exercise, and continuation of prescribed medication therapy.

Expectations of Therapy

Discuss expectations of therapy with the patient (i.e., level of exercise, degree of pain relief, frequency of medication use, relief of dyspnea, sexual activity, maintenance of mobility, ability to maintain activities of daily living and/or work).

Changes in Expectations

Assess changes in expectations as therapy progresses and the patient gains understanding and skill in the management of the diagnosis.

Changes in Therapy through Cooperative Goal-Setting

Work with the patient to encourage adherence to the prescribed treatment. When the patient feels that a change should be made in a treatment plan, encourage discussion first with the physician.

Written Record

Enlist the patient's aid in developing and maintaining a written record of monitoring parameters (i.e., blood pressure, pulse, daily weights, degree of pain relief, exercise tolerance) and response to prescribed therapies for discussion with the physician. Patients should be encouraged to take this record on follow-up visits.

Fostering Compliance

Throughout the patient's hospitalization, discuss medication information and how it will benefit the course of treatment. Seek cooperation and understanding of the following points so that medication compliance may be enhanced:

1. Name
2. Dosage
3. Route and administration times
4. Anticipated therapeutic response
5. Side effects to expect
6. Side effects to report
7. What to do if a dosage is missed
8. When, how, or if to refill the medication prescription

Difficulty in Comprehension

If it is evident that the patient and/or family does not understand all aspects of continuing therapy being prescribed (i.e., administration and monitoring of medications, exercises, diets, follow-up appointments) consider the use of social service or visiting nurse agencies.

Associated Teaching

Give patients the following instructions:
Always inform the physician or dentist of any prescription or over-the-counter medication being taken.

Over-the-counter medications should not be taken without first discussing with a physician or pharmacist.

Always report side effects of rash, itching, or hives immediately. Nausea, vomiting, or diarrhea should also be reported for the physician's evaluation if it is a new symptom.

Take all of the medication as prescribed for the full course of treatment. Do not discontinue use when feeling improved; do not save for future use; do not give your medicine to another individual. Sudden discontinuation of certain medications may produce harmful effects.

Keep all medications out of reach of children.

If pregnancy is suspected, consult an obstetrician as soon as possible about continuation of medication therapy.

At Discharge

Items to be sent home with the patient should

1. Have written instructions for use.
2. Be labeled in a level of language and size of print appropriate for the patient.
3. If needed, include identification cards or bracelets.
4. Include a list of additional supplies to be purchased after discharge (e.g., syringes, dressings).
5. Include a schedule of follow-up appointments.

Allopurinol (al-o-pu′ri-nol) *(Zyloprim)* (zy′lo-prim)

Allopurinol represents an entirely different approach to the treatment of gout. It blocks the terminal steps in uric acid formation by inhibiting the enzyme xanthine oxidase. This agent can be used for the treatment of primary gout or gout secondary to antineoplastic therapy. It is not effective in treating acute attacks of gouty arthritis.

Allopurinol has an advantage over uricosuric agents in that gouty nephropathy and the formation of urate stones are less likely with allopurinol because the drug reduces the amount of uric acid produced. It may also be used in patients with renal failure, whereas uricosuric agents should not be.

Side Effects

The number of gouty attacks may increase during the first 6 to 12 months of treatment. Continue allopurinol therapy without changing doses during these attacks. Treat the acute attack with colchicine or anti-inflammatory agents.

General side effects are nausea, vomiting, headache, diarrhea, drowsiness, and a metallic taste in the mouth.

Rarely, allopurinol may produce hepatotoxicity or blood dyscrasias. Periodic laboratory tests, including blood counts and liver function tests, are recommended to avoid complications.

Patients may develop a hypersensitivity to allopurinol manifested by fever, pruritus, and rashes. If these symptoms develop, discontinue therapy.

Availability

PO—100 and 300 mg tablets.

Dosage and Administration

Adult
PO—Initially 100 mg daily. Increase the daily dosage by 100 mg/week until the serum urate level falls to 6 mg/100 ml or a maximum dosage of 800 mg daily is achieved.

- The average maintenance dose is 300 mg daily.
- Therapy is better tolerated if the drug is taken with meals.
- Maintain fluid intake at 2 to 3 liters daily.

**PATIENT CONCERNS:
NURSING INTERVENTION/RATIONALE**

Side Effects to Expect

Acute Gout Attacks

Patients should be told that the frequency of gout attacks may increase for the first few months of therapy. The patient should continue therapy without changing the doses during the attacks.

Nausea, Vomiting, Diarrhea, Dizziness, Headache

These side effects are usually mild and tend to resolve with continued therapy. Encourage the patient not to discontinue therapy without consulting the physician first.

Side Effects to Report

Hepatotoxicity

The symptoms of hepatotoxicity are anorexia, nausea, vomiting, jaundice, hepatomegaly, splenomegaly, and abnormal liver function tests (elevated bilirubin, SGOT, SGPT, alkaline phosphatase, prothrombin time).

Blood Dyscrasias

Routine laboratory studies (RBC, WBC, and differential counts) should be scheduled. Stress returning for this laboratory work.

Monitor for the development of a sore throat, fever, purpura, jaundice, or excessive, progressive weakness.

Fever, Pruritus, Rash

Report symptoms for further evaluation by the physician.

Pruritus may be relieved by adding baking soda to the bath water.

Dosage and Administration

Gastric Irritation

If gastric irritation occurs, administer with food or milk. If symptoms persist or increase in severity, report for physician evaluation.

Fluid Intake

Maintain fluid intake at 8 to 12 8-ounce glasses daily.

Drug Interactions

Theophylline Derivatives

Allopurinol, when given with theophylline derivatives, may result in theophylline toxicity. Observe for vomiting, dizziness, restlessness, and cardiac arrhythmias. The dosage of theophylline may need to be reduced.

Dicumarol (Possibly Warfarin)

This medication may enchance the anticoagulant effects of dicumarol. Observe for the development of petechiae, ecchymoses, nosebleeds, bleeding gums, dark tarry stools, and bright red or "coffee-ground" emesis. Monitor the prothrombin time and reduce the dosage of dicumarol if necessary.

Chlorpropamide

Allopurinol may reduce the metabolism of chlorpropamide. Monitor for hypoglycemia: headache, weakness, decreased coordination, general apprehension, diaphoresis, hunger, blurred or double vision.

The dosage of the hypoglycemic agent may need to be reduced. Notify the physician if any of the above symptoms appears.

Azathiprine, Mercaptopurine

When initiating therapy with azothioprine or mercaptopurine, start at one-fourth to one-third of the normal dosage and adjust subsequent dosages to the patient's response.

Vidarabine

Allopurinol alters the metabolism of vidarabine. Monitor closely for signs of neurotoxicity: pain, itching, tremors of the extremities and facial muscles, and impaired mentation.

Perform a baseline assessment of the patient's degree of alertness and orientation to name, place, and time *before* initiating therapy. Make regularly scheduled subsequent mental status evaluations and compare findings. Report development of alterations.

Ampicillin

There is a high incidence of rash when patients are taking both allopurinol and ampicillin. Do not label the patient allergic to either drug until sensitivity tests identify a hypersensitivity reaction.

Cyclophosphamide

There is a greater frequency of bone marrow depression in patients receiving these agents concurrently. Monitor for the development of a sore throat, fever, purpura, jaundice, or excessive, progressive weakness.

Colchicine (kol'chi-sin) (Colsalide) (kol'sa-lyd)

Colchicine is an alkaloid that has been used for hundreds of years to prevent or relieve acute attacks of gout. The exact mechanism of action is not known, but colchicine does interrupt the cycle of urate crystal deposition in the tissues that results in an acute attack of gout. It does not affect the amount of uric acid in the blood or urine, so it is not a uricosuric agent.

Side Effects

Nausea, vomiting and diarrhea are common adverse effects of colchicine therapy. Discontinue therapy when gastrointestinal symptoms develop.

Serious, potentially fatal blood dyscrasias including anemia, agranulocytosis, and thrombocytopenia have been associated with colchicine therapy. Although the development of blood dyscrasias is quite rare, periodic differential blood counts are recommended if the patient requires prolonged treatment.

Availability

PO—0.432 and 0.6 mg tablets, 0.5 mg granules.
IV—1 mg/2 ml ampules.

Dosage and Administration

Note: Use with extreme caution in elderly or debilitated patients and in those patients with impaired renal, cardiac, or gastrointestinal function.

Adult
PO—Acute gout: initially 0.5 to 1.2 mg, followed by 0.6 mg every 1 to 2 hours until pain subsides or nausea, vomiting, and diarrhea develop. A total dosage of 4 to 10 mg may be required. After the acute attack, 0.5 to 0.6 mg should be administered every 6 hours for a few days to prevent relapse. Do not repeat high-dose therapy for at least 3 days. Prophylaxis for recurrent gout: 0.5 to 0.6 mg every 1 to 3 days depending on the frequency of gouty attacks.

IV—Acute gout: initially 2 mg diluted in 20 ml of saline solution. Follow with 0.5 mg every 6 to 12 hours to a maximum of 4 mg in 24 hours. If pain recurs, daily doses of 1 to 2 mg may be administered for several days. Do not repeat high-dosage therapy for at least 3 days. *Avoid extravasation.*
DO NOT ADMINISTER SC OR IM!

PATIENT CONCERNS: NURSING INTERVENTION/RATIONALE

Side Effects to Expect

Nausea, Vomiting, Diarrhea

Discontinue therapy when gastrointestinal symptoms develop. Always report bright blood or "coffee-ground" appearing vomitus or dark tarry stools.

Therapeutic Effects

Joint pain and swelling begin to subside within 12 hours and are usually gone within 48 to 72 hours following initiation of therapy.

Side Effects to Report

Blood Dyscrasias

Routine laboratory studies (RBC, WBC, and differential counts) should be scheduled. Stress returning for this laboratory work.

Monitor for the development of a sore throat, fever, purpura, jaundice, or excessive, progressive weakness. Report immediately.

Dosage and Administration

IV

Dilute 2 mg in 20 ml of saline solution and administer slowly over 5 minutes.

Extravasation

Observe IV site for any change in the color, size, or skin integrity. Pain, swelling, or erythema signify infiltration.

- Clamp, report, and follow hospital protocol for extravasation.
- Elevate the infiltrated area.
- Prepare to assist with administration of drugs to counteract the necrotizing effects.

SC, IM

Do not administer via these routes.

Fluid Intake

Monitor intake and output during therapy. Maintain fluid intake at 8 to 12 8-ounce glasses daily.

Disulfiram (di-sul'fi-ram) *(Antabuse)* (an'tah-byuse)

Disulfiram is an agent that, when ingested before any form of alcohol, produces a very unpleasant reaction to the alcohol. It is used in alcohol rehabilitation programs for chronic alcoholic patients who want to maintain sobriety. It should be used only in conjunction with other rehabilitative therapy.

The disulfiram–alcohol reaction is manifested by nausea, severe vomiting, sweating, throbbing headache, dizziness, blurred vision, and confusion. The intensity of the reaction is somewhat dependent on the sensitivity of the individual and the amount of alcohol consumed. The duration of the reaction depends on the presence of alcohol in the blood. Mild reactions may last from 30–60 minutes, whereas more severe reactions may last for several hours.

Patients must be fully informed of the consequences of drinking alcohol while receiving disulfiram therapy. As little as 10 to 15 ml of alcohol may produce a reaction. Patients must not drink alcohol in any form, including over-the-counter products such as sleep aids, cough and cold products, after-shave lotions, mouthwashes, and rubbing lotions. Dietary sources, such as sauces and vinegars containing alcohol, are prohibited. A disulfiram–alcohol reaction may occur with the ingestion of any alcohol for 1 to 2 weeks after the discontinuation of disulfiram therapy.

Side Effects

Disulfiram generally does not induce many side effects; however, some patients have reported drowsiness, fatigability, impotence, headache, acne, or metallic or garlic taste. These side effects are generally mild and transient. Hypersensitivity reactions manifested by rashes have been reported.

Hepatotoxicity has been reported with disulfiram therapy. Baseline liver function tests are recommended, with follow-up in 10 to 14 days, to detect hepatic dysfunction. Routine liver and kidney function tests, as well as measurement of electrolytes, are recommended every 6 months.

Because of the consequences of a disulfiram–alcohol reaction on other disease states, use disulfiram therapy very cautiously in patients with diabetes mellitus, hypothyroidism, epilepsy, cerebral damage, chronic and acute nephritis, hepatic cirrhosis, or hepatic insufficiency.

Availability

PO—250 and 500 mg tablets.

Dosage and Administration

Note: Disulfiram must never be administered to patients when they are in a state of intoxication or when they are unaware they are receiving therapy. Family members should also be told of the treatment to help provide motivation and support and to help avoid accidental disulfiram–alcohol reactions.

Do not administer disulfiram until the patient has abstained from alcohol for at least 12 hours.

Adult

PO—Initially a maximum of 500 mg once daily for 1 to 2 weeks. The maintenance dose is usually 250 mg daily (range: 125 to 500 mg). Do not exceed 500 mg daily.

PATIENT CONCERNS: NURSING INTERVENTION/RATIONALE

Side Effects to Expect

Drowsiness, Fatigue, Headache

These side effects are usually mild and tend to resolve with continued therapy. Encourage the patient not to discontinue therapy without consulting the physician first.

Side Effects to Report

Hepatotoxicity

The symptoms of hepatotoxicity are: anorexia, nausea, vomiting, jaundice, hepatomegaly, splenomegaly, and abnormal liver function tests (elevated bilirubin, SGOT, SGPT, alkaline phosphatase, prothrombin time).

Nephrotoxicity

Monitor urinalysis and kidney function tests for abnormal results. Report an increasing BUN and creatinine, decreasing urine output and/or decreasing specific gravity (despite amount of fluid intake), casts or protein in the urine, frank blood or smoky-colored urine, or RBCs in excess of 0–3 on the urinalysis report.

Hives, Pruritus, Rash

Report symptoms for further evaluation by the physician.

Pruritus may be relieved by adding baking soda to the bath water.

Dosage and Administration

PO

Administer at bedtime to avoid the complications of sedative side effects.

Drug Interaction

Warfarin

This medication may enhance the anticoagulant effects of warfarin. Observe for the development of petechiae, ecchymoses, nosebleeds, bleeding gums, dark tarry stools, and bright red or "coffee-ground" emesis. Monitor the prothrombin time and reduce the dosage of warfarin if necessary.

Phenytoin

Disulfiram inhibits the metabolism of phenytoin. Monitor patients with concurrent therapy for signs of phenytoin toxicity: nystagmus, sedation, lethargy. Serum levels may be ordered and the dosage of phenytoin may be reduced.

Isoniazid

Disulfiram alters the metabolism of isoniazid. Perform a baseline assessment of the patient's degree of alertness (orientation to name, place, and time) and of coordination *before* initiating therapy. Make regularly scheduled subsequent mental status evaluations and compare findings. Report development of alterations.

Metronidazole

Concurrent administration of disulfiram and metronidazole may result in psychotic episodes and confusional states. Concurrent therapy is not recommended.

Lactulose (lak'tu-los)
(Cephulac) (sef'u-lak) (Duphalac) (du'fah-lak)

Lactulose is a sugar used to treat portal-systemic (hepatic) encephalopathy and hepatic coma by reducing blood ammonia levels. It acts by acidifying the colon, thus preventing the absorption of ammonia, which is implicated as a cause of hepatic encephalopathy and coma. Lactulose may also be used as a laxative.

Side Effects

Common adverse effects frequently observed in the early stages of therapy are belching, gaseous distension, flatulence, and cramping. These side effects resolve with continued therapy, but dosage reduction may also be necessary. Diarrhea is a sign of overdosage and responds to dosage reduction.

Use with caution in patients with diabetes mellitus. Lactulose syrup contains small amounts of free lactose, galactose, and other sugars.

Patients who use lactulose chronically for 6 months or longer should have serum potassium and chloride levels measured periodically.

Availability

PO—10 g of lactulose per 15 ml of syrup.

Dosage and Administration

Adult
Laxative:
PO—Initially 15 to 30 ml daily. Increase to 60 ml daily if necessary.
Portal-systemic encephalopathy:
PO—Initially 30 to 45 ml every hour for rapid laxation. Once the laxative effect is achieved, the dosage is reduced to 30 to 45 ml 3 to 4 times daily. Adjust the dose to produce 2 or 3 soft, formed stools daily.
Rectal—Mix 300 ml of syrup with 700 ml of water or normal saline. Instill rectally every 4 to 6 hours with a rectal balloon catheter. Have the patient attempt to retain for 30 to 60 minutes.

• Do not use soap suds or cleansing enemas.

PATIENT CONCERNS:
NURSING INTERVENTION/RATIONALE

Side Effects to Report

Electrolyte Imbalance, Dehydration

These effects may result from diarrhea. The electrolytes most commonly altered are potassium (K^+) and chloride (Cl^-). *Hypokalemia* is most likely to occur.

Many symptoms associated with altered fluid and electrolyte balance are subtle and resemble general symptoms of drug toxicity or the disease process itself.

Gather data relative to changes in the patient's mental status (i.e., alertness, orientation, confusion), muscle strength, muscle cramps, tremors, nausea, and general appearance (drowsy, anxious, lethargic).

Always check the electrolyte reports for early indications of electrolyte imbalance.

Keep accurate records of I/O, daily weights, and vital signs.

Dosage and Administration

PO

Twenty-four to forty-eight hours may be required to produce a normal bowel movement. Administer with fruit juice, water, or milk to make the syrup more palatable.

Rectal

See instructions above.

Drug Interactions

Laxatives

Do not administer with other laxatives. Diarrhea makes it difficult to adjust to a proper dosage of lactulose.

Antibiotics

Antibiotic therapy may destroy too much of the bacteria in the colon that are necessary for lactulose to work. Monitor patients closely for reduced lactulose activity when concurrent antibiotic therapy is prescribed.

Appendixes

Appendix A

Common Medical Abbreviations

A	Assessment (POMR)	BAL	British anti-lewisite (dimercaprol)	CHF	Congestive heart failure
A$_2$	Aortic second sound	bands	Banded neutrophils	CHO	Carbohydrate
A$_2$>P$_2$	Aortic sound larger than second pulmonary sound	BBB	Bundle branch block; blood-brain barrier	Chol	Cholesterol
AAL	Anterior axillary line	BBT	Basal body temperature	CI	Color index; contraindication
Ab	Abortion	BE	Barium enema; base excess	CK	Check
Abd	Abdomen, abdominal	BEI	Butanol-extractable iodine	CLL	Chronic lymphocytic leukemia
ABE	Acute bacterial endocarditis	bili	Bilirubin	CNS	Central nervous system
ABG	Arterial blood gases	BJ	Biceps jerk; bone and joint	COAP	Cyclophosphamide, Oncovin, Ara-C, Prednisone
ACD	Anterior chest diameter	BK	Below knee (amputation)		
ADH	Antidiuretic hormone	BLB	A type of oxygen mask	C/O	Complains of
ADT	Alternate-day therapy	BLOBS	Bladder observation	Cong	Congenital
AF	Atrial fibrillation; acid fast	BM	Bowel movement; basal metabolism	COP	Cyclophosphamide, Oncovin, Prednisone
AFB	Acid-fast bacteria; acid-fast bacilli	BMR	Basal metabolic rate		
A/G	Albumin to globulin ratio	B & O	Belladonna and opium	COPD	Chronic obstructive pulmonary disease
AGN	Acute glomerular nephritis	BP	Blood pressure; British Pharmacopoeia		
AHF	Antihemophilic factor			CPK	Creatine phosphokinase
AHFS	American Hospital Formulary Service	BPH	Benign prostatic hypertrophy	C & P	Cystoscopy and pyelography
		BRP	Bathroom privileges	CP	Cerebral palsy; cleft palate
AHG	Antihemophilic globulin	BS	Bowel sounds; breath sounds	CPR	Cardiopulmonary resuscitation
AI	Aortic insufficiency	BSO	Bilateral salpingo-oophorectomy	CR	Cardiorespiratory
AJ	Ankle jerk	BSP	Bromsulphalein	CRF	Chronic renal failure
AK	Above knee (amputation)	BT	Breast tumor; brain tumor	CRP	C-reactive protein
ALD	Alcoholic liver disease	BTL	Bilateral tubal ligation	CS	Coronary sclerosis
ALL	Acute lymphocytic leukemia	BTFS	Breast tumor frozen section	C & S	Culture and sensitivity
ALS	Amyotrophic lateral sclerosis	BU	Bodansky unit	CSF	Cerebrospinal fluid
AMA	Against medical advice	BUN	Blood urea nitrogen	C sect	Cesarean section
AMI	Acute myocardial infarction	BVL	Bilateral vas ligation	CT	Circulation time
ANA	Antinuclear antibodies	BW	Body weight	CV	Cardiovascular; costovertebral angle
AODM	Adult-onset diabetes mellitus	Bx	Biopsy	CVA	Cerebrovascular accident
A & P	Anterior and posterior; auscultation and percussion			CVP	Central venous pressure
				CX	Cervix, cervical
ASAP	As soon as possible	C	Centigrade, Celsius	CXR	Chest X-ray
AP	Apical pulse, anteroposterior	C$_2$	Second cervical vertebra		
APB	Atrial premature beats	CA	Carbonic anhydrase		
AS	Anal sphincter; arteriosclerosis	Ca	Cancer, calcium	DC (D/C)	Discontinue
ASCVD	Arteriosclerotic cardiovascular disease	C & A	Clinitest and Acetest	D & C	Dilatation and curretage
		CAD	Coronary artery disease	DD	Differential diagnosis
ASHD	Arteriosclerotic heart disease	CBC	Complete blood count	DDD	Degenerative disc disease
ASO	Antistreptolysin titer; arteriosclerosis obliterans	CC	Chief complaint	DIC	Disseminated intravascular coagulation
		CCR	Creatinine clearance		
ATN	Acute tubular necrosis	CCU	Coronary care unit	Diff	Differential blood count
AV	Arteriovenous; atrioventricular	Ceph floc	Cephalin flocculation	DJD	Degenerative joint disease
A & W	Alive and well	CF	Complement fixation	DM	Diabetes mellitus
				DOA	Dead on arrival

DOE	Dyspnea on exertion	HTVD	Hypertensive vascular disease	M
DPT	Diphtheria, pertussis, and tetanus	Hx	History	m²
DSD	Dry sterile dressing			M₁
DT	Delirium tremens	IASD	Intraatrial septal defect	MCH
DTR	Deep tendon reflex	IBC	Iron-binding capacity	MCHC
Dx	Diagnosis	IBI	Intermittent bladder irrigation	

DOE — Dyspnea on exertion
DPT — Diphtheria, pertussis, and tetanus
DSD — Dry sterile dressing
DT — Delirium tremens
DTR — Deep tendon reflex
Dx — Diagnosis
D₅W — Dextrose 5% in water

E — Enema
EBL — Estimated blood loss
ECF — Extracellular fluid
ECG — Electrocardiogram
ECT — Electroconvulsive therapy
ECW — Extracellular water
EDC — Expected date of confinement (obstetrics)
EEG — Electroencephalogram
EENT — Eyes, ears, nose, throat
EFA — Essential fatty acids
EH — Enlarged heart
EKG — Electrocardiogram
EM — Electron microscope
EMG — Electromyography
ENT — Ears, nose, and throat
ER — Emergency room
ESR — Erythrocyte sedimentation rate (sed rate)
EST — Electroshock therapy
EUA — Examine under anesthesia

F — Fahrenheit
FB — Finger breadths; foreign bodies
FBS — Fasting blood sugar
FEV₁ — Forced expiratory volume in one second
FF — Filtration fraction
FFA — Free fatty acids
FH — Family history
FLK — Funny looking kid
FP — Family practice; family planning
FSH — Follicle-stimulating hormone
FTA — Fluorescent treponemal antibody
FUO — Fever of undetermined origin
Fx — Fracture; fraction

G — Gravida
GA — General appearance
GB — Gallbladder
GC — Gonococcus; gonorrhea
GFR — Glomerular filtration rate
GI — Gastrointestinal
G6PD — Glucose-6-phosphate dehydrogenase
G-P- — Gravida-; para-
GU — Genitourinary
GYN — Gynecology

H — Hypodermic; heroin
HA — Headache
HAA — Hepatitis-associated antigen
HBP — High blood pressure
Hct — Hematocrit
HCVD — Hypertensive cardiovascular disease
HEENT — Head, eyes, ears, nose, throat
Hgb — Hemoglobin
HHD — Hypertensive heart disease
HO — House officer
HOB — Head of bed
HPF — High power field
HPI — History of present illness
HSA — Human serum albumin
HTN — Hypertension

HTVD — Hypertensive vascular disease
Hx — History

IASD — Intraatrial septal defect
IBC — Iron-binding capacity
IBI — Intermittent bladder irrigation
ICF — Intracellular fluid volume
ICM — Intracostal margin
ICS — Intercostal space
ICU — Intensive care unit
ICW — Intracellular water
ID — Initial dose; intradermal
I & D — Incision and drainage
IDU — Idoxuridine
I & O — Intake and output
IHSS — Idiopathic hypertrophic subaortic stenosis
IM — Intramuscular
Imp — Impression
Int — Internal
IP — Intraperitoneal
IPPB — Intermittent positive pressure breathing
ISW — Interstitial water
ITh — Intrathecal
IU — International unit
IUD — Intrauterine device (contraceptive)
IVP — Intravenous pyelogram
IVPB — Intravenous piggyback
IVSD — Intraventricular septal defect

JRA — Juvenile rheumatoid arthritis
JVD — Jugular venous distension

K⁺ — Potassium
KO — Keep open
17-KS — 17-Ketosteroids
KUB — Kidney, ureter, and bladder
K.W. — Keith Wagner (ophthalmoscopic findings)

L₂ — Second lumbar vertebra
LA — Left atrium
Lap — Laparotomy
LATS — Long-acting thyroid stimulator
LBBB — Left bundle branch block
LCM — Left costal margin
LD — Longitudinal diameter (of heart)
LDH — Lactic dehydrogenase
LDL — Low density lipoproteins
LE — Lupus erythematosus
LFTs — Liver function tests
LHF — Left heart failure
LKS — Liver, kidneys, and spleen
LLE — Left lower extremity
LLL — Left lower lobe
LLQ — Left lower quadrant (abdomen)
LMD — Local medical doctor
LML — Left middle lobe (lung)
LMP — Last menstrual period
LOA — Left occipital anterior
LOM — Limitation of motion
LOP — Left occipital posterior
LP — Lumbar puncture
lpf — Low power field
LUQ — Left upper quadrant
LVH — Left ventricular hypertrophy
L & W — Living and well
LWCT — Lee-White clotting time
lytes — Electrolytes

M — Murmur
m² — Square meters of body surface
M₁ — First mitral sound
MCH — Mean corpuscular hemoglobin
MCHC — Mean corpuscular hemoglobin concentration
MCL — Midclavicular line
MCV — Mean corpuscular volume
MF — Myocardial fibrosis
MH — Marital history; menstrual history
MI — Myocardial infarction; mitral insufficiency
MIC — Minimum inhibitory concentration
MJT — Mead Johnson tube
ML — Midline
MOM — Milk of Magnesia
MS — morphine sulfate; multiple sclerosis; mitral stenosis
MSL — Midsternal line

N — Normal; Negro
NAD — No acute distress; no apparent distress
NG — Nasogastric
NM — Neuromuscular
NPN — Nonprotein nitrogen
NPO — Nothing by mouth
NR — No refill
NS — Normal saline
NSFTD — Normal spontaneous full-term delivery
NSR — Normal sinus rhythm
NTG — Nitroglycerin
NVD — Nausea, vomiting, diarrhea; neck vein distension
NYD — Not yet diagnosed

O₂ — Oxygen
O — Objective data (POMR)
OB — Obstetrics; occult blood
OOB — Out of bed
OOBBRP — Out of bed with bathroom privileges
OD — Overdose
OR — Operating room
OT — Occupational therapy

P — Plan (POMR), pulse
P & A — Palpation and auscultation
PA — Posteroanterior
PAT — Paroxysmal atrial tachycardia
PBI — Protein-bound iodine
PC — After meals
PCN — Penicillin
PCV — Packed cell volume (hematocrit)
PE — Physical examination
PEEP — Positive end expiratory pressure
PEG — Pneumoencephalogram
PERRLA — Pupils equal, round, react to light and accommodation
PH — Past history
PI — Present illness
PID — Pelvic inflammatory disease
PIE — Pulmonary infiltration with eosinophilia
PKU — Phenylketonuria
PMH — Past medical history
PMI — Point of maximal impulse or maximum intensity
PMN — Polymorphonuclear neutrophil
PMT — Premenstrual tension
PND — Paroxysmal nocturnal dyspnea
PNX — Pneumothorax
POMR — Problem-oriented medical record

Postop	After surgery	S₂	Second heart sound	TP	Total protein; thrombophlebitis
PO	By mouth	SA	Sinoatrial	TPI	*Treponema pallidum* immobilization
PP	Postpartum; postprandial	SBE	Subacute bacterial endocarditis	TPN	Total parenteral nutrition
PPD	Purified protein derivative	SC	Subclavian, subcutaneous	TPR	Temperature, pulse, and respiration
PPL	Penicilloyl-polylysine conjugate	Sed rate	Erythrocyte sedimentation rate	TRA	To run at
P & R	Pulse and respiration	Segs	Segmented neutrophils	T-set	Tracheotomy set
Preop	Before surgery	SGOT	Serum glutamic oxaloacetic trans-	TSH	Thyroid-stimulating hormone
PT	Physical therapy; prothrombin time		aminase	TUR	Transurethral resection
PTA	Prior to admission	SGPT	Serum glutamic pyruvic transaminase	TV	*Trichomonas vaginalis*
PUD	Peptic ulcer disease	SH	Social history; serum hepatitis		
PVC	Premature ventricular contraction	SID	Sudden infant death	UA (U/A)	Urinalysis
PZI	Protamine zinc insulin	SL	Sublingual	U & C	Urethral and cervical
		SLE	Systemic lupus erythematosus	UCHD	Unusual childhood diseases
R	Respiration	SLDH	Serum lactic dehydrogenase	UGI	Upper gastrointestinal
RA	Rheumatoid arthritis; right atrium	SMA	Serial multiple analysis	URI	Upper respiratory infection
RBC	Red blood cell	SOAP	Subjective, objective, assessment	UTI	Urinary tract infection
RBF	Renal blood flow		plan (POMR)		
RCM	Right costal margin	SOB	Shortness of breath	V	Vein
RF	Rheumatoid factor	S/P	Status post	Vag hyst	Vaginal hysterectomy
RHD	Rheumatic heart disease; renal hy-	SR	Sedimentation rate (ESR)	VAH	Veterans' Administration Hospital
	pertensive disease	SSE	Saline solution enema; soapsuds	VC	Vena cava
RISA	Radioactive iodine serum albumin		enema	VCU	Voiding cystourethrogram
RLL	Right lower lobe	SSPE	Subacute sclerosing panencephalitis	VDRL	Venereal Disease Research Labora-
RLQ	Right lower quadrant	STD	Skin test dose		tories (for syphilis)
RO	Rule out	STS	Serologic test for syphilis	VF	Ventricular fibrillation
ROM	Range of motion	SVC	Superior vena cava	VMA	Vanillylmandelic acid
ROS	Review of systems; review of symp-			VP	Venous pressure
	toms	T	Temperature	VPC	Ventricular premature contraction
RPF	Renal plasma flow; relaxed pelvic	T₃	Triiodothyronine	VS	Vital signs
	floor	T₄	Thyroxin	VSD	Ventricular septal defect
RQ	Respiratory quotient	T & A	Tonsillectomy and adenoidectomy	VT	Ventricular tachycardia
RR	Recovery room; respiratory rate	TAH	Total abdominal hysterectomy		
RSR	Regular sinus rhythm	TAO	Thromboangiitis obliterans	W	White; widow
RTA	Renal tubular acidosis	TB	Tuberculosis	WBC	White blood cell; white blood count
RTN	Renal tubular necrosis	TBW	Total body water	WDWN-	Well-developed, well-nourished,
RUL	Right upper lobe	TD	Transverse diameter (of heart)	WF	white female
RUQ	Right upper quadrant	TEDS	Elastic stockings	WDWN-	Well-developed, well-nourished,
RV	Right ventricle	TIA	Transient ischemic attack	WM	white male
RVH	Right ventricular hypertrophy	TIBC	Total iron-binding capacity	WNL	Within normal limits
		TKO	To keep open	Wt	Weight
S	Subjective data (POMR)	TLC	Tender loving care		
S₁	First heart sound	TM	Tympanic membrane		

Appendix B

Prescription Abbreviations

aa, a̅a̅	of each (equal parts)	fl	fluid	q.i.d.	four times daily
a.c.	before meals	gtt	a drop	qod	every other day
ad	to; up to	h.s.	at bedtime	s̄	without
ad lib	as much as desired	o.d.	right eye	sig.	label
b.i.d.	twice daily	o.s.	left eye	ss	one-half
c̄, c	with	o.u.	both eyes	stat	at once
caps	capsules	p.c.	after meals	t.i.d.	three times daily
d	day	p.r.n.	as needed	ung	ointment
et	and	q	every	ut dict.	as directed
ext	an extract	qd	once daily		

Appendix C

Derivatives of Medical Terminology

adeno-	gland	*homo-*	same	*osteo-*	bone
adreno-	adrenal gland	*hydro-*	wet, water	*-ostomy*	opening
-algia	pain	*hystero-*	uterus	*-otomy*	into
angio-	vessel	*ileo-*	ileum	*patho-*	disease
arterio-	artery	*-itis*	inflammation	*phago-*	eat
arthro-	joint	*jejuno-*	jejunum	*phlebo-*	vein
auto-	self	*laparo-*	loin or flank	*-phobia*	fear
broncho-	bronchus	*laryngo-*	larynx	*pilo-*	hair
brachy-	short	*leuko-*	white	*-plegia*	paralysis
brady-	slow	*lipo-*	fat	*pneumo-*	lungs; air
carcino-	cancer	*litho-*	stone	*procto-*	rectum
cardio-	heart	*lympho-*	lymph	*ptosis*	fall
-cele	herniation	*macro-*	large	*pyelo-*	pelvis of kidney
-centesis	puncture	*masto-*	breast	*pyo-*	pus
chole-	bile	*medius*	middle	*rhino-*	nose
chondro-	cartilage	*megalo-*	huge	*-rrhagia*	burst forth
costo-	ribs	*meningo-*	meninges	*-rrhaphy*	suture
cranio-	head	*metra-, metro-*	uterus	*-rrhea*	flow; discharge
cysto-	bladder	*micro-*	small	*sero-*	serum
cyto-	cell	*myco-*	fungus	*splanchno-*	viscera
derma-	skin	*myelo-*	bone marrow; spinal cord	*spleno-*	spleen
diplo-	double	*myo-*	muscle	*-stasis*	stop
-ectomy	out	*necro-*	death	*stoma-*	mouth
edem-	swell	*neo-*	new	*tachy-*	fast; swift
entero-	intestines	*nephro-*	kidney	*thrombo-*	clot
erythro-	red	*neuro-*	nerve	*thyro-*	thyroid
gastro-	stomach	*oculo-*	eye	*tom-*	cut
glomerulo-	glomerulus	*oligo-*	few	*tricho-*	hair
glyco-	sweet	*-oma*	tumor	*uretero-*	ureter
hem-, hemato-	blood	*oophoro-*	ovary	*urethro-*	urethra
hepato-	liver	*orchio-, orchido-*	testes	*uro-*	urine
-hesion	joint together	*os*	mouth; bone	*vaso-*	vessel
hetero-	different	*-osis*	condition	*veno-*	vein

Appendix D

Mathematic Conversions

Abbreviations

kg = kilograms	ng = nanograms	mEq = milliequivalent
g = grams	m = meter	μm = micron
mg = milligrams	cm = centimeter	L = liter
μg = micrograms	mm = millimeter	ml = milliliter

Metric system	*Common system*

Metric system

WEIGHT

1 kilogram	= 1000 grams
1 gram	= 1000 milligrams
1 milligram	= 1000 micrograms
1 microgram	= 0.001 milligram
1 milligram	= 0.001 gram
1 gram	= 0.001 kilogram

VOLUME

1 deciliter	= 100 milliliters
1 liter	= 1000 milliliters
1 milliliter	= 0.001 liter
1 deciliter	= 0.1 liter

LENGTH

1 centimeter	= 10 millimeters
1 decimeter	= 10 centimeters
1 meter	= 10 decimeters
1 kilometer	= 1000 meters
1 millimeter	= 0.1 centimeter
1 centimeter	= 0.1 decimeter
1 decimeter	= 0.1 meter
1 meter	= 0.001 kilometer

Common system

APOTHECARY WEIGHT

1 scruple(Э)	= 20 grains (gr)
60 grains	= 1 dram (ʒ)
8 drams	= 1 ounce (ʒ)
1 ounce	= 480 grains
12 ounces	= 1 pound

AVOIRDUPOIS WEIGHT

1 ounce (oz)	= 437.5 grains
1 pound (lb)	= 16 ounces

APOTHECARY VOLUME

60 minims (ṃ)	= 1 fluidram (flʒ)
8 fluidrams	= 1 fluid ounce (flʒ)
1 fluid ounce	= 480 minims
16 fluid ounces	= 1 pint (pt)

LENGTH

12 inches	= 1 foot
36 inches	= 1 yard
3 feet	= 1 yard
5280 feet	= 1 mile
1760 yards	= 1 mile

Metric and common system equivalents

MILLIGRAMS	GRAMS	GRAINS		
			1 gram	= 15.4 grains
			1 grain	= 64.8 milligrams
.1	.0001	1/600	1 ounce (ʒ)	= 31.1 grams
.2	.0002	1/300	1 ounce (oz)	= 28.3 grams
.3	.0003	1/200	1 pound (lb)	= 453.6 grams
.4	.0004	1/150	1 kilogram (kg)	= 2.2 pounds
.5	.0005	1/120	1 milliliter (ml)	= 16.23 minims
.6	.0006	1/100	1 minim (ṃ)	= 0.06 ml
1.0	.001	1/60	1 fluid ounce (flʒ)	= 29.5 ml
2.0	.002	1/30	1 pint	= 473 ml
10	.01	1/6	1 meter	= 39.3 inches
15	.015	1/4	1 kilometer	= .6 mile
30	.03	1/2	1 mile	= 1.6 mile
45	.045	3/4	1 inch	= 2.54 cm
60 (65)	.06	1	1 foot	= 30 cm
300 (330)	.3	5	1 yard	= .9 meter
600 (650)	.6	10		
1000	1.0	15		
2000	2.0	30		
3000	3.0	45		

Approximate household measurements

1 teaspoonful		5 ml
1 dessertspoonful		10 ml
1 tablespoonful	½ fl oz	15 ml
1 jigger	1½ fl oz	45 ml
1 wineglassful	2 fl oz	60 ml
1 teacupful	4 fl oz	120 ml
1 glassful (tumblerful)	8 fl oz	240 ml

Appendix E

Formulas for the Calculation of Infants' and Children's Dosages

CHILDREN'S DOSAGES

Bastedo's rule:

$$\text{Child's approximate dose} = \frac{\text{age in years} + 3}{30} \times \text{adult dose}$$

Clark's rule:

$$\text{Child's approximate dose} = \frac{\text{weight of child (lb)}}{150} \times \text{adult dose}$$

Cowling's rule:

$$\text{Child's approximate dose} = \frac{\text{age (on next birthday)}}{24} \times \text{adult dose}$$

Dilling's rule:

$$\text{Child's approximate dose} = \frac{\text{age (in years)}}{20} \times \text{adult dose}$$

Young's rule:

$$\text{Child's approximate dose} = \frac{\text{age of child (in years)}}{\text{age} + 12} \times \text{adult dose}$$

INFANTS' DOSAGES (YOUNGER THAN 1 YEAR OF AGE)

Fried's rule:

$$\text{Infant dose} = \frac{\text{age (in months)}}{150} \times \text{adult dose}$$

Appendix F

Weight Conversion Table

lb	kg	lb	kg	lb	kg
5	2.3	105	47.7	210	95.5
10	4.5	110	50	220	100
15	6.8	115	52.3	230	104.5
20	9.1	120	54.5	240	109
25	11.4	125	56.8	250	113.6
30	13.6	130	59	260	118.2
35	15.9	135	61.4	270	122.7
40	18.1	140	63.6	280	127.2
45	20.4	145	66	290	131.8
50	22.7	150	68.1	300	136.4
55	25	155	70.5	310	140.9
60	27.3	160	72.7	320	145.5
65	29.5	165	75	330	150
70	31.8	170	77.3	340	154.5
75	34.1	175	79.5	350	159
80	36.4	180	81.8	360	163.6
85	38.6	185	84.1	370	168.2
90	40.9	190	86.4	380	172.7
95	43.2	195	88.6	390	177.2
100	45.4	200	90.9	400	181.8

1 lb = 0.454 kg; 1 kg = 2.2 lb

Appendix G

Temperature Conversion Table

F	C	F	C	F	C
95.0	35.0	98.4	36.9	101.8	38.7
.2	35.1	.6	37.0	102.0	38.8
.4	35.2	.8	37.1	.2	38.9
.6	35.3	99.0	37.2	.4	39.1
.8	35.4	.2	37.3	.6	39.2
96.0	35.5	.4	37.4	.8	39.3
.2	35.6	.6	37.5	103.0	39.4
.4	35.7	.8	37.6	.2	39.5
.6	35.9	100.0	37.7	.4	39.6
.8	36.0	.2	37.8	.6	39.7
97.0	36.1	.4	37.9	.8	39.8
.2	36.2	.6	38.1	104.0	40.0
.4	36.3	.8	38.2	.2	40.1
.6	36.4	101.0	38.3	.4	40.2
.8	36.5	.2	38.4	.6	40.3
98.0	36.6	.4	38.5	.8	40.4
.2	36.7	.6	38.6	105.0	40.5

$C° = \frac{5}{9}(F° - 32°); F° = \frac{9}{5}C° + 32°$

Appendix H

Nomogram for Calculating the Body Surface Area of Adults and Children

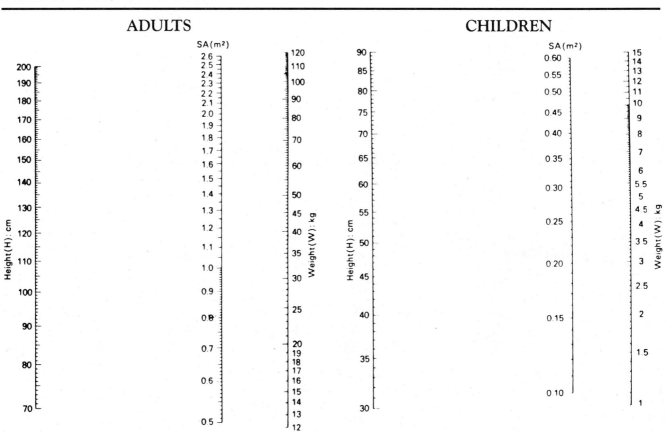

Align a ruler with the height and weight. The point at which the center line is intersected gives the corresponding value for surface area (SA). (From Haycock, G. B.: *J. Pediatr.* 93:62–66, July 1978.)

Appendix I

Commonly Used Laboratory Test and Drug Values

TEST	NORMAL VALUE
Albumin, serum	Adult: 3.4–5.2 g/dl Newborn: 2.9–5.5 g/dl
Alkaline phosphatase	Adult: 15–80 units <16 yrs: <250 units
Bilirubin	Adult: Direct < 0.3 mg/dl Total < 1.2 mg/dl Newborn: Total, 24 hr: 2–6 mg/dl 48 hr: < 7 mg/dl 3–5 day: < 12 mg/dl
BUN (blood urea nitrogen)	5–22 mg/dl
Calcium	Adult: 8.4–10.4 mg/dl Birth to 1 wk: 6.5–11 mg/dl
CBC (complete blood count)	
White blood count	4000–11,000/mm^3
Hemoglobin	Males: 13–17 g/dl Females: 11.5–15.5 g/dl Newborn: 14–25 g/dl
Differential white count	
	Segs: 43–74% Bands: 0–10% Lymphocytes: 13–43% Monocytes: 2–12% Eosinophils: 0–6 % Basophils: 0–2 % Metamyelocytes: 0–1 %
Chloride, serum	95–110 mEq/L
Cholesterol	Adult, >30 yr: <300 mg/dl 17–30 yr: <270 mg/dl
Coombs test, direct	Negative
Coombs test, indirect Creatine phosphokinase (CPK)	Negative

TEST	NORMAL VALUE		
Isoenzymes	CPK3 (MM)	CPK2 (MB)	CPK1 (BB)
Adult male	<75 U	<10 U	absent
Adult female	<70 U	<10 U	absent
	(Greater than 10 CPK2 units suggests myocardial damage)		

Creatinine, serum — <1.4 mg/dl

Creatinine clearance — Males: 117 ± 20 ml/min
Females: 108 ± 20 ml/min

Dif (differential white count) — See CBC

Erythrocyte count (RBC) — Spinal fluid: none
Whole blood:
  Males: 4.4–5.8 × 106/mm^3
  Females: 3.8–5.2 × 106/mm^3

Folic acid — 3–25 ng/ml

Gamma glutamyl transpeptidase (GTT) — Adult male: 15–85 IU/L
Adult female: 5–55 IU/L

Glucose
  Plasma, fasting — 60–115 mg/dl
  Plasma, 2 hr postprandial — 60–140 mg/dl

Glucose-6-phosphate dehydrogenase (G6PD) — 7–16 U/g hemoglobin

Hematocrit — Males: 37–51%
Females: 35–46%

Hemoglobin — See CBC

Iron, serum — Adult: 50–190 µg/dl

Iron binding capacity, total (TIBC) — Adult: 230–400 µg/dl

Lactic dehydrogenase (LDH)
  Serum — Adult: 0–110 units
  Cardiac Isoenzyme — 0–40 units
  Isoenzymes — Total: 0–110 units
Fraction 1: 10–35 units
Fraction 2: 20–55 units
Fraction 3: 5–18 units
Fraction 4: 0–10 units
Fraction 5: 0–14 units

Magnesium, serum — Adults: 1.6–2.4 mg/dl
Newborn: 1.7–3.0 mg/dl

Mean corpuscular hemoglobin (MCH) — 27–33 µg

Mean corpuscular hemoglobin concentration (MCHC) — 32–36%

Mean corpuscular volume (MCV) — 82–98 cubic microns (µm^3)

Occult blood
  Urine — Negative
  Stool — Negative

Partial thromboplastin time (PTT) — 25–37 sec

Potassium, serum — Adult: 3.5–4.7 mEq/liter
Newborn: 4.0–7.5 mEq/liter

TEST	NORMAL VALUE
Prothrombin time (PT)	9–12 sec
Red blood cell count (RBC)	See erythrocyte count
Reticulocyte count	Adults: 0.4–2.7% Newborn: 2–6%
Sedimentation rate	Male: 0–13 mm/hr Female: 0–24 mm/hr
SGOT	Adult: <25 units
SGPT	<30 units
Sodium, serum	135–145 mEq/liter
T_3 Serum (RIA)	80–170 ng/dl
T_3 Uptake (thyrobinding index)	35–46% uptake
T_4 (thyroxine)	> 1 yr: 5–12 μg/dl
T_7, Free thyroxine index	1.7–4.5
Thyroid stimulating hormone (TSH)	2–10 μIU/ml
Urea nitrogen, serum	See BUN
Uric acid	Males: 2–7.5 mg/dl Females: 1.4–6.6 mg/dl

Urinalysis, routine	Male	Female
Protein	neg	neg
Glucose	neg	neg
Ketone	neg	neg
Occult blood	neg	neg
Epith cells/LPF	Rare	Rare-mod
RBC/HPF	<3	<3
WBC/HPF	<15	<5
Casts/LPF	<3 hyaline and/or granular	
Bacteria/HPF	Rare	Rare-mod

White blood cell count (leukocyte)	
Spinal fluid	Adult: 0–8 mononuclear cells/mm³ 0 polymorphonuclear cells
Whole blood	4000–11,000/mm³

DRUG	THERAPEUTIC LEVEL
Alcohol	Negative
Aminophylline	See Theophylline
Carbamazepine (Tegretol)	8–12 μg/ml
Digitoxin (Purodigin)	9–25 ng/ml
Digoxin (Lanoxin)	Adult: 1.0–2.0 ng/ml
Dilantin	See Phenytoin
Ethosuximide (Zarontin)	40–100 μg/ml
Gentamicin (Garamycin)	Peak level: 4–12 μg/ml Trough level: <2 μg/ml
Lidocaine (Xylocaine)	1.2–5 μg/ml
Lithium	0.6–1.2 mEq/liter
Phenobarbital	15–40 μg/ml
Phenytoin (Dilantin)	10–20 μg/ml

DRUG	THERAPEUTIC LEVEL
Primidone (Mysoline)	5–12 μg/ml
Propranolol (Inderal)	50–100 ng/ml
Quinidine	2–4 μg/ml
Salicylate	2–29 mg/dl
Theophylline	Adult: 10–20 μg/ml Newborn: 6–11 μg/ml
Tobramycin (Nebcin)	Peak level: 4–10 μg/ml Trough level: <2 μg/ml
Valproic acid (Depakene)	50–120 μg/ml

Appendix J

Directory of United States and Canadian Poison Control Services (1983)

STATE, TERRITORY, OR PROVINCE	ADDRESS	PHONE
Alabama	Department of Public Health Montgomery, AL 36117	(205) 832-3194 (205) 832-3935
Alaska	Department of Health and Social Services Juneau, AK 99811	(907) 465-3100
Arizona	Arizona Poison Control System University of Arizona College of Pharmacy Tucson, AZ 87524	(602) 626-6016 (800) 362-0101 (Statewide)
Arkansas	Division of Environmental Health Protection Arkansas Department of Health Little Rock, AR 72201	(501) 661-2301
California	Emergency Medical Services Authority 1600 Ninth St, Room 460 Sacramento, CA 95814	(916) 322-4336
Colorado	Department of Health Emergency Medical Services Division 4210 E 11th Avenue Denver, CO 08220	(303) 320-8476
Connecticut	University of Connecticut Health Center Farmington, CT 06032	(203) 674-3456
Delaware	Wilmington Medical Center Delaware Division Wilmington, DE 19801	(302) 655-3389
District of Columbia	Department of Human Services Washington, DC 20009	(202) 673-6741 (202) 673-6736
Florida	Department of Health and Rehabilitative Services Office of Emergency Medical Services Tallahassee, FL 32301	(904) 487-1566

STATE, TERRITORY, OR PROVINCE	ADDRESS	PHONE
Georgia	Department of Human Resources Emergency Health Section Atlanta, GA 30303	(404) 894-5170
Guam	Guam Memorial Hospital PO Box AX Agana, Guam 96910	646-5801
Hawaii	Department of Health Honolulu, HI 96801	(808) 531-7776
Idaho	Department of Health and Welfare Boise, ID 83720	(208) 334-4245
Illinois	Division of Emergency Medical Services & Highway Safety Springfield, IL 62761	(217) 785-2080
Indiana	Indiana State Board of Health Hazardous Products Section and Division of Drug Control PO Box 1964 Indianapolis, IN 46206	(317) 633-0332
Iowa	Department of Health Des Moines, IA 50319	(515) 281-4964
Kansas	Kansas Department of Health and Environment Bureau of Food and Drug Forbes Field Topeka, KS 66620	(913) 862-9360 Ext. 541
Kentucky	Department for Human Resources Frankfort, KY 40601	(502) 564-3970
Louisiana	LSU Poison Control & Drug Abuse Information Center Louisiana State University PO Box 33932 Shreveport, LA 71130	(318) 425-1524
Maine	Maine Poison Control Center Portland, ME 04102	(207) 871-2950
Maryland	Maryland Poison Center University of Maryland School of Pharmacy Baltimore, MD 21201	(301) 528-7604 (Statewide)
Massachusetts	Department of Public Health Boston, MA 02111	(617) 727-2700
Michigan	Department of Public Health Emergency Medical Services Lansing, MI 48909	(517) 373-1406
Minnesota	EMS Section Minnesota Department of Health 717 Delaware Street SE Minneapolis, MN 55404	(612) 623-5284
Mississippi	State Board of Health Jackson, MS 39205	(601) 354-7660
Missouri	Bureau of EMS Missouri Division of Health Jefferson City, MO 65102	(314) 751-2713

STATE, TERRITORY, OR PROVINCE	ADDRESS	PHONE
Montana	Department of Health and Environmental Sciences Helena, MT 59620	(406) 449-3895
Nebraska	Department of Health Lincoln, NE 68502	(402) 471-2122
Nevada	Department of Human Resources Carson City, NV 89710	(702) 885-4750
New Hampshire	New Hampshire Poison Center Dartmouth-Hitchcock Medical Center 2 Maynard St Hanover, NH 03756	(603) 646-5000 (800) 562-8236 (Statewide)
New Jersey	Department of Health Accident Prevention and Poison Control Program Trenton, NJ 08625	(609) 292-5666
New Mexico	New Mexico Poison Drug Information & Medical Center University of New Mexico Albuquerque, NM 87131	(505) 843-2551 (800) 432-6866 (Statewide)
New York	Department of Health Albany, NY 12237	(518) 474-3785
North Carolina	Duke University Medical Center Durham, NC 27710	(919) 684-8111 (800) 672-1697 (Statewide)
North Dakota	Department of Health Bismarck, ND 58505	(701) 224-2388
Ohio	Department of Health Columbus, OH 43216	(614) 466-5190
Oklahoma	Oklahoma Poison Control Center Oklahoma Children's Memorial Hospital PO Box 26307 Oklahoma City, OK 73126	(405) 271-5454 (800) 522-4611 (Statewide)
Oregon	Oregon Poison Control and Drug Information Center University of Oregon Health Sciences Center Portland, OR 97201	(503) 225-8968 (800) 452-7165 (Statewide)
Panama	USA MEDDAC Panama Gorgas US Army Hospital Ancon, Panama APO Miami 34004	(507) 252-7500
Pennsylvania	Director, Division of Drugs, Devices and Cosmetics Department of Health PO Box 90 Harrisburg, PA 17108	(717) 787-2307
Puerto Rico	University of Puerto Rico Rio Piedras, PR	(809) 765-4880 (809) 765-0615
Rhode Island	Rhode Island Poison Center Rhode Island Hospital 593 Eddy Street Providence, RI 02902	(401) 277-5727

STATE, TERRITORY, OR PROVINCE	ADDRESS	PHONE
South Carolina	Department of Health and Environmental Control Columbia, SC 29201	(803) 758-5654
South Dakota	Department of Health Pierre, SD 57501	(605) 773-3361
Tennessee	Department of Public Health Division of Emergency Services Nashville, TN 37216	(615) 741-2407
Texas	Texas Department of Health Division of Occupational Health Austin, TX 78756	(512) 458-7254
Utah	Utah Department of Health Division of Family Health Services Salt Lake City, UT 84113	(801) 533-6161
Vermont	Department of Health Burlington, VT 05401	(802) 862-5701
Virginia	Division of Emergency Medical Services Room 1102 109 Governor Street Richmond, VA 23219	(804) 786-5188
Virgin Islands	Department of Health St Thomas, VI 00801	(809) 774-6097 (809) 774-0117
Washington	Department of Social and Health Services Seattle, WA 98115	(206) 522-7478
West Virginia	The West Virginia Poison System West Virginia University School of Pharmacy 3110 MacCorkle Ave SE Charleston, WV 25304	(304) 348-4211 (800) 642-3625 (Statewide)
Wisconsin	Department of Health and Social Services Division of Health Madison, WI 53701	(608) 267-7174
Wyoming	Office of Emergency Medical Services Department of Health and Social Services Cheyenne, WY 82002	(307) 777-7955

CANADA

Alberta	Calgary General Hospital 841 Centre Ave, E Calgary, Alberta T2E 0A1	(403) 262-5982
	Royal Alexandria Hospital 10240 Kingsway Avenue Edmonton, Alberta T5H 3V9	(403) 474-3431
British Columbia	BC Drug and Poison Information Centre St Paul's Hospital 1081 Burrard St Vancouver, British Columbia V6X 1Y6	(604) 682-5050

STATE, TERRITORY, OR PROVINCE	ADDRESS	PHONE
	Emergency Department Royal Jubilee Hospital Poison Control Centre 1900 Forte St Victoria, British Columbia V8R 1J8	(604) 595-9212
Manitoba	Health Sciences Children's Centre 685 Bannatyne Avenue Winnipeg, Manitoba R3E 0W1	(204) 787-2444
New Brunswick	Dr Everett Chalmers Hospital Poison Control Centre Box 9000 Fredericton, Nova Scotia E3B 5N5	(506) 452-5400
Newfoundland and Labrador	Provincial Poison Control Centre The Dr Charles A Janeway Child Health Centre Newfoundland Drive St John's, Newfoundland 81A 1R8	(709) 722-1110
Nova Scotia	The Izaak Walton Killam Hospital for Children Poison Control Centre PO Box 3070 Halifax, Nova Scotia B3J 3G9	(902) 424-6161
Ontario	Hospital for Sick Children Poison Control Centre 401 Smythe Road Ottawa, Ontario K1H 8L1	(416) 598-5900 (800) 268-9017
Ontario	Children's Hospital of Eastern Ontario Poison Control Centre 555 Univero Avenue Toronto, Ontario M5G 1X8	(613) 521-4040 (800) 267-1373
Prince Edward Island	Queen Elizabeth Hospital PO Box 6600 Riverside Drive Charlottetown, PEI C1A 8T5	(902) 566-6250
Quebec	Hôpital Sainte-Justine Poison Control Centre 3175 St Catherine Road Montreal, Quebec H3T 1C5	(514) 731-4931
	Central Hospitalier del'Université Laval 2705 Laurier Blvd. Ste. Foy Quebec City, Quebec 61V 4G2	(418) 656-8090
Saskatchewan	Regina General Hospital Poison Control Centre Regina, Saskatchewan S4P 0W5	(306) 359-4545
	Saskatoon University Hospital Poison Control Centre Saskatoon, Saskatchewan S7N 0W0	(306) 343-3323

(Adapted from *Directory of United States Poison Control Centers and Services, 1983.* Rockville, Md, US Department of Health and Human Services, 1983.)

Appendix K

Sodium, Potassium, and Caloric Content of Selected Foods

FOOD	PORTION	CALORIES	POTASSIUM	SODIUM
Fruits			(mg)	(mg)
Apricots, fresh	3	55	301	1
Apricots, large, dried	10 halves	125	470	12
Banana, large	1 large	116	503	1
Breadfruit, raw	3½ oz	103	439	15
Cantaloupe, medium	¼ melon	41	341	17
Casaba, medium	⅒ melon	40	351	17
Dates, dried	10	219	518	1
Elderberries, raw	3½ oz	72	300	—
Figs, dried	7–10	274	640	34
Grapefruit, medium	1 whole	82	270	2
Honeydew, medium	⅒ melon	40	351	17
Lychees, dried	3½ oz	277	1100	—
Orange, 3″ diam. size #72	1 large	87	333	2
Papaya, 1 lb medium	1 whole	119	711	7
Peaches, dried	5	170	618	11
Prunes, cooked dried	½ c	126	347	4
Prunes, pitted uncooked	10	260	708	8
Raisins, dried	½ c	268	553	18
Watermelon, slice	1	108	454	5
Fruit juice				
Apricot nectar	1 c	143	379	trace
Blackberry juice	1 c	74	340	2
Grapefruit juice	1 c	84	324	2
Orange-grapefruit juice	1 c	86	364	2
Orange juice	1 c	112	496	2
Pineapple juice	1 c	138	373	3
Prune juice	1 c	197	602	5
Tangerine juice	1 c	106	440	2
Meat and fish (unsalted)				
Beef meat, cooked	3½ oz	245	370	60
Chicken and turkey (light meat)	3½ oz	182	422	66
Flounder, cooked (baked with margarine)	4 oz	228	664	268
Halibut, cooked	4 oz	192	596	152
Rockfish, steamed	4 oz	120	504	76
Nuts and seeds (unsalted)				
Almonds, whole shelled	½ c	425	549	3
Brazil nuts, whole shelled	½ c	458	500	1

FOOD	PORTION	CALORIES	POTASSIUM	SODIUM
Cashew nuts	½ c	392	325	11
Hazel nuts, whole shelled	½ c	428	475	1
Peanuts, unsalted shelled	⅓ c	332	382	3
Pecans, whole shelled	½ c	371	326	1
Sunflower seeds, hulled	½ c	406	667	22
Milk				
Milk, nonfat	1 c	89	355	127
Vegetables (unsalted)				
Avocado, raw medium	½	188	680	5
Bamboo shoots, raw	1 c	41	806	—
Beans, baby lima cooked	1 c	118	394	129
Beans, lima frozen cooked	½ c	111	426	101
Beans, red cooked	½ c	118	340	3
Beans, soy cooked	1 c	234	972	4
Beans, white cooked	½ c	118	416	7
Chard, Swiss cooked	1 c	26	465	125
Collards	1 c	63	498	—
Cress, garden cooked	1 c	31	477	11
Mustard greens	1 c	32	308	25
Okra, cooked	1 c	70	303	4
Parsnips, cooked	1 c	139	587	12
Peas, black eye, frozen cooked	1 c	210	619	80
Peppers, green raw	1 whole	36	349	21
Potato, baked	1 medium	122	536	4
Potato, baked, with skin	1 medium	145	782	6
Spinach, cooked New Zealand	1 c	23	833	166
Spinach, frozen cooked	1 c	47	683	107
Split peas, cooked	1 c	230	592	26
Squash, butternut, baked, mashed	1 c	139	1248	2
Squash, Hubbard baked	1 c	103	556	2
Tomato juice	1 c	46	552	486
Tomatoes, canned	1 c	51	523	313
Tomatoes, fresh	1	27	300	4
Turnips, frozen, drained	1 c	38	246	28
Turnips, green, canned with liquid	1 c	42	564	548
Miscellaneous				
Molasses, blackstrap	1 T	43	585	19
Salt substitute	¼ t		500	

In general potassium values for all foods are higher for raw than for cooked, as soaking and/or cooking in water tends to reduce K$^+$ unless the cooking water is used.

c = cup, T = tablespoon, t = teaspoon

(Adapted from McRae, P. M.: Foods high in potassium. *Hospital Pharmacy* 14:730–1, 1979.)

Appendix L

Template for Developing a Written Record for Patients to Monitor Their Own Therapy

(Physicians, pharmacists, nurses, and other health practitioners are given permission to reproduce a limited number of this template for direct distribution, without charge, to their patients to aid in monitoring therapy.)

Medications	Color	To be taken

Name _____

Physician _____

Physician's phone _____

Next appt.* _____

Parameters	Day of discharge							Comments

*Please bring this record with you to your next appointment.
Use the back of this sheet for additional information.

555

Bibliography

Abrams, A. C., et al.: *Clinical Drug Therapy*. New York, J. B. Lippincott Co., 1983.

Anderson, L., et al.: *Nutrition in Health and Disease*, ed. 17. Philadelphia, J. B. Lippincott Co., 1982.

Barry, P. D.: *Psychosocial Nursing Assessment and Intervention*. Philadelphia, J. B. Lippincott Co., 1984.

Beardsley, R. S., et al.: Elder-ed: Consumer drug education to older persons. *American Journal of Pharmacological Education* 45(2):36–39, 1981.

Billups, N. F.: *American Drug Index*, ed. 23. Philadelphia, J. B. Lippincott Co., 1984.

Billings, D. M., and Stokes, L. G.: *Medical-Surgical Nursing: Common Health Problems of Adults and Children Across the Life Span*. St. Louis, The C. V. Mosby Co., 1982.

Centers for Disease Control: *Morbidity and Mortality Weekly Reports* 32:2–16, 1983.

Chyun, D. A.: Intravenous nitroglycerin in ischemic heart disease. *Dimensions of Critical Care Nursing* 2(1):10–22, 1983.

Cibulskis, M. M.: *Essentials of Pharmacology*. Philadelphia, J. B. Lippincott Co., 1982.

Clark, J. B., et al.: *Pharmacological Basis of Nursing Practice*. St. Louis, The C. V. Mosby Co., 1982.

Clayton, B. D.: *Handbook of Pharmacology in Nursing*, ed. 3. St. Louis, The C. V. Mosby Co., 1984.

Conley, S. K., and Small, R. E.: Administering IV nitroglycerin—Nursing implications. *Dimensions of Critical Care Nursing* 2(1):18–19, 1983.

DeAngelis, R., and Brot, W. H.: The "Factor 15" method. *Dimensions of Critical Care Nursing* 1(6):334–337, 1982.

DeLand, L. A.: The patient care unit, in Blissitt, C. W., et al., eds.: *Clinical Pharmacy Practice*. Philadelphia, Lea & Febiger, 1972.

Directory of United States Poison Control Centers and Services, 1983. Rockville, Md., U.S. Department of Health and Human Services, 1983.

Evaluations of Drug Interactions, ed. 2. Washington, D.C., American Pharmaceutical Association, 1976.

Garrison, T. J.: Medication distribution systems, in Smith, M. C., and Brown, T. R., eds.: *Handbook of Institutional Practice*. Baltimore, Williams & Wilkins Co., 1979.

Goodman, L. S., and Gilman, A., eds.: *The Pharmacological Basis of Therapeutics*, ed. 6. New York, Macmillan, Inc., 1980.

Guyton, A. C.: *Textbook of Medical Physiology*, ed. 6, Philadelphia, W. B. Saunders Co., 1981.

Hahn, A. B., et al.: *Pharmacology in Nursing*, ed. 15. St. Louis, The C. V. Mosby Co., 1982.

Hansten, P. D.: *Drug Interactions*, ed. 4. Philadelphia, Lea & Febiger, 1979.

Hansten, P. D., ed.: *Drug Interactions Newsletter*. San Francisco, Applied Therapeutics, Inc., 1981–84.

Hatcher, R. A., et al.: *Contraceptive Technology, 1982–83*, ed. 11. New York, Irvington Publishers, 1982.

Hill, M., and Fink, J. W.: In hypertensive emergencies act quickly but also act cautiously. *Nursing 83* 13(2):34–41, 1983.

Jacobsen, M. F.: The caffeine catch. *Family Health* 3:20–23, 1981.

Jones, D. A., et al.: *Medical Surgical Nursing, a Conceptual Approach*, ed. 2. New York, McGraw-Hill Book Co., 1982.

Jones, D. A., et al.: *Health Assessment Across the Life Span*. New York, McGraw-Hill Book Co., 1984.

Kastrup, E. K., and Boyd, J. R., eds.: *Facts and Comparisons*. St. Louis, Facts and Comparisons, Inc., 1984.

Katcher, B., et al., eds.: *Applied Therapeutics*, ed. 3. San Francisco, Applied Therapeutics, Inc., 1983.

Keenan, P. A.: The "key number" conversion method. *Dimensions of Critical Care Nursing* 1(6):332–333, 1982.

Kirschenbaum, H. L., and Rosenberg, J. M.: Hydralazine and minoxidil. *R.N.* 45(12):42–43, 1982.

Kreigh, H. Z., and Perko, J. E.: *Psychiatric and Mental Health Nursing: A Commitment to Care and Concern*. Reston, Va., Reston Publishing Company, Inc., 1983.

Kozier, B., and Erb, G.: *Fundamentals of Nursing*, ed. 2. Menlo Park, Addison-Wesley Publishing Co., Inc., 1983.

Kozier, B., and Erb, G.: *Techniques in Clinical Nursing, a Comprehensive Approach*. Menlo Park, Addison-Wesley Publishing Company, Inc., 1983.

Levine, R. R.: *Pharmacology, Drug Actions, and Reactions*. Boston, Little, Brown and Co., 1973.

Lindberg, J.: *Introduction to Person-centered Nursing*. Philadelphia, J. B. Lippincott Co., 1983.

Loebl, S., et al.: *The Nurse's Drug Handbook*, ed. 3. New York, John Wiley & Sons, Inc., 1983.

Malseed, R.: *Quick Reference to Drug Therapy and Nursing Considerations*. Philadelphia, J. B. Lippincott Co., 1983.

Mangini, R. J., ed.: *Drug Interaction Facts*. St. Louis, Facts and Comparisons, Inc., 1984.

Marra, S., et al.: Acute effects of chewable nifedipine on hemodynamic responses to upright exercise in patients with prior myocardial infarction and effort angina. *Chest* 83(1):50–55, 1983.

Medical Letter. New Rochelle, N.Y., The Medical Letter, Inc., 1984.

McEvoy, G., ed.: *American Hospital Formulary Service*. Washington, D.C., American Society of Hospital Pharmacists, Inc., 1983.

Nemchik, R.: The news about insulin. *R.N.* 45(12):49–54, 1982.

Nemchik, R.: The new insulin pumps: Tight control at a price. *R.N.* 46(5):52–59, 1983.

Oppeneer, J. E., and Vervoeen, T. M.: *Gerontological Pharmacology*, *a Resource for Health Practitioners.* St. Louis, The C. V. Mosby Co., 1983.

Pagliaro, L. A.: *Pharmacologic Aspects of Aging.* St. Louis, The C. V. Mosby Co., 1983.

Pagliaro, L. A., et al.: *Pediatric Drug Therapy.* Hamilton, Ill., Drug Intelligence Publications, Inc., 1979.

Phipps, W. J., et al.: *Medical-Surgical Nursing: Concepts and Clinical Practice,* ed. 2. St. Louis, The C. V. Mosby Co., 1983.

Physician's Desk Reference. Oradell, N.J., Medical Economics Co., 1984.

Ray, O.: *Drugs, Society and Human Behavior,* ed. 3. St. Louis, The C. V. Mosby Co., 1983.

Reeder, S. J., et al.: *Maternity Nursing,* ed. 15. Philadelphia, J. B. Lippincott Co., 1983.

Reiss, B. S., and Melick, M. E.: *Pharmacological Aspects of Nursing Care.* Albany, Delmar Publishers, Inc., 1984.

Rodman, M. J., and Smith, D. W.: *Pharmacology and Drug Therapy in Nursing,* ed. 2. New York, J. B. Lippincott Co., 1979.

Ronshausen, R. G.: *Quick Reference to Nursing Implications of Diagnostic Tests.* Philadelphia, J. B. Lippincott Co., 1983.

Rosenthal, K. A.: Converting micrograms/kilograms/minute to microdrops, 1. Chart vs. formula method. *Dimensions of Critical Care Nursing* 1(6):326-331, 1982.

Rossi, L. P., and Antman, E. M.: Calcium channel blockers—new treatment for cardiovascular disease. *American Journal of Nursing* 83(3):382-387, 1983.

Scherer, J. C.: *Introductory Clinical Pharmacology,* ed. 2. Philadelphia, J. B. Lippincott, Co., 1982.

Smith, D. L.: Patient education—its time has come. *American Pharmacy* NS21(7):14-19, 1981.

Smith, S., and Duell, D.: *Nursing Skills and Evaluation, a Nursing Process Approach.* Copyright 1982 by National Nursing Review, Inc. St. Louis, The C. V. Mosby Co., 1982.

Stuart, G. W., and Sundeen, S. J.: *Principles and Practices of Psychiatric Nursing,* ed. 2. St. Louis, The C. V. Mosby Co., 1983.

Tester, W. W.: Recent advances in drug distribution systems and their economic feasibility, in Franke, D. E., and Whitney, H.A.K. Jr., eds.: *Perspectives in Clinical Pharmacy.* Hamilton, Ill., Drug Intelligence Publications, 1972.

Trifiletti, P. E.: Nitroglycerin ointment application and use. *Critical Care Nurse* 2(5):46-48, 1982.

Trissel, L. A.: *Handbook on Injectable Drugs,* ed. 3. Bethesda, Md., American Society of Hospital Pharmacists, 1983.

USAN and USP *Dictionary of Drug Names.* Rockville, Md., United States Pharmacopeial Convention, Inc., 1978.

U.S. Pharmacopeia, ed. 20. Easton, Pa., The Mack Publishing Co., 1980.

U.S. Pharmacopeial Convention, Inc.: *1983 USP-DI.* St. Louis, The C. V. Mosby Co., 1983.

Weiner, M. B., et al.: *Clinical Pharmacology and Therapeutics in Nursing.* New York, McGraw-Hill Book Co., 1979.

Whaley, L. F., and Wong, D. L.: *Nursing Care of Infants and Children,* ed. 2. St. Louis, The C. V. Mosby Co., 1983.

Glossary

abruptio placentae Premature separation of the placenta from the uterus.

absorbent Medicine or substance that absorbs liquids or other secretion products; a substance that takes in, or picks up, such as a blotter that absorbs ink.

pathologic The absorption into the blood of any bodily excretion or morbid product, such as the bile or pus.

acceleration Quickening, as of the pulse rate or respiration.

accommodation Adjustment, especially that of the eye for various distances.

absolute The accommodation of either eye separately.

binocular The convergence of the two eyes so as to bring the image of the object seen on each retina.

acetylation Introduction of an acetyl group into an organic molecule.

acetylcholine Acetic acid ester of choline chloride, normally present in many parts of the body and having many important physiologic functions. For example, in the central nervous system it is for the purpose of transmission of nerve impulses. It is used subcutaneously and intravenously to relax peripheral blood vessels.

acetylcholinesterase An esterase in the blood that hydrolyzes any excess of acetylcholine, splitting it into acetic acid and choline.

achlorhydria Absence of hydrochloric acid from the gastric secretions.

acidosis Condition of lessened alkalinity in the body, caused by formation of excess amounts of acid or by lessened amounts of base.

acne Any inflammatory disease of the sebaceous glands, especially acne vulgaris, or common acne. It is chronic and commonly occurs on the chest, back, and face.

acromegaly Enlargement of the bony structure characterized by gigantism and caused by a tumor of the pituitary gland with increased secretion from the gland.

Addison's disease Disease characterized by a bronze-like pigmentation of the skin, severe prostration, progressive anemia, low blood pressure, diarrhea, and digestive disturbances. This condition is caused by lack of function of the adrenal (suprarenal) glands located on top of each kidney and by initial tuberculous infiltration (the last in less than half of the cases today). It is treated with cortisone or hydrocortisone and other hormones and a high-carbohydrate, high-protein diet.

adrenal cortex Outer layer of adrenal gland that manufactures specific hormones.

adrenal gland Gland of internal secretion situated on top of the kidney; also called the suprarenal gland.

adrenalectomy Removal of adrenal bodies.

adrenergic Activated or transmitted by epinephrine (adrenalin); a term applied to that form of autonomic nerves that acts by setting free acetylcholine from their nerve terminations.

adsorbent Substance that acts by gathering up another substance on its surface in a condensed layer.

aerobe A microorganism that can live and grow in the presence of free oxygen.

afferent Carrying, for example, of blood or impulses from the periphery to the center.

aggravate To make worse or to irritate.

aggregation Crowding or clustering together.

agranulocytopenia See *agranulocytosis*.

agranulocytosis Complete or nearly complete absence of the granular leukocytes (granulocytes) from the bone marrow and blood; also called agranulocytopenia.

albumin Protein found in nearly every animal and in many vegetable tissues and characterized by being soluble in water and coagulable by heat. It contains carbon, hydrogen, nitrogen, oxygen, and sulfur.

albumin A A certain constituent of the blood serum, reduced in amount in cancer patients but increased in cancer cells.

acetosoluble A form of albumin soluble in acetic acid; sometimes found in urine.

albuminuria The presence of albumin in the urine, indicating either a simple mixture of albuminous matters, such as blood, with the urine or a morbid state of the kidneys that is permitting albumin to pass from the blood.

alkalosis Excessive alkalinity of the body fluids; increased alkali reserve in the blood and other body tissues.

allergy Unusual reaction to a substance that in similar amounts is harmless to most persons.

alopecia Baldness, deficiency of hair, natural or abnormal.

amebiasis State of being infected with amebae.

amenorrhea Absence or abnormal stopping of menstrual flow.

amide Any compound derived from ammonia by substituting an acid radical for hydrogen.

amine Class of compounds derived from ammonia.

amino acids Organic acids in which one or more hydrogen atoms have been replaced by the amino group NH_2. The amino acids are the building blocks of the protein molecule and the end product of protein digestion.

anabolism, anabolic To build up; any constructive process by which simple substances are converted by living cells into more complex compounds; constructive metabolism and assimilation.

anaerobe Any microorganism having the power to live without either air or free oxygen.

analeptic Restorative medicine or agent. Central nervous system stimulants used to antagonize depressant drugs are called analeptics; they restore consciousness and mental alertness.

analgesic Medication to relieve pain, such as aspirin or morphine.

analogue Part or organ having the same function as another, but of a different structure.

analogy Resemblance in structure caused by similarity of function.

anaphylaxis Unusual or exaggerated reaction of an organism or individual to foreign proteins or other substances. These reactions are immediate, shock-like, and frequently fatal within minutes. They include symptoms such as apprehension, burning, prickling sensations, generalized urticaria or hives, edema, choking sensation, cyanosis, wheezing, cough, incontinence, shock, fever, dilation of pupils, loss of consciousness, and convulsions. Reaction to penicillin is an example. Emergency drugs should always be available whenever injections are administered.

androgen Male sex hormones.

anemia Insufficient blood cells or iron.

anesthetic Drug causing a temporary loss of sensation.

angina pectoris Severe, cramp-like pain of the chest, caused by insufficient circulation and characterized by spasms of the muscles of the coronary arteries surrounding and entering the heart.

angioneurotic edema Giant hives characterized by large wheals or pinkish elevations similar to hives on the skin, with marked itching, nausea, fever, and malaise; generally caused by sensitivity to a food or foods.

anhydrase An enzyme that catalyzes anhydration.

carbonic An enzyme that catalyzes the release of carbon dioxide from the blood in the tissues and the lungs.

anion Ion carrying a negative charge. They include all the non-metals, the acid radicals, and the hydroxyl ion.

anomalies *(anomaly)* Marked deviations from the normal standard.

anorexia Lack or loss of appetite for food.

anthelmintic Agent to destroy worms.

anthrax Carbuncle or other infection caused by the anthrax bacillus.

malignant A fatal infectious disease of cattle and sheep caused by the anthrax bacillus and characterized by formation of hard edema or ulcers at the point of inoculation and by collapse symptoms. It may occur in humans.

anti Against.

antibiotic Against life.

antibiotics Medications used to kill living microorganisms that cause infection.

antibodies Substances in the body that react with a specific antigen. They may be present under apparently normal conditions but develop anew in response to the introduction of specific antigen into the tissues or blood. Antibodies include, among others, agglutinins, antienzymes, and antitoxins.

anticoagulant Substance used to prevent blood clotting.

antiemetic Arresting or preventing emesis or vomiting, relieving nausea.

antigen Any substance that will lead to the development of antibodies.

antihistamine Agent given to neutralize histamine produced by the body.

antipyretic Relieving fever; cooling.

antiseptic Drug that tends to prevent or lessen the activity of infection by slowing the growth of microorganisms.

antispasmodic Agent used in relieving muscular contractions, spasms, and convulsions.

antitoxin Serum used to lessen the effects of the toxins or poisons produced by bacteria.

antitussive Relieving or preventing cough.

anuria, anuresis Absolute suppression of urinary secretion.

apical pulse Heartbeat taken with a stethoscope, the bell or disc of the stethoscope being placed over the apex or pointed extremity of the heart.

aplastic anemia Rare condition in which the bone marrow cells cease to produce leukocytes in sufficient amounts to compensate for their destruction.

apnea The transient cessation of breathing that follows forced respiration; asphyxia.

apoplexy Stroke or paralysis caused by rupture of a blood vessel.

apothecary Druggist or pharmacist.

appendicitis Inflammation of the appendix.

appetite Hunger, natural longing, or desire, especially for food.

aqueous humor Fluid filling the anterior and posterior chambers of the eye in front of the lens.

arrhythmia Any variation from the normal rhythm of the heartbeat; irregularities. Some various forms of arrhythmias include sinus arrhythmia, extrasystole, heart block, auricular fibrillation, auricular flutter, and paroxysmal tachycardia.

arteriole Any minute arterial branch.

arteriosclerosis Scarring or hardening of the arteries that results from disease of the arterial walls.

obliterans Proliferation of the intima, or innermost of the three coats of the artery, causing complete obliteration or closing of the lumen of the artery.

arthralgia Neuralgia or pain in a joint.

arthritis Rheumatism characterized by symptoms such as pain, swelling, inflammation, and stiffness of joints.

ascites Accumulation of serous fluid in the peritoneal cavity; dropsy of the abdominal cavity; painless swelling of the abdomen that gives a dull sound on percussion. Causes include local inflammation of the peritoneum and obstruction of the venous circulation by disease of the heart, kidney, or liver.

asphyxia Suffocation or a deficiency of oxygen in the blood.

neonatorum Suffocation in the newborn.

asthma Disease of the bronchi, with difficulty and shortness of breath; often caused by allergies.

asystole Imperfect or incomplete systole; inability of the heart to perform a complete systole.

ataxia Failure of muscular coordination; irregularity of muscular action.

atelectasis Partial collapse of the lung; imperfect expansion of the lung in the newborn.

atherosclerosis Form of arteriosclerosis with marked degenerative changes and fatty degeneration of the connective tissue of the arterial walls.

athetosis A derangement marked by constant recurring series of slow, vermicular movements of the hands and feet, occurring chiefly in children and resulting principally from a brain lesion.

athlete's foot Ringworm of the feet; fungus infection.

atonic Characterized by lack of normal tone, for example, lack of muscle tone.

atrioventricular heart block A blocking at the atrioventricular or auriculoventricular junction (the auricles and ventricles beat independently of each other).

atrium See *auricle.*

atrophy Change or degeneration in a part.

attenuation Act or process of thinning or weakening, especially the weakening of the toxicity of a virus or a microorganism by repeated inoculation and successive culture, adding an agent such as formaldehyde.

auricle Atrium of the heart; chamber at the apex of the heart on either side above the ventricle; divided into right and left auricle or atrium.

autoimmunization Immunization effected by processes within the body.

autonomic Self-governing; independent in function.

azotemia The presence of urea or other nitrogenous bodies in the blood.

chloropenic Condition characterized by deficiency of sodium chloride, fixation of chlorine in the tissues, and azoturia (excess urea and other nitrogenous bodies in the urine).

bactericidal Able to kill bacteria.

bacteriostasis Condition in which bacteria are prevented from growing and spreading. *Bacteriostatic* is more general in its meaning than *antiseptic.*

beriberi An endemic form of polyneuritis prevalent chiefly in Japan, India, China, the Philippines, and the Malay peninsula and often fatal. Characteristic symptoms: spasmodic rigidity of the lower limbs, with muscular atrophy, paralysis, anemia, and neuralgic pains. The disease is thought to result from an almost exclusive diet of overmilled or highly polished rice or other carbohydrate food, which is deficient in the accessory food factor known as antineuritic vitamin.

bilateral Having two sides or pertaining to two sides.

biliary colic Spasm of the gallbladder, hepatic ducts, common bile duct, and cystic duct.

blepharitis Inflammation of the eyelids.

blood pressure Pressure of the blood on the wall of the arteries, dependent on the energy of the heart action, the elasticity of the walls of the arteries, the resistance in the capillaries, and the volume and the viscosity of the blood.

basic That pressure exerted on the blood by the contractile walls independent of the additional pressure caused by the systolic contraction of the heart.

diastolic The lowest arterial pressure at any one time during the cardiac cycle. It results from the recoil of the elastic walls of the aorta and arteries and the pressure this recoil exerts on the blood. It is known as the resting pressure that is being constantly exerted by the aorta and arteries and which the left ventricle must overcome before blood can be ejected into the aorta. This pressure represents the constant minimal load that the arteries must bear at all times.

pulse pressure The difference between systolic and diastolic pressures. Pulse pressure is an important indication of cardiac output and peripheral resistance shown by the width of pulse pressure. A wide pulse pressure is a normal finding if there is bradycardia, and a narrow pulse pressure is normal if there is tachycardia. In hemorrhage, systolic level may fall, but the diastolic level tends to rise. The result is a narrow pulse pressure indicating decreased cardiac output. A pulse pressure as low as 20 mm Hg or as high as 50 mm Hg is pathologic.

systolic The highest arterial pressure at any one time during the cardiac cycle. It is a combination of the ejection of blood from the ventricles during systole and the blood pushing against the elastic walls of the aorta and arteries. It is also known as the active or working pressure. Normal range is about 110 to 140 mm Hg.

blood sugar A simple sugar normally found in the blood.

bolus A rounded mass; a mass of food ready to be swallowed or a mass passing along the intestines. In pharmacy, a rounded mass larger than a pill.

botulism A type of food poisoning caused by a toxin produced by *Clostridium (Bacillus) botulinum* in improperly canned or preserved foods and characterized by vomiting, abdominal pain, disturbances of secretion, motor disturbances, dryness of the mouth and pharynx, dyspepsia, barking cough, mydriasis, paralytic drooping of the eyelid, and prolapse of other parts or organs. It requires immediate medical attention; death can often occur without treatment.

Bowman's capsule Globular dilation that forms the beginning of a uriniferous tubule within the kidney. Each nephron begins as a Bowman's capsule.

bradycardia Abnormal slowness of the heartbeat, as evidenced by slowing of the pulse rate to 60 or less.

broad-spectrum Usually refers to antibiotics and

their ability to kill a wide variety of gram-positive and gram-negative bacteria.

bronchial asthma Disease of the bronchi with difficulty and shortness of breath.

bronchiectasis Dilation of the bronchi or of a bronchus, marked by foul breath, paroxysmal coughing, and expectoration of mucopurulent matter.

bronchogenic Originating in a bronchus.

bronchoscopy Examination of the bronchi through a tracheal wound or through an instrument called a bronchoscope.

bronchus Tube-like structure leading to the lung; located between trachea, or windpipe, and lung. There is a left and right bronchus (bronchi).

brucellosis The disease produced by *Brucella*, a bacteria; undulant fever characterized by wave-like changes in fever.

buccal Pertaining to the cheek. In drug administration the mucous-membrane side of the inner cheek.

Buerger's disease Chronic inflammation of the arteries of the extremities with eventual thrombus or clot formation and blocking or occlusion of the blood vessel and gangrene.

buffer Any substance in a fluid that tends to lessen the change in hydrogen ion concentration (reaction), which otherwise would be produced by adding acids or alkalis; any substance that decreases or prevents the reaction that a chemotherapeutic agent would produce if administered alone; the action produced by a buffer.

BUN A laboratory blood: blood urea nitrogen.

Burkitt's lymphoma A rapidly progressive lymphatic tumor that occurs most commonly in the jaw, abdominal cavity, and meninges. Spontaneous regressions have been observed, and many patients are highly responsive to chemotherapy.

bursitis Inflammation of the bursae, or small sacs of tissue, some of which are found in the shoulder and knee.

caduceus Emblem of the medical profession; a wand with wings at the top and two serpents twisted around it.

calcinosis Condition marked by the disposition of calcium salts in nodules under the skin and in the muscles, tendons, nerves, and connective tissue.

Candida, candidal A genus of yeast-like fungi of the family Cryptococcaceae, various species of which have been isolated from pulmonary lesions in man.

Candida albicans A yeast-like fungus that causes an inflammation of the corners of the mouth.

Candida vulva Inflammation of the vulva or external part of the organs of generation in the female, caused by a yeast-like fungus *Candida vulva*.

capillary One of the microscopic blood vessels connecting arteries and veins.

carcinoma Malignant tumor or cancer; new growth made up of epithelial cells that tend to infiltrate and metastasize.

cardiac insufficiency Inability of the heart to perform its function properly.

cardiogenic shock Shock resulting from diminution of cardiac output in heart disease.

cardiospasm Spasm of the cardiac sphincter of the stomach.

carminative Medicine that expels gas from the stomach and intestines.

carotene Yellow pigment found in carrots, sweet potatoes, other vegetables, milk fat, body fat, and egg yolk. It may be converted in the body into vitamin A.

carotenoid Marked by a yellow color resembling that produced by carotene.

catabolism Destructive metabolism; passage of tissue material from a higher to a lower plane of complexity or specialization.

cataract An opacity of the crystalline eye lens or of its capsule.

catecholamines Dopamine, norepinephrine, and epinephrine synthesized, stored, and metabolized in the brain and affecting the central nervous system slightly and the autonomic nervous system to a greater degree.

cation Element or elements of an electrolyte that appears at the negative pole or cathode. Cations include all metals and hydrogen.

cationic See *cation*.

causalgia, causalgic Neuralgia characterized by intense local sensation, as of burning pain.

celiac disease Childhood form of sprue characterized by impaired absorption of fats, perhaps glucose, and with such symptoms as diarrhea (with bulky, pale, frothy, foul-smelling stools), weight loss, vitamin deficiencies, anemia, infantilism, tetany, rickets, and sometimes dwarfism. The disease responds to the elimination of wheat gluten from the diet, administration of oral iron for hypochromic anemia, and vitamin B_{12} for macrocytic anemia. Diet in celiac disease should be high calorie, high protein, low fat, and gluten free.

cellulitis Inflammation of the cellular tissue, especially purulent inflammation of the loose subcutaneous tissue.

cerebellum That division of the brain behind the cerebrum and above the pons and fourth ventricle; it is concerned with the coordination of movements.

cerebrum Main portion of the brain occupying the upper part of the cranium and consisting of two equal portions called hemispheres, which are united at the bottom by a mass of white matter called the corpus callosum. The cerebrum is the organ of associative memory, reasoning, and judgment.

cervix Lower, neck-like portion of the uterus.

cheilitis Inflammation of the lip.

chemoreceptor Receptor adapted for excitation by chemical substances, such as olfactory and gustatory receptors; a supposed group of atoms in cell protoplasm having the ability to fix chemicals in the same way as bacterial poisons are fixed.

chemotherapeutic agent Agent of chemical nature used in the treatment of disease.

chilblains Inflammation and swelling of the toes, feet, or fingers caused by cold.

cholestatic Resulting from stoppage of bile flow.

cholesterol Fat-like, pearly substance crystallizing in the form of leaflets or plates and found in all animal fats and oils, in bile, blood, brain tissue, milk, egg yolk, kidneys, and suprarenal bodies. It constitutes a large part of the most frequently occurring gallstones and appears in atheroma of the arteries.

cholinergic Stimulated, activated, or transmitted by choline (acetylcholine); term applied to nerve fibers whose activity is transmitted by acetylcholine; drugs that cause effects in the body similar to those produced by acetylcholine.

cholinesterase Enzyme that hydrolyzes or destroys acetylcholine.

chorea (St. Vitus' dance) Convulsive nervous disease with involuntary and irregular jerking movements and attended with irritability, depression, and mental impairment; it occurs in early age, more commonly in girls than boys, and may be hereditary.

choriocarcinoma Carcinoma (cancer) developed from the epithelium.

chorion The outermost envelope of the growing zygote or fertilized ovum that serves as a protective and nutritive covering.

cicatric, cicatrix A scar; the mark left by a sore or wound.

ciliary Pertaining to or resembling the eyelashes.

cirrhosis Disease of the liver marked by thickening, atrophy, degeneration, and a granular yellow appearance to the organ caused by coloring from bile pigments.

climacteric Time in life when the body undergoes marked changes and the reproductive organs no longer fully function; menopause.

clitoris A small, elongated, erectile body or organ of the female, situation at the anterior angle of the vulva and homologous with the penis in the male.

clonus Spasm in which there is alternate rigidity and relaxation in rapid succession.

foot A series of convulsive movements of the ankle, induced by suddenly pushing up the foot while the leg is extended.

toe Rhythmic contractions of the great toe, induced by suddenly extending the first phalanx.

wrist Spasmodic contractions of the hand muscles, induced by forcibly bending the hand backward.

Clostridium Genus of Bacillaceae that are anaerobic or microaerophilic and that form clostridial spore forms.

Clostridium oedematiens Strictly anaerobic organism isolated from war wounds in about 40% of the cases. It is gram-positive and forms large subterminal spores.

Clostridium septicum (Clostridium oedematis maligni) Moderately large, motile, gram-positive, rod-shaped organism with rounded ends and oval subterminal spores; infectious for humans only through wounds.

coagulant Agent causing blood or fluid to clot.

coalesce The fusing or blending of parts.

coarctation A straightening or pressing together; a condition of stricture or contraction; for example, of the aorta, with usually severe narrowing of the vessel lumen.

coenzyme A noncolloidal substance that combines with an inactive enzyme to produce activation of the enzyme.

colectomy Excision of a portion of the colon.

colitis Inflammation of the colon.

colloid Glutinous or resembling glue; a state in which the matter is distributed through some form of dispersing medium.

emulsion The dispersing medium is usually water, and the disperse phase consists of highly complex organic substances such as starch or glue, which absorb much water, swell, and become uniformly distributed throughout the dispersion medium.

suspension The disperse or distributing phase consists of particles of any insoluble substance such as metal, and the medium may be gaseous, liquid, or solid.

colostomy The formation of a permanent artificial opening (artificial anus) into the colon.

conduction Transfer of sound waves, heat, nerve influences, or electricity.

conductivity Capacity of a body to conduct a current.

congestive heart failure Result of the inability of the heart to expel sufficient blood for the metabolic demands of the body. Most common causes are hypertension, coronary atherosclerosis, and rheumatic heart disease. Less common causes include chronic pulmonary disease, congenital heart disease, syphilitic aortic insufficiency, calcific aortic stenosis, and bacterial endocarditis.

conjunctiva Mucous membrane lining the inner surface of the eyelids and covering the forepart of the eyeball.

conjunctivitis Inflammation of the mucous membrane conjunctiva. See *conjunctiva*.

constipation Infrequency or difficulty in movements of the bowels.

constriction A constricted part or place, a narrowing.

contract To decrease in size, as muscle tissue.

contractility Capacity for becoming short in response to a suitable stimulus.

cornea Transparent membrane forming the anterior or front part of the outer layer of the eyeball.

coronary occlusion The formation of a clot in a branch of the coronary arteries, which supply blood to the heart muscle, resulting in obstruction of the artery and infarction of the area of the heart supplied by the occluded vessel. Also called cardiac infarction and coronary thrombosis.

cortex Outer part of a gland or structure, such as the rind or bark.

craniotomy Operation on the cranium.

creatine Crystallizable nitrogenous principle, or methyl-guanidine-acetic acid, derived from the juice of muscular tissue; therapeutically, a cardiac, muscular, and digestive tonic.

creatinine Basic substance called creatine anhydride, procurable from creatine and from urine.

cretinism A chronic condition, congenital or developed before puberty, characterized by arrested physical and mental development, with dystrophy of the bones and soft parts. It is regarded as a form of myxedema and is probably caused by deficient thyroid activity.

cryptorchidism Undescended testicle.

crystalluria Formation of crystals in the urine or in the kidneys.

curie Standard unit for measuring the amount of radium emanation. The word curie comes from the discoverer of radium, Marie Sklodowska Curie, a Polish chemist in Paris, who lived 1867-1934.

Cushing's disease Disease caused by overgrowth of the basophil cells of the anterior lobe of the pituitary gland and marked by rapidly developing obesity of the face, neck, and trunk, decreased sexual activity, abnormal growth of hair, abdominal pain, weakness, and sometimes supraclavicular fat pads, striae, and acne.

cutaneous Pertaining to the skin.

cyanosis Blueness of the skin, lips, and often fingernails resulting from cardiac malformations causing insufficient oxygenation of the blood.

cycloplegia Paralysis of the ciliary muscle of the eye.

cystic fibrosis An infant and childhood disease probably inherited with pancreatic pathology and digestive and respiratory difficulties. Respiratory failure is most frequently the eventual cause of death. Characteristic symptoms are changes in the activity of the exocrine glands, including sweat (with a salty taste to the skin), salivary, and mucus-producing glands; the newborn manifest meconium ileus, with thick meconium obstructing the lower digestive tract, resulting in the need for emergency surgery. Other infant and childhood symptoms include bulky, offensive stools, protruding abdomen, spindly arms and legs, emaciation of the buttocks, and growth retardation. Foodstuffs, especially proteins and fats, are poorly digested and assimilated; pancreatic digestive enzymes are reduced or absent. Digestive problems improve with additional pancreatic enzymes in the diet. Blocking of the bronchioles, which results from extremely thick and tenacious secretions of the mucus-producing glands of the bronchi, are serious problems, causing cough, wheezing, respiratory obstruction, emphysema, and frequently infection. The lungs are usually defenseless against microbes. In severe, chronic cases of the disease, patients manifest heart problems, a barrel-like, deformed chest, cyanosis, and clubbing of fingers and toes.

cystitis Inflammation of the bladder.

cystoscopy Examination of the bladder with an instrument called a cystoscope.

cytotoxic Having the action of a cytotoxin.

cytotoxin Toxin or antibody that has a specific toxic action on cells of special organs.

debilitated, debility Lack or loss of strength.

decrease To lessen or diminish.

defecation The discharge of fecal matter from the bowel.

degradation Reduction of a chemical compound to one less complex, as by splitting off one or more groups.

dehydration Removal of water from a substance or compound; also removal of water from the body; restriction of the water intake.

delirium tremens Condition marked by great excitement with anxiety and mental distress; caused by overuse of alcoholic drinks and characterized by hallucinations.

dementia Insanity characterized by loss or serious impairment of intellect, will, and memory.

demulcent substance Soothing preparation.

deodorant Medicine or substance that covers up, absorbs, or destroys objectionable odors.

depolarization Process or act of neutralizing polarity.

depressor Agent that causes a slowing-up action when applied to nerves and muscles.

derivative Agent that withdraws blood from the seat of a disease; anything that is obtained from another.

dermatitis Inflammation of the skin. Contact dermatitis is caused by contact with an irritating substance followed by an allergic response such as skin reddening, rash, itching, and scaling.

dermatomyositis An inflammatory disease of the voluntary muscles accompanied by characteristic skin lesions. It is attended by violent pains, swellings in the muscles, inflammation of the skin, and edema. Also called multiple myositis.

dermatophyte A plant growth, or species of plant, parasitic on the skin.

dermatoses Skin diseases.

detergent Cleansing agent.

diabetes insipidus Chronic disease, usually of young male adults, characterized by great thirst and the passage of a large amount of urine with no excess of sugar. Huge appetite, loss of strength, and emaciation are often noted. Causes include a deficiency of pitressin secretion from the posterior pituitary gland, impaired function of the supraoptic pathways regulating water metabolism, and, rarely, unresponsiveness of the kidney to pitressin.

diabetes mellitus Metabolic disorder marked by inability of the body to store or utilize carbohydrate.

diaphoresis, diaphoretic Profuse perspiration.

diarrhea Loose, watery bowel movements.

diastolic blood pressure See *blood pressure*.

diffuse Process of becoming widely spread, as through a membrane or fluid.

dilate To enlarge or stretch beyond normal measurements.

diplopia The seeing of single objects as double or two.

disinfectant An agent that destroys disease-producing substances or organisms.

disk (disc) A circular or rounded flat plate or organ.

choked An inflamed and edematous optic disk, resulting from increased intracranial pressure. Called also papilledema.

interarticular An interarticular fibrocartilage.

intervertebral intervertebral A layer of fibrocartilage between adjacent vertebrae.

distal Remote, farthest from the center, origin, or head; opposed to proximal.

diuresis Increased secretion of urine.

diuretic Drug that increases the flow of urine.

diverticulitis Inflammation of a diverticulum.

diverticulum Sac or pouch protruding from the wall of a tube or hollow organ, for example, from the intestine.

dosage Determination of the amount of medication to be administered to a patient, depending on the patient's weight and age.

ductless Having no excretory duct, as in ductless glands.

duodenum Portion of the small intestine leading from the stomach.

dyscrasias Abnormal composition of the blood.

dysentery Infection of the bowel characterized by inflammation, discharge of liquid and bloody stools, and pain, especially during discharge.

dysmenorrhea Painful menstruation.

dysphoria Disquiet; restlessness; feeling of ill-being; malaise.

dyspnea Difficult or labored breathing.

ecchymosis A discharge or escape of blood; a discoloration of the skin caused by discharge or extravasation of blood.

eclampsia Toxic or poisonous condition usually observed during the last 3 months of pregnancy and characterized by edema or fluid in the tissues, rapid weight gain from the edema, increase in blood pressure, albumin in urine, headache, possible convulsions, and other symptoms.

ectopic Out of the normal place.

edema Increase of tissue fluid in the tissue space; often noticed in the face, hands, fingers, abdomen, ankles, and feet.

efferent Carrying blood or secretion away from a part; carrying impulses away from a nerve center.

effusion Escape of fluid into a part or tissue.
pleural Presence of fluid in the pleural space or area occupied by the lungs.

electrocardiogram Graphic tracing of the heart action produced by electrocardiography.

electrocardiography Recording of the electric currents in the heart through leads placed on various parts of the body.

electroencephalogram Recording made of the electric currents developed in the cortex by brain activity.

electrolytes Solution that is a conductor of electricity; acids and salts are common electrolytes.

embolism Condition of plugging of an artery or vein by a clot or obstruction that has been brought to its place by the blood current.

embolus Clot or other plug brought by the blood current from a distant vessel and forced into a smaller one, obstructing the circulation.

embryoma A tumor containing embryonic elements or those derived from a rudimentary retained twin parasite.

emetic Substance that causes vomiting, such as mustard and water or the drug apomorphine.

emphysema Presence of air in the alveolar (air sac) tissue of the lungs; distension of the alveoli with air. A few symptoms are exertional dyspnea, prolonged expiratory phase, wheezing, productive cough with difficulty in clearing the bronchi, barrel chest, overuse of accessory muscles of respiration, overaerated lung fields, and flattened diaphragm (only last two indicated in X-rays).

endocarditis Inflammation of the endocardium or epithelial lining membrane of the heart.
bacterial Endocarditis caused by bacterial infection developing as a complication of some infectious diseases.

endometriosis Presence of endometrial tissue in abnormal situations.
internal Occurring in the wall of the uterus or fallopian tube.
external Occurring on the external surface of the uterus, in the ovary, bladder, or intestine, or extraperitoneally.
vesicae Endometriosis involving the bladder.

endometrium Mucous membrane lining of the uterus.

endoscopy Inspection of any cavity of the body, such as the bladder, by means of an endoscope.

endotracheal intubation Insertion of a tube into the larynx through the glottis or into the trachea for the introduction of air; often used during anesthesia to introduce an anesthetic and to keep a proper airway; also used in diphtheria and edema of the glottis to aid breathing.

enhance, enhancing Increasing.

enteric coating Type of coating for tablets and capsules to prevent dissolving until medication reaches intestines, thus preventing stomach juices from destroying certain drugs.

enteritis Inflammation of the intestine, chiefly the small intestine.

enterocolitis Inflammation of the small and the large intestines.

enzymatic Relating to enzyme.

enzyme A chemical ferment formed by living cells. Enzymes are complex organic chemical compounds capable of producing by catalytic action the transformation of some other compound or compounds.

eosinophil Structure, cell, or histologic element readily stained by eosins; particularly an eosinophilic leukocyte or white cell.

eosins Rose-colored stains or dye, the potassium and sodium salts of tetrabromofluorescein. Several other red coal-tar dyes are also called eosins.

epidemic Disease that affects a large group of people in a certain locality at about the same time.

epidermophytosis Fungous infection of the skin.

epigastric Pertaining to epigastrium.

epigastrium The upper middle portion of the abdomen over or in front of the stomach.

epilepsy Nervous system disease with convulsive seizures.
grand mal Epilepsy in which there are severe convulsions and loss of consciousness, or coma; also called *haut mal*.
Jacksonian A form of epilepsy marked by localized spasm, mainly limited to one side and often to one group of muscles.
petit mal Epilepsy with no decided period of unconsciousness and no obvious spasm or only a slight one.

epistaxis Nosebleed; hemorrhage from the nose.

epithelium Covering of the skin and mucous membranes consisting wholly of cells of varying form and arrangement. The four principal varieties, named according to the shape of the cells, are modified, specialized, columnar, and squamous.

eructate The act of belching; casting up wind from the stomach.

erythema Morbid redness of the skin of many varieties caused by congestion of the capillaries; rose rash.

erythroblastosis fetalis A disease of early infancy showing marked disturbance in the formation of blood.

erythrocytes Red blood corpuscles, circular biconcave disks containing hemoglobin, that carry the oxygen of the blood. Normal red blood cell count (RBC) is 4 ½ to 5 million/cu ml of blood.

erythrocytosis Increase in the number of red blood corpuscles in the circulation.

eschar A slough produced by burning or by a corrosive application.

esophagitis Inflammation of the esophagus or gullet, which is a musculomembranous canal extending from the pharynx to the stomach.

esterase An enzyme that splits esters.

estrogen Generic term for many compounds having estrogenic activity; producing effects similar to estrin; a female sex hormone.

eunuch Man or boy deprived of the testes or external genital organs.

eunuchism Condition of a castrated male.

eunuchoidism A defective state of the testicles or of the testicular secretion, with impaired sexual power and eunuch-like symptoms.

euphoria Bodily comfort; well-being; absence of pain or distress.

Ewing's tumor (endothelial myeloma) A form of bone sarcoma that usually involves widening the shaft of long bones by spreading the lamellae apart.

exacerbation Increase in the severity of any symptoms or disease.

excitation Act of irritation or stimulation; a condition of being excited.

excreta Waste matter discharged from the body, particularly fecal matter.

exfoliative dermatitis Inflammation of the skin characterized by a falling off of scales or skin layers and resembling pityriasis rubra, a skin disease.

exophthalmic, exophthalmos Protruding of the eyeballs, sometimes caused by pressure of a goiter on the vessels in the neck leading to the face.

expectorant Medication used to increase secretion and aid in expelling mucus from the respiratory tract or to modify such secretions.

extravasation Discharge or escape, as of blood, from a vessel into the tissues.

fenestration The act of perforating, or the condition of being perforated with openings.

fibrillation Condition in which the groups of muscle fibers of the heart do not contract in unison, causing a rapid and irregular pulse.

fibrin Whitish, insoluble protein formed from fibrigen by the action of thrombin (fibrin ferment), as in the clotting of blood. Fibrin forms the essential portion of the blood clot.

fibrinogen Soluble protein in the blood plasma that is converted into fibrin by the action of thrombin (fibrin ferment), thus producing clotting of the blood.

fibromyositis Inflammation of fibromuscular tissue.

fibrositis Inflammation of muscle fibers.

fimbriae Fringe-like, finger-like tissue projections at the ends of the fallopian tubes of the female reproductive system.

fissure
abnormal Cleft-shaped sore.
normal Groove or cleft, such as one of the fissures of the brain.

flatulence Distension of the stomach or intestines with air or gases.

flexion The act of bending or condition of being bent.

follicle A very small excretory or secretory sac or gland.
graafian Any one of the small spherical vesicular sacs embedded in the cortex of the ovary, each of which contains an egg cell, or ovum. Each follicle contains a liquid supplied with the hormone folliculin, or estrin.

frostbite Condition produced by the freezing of a part, such as fingers, toes, or feet.

fulminant, fulminating Sudden; severe; coming on suddenly with intense severity.

fungus Plant organism characterized chiefly by the absence of chlorophyll.

galactorrhea Excessive or spontaneous secretion of milk.

gallbladder Muscular sac that contains bile; located under the right lobe of the liver.

ganglia Plural of ganglion; any collection or mass or nerve cells that serves as a center of nervous influence.

gangrene Necrosis of tissue combined with invasion by saprophytic organisms.

gastrectomy Removal of the stomach or a portion of it.

gastritis Inflammation of the stomach.

gastroenteritis Inflammation of the stomach and the intestines.

gastrointestinal Pertaining to the stomach and the intestines.

gastroparesis A mild form of paralysis of the stomach. Reversible to some extent.

genetic Congenital or inherited.

geriatrics That branch of medicine that treats the diseases of old age.

gestation Pregnancy; gravidity.

glaucoma A disease of the eye marked by intense intraocular pressure, resulting in hardness of the eye, atrophy of the retina, cupping of the optic disk, and blindness.

globulin Protein substance similar to albumin; examples include cell globulin, fibrinogen, lactoglobulin, and serum globulin.

glomerulonephritis Inflammation of the glomeruli of the kidney.

glomerulus Tuft or cluster; a coil of blood vessels projecting into the expanded end or capsule of each of the uriniferous tubules (channels for the passage of urine).

glossitis Inflammation of the tongue.

gluteus, gluteal Muscles of the buttock commonly used as sites for intramuscular injection of medications.

glycosuria Sugar in the urine.

goiter Enlargement of the thyroid gland, located in the neck.

   exophthalmic Enlargement of the thyroid gland, with such symptoms as rapid pulse, sweating, nervousness, muscular tremors, psychic disturbance, emaciation, and increased basal metabolism.

gonads Sex glands; testes in male, ovaries in the female.

gonioscope A kind of ophthalmoscope for examining the angle of the anterior chamber of the eye and for demonstrating ocular motility and rotation.

gonioscopy An examination of the eye with a gonioscope. See *gonioscope*.

gonorrhea Venereal disease of the mucous membrane of the genitalia; can affect the mucous membrane of the eyes.

gout A metabolic disease in which purine substances are deposited in the body, with excess uric acid in the blood, chalky deposits in the cartilages of body joints, and acute arthritis. Characteristic symptoms are acute pain, tenderness, and swelling in body joints, such as in the large toe, ankle, instep, knee, and elbow; elevation of uric acid in the blood; and formation of uric-acid or urate deposits in the cartilage of various parts of the body. These tophi ("chalk stone" or calcareous matter) increase in size and are most often seen along the edge of the ear.

graafian follicle See *follicle, graafian*.

gram-negative Bacteria or tissues that lose the stain or become decolorized by alcohol in Gram's method of staining.

gram-positive Bacteria or tissues that retain the stain in Gram's method of staining.

granulocytes Cells containing granules.

granulocytopenia Abnormal reduction of granulocytes or white blood cells in the blood. See *agranulocytosis*.

Graves' disease See *goiter, exophthalmic*.

gravid Pregnant; with child; containing a fetus.

gripes, gripping Severe and often spasmodic pain in the bowel.

hallucination A sense perception not founded on an objective reality.

hay fever Acute seasonal disease usually caused by an allergy to pollen with characteristic symptoms similar to those of a cold.

heart failure Failure of the heart to work as a pump; characteristic symptoms are fluid in the lungs, ankles, and abdomen.

hemagglutinin Substance that causes agglutination or clumping of red blood corpuscles.

hematocrit Centrifuge for separating corpuscles from plasma or serum of blood.

hematoma Tumor containing effused (spread out, profuse) blood.

hematopoietic Pertaining to or concerned with the formation of blood.

hematuria Discharge of bloody urine.

hemiplegia Loss of function and movement of one side of the body with paralysis.

hemodialysis Installation of an arterial-venal shunt that is connected to the dialyzing machine; the blood is pumped through the dialyzing fluid with a partially porous (semipermeable) plastic membrane to protect the cells. Dialysis is usually performed three times a week for 8 hours each time, but this may vary. It is extremely expensive but lifesaving in chronic renal failure (chronic uremia).

hemoglobin Iron content of the red blood cell.

hemoglobinuria The presence of hemoglobin in the urine resulting from destruction of the blood corpuscles in the vessels or in the urinary passages.

hemolysis Separation of the hemoglobin from the corpuscles and its appearance in the fluid in which the corpuscles are suspended. A few common causes include hemolysins, chemicals, freezing, heating, and placing in distilled water.

hemolytic Causing hemolysis.

hemoperitoneum The presence of extravasated (discharged or escaped) blood into the peritoneal cavity.

hemophilia Congenital condition characterized by delayed clotting of the blood and consequent difficulty in checking hemorrhage; inherited by males through the mother as an x-linked recessive trait.

hemorrhage Massive loss of blood from the body.

hemorrhoids Varicose veins or dilated blood vessels in the anal area.

hemostatic Checking the flow of blood; an agent that arrests the flow of blood.

Henle's loop A U-shaped turn in a uriniferous tubule of the kidney.

hepar Liver.

hepatic Referring to hepar or liver.

hepatitis Infectious inflammation of the liver; a viral infection transmitted by the intestinal-oral route and characterized by symptoms such as anorexia, malaise, nausea, vomiting, fever, enlarged tender liver, jaundice, normal to low white blood cell count, and abnormal hepatocellular liver function tests. The virus is present in the feces and blood during prodromal and acute phases and often in asymptomatic carriers; it may persist for long periods without symptoms after the acute phase. Incubation period is 2 to 6 weeks.

hepatotoxicity Poisoning or toxins destructive to liver cells and originating in the liver.

herpes simplex Skin disease marked by the formation of one or more vesicles on the border of the lip, eye, external nares, or mucous surface of the genitals.

Hg Symbol for mercury; abbreviation for hemoglobin.

hiatus hernia, or **hiatal hernia** Protrusion of any structure through the esophageal hiatus of the diaphragm.

hirsutism Abnormal hairiness, especially in women.

histamine Substance found in the body and in nearly all plant tissues wherever protein is broken down or there is tissue damage.

Hodgkin's disease Characterized by an infectious granulomatous condition (inflammatory enlargement) involving particularly the lymphadenoid tissues of the body. Eosinophils, fibroblasts, giant cells, and frequently *Corynebacterium* organisms, which may be causative agents of the disease, may be found. The glandular enlargement begins at the side of the neck and then extends to the axillary, inguinal, and mediastinal glands and spleen. There is usually a relapsing fever. The disease is called by many names. A few are infectious granuloma, malignant granuloma, malignant lymphoma, lymphadenoma, and lymphosarcoma.

homologous Of similar structure or situation, but not necessarily of similar function.

hormone Chemical product manufactured by some tissue, such as a gland, which is carried by the blood and acts as a messenger to control other tissues, for example, by stimulation or depression, by control of growth sex characteristics, or by effects on the heartbeat.

hydrocholeretics Drugs stimulating the production of bile of a low specific gravity.

hydrogen ion concentration Acidic concentration of hydrogen ions that were formed and given their acid character by acid; has a vital effect on all life processes.

hydrolization, hydrolysis Decomposition resulting from the incorporation of water. The two resulting products divide the water, the hydroxyl group being attached to one and the hydrogen atom to the other.

hydrolyze To subject to hydrolysis.

hydrostatic Pertaining to the pressure exerted by liquids and on liquids; medically, stagnation of fluids.

hydrotropic Chemotropism produced by water; tendency of cells to turn or move in a certain direction under the influence of chemical stimuli.

hyper- A prefix indicating above, beyond, or excessive.

hyperacidity Excessive degree of acidity, often in the stomach.

hyperadrenalism Abnormally increased activity of adrenal gland secretion.

hypercalcemia Abnormally high calcium content in the blood.

hyperchlorhydria Excessive secretion of hydrochloric acid by stomach cells.

hypercholesterolemia Excess of cholesterol in the blood.

hyperflexia, hyperflexion Forcible overflexion or bending of a limb.

hyperglycemia Excess sugar in the blood.

hyperkalemia Abnormally high potassium content in the blood.

hyperoxemia Excessive acidity of the blood.

hyperoxia High oxygen tension in the blood.

hyperplasia Abnormal multiplication or increase in the number of normal cells in normal arrangement in a tissue.

hyperprolactinemia Elevated blood levels of prolactin, the pituitary hormone that causes lactation.

hyperpyrexia A high degree of fever.

hypertension Abnormally high tension, especially high blood pressure.

benign Essential hypertension that exists for years without producing any symptoms; fluctuating type. Elevation of blood pressure tends to return to normal with rest or sedation.

essential, primary High blood pressure without previous inflammatory disease of the kidney or urinary tract or any other known cause. A systolic pressure above 150 mm Hg and a diastolic pressure of 100 mm Hg is abnormal at all ages. The upper limit for normal blood pressure, as established by insurance companies, is 140/90 mm Hg.

malignant Essential hypertension with an acute, stormy onset, development of neuroretinitis, a progressive course, a sustained elevation of blood pressure, and a poor prognosis.

secondary Elevation of the blood pressure for which the cause is known, such as endocrine, cardiovascular, renal, or neural origin.

hypertensive encephalopathy A complex of cerebral symptoms, including headache, convulsions, and coma, occurring in the course of glomerulonephritis.

hyperthyroid Abnormal condition caused by overactivity of the thyroid gland.

hypertonic Excessive tone, tension, or activity.

hypertrophic, hypertrophy Morbid enlargement or overgrowth of an organ or part.

hypertrophic gastritis Enlargement and inflammation of the stomach.

hyperuricemia Excess of uric acid in the blood.

hyperventilation Abnormally prolonged and deep breathing.

hypnotic Any agent that will produce sleep.

hypo- A prefix denoting a lack or deficiency; also a position under or beneath.

hypocalcemia Reduction of blood calcium below normal.

hypochloremic Pertaining to or characterized by lowered chloride content of the blood.

hypochlorhydria Too small a proportion of hydrochloric acid in the gastric juice.

hypodermic Any method that employs the use of a needle and syringe to place medication under the skin.

hypogenitalism Eunuchoid condition caused by defect of the internal secretion of the testicle or the ovary.

hypoglycemia Deficiency of sugar in the blood.

hypogonadism Decrease of the internal secretion of the gonads; eunuchoidism.

hypokalemia Abnormally low potassium content of blood.

hyponatremia Deficiency of sodium in the blood.

hypoparathyroidism Insufficiency of the parathyroid hormone secretion.

hypopituitarism Condition caused by pathologically diminished activity of the hypophysis or pituitary body and marked by excessive deposits of fat and persistence or acquisition of adolescent characteristics.

hypotassemia Deficiency of potassium in the blood.

hypotension Diminished tension, lowered blood pressure.

hypothalamus The ventral subdivision of the diencephalon or forebrain.

hypothermia Abnormally low temperature.

hypothyroidism Underactivity of the thyroid gland in the neck.

hypoventilation Decrease of the air in the lungs below the normal amount.

hypoxia (hypoxemia) Lack of oxygen and deficient oxygenation of the blood.

idiopathic Morbid state of spontaneous origin; neither sympathetic nor traumatic.

idiosyncrasy Peculiar susceptibility to some drug protein or other substance; exaggerated reaction to drugs.

ileitis Inflammation of the ileus, part of the small intestine.

ileostomy The making of an artificial opening into the ileum.

ileum The distal portion of the small intestine, extending from the jejunum to the cecum.

immunization Method of preventing a first or a second attack of a certain disease.

impacted Driven firmly in, closely lodged.

impermeable Not permitting a passage, as for fluid.

impetigo Low-grade skin infection with small pustules.

incipient Beginning to exist; coming into existence.

increase To enlarge, to grow.

infantilism Condition in which the characters of childhood persist in adult life; marked by mental retardation, underdevelopment of the sexual organs, and often dwarfism.

infarct Area of coagulation necrosis in a tissue caused by local anemia resulting from obstruction of circulation to the area.

inhibits Lessens, decreases.

innervation Distribution or supply of nerves to a part; supply of nervous energy or of nerve stimulus sent to a part.

inoculation Topical or subcutaneous (under the skin) application of bacteria into a human being to produce a mild form of a disease for the purpose of creating an immunity to future attacks.

inotropic To turn or influence; affecting the force or energy of muscular contractions.

negative Weakening the force of muscular action.

positive Increasing the strength of muscular contraction.

in situ In the natural or normal place.

insomnia Inability to sleep.

insulin Hormone drug used in the treatment of diabetes mellitus; extract of the islands of Langerhans of the pancreas.

intestines The small and large bowels.

intracranial Within the cranium or skull or brain pan.

intramuscular Into or within the muscle.

intraocular Into or within the eye.

intravenous Into or within the vein.

intrinsic Situated on the inside; situated entirely within or pertaining exclusively to a part.

inulin Polysaccharide found in Inula, Dahlia, and other plants that yield levulose on hydrolysis; also a concentration of resinoid from elecampane root; an aromatic and tonic expectorant.

involution A rolling or turning inward; the return of the uterus to its normal size after childbirth; a retrograde change; the reverse of evolution; involutional, pertaining to, due to, or occurring in involution.

senile the shriveling of an organ in aged people.

ion Atom or group of atoms having a charge of positive (cation) or negative (anion) electricity.

ionization Dissociation of a substance in solution into its constituent ions.

ionize To separate into ions.

iris Circular pigmented membrane behind the cornea of the eye, perforated by the pupil; made up of circular muscular fibers surrounding the pupil and a band of radiating fibers by which the pupil is dilated.

irradiation Treatment by roentgen rays or other forms of radioactivity.

ischemia Local and temporary deficiency of blood, caused chiefly by contraction of a blood vessel.

isotonic Having a uniform tension. Isotonic solutions are those that have the same osmotic pressure.

isotonic salt solution Solution having the same amount of salt substance as the blood (approximately 0.9% sodium chloride).

isotope Either of two substances chemically identical but with differing atomic weights.

isthmus A narrow strip of tissue or a narrow passage connecting two larger parts; of the thyroid, the band or strip of tissue that connects the lobes of the thyroid gland.

jaundice (icterus) Condition characterized by the presence of bilirubin, a red bile pigment, and deposition of the bile pigment in the skin and mucous membranes, with resulting yellow appearance of the skin and yellow whites of the eyes. It may be caused by obstruction in the biliary system, blockage from a stone that obstructs the passage of bile from the liver to the intestines, or impairment of the liver itself, which produces the bile to aid in the digestion of fats.

juxta Situated near or in the region of, such as juxtaglomerular—near or in the region of a glomerulus.

keratitis Inflammation of the cornea of the eye.

ketoacidosis A condition of metabolism in which abnormal quantities of acetone bodies are present in the body.

kilogram Unit of weight equal to 1,000 g or 2.2

pounds avoirdupois (the ordinary system of weights in the United States).

labyrinthitis Inflammation of the labyrinth or the intercommunicating cavities or canals of the internal ear: cochlea, vestibule, and canals.

laceration Mangled or torn skin or tissue.

lacrimal canaliculi Tear channels or canals of the eye.

lactation The secretion of milk; the period of the secretion of milk; suckling.

laity The nonprofessional segment of the population.

laryngeal Pertaining to the larynx.

laryngitis Inflammation of the larynx.

larynx Musculocartilaginous, box-like structure, lined with mucous membrane, situated at the top of the trachea and below the root of the tongue and the hyoid bone; located in the midline of the neck. It is the organ of the voice, or voice box.

lateral Pertaining to a side.

laxative Drug having the property of overcoming constipation.

lecithin A monoaminomonophosphatide containing fatty acids and found in animal tissues, especially nerve tissue, semen, yolk of egg, and in smaller amount in bile and blood. Lecithins are said to have the therapeutic properties of phosphorus and have been given in rickets, dyspepsia, neurasthenia, diabetes, anemia, and tuberculosis; lecithins also are said to be antivenomous.

lens A transparent gelatinous mass of fibers situated behind the iris and pupil of the eye and having the function of giving the image on the retina a sharp focus and of converging or scattering the rays of light.

leprosy Chronic infectious disease caused by a specific microbe (Hansen's bacillus) and marked by a very gradual onset, malaise, headache, formation of nodules, ulcerations, and deformities, and loss of sensation in affected parts; often called Hansen's disease.

lethargy Condition of drowsiness of mental origin.

leukemia Often fatal disease with a marked increase in the number of leukocytes in the blood, with enlargement and proliferation of the lymphoid tissue of the spleen, bone marrow, and lymphatic glands. A few characteristic symptoms include progressive anemia, internal hemorrhage, and increasing exhaustion.

leukocyte Any colorless, ameboid cell mass, such as a white blood corpuscle, pus corpuscle, lymph corpuscle, or wandering connective tissue cell, consisting of a colorless granular mass of protoplasm having ameboid movements and varying in size. Normal white blood cell count (WBC) is 5,000 to 10,000/cu ml of blood.

leukocytosis Increase in the number of leukocytes in the blood, generally caused by the presence of infection.

leukopenia Reduction in the number of leukocytes in the blood to 5,000/cu ml of blood or less.

lipids Any one of a group of substances that include the fats and the esters having corresponding properties. The American usage of the term includes fatty acids and soaps, neutral fats, waxes, sterols, and phosphatides. Lipids have a greasy feel.

liver Largest gland of the body, located in the right upper part of the abdomen. It has many functions, including formation and secretion of bile to aid in fat digestion, storage of sugar in the form of glycogen, formation of vitamin A from carotene, and storage of vitamins A and D_2. As a drug it is produced in many forms and has lifesaving properties for many types of anemia.

local Limited to, or pertaining to, one part or spot.

lumen Transverse section of the clear space within a tube; an opening.

lupus erythematosus Chronic, nontuberculous disease of the skin marked by disk-like patches with raised reddish edges and depressed centers and covered with scales or crusts that fall off, leaving off-white scars.

lymphangitis Inflammation of a lymphatic vessel or vessels.

lymphatic system System of vessels carrying lymph (a transparent, slightly yellow liquid, alkaline in reaction) to parts of the body.

lymphocyte Variety of white blood corpuscle with a single nucleus and increased cytoplasm. These corpuscles arise in the reticular tissue of the lymph glands and lymph nodes.

lymphocytic Pertaining to lymphocytes.

lymphoma Any tumor made up of lymphoid tissue.

lymphopenia Decrease in the proportion of lymphocytes in the blood.

lymphosarcoma Malignant neoplasm arising in lymphatic tissue from proliferation of atypical lymphocytes.

lysozyme A mucolytic lubrication for eyelid movements.

macrocytic Condition referring to abnormally large erythrocytes, or red blood corpuscles.

malabsorption Disorder of normal nutritive absorption; disordered anabolism.

malaise Feeling of ill-being; not feeling well.

malignant Virulent; tending to go from bad to worse; progressive.

manic-depressive Insanity in which mania and melancholia alternate.

meconium The fecal matter of the newborn; it consists of a green, sticky substance containing mucus, bile, and epithelial threads.

medulla oblongata Cone of nervous tissue continuous above with the pons of the brain and below with the spinal cord, lying ventral to the cerebellum and forming the floor of the fourth ventricle, with its back; continuation of the spinal cord within the cranium.

megaloblast An erythroblast or primitive red blood corpuscle of large size found in the blood of pernicious anemia.

Ménière's syndrome Disease or inflammatory process and congestion of the semicircular canals in the inner ear with symptoms such as pallor, vertigo, nausea, lack of balance, and several ear and eye disturbances.

meninges The three membranes that envelop the brain and spinal cord, including the dura, the pia, and the arachnoid.

meningitis Inflammation of the meninges of the brain.

menopause Cessation of menstruation; often called "the change of life."

menorrhagia Abnormally profuse menstruation.

menstruation Monthly bloody discharge from the uterus.

mesial Situated in the middle; median; toward the middle line of the body or toward the center line of the dental arch.

metabolism Tissue change; the sum of all the physical and chemical processes by which living organized substance is produced and maintained; the transformation by which energy is made available for the uses of the organism.

metastasis The moving or spreading of infection or cell growth from one area to another.

metorrhagia Profuse bleeding from the uterus at times other than during the menstrual period.

microcurie One-millionth of a curie.

microgram One-millionth part of a gram.

migraine Periodic headache, usually on one side, with such severe symptoms as nausea, vomiting, and light sensitivity.

millicurie One-thousandth of a curie, which is a unit of radiation energy.

milliequivalent One-thousandth of an equivalent combining weight of an atom or ion; an equivalent combining weight, as the weight of an element (in grams) that will combine with 1.008 g of hydrogen.

miosis Excessive contraction of the pupil of the eye.

miotic, myotic Drug that causes the pupil to contract, such as morphine, nicotine, physostigmine, and pilocarpine.

mittelschmerz Intermenstrual pain occurring about halfway through the menstrual cycle, generally during ovulation.

molecule Very small mass of matter; a gathering together or clumping of atoms.

motion sickness Nausea, dizziness, and often vomiting caused by motion of the body when riding in a ship, airplane, automobile, or train.

multipara A woman who has borne several children.

multiple myeloma Tumor composed of cells of the type normally found in the bone marrow; a primary malignant tumor of bone marrow marked by circumscribed or diffuse, tumor-like hyperplasia (abnormal multiplication or increase in number of normal cells in normal arrangement in a tissue) of the bone marrow. It is usually associated with anemia and with Bence Jones protein in the urine. Neuralgic pains and painful swellings on the ribs and skull occur, along with spontaneous fractures.

multiple sclerosis Nervous system disease characterized by scarring of brain and spinal cord that occurs in scattered patches. Patient shows progressive weakness, paralysis, muscle contraction, and muscle cramps. The cause is unknown, and the treatment limited.

multisynaptic See *synapse.*

myalgia Pain in a muscle or muscles.

myasthenia gravis Disease characterized by an abnormal weakness of muscles.

mycosis fungoides Fatal fungous skin disease marked by the development of firm, reddish tumors on the scalp, face, and chest that are painful and have a tendency to spread and ulcerate. The disease may last several years.

mydriasis Extreme or morbid dilation of the pupil of the eye.

mydriatic Drug that dilates the pupil of the eye, such as atropine, homatropine, cocaine, phenacaine, hyoscyamine, and ephedrine.

myelin The fat-like substance forming a sheath around the medullated (myelinated) nerve fibers.

myocardium Heart muscle; myocardial infarct; a blockage or clot in the heart muscle.

myoma Any tumor made up of muscular elements; if they are striated, it is a rhabdomyoma, if not, it is a leiomyoma.

myositis Inflammation of muscle.

myxedema Hypothyroid condition causing an edema of tissues, loss of hair, and physical and mental sluggishness in adults.

narcotic Drug that produces sleep or stupor and relieves pain.

nausea Inclination to vomit.

nebulae Very small droplets of water or oil, usually sprayed from an atomizer.

necrosis Death of a circumscribed portion of tissue.

neoplasm Any new and abnormal formation, such as a tumor.

nephritis Inflammation of the kidney.

nephrons Multifunctional units; the renal unit consists of Bowman's capsule, the globular upper end of the tubule, and the tubule, which is concerned with kidney circulation.

nephropathy Disease of the kidneys.

nephrosis Degenerative changes in the kidney without inflammation.

nephrotoxic Toxic or destructive to the kidneys.

neuralgia Nerve pain.

neuritis Inflammation of a nerve, or nerves, with pain.

neuroblasts Any embryonic cell that develops into a nerve cell or neuron; an immature nerve cell.

neuroblastomas Malignant tumors of the nervous system composed chiefly of neuroblasts.

neurogenic Forming nervous tissue, or stimulating nervous energy; originating in the nervous system.

nocturnal Pertaining to, occurring at, or active at night.

node Swelling or protuberance.

auriculoventricular Remnant of primitive fibers found in all mammalian hearts at the base of the intraauricular septum (separation or partition) and forming the beginning of the bundle of His.

normotensive Characterized by blood pressure within the normal range.

nucleic acid Acid obtained from nuclein, a decomposition product of nucleoprotein.

occlusion Act of closure or state of being closed.

occlusive Effecting a complete occlusion or closure.

occult Obscure, difficult to be observed, hidden.

oculogyric crisis A painful spasm of the eye muscles.

Ocusert A method of administration of eye drops over a continuous, extended period.

oligomenorrhea Scanty or infrequent menstrual flow.

oliguria Deficient secretion of urine.

ophthalmic Pertaining to the eye.

optic Of or pertaining to the eye.

orthopnea Inability to breathe except when sitting up.

orthostatic hypotension Blood pressure lower than normal when the individual is standing or in upright position.

osmosis Passage of pure solvent (liquid used to dissolve) from the lesser to the greater concentration when two solutions are separated by a membrane that selectively prevents the passage of solute (dissolved substance) molecules but that is permeable to the solvent.

osteoarthritis Inflammation of a bony union or joint; it is not as crippling and causes less inflammation than rheumatoid arthritis.

osteomalacia An adult disease marked by increasing softness of the bones so that they become flexible and brittle and attended by rheumatic pains, weakness, and exhaustion, with the patient dying eventually from exhaustion.

osteomyelitis Inflammation of the bone marrow, or bone, or medullary cavity of bone.

osteoporosis Abnormal porousnes or loss of density of bone by enlargement of its canals or the formation of abnormal spaces; softening of bone.

otitis media Inflammation of the middle ear.

ototoxicity Poisonous or deleterious to the organs of hearing and balance.

ovary Female sex organ in which ova, or eggs, develop and mature.

palliative Alleviating medicine or treatment offering relief or reducing the severity of pain but not curing the cause.

palpitation Unduly rapid action of the heart felt by the patient.

pancreas Gland of the endocrine system lying behind the stomach and containing the islands of Langerhans, which produce insulin, an internal secretion that reduces the blood and urinary sugar to normal. The pancreas also produces enzymes to aid in the digestion of proteins, carbohydrates, and fats.

pancreatitis Inflammation of the pancreas marked by abdominal pain, pain around the umbilicus or navel, abdominal distension, nausea, and vomiting.

papilla Any small, nipple-shaped elevation.

optic The optic disk, a round white disk in the fundus oculi medial to the posterior pole of the eyes; corresponds to the entrance of the optic nerve and retinal blood vessels.

papilledema Edema of the optic papilla; a choked disk; optic neuritis caused by intracranial pressure and without inflammatory manifestations.

paralytic ileus Paralysis of the muscular coats of the ileum, a part of the small intestine characterized by possible obstruction of intestinal contents, continuous abdominal pain, distension, vomiting, severe constipation, peritonitis, minimal abdominal tenderness, decreased or absent bowel sounds, history of surgery, and X-ray evidence of gas and fluid in the bowel.

parasympathetic nervous system Part of the autonomic nervous system, including certain nerves whose fibers start from the midbrain, hindbrain, and sacral parts of the spinal cord.

parasympathomimetic drugs Drugs that cause effects in the body similar to those produced by acetylcholine; cholinergic drugs.

parathyroid gland Four small glands, two of which are found on the surface of each lateral lobe of the thyroid. These glands secrete a hormone that regulates calcium-phosphorus metabolism.

parenteral, parenterally Subcutaneous, intramuscular, or intravenous method of administration; treatment by injection.

paresthesia An abnormal sensation, such as burning or prickling.

Parkinson's disease Disease marked by slowing and weakness of voluntary movement, muscular rigidity, and tremor; also known as palsy and paralysis agitans.

paroxysm Sudden recurrence or intensification of symptoms.

patent Wide open.

pathogen Any disease-producing microorganism or material.

pathology The branch of medicine that treats the essential nature of disease, especially the structural and the functional changes caused by disease.

pediculicide Destroying lice; Pediculin is a proprietary remedy for killing lice.

pellagra Endemic skin and spinal disease occurring in southern Europe and southern and central parts of the United States; thought to be caused by deficiency of vitamins B_2 or G, which are found in lean meat, milk, yeast, and other foods. Characteristic symptoms includ recurring reddening of the body surface followed by falling off of the skin in layers, along with weakness, debility, digestive disturbances, spinal pain, convulsions, melancholia, and idiocy.

pentagastrin A synthetic peptide that stimulates gastric acid without producing the undesirable side effects of histamine.

peptic ulcer Stomach ulcer.

peptide A compound formed by the union of two or more amino acids. When two amino acids unite, the result is a dipeptide; three form a tripeptide; and more than three form a polypeptide.

perfusion Pouring through or into.

peripheral, periphery Outward part or surface.

blood vessels Blood vessels near the skin or surface of the body.

neuropathy Any disease affecting peripheral nerves.

resistance Ratio of pressure to flow. It is not constant along vessels because of the plastic nature of blood. Resistance is influenced by pressure, viscosity, and vessel lumen size.

peristalsis Worm-like contraction of the muscle tissue of the intestines or certain other organs.

peritoneal cavity Space between the visceral and parietal peritonea.

peritoneum Serous membrane that lines the abdominal walls and invests the contained viscera; holds viscera in place.

parietal Membrane that lines the abdominal walls, pelvic walls, and undersurface of the diaphragm.

visceral Membrane reflected at various places over the viscera, forming a complete covering for the stomach, spleen, liver, and many parts of the small and the large intestines.

perlèche Inflammation of the corners of the mouth caused by a yeast-like fungus, *Candida albicans.*

permeability Property or state of being permeable; may be traversed or passed through.

pernicious anemia Chronic disease characterized

by a progressive decrease in the number of red corpuscles.

petechiae, petechia Small spots formed by the escape of blood into a part or tissue, as seen in typhus or purpura. See *purpura*.

pH The symbol commonly used in expressing hydrogen ion concentration.

phagocyte Any cell that ingests microorganisms or other cells and substances. The ingested material is often, but not always, digested within the phagocyte. Phagocytes are either fixed, such an endothelial cells, or free, such as leukocytes. The two forms of leukocytes that are phagocytic are the large lymphocyte (macrophage) and the polymorphonuclear leukocyte (microphage). *Polymorphonuclear* means many-shaped nucleus.

pharyngitis Inflammation of the pharynx.

pharynx Tube-shaped passage or musculomembranous sac between the mouth and nares and the esophagus. It is continuous below with the esophagus and above it communicates with the larynx, mouth, nasal passages, and eustachian tubes. It is a passage for both air and food.

pheochromocytoma Tumor of the kidney or adrenal gland consisting of chromaffin cells, which secrete epinephrine.

phlebitis Inflammation of a vein, marked by infiltration of the coats of the vein and the formation of a thrombus of coagulated blood.

phobia Any persistent insane dread or fear.

phosphatide, phosphotidate Phospholipid from which choline or colamine has been split off.

phospholipid Lipin containing phosphorus that yields fatty acids and glycerin on hydrolysis. Lecithin is the best-known example.

photophobia Abnormal sensitivity to or intolerance of light.

pituitary gland (or **body**) Small, bean-shaped body located in a depression of the sphenoid bone in the skull. It is divided into anterior and posterior lobes, each of which gives off several hormones.

placenta Any cake-like mass; the round, flat organ about 1 inch thick and 7 inches in diameter within the uterus that establishes communication between the mother and child by means of the umbilical cord.

placenta previa A condition in which the placenta is implanted in the lower uterine segment, partially or completely covering the cervical outlet.

platelets Oval disks without hemoglobin found in the blood; they are essential for clotting. Platelets, or thrombocytes, may be manufactured in the red bone marrow. There is wide variance in platelet count, but normal count may be 250,000 to 500,000/cu ml of blood.

pleura The serous membrane that invests the lungs, lines the thorax, and is reflected on the diaphragm. There are two pleurae, right and left, entirely shut off from each other. The pleura is moistened with a serous secretion that eases the movements of the lungs in the chest.

pleural effusion A second stage inflammation of the pleura in which exudation of copious amounts of serum occurs. The inflamed surfaces of the pleura may become united by adhesions, which are usually permanent. Symptoms include a "stitch" in the side, and a chill followed

by a fever, a dry cough, and pain during breathing. As effusion occurs, there is an onset of dyspnea and a lessening of pain. The patient lies on the affected side.

pleurisy A disease marked by inflammation of the pleura, with exudation into its cavity and on its surface.

polarity Fact or condition of having poles; exhibition of opposite effects at two extremities.

polycythemia vera A disease lasting many years and marked by a persistent increase in the red blood corpuscles (polycythemia), resulting from excessive formation of erythroblasts by the bone marrow and characterized by increased viscosity of the blood, enlargement of the spleen, and cyanotic appearance of the patient.

polymer Any member of a series of substances concerned with, derived from, or pertaining to several pigments.

polymorphonuclear Having nuclei of many forms or shapes, as in certain leukocytes.

polysaccharides Group of carbohydrates that contain more than three molecules of simple carbohydrates combined with each other. They comprise dextrins, starches, glycogens, cellulose, gums, inulin, and pectose.

polyuria Excessive secretion and discharge of urine containing increased amounts of solid constituents.

postpartum Period occurring after delivery or childbirth.

potency Power, strength, as of medicines.

potential Existing and ready for action but not yet active.

precordial Pertaining to the precordium, the region over the heart or stomach; the epigastrium and lower part of the thorax.

precursor Something that precedes or goes before.

priapism Abnormal, painful, and continuous erection of the penis due to disease, usually without sexual desire.

prognosis Forecast as to the probable result of a disease attack; the prospect of recovery from a disease gained through the nature and the symptoms of the case.

proliferation, proliferating Reproduction or multiplication of similar forms, especially of cells and morbid cysts.

prostaglandin A series of chemicals that have pressor, vasodilator, and stimulant effects on the intestinal and uterine muscles.

prostate A gland in the male that surrounds the neck of the bladder and the urethra. It consists of a median lobe and two lateral lobes and is made up of glandular matter, the ducts that empty into the prostatic portion of the urethra, and the muscular fibers that encircle the urethra.

prostatectomy Surgical removal or the prostate or a part of it.

prostatic hypertrophy An enlargement of the prostate gland.

protein Any one of a group of nitrogenized compounds, similar to each other, widely distributed in the animal and vegetable kingdoms, and forming the characteristic constituents of the tissues and fluids of the animal body. They are essentially combinations of α-amino acids and their derivatives.

proteinuria The presence of protein in the urine.

prothrombin Fibrin factor in blood plasma that

is supposed to be a precursor of thrombin; also called thrombogen and thrombinogen.

proximal Nearer to or on the side toward the body; opposed to distal.

pruritus Intense itching; a symptom of many skin and other diseases.

psoriasis Chronic inflammatory skin disease marked by the formation of scaly red patches on the surface of the body.

psychomotor Pertaining to or causing voluntary movements.

psychoneurosis Borderline disorder of the mind that is not a true insanity, such as hysteria and neurasthenia.

psychosis Disease or disorder of the mind.

pulmonary embolism Blood clot or foreign material that travels through the circulation and finally lodges in a blood vessel of the lungs.

pulmonary wedge pressure A Swan-Ganz catheter or a special, pliable, multiple-lumen, balloon-tipped catheter is inserted by a highly skilled physician under sterile technique into the subclavian, jugular, or femoral vein and on through the vena cava, the right atrium, and the right ventricle to the pulmonary artery. The large or major lumen of the catheter terminates at the catheter tip and measures pulmonary artery pressure. The small lumen terminates in a latex balloon that can be inflated to surround, but not occlude, the tip of the catheter. When the balloon is inflated and wedged against the pulmonary artery, it continuously measures pulmonary pressure and transmits the measurements to an oscilloscope at the bedside. This procedure is used in congestive heart failure, in myocardial infarction, in measuring left heart pressures and function, and in many other conditions. It is a lifesaving procedure.

pulse pressure See *blood pressure*.

pulvule Proprietary capsule containing a dose of a powdered drug.

pupil Opening in the center of the iris of the eye for the passage of light rays to the retina.

purgative Strong medication administered by mouth to produce bowel evacuation or several movements of the bowels.

purpura Disease characterized by the formation of purple patches on the skin and mucous membranes, caused by the escape of blood into a part or tissue.

purulent Consisting of or containing pus.

pyelitis Inflammation of the pelvis of the kidney; it may be caused by a renal stone, extension of inflammation from the bladder, or stagnation of urine. Symptoms include pain and tenderness in the loins, irritability of the bladder, remittent fever, blood or purulent urine, diarrhea, vomiting, and peculiar pain on flexion of the thigh.

pyelonephritis Inflammation of the kidney and its pelvis.

pyloric spasm Contraction of the pylorus or pyloric sphincter caused by muscle spasm; this will not allow the pylorus to relax and the stomach to empty.

pylorus Gate to the outlet of the stomach; a ring-like band of muscle tissue between the opening of the stomach and the duodenum, or the first part of small intestine.

pyrogen A fever-producing substance.

pyrogenic Inducing fever, also caused by or resulting from fever.

rabies (or hydrophobia, fear of water) Filtrable infectious disease of certain animals, especially dogs, wolves, and squirrels; communicated to man by direct inoculation from the bite of the infected animal—the virus is in the saliva. Incubation period is 1 to 6 months. Symptoms include malaise, depression of spirits, swelling of lymphatics in the region of the wound, choking, spasmodic breathing, and increasing tetanic muscle spasms, especially of respiratory and swallowing muscles, which are increased by attempts to drink water or even by the sight of water. Fever, mental derangement, vomiting, profuse secretion of a sticky saliva, and albuminuria also occur. Disease is almost 100% fatal within 2 to 5 days after onset of symptoms unless rabies vaccine is administered within a short period after the bite occurs.

Raynaud's disease Disease characterized by disturbances in circulation in the blood vessels of the extremities, with the possibility of gangrene and amputation of a limb.

reflux A backward or return flow.

refractory Not readily yielding to treatment.

regurgitation The casting up of undigested food; a backward flowing of the blood through the left atrioventricular opening resulting from imperfect closure of the mitral valve.

remission Period during which symptoms of a disease are abated or lessened in severity.

renal Pertaining to the kidney.

resection Excision of a part of an organ; excision of the ends of bones and other structures forming a joint.

reticulin Albuminoid substance from the connective fibers of reticular tissue; a net-like tissue.

reticulocyte Young red blood cell showing a reticulum or protoplasmic network construction under vital staining.

retina, retinal The innermost tunic (coat, membrane) and perceptive structure of the eye, formed by the expansion of the optic nerve and covering the back part of the eye as far as the ora serrata (the zigzag anterior edge of the retina); often called the nerve of the sense of sight.

retinoblastoma A tumor arising from retinal germ cells.

retinopathy Disease of the retina of the eye.

rhabdomyoma A tumor (myoma) composed of striated muscular fibers.

rhabdomyosarcoma A combined sarcoma and rhabdomyoma.

rheumatic fever Inflammatory joint disease that usually occurs following a streptococcal infection and that is characterized by fever, malaise, joint inflammation and swelling, and transitory pain in the joints. It is usually recurrent and may damage the heart valves.

rheumatic heart disease Chronic disease of the heart valve or valves caused by rheumatic fever.

rheumatoid arthritis Type of arthritis marked by joint pain, swelling of joints, fever, malaise, and crippling of joints.

rhinitis Inflammation of the mucous membrane of the nose; a cold.

rhinorrhea Free discharge of a thin nasal mucus.

rickets Softness of bones in childhood caused by lack of calcium salts, which results in a slowing of the bone-hardening process; lack of vitamin D is a contributing cause.

rickettsiae (Howard Taylor Ricketts' organism) group of bacteria-like microorganisms that may be transmitted to humans by lice or other parasites. Some diseases caused by rickettsiae include Brill's disease (a form of typhus fever), endemic typhus fever, epidemic typhus fever, and Rocky Mountain spotted fever.

ringworm Parasitic fungus causing a contagious skin disease marked by ring-shaped colored patches; usually on the scalp but can appear on other parts of the body.

roentgen The international unit of roentgen radiation.

roentgen rays Electromagnetic vibrations of waves of very short wavelengths, set in motion when electrons, moving at high velocity, impinge on certain substances, especially the heavy metals. They are able to penetrate most substances, to affect a photographic plate, to bring about chemical reactions, and to produce changes in living matter. They are used in taking photographs of the human body (roentgenograms) or in visualizing portions of the body (fluoroscopy). They reveal foreign bodies in the human body such as calculi (stones) and bullets, as well as fractures of the bone and the functions of such organs as the heart, stomach, and intestines. They are also used in treating various diseases, such as lupus, cancer, and eczema. Also called X-rays.

rubella German measles; an acute eruption rash and febrile disease not unlike measles. After an incubation period of 1 to 3 weeks, the disease begins with slight fever and catarrhal symptoms, sore throat, pains in the limbs, and the eruption of red papules similar to those appearing in measles but lighter in color, not arranged in crescentic masses, and disappearing without peeling or skin flaking within a week.

rubeola A viral disease or measles, characterized by fever, coryza, cough, conjunctivitis, photophobia, and Koplik's spots; the latter usually appear about 2 days before the rash and last 4 days as tiny "table-salt crystals" on the dull-red mucous membranes of the inner aspects of the cheeks and often on the inner conjunctival folds and vaginal mucous membranes. Exposure occurs 14 days before the rash. The rash is brick-red, irregular, and maculopapular, with onset 4 days after initial symptoms, appearing on the face first, then on the chest, the extremities, and the back. The rash begins fading on the third day in the order that it appeared. Slight desquamation (peeling and flaking of skin) also occurs.

sacroiliac Referring to the sacrum and the ilium bones of the pelvis.

salivation Process of secreting saliva from the salivary glands in the mouth.

salpinx Fallopian or eustachian tube.

saphenous Veins in the legs.

   magna The longest vein in the body, extending from the dorsum of the foot to just below the inguinal ligament, where it opens into the femoral vein.

   parva Continues the marginal vein from behind the malleolus (ankle joint) and passes up the back of the leg to the knee joint, where it opens into the popliteal vein.

scabies Communicable skin disease caused by the itch mite and attended with intense itching.

schizoid Resembling schizophrenia; reclusive, unsocial, introspective type of personality.

schizophrenia Dementia praecox; adolescent insanity; the term includes a large range of mental disorders that occur early in life and are marked by melancholia, self-absorption, reclusive, unsocial, introspective, withdrawn type of personality, and general mental weakness.

sciatica Inflammation of the sciatic nerve, usually a neuritis. Symptoms include abnormal burning, prickling sensation (paresthesia) of the thigh and leg, tenderness along the course of the nerve, pain that is usually constant, and sometimes a wasting of the calf muscles. It may recur.

sciatic nerve Long nerve with many branches originating in the sacral plexus (a network or tangle of nerves) and distributing through the skin of muscles in thigh, leg, and foot.

sclera The tough, white supporting tunic of the eyeball, covering it entirely except for the segment covered by the cornea; continuous with the cornea; nontransparent; the white portion of the eye.

scurvy Nutritional disease caused by dietetic errors, marked by weakness, anemia, spongy gums, tendency to mucocutaneous hemorrhage, and hardening of the muscles of the calves and legs. Treatment consists of eating fresh potatoes, scurvy grass, onions, lime juice, other citrus fruits such as oranges and lemons, and vitamin C.

sebaceous gland Any gland secreting sebaceous matter (sebum, or a greasy, lubricating substance); chiefly situated in the corium, or true skin.

sedative Quieting or calming type of drug.

serum Watery fluid of the body, especially the fluid left after removal of solid materials of the blood.

SGOT A laboratory blood test: serum glutamic-oxaloacetic transaminase.

smallpox Infectious viral disease marked by a rash that passes through several successive stages.

somatic Pertaining to the body tissues, as opposed to reproductive tissues and as distinguished from the psyche.

sperm Mature male cells found in the semen or testicular secretion.

sphincter Ring-like muscle that closes a natural orifice, for example, the pyloric sphincter or the anal sphincter.

spinal cord Cord-like structure contained in the spinal canal and extending from the foramen magnum to the second lumbar vertebra. It is a center for reflex activity and also functions in the transmission of impulses to and from the higher centers in the brain.

splenic flexure syndrome Discomfort originating from the bend of the colon at the junction of the transverse and descending portions.

spondylitis Inflammation of one or more vertebrae.

sprue Chronic disease of disturbed small intestine function characterized by impaired absorption, particularly of fats, and motor abnormalities. Symptoms include bulky, pale, frothy, foul-smelling, greasy stools; weight loss; vitamin deficiencies; impaired intestinal absorption of glucose, vitamins, and fat; large amounts of free fatty acids and soaps in the stool; sore mouth and raw-looking tongue; gastrointestinal catarrh with periodic diarrhea; and change in liver size. The anemia is treated with oral iron for hypochromic anemia and vitamin B_{12} for macrocytic anemia. Therapeutic diet should be high-calorie, high-protein, low-fat, and gluten-free. Sprue occurs mostly in hot countries and is known as tropical sprue. Nontropical sprue is also called intestinal infantilism. See *celiac disease* and *infantilism*.

sputum Substance sent forth from the bronchial tubes and the mouth containing saliva, mucus, and sometimes pus; phlegm.

squamous cell A flat, scale-like epithelial cell.

stasis Stoppage of the flow of blood in any part of the body.

status asthmaticus State or condition of asthma.

status epilepticus A series of rapidly repeated epileptic convulsions with no periods of consciousness.

steatorrhea Presence of excess fat in the stools. *idiopathic* Intestinal infantilism.

stenosis Narrowing or stricture of a duct or canal.

sterol A monohydroxy alcohol of high molecular weight; one of a class of compounds widely distributed in nature, which, because their solubilities are similar to those of fats, have been classified with the lipins. Cholesterol is the best-known member of the group.

stimulant Type of drug that increases activity and hastens action in the body.

stomatitis Inflammation of the mouth.

stratum A layer or set of layers, as in the epidermis, or outermost and nonvascular layer of the skin.

Stria (striae atrophicae) Streak or line on the skin. Many of these are often seen on the abdomen of pregnant women or after childbirth, first as reddish streaks, gradually fading to white. They are permanent and caused by atrophy or stretching of the skin.

stricture The abnormal narrowing of a canal, duct, or passage, either from cicatric contraction or the deposit of abnormal tissue.

stye Inflammation of an oil gland of the eyelid.

subaortic Situated below the aorta or the main blood vessel trunk from which the entire systemic arterial system proceeds.

subcapsular cataract Opacity or cloudiness situated beneath the anterior or posterior capsule of the eye lens.

subcutaneous Beneath the skin or in the tissues.

sublingual Beneath the tongue.

substrate A substratum, or lower stratum; the term is applied to the substance on which a ferment or enzyme acts.

supraclavicular Situated above the clavicle, or collar bone.

sympathectomy Surgical removal of a part of a sympathetic nerve, especially the superior cervical sympathetic ganglion.

sympathetic nervous system Part of the autonomic nervous system; also known as the vegetative or visceral nervous system because the organs controlled by it function unconsciously.

sympathomimetic Resembling the effects produced by disturbance of the sympathetic nervous system. Sympathomimetic drugs relieve the symptoms.

symptom Any disorder of function, appearance, or sensation that the patient experiences.

synapse Anatomic relation of one nerve cell to another; the point of contact between processes of two adjacent neurons, forming the place where a nervous impulse is transmitted from one neuron to another; also called synaptic junction.

syndrome Set of symptoms that occur together.

synovial fluid Fluid secreted by the synovial membrane and contained in joint cavities.

synovitis Inflammation of the synovial membrane, or the covering around joints.

synthesis The artificial building up of a chemical compound by the union of its elements.

syphilis A contagious venereal disease leading to many structural and cutaneous lesions, resulting from a microorganism, the *spirochete pallida*, or *Treponema pallidum*. It is generally propagated by direct venereal contact or by inheritance. Its primary site is a hard or true chancre, whence it extends by means of the lymphatics to the skin, mucosa, and nearly all the tissues of the body, even to the bones and periosteum (the tough, fibrous membrane surrounding bone).

systolic blood pressure See *blood pressure*.

tachycardia Excessive rapidity in the action of the heart, with usually a pulse rate greater than 130 beats per minute.

tachyphylaxis Rapid immunization from the effects of toxic doses of an extract by previous injection of small doses.

tapeworm Flat, tape-like, segmented parasite sometimes found in the intestines of man.

tenacious Holding fast, thick, sticky, adhesive; for example, mucus and sputum.

tenosynovitis Tendon inflammation.

teratogenic Tending to produce fetal monstrosity.

testes Male gonads; organ in reproduction.

tetanus (lockjaw) Acute infectious disease caused by a toxin related by the *Clostridium tetani* (tetanus bacillus) and characterized by more or less persistent tonic spasm of some of the voluntary muscles. Continuous spasm or steady contraction of a muscle without distinct twitching can occur. Spasm can cause locking of the jaw muscles so jaws cannot open, hence its common name.

tetany Nervous affection characterized by muscle twitching, cramps, muscle pains, and convulsions.

thalamus Mass of gray matter at the base of the brain projecting into and bounding the third ventricle.

thrombin The hypothetical fibrin ferment of the blood; the enzyme, present in clotted but not in circulating blood, that converts fibrinogen into fibrin; also called thrombase, fibrin ferment, and fibrinogen.

thromboangiitis obliterans Form of gangrene attributed to a thromboangiitis occurring generally in the larger arteries and veins of the leg, although it may appear in the upper extremity. Also called Buerger's disease and presenile spontaneous gangrene.

thrombocytes Blood platelets.

thrombocytopenia Decrease in the number of blood platelets; same as thrombopenia.

thrombocytopenic purpura Severe form of purpura, with copious hemorrhages from the mucous membranes, marked lessening of the number of blood platelets, marked loss of nuclear substance of blood platelets, and severe constitutional symptoms.

thrombophlebitis Inflammation of a vein or veins resulting from an infection or clot.

thromboplastin Substance existing in the tissue that causes clotting of the blood.

thrombosis Formation or development of a thrombus or clot in a blood vessel and remaining at its point of formation.

thyroid gland Gland of internal secretion found in the neck.

thyrotoxicosis Severe condition resulting from abnormal increase of thyroid activity.

tinea corporis Ringworm of the body.
cruris Ringworm of the groin.
pedis Ringworm of the feet, or athlete's foot.

tinnitus Ringing or singing sound heard in the ears; also a clicking sound in the ear heard in chronic catarrhal otitis media or inflammation of the middle ear.

titer Quantity of a substance required to produce a reaction with a given amount of another substance.
agglutination The highest dilution of a serum that causes clumping of bacteria.
colon The smallest amount of a certain substance that indicates the presence of the colon bacillus under standard conditions.

tone In the circulatory system, the factor responsible for a small blood vessel being stiffer or showing more resistance to stretching than a larger vessel, even though the wall material of both small and large vessels possesses exactly the same mechanical properties.

tonometry The measurement of tension, especially intraocular tension.

topical Pertaining to a particular spot; local; medicine for local application, for example, eye drops.

torticollis Wryneck; a contracted state of the cervical or neck muscles producing twisting of the neck and an unnatural position of the head.

trachea Windpipe; the cartilaginous and membranous tube descending from the larynx to the bronchi.

tracheitis Inflammation of the trachea.

tracheostomy Operative formation of an opening into the trachea (windpipe) through the neck and insertion of a trachea tube to aid breathing.

transient Temporary, passing through or over.

trauma Wound or injury.

trifacial neuralgia Pain in the fifth cranial nerve, a nerve of the face. Pain is very severe, shooting, stabbing, searing, or burning in the area of one or more branches of the nerve. Attack frequency varies from many times a day to several times a month or year. Also known as trigeminal neuralgia or tic douloureux.

trigonum vesicae Triangular area of the interior of the bladder between the opening of the ureters and the orifice of the urethra. Called also trigone of bladder and vesical trigone.

trophic Of or pertaining to nutrition.

tuberculosis Infectious disease caused by the tubercle bacillus and marked by presence of tubercles in the affected tissues; most common site is in the lungs.

typhoid fever Contagious disease marked by fever, diarrhea that is sometimes bloody, and malaise. The typhoid bacillus enters the body with food such as milk, watery vegetables such as lettuce, and drinking water.

typhus fever Rickettsial infectious disease characterized by symptoms such as petechial eruptions, high temperature, chills, backache, headache, and great prostration. See *rickettsia*.

urate Any salt or uric acid. Urates, especially that of sodium, are constituents of urine, blood, and tophi or calcerous concretions (a stone or mass containing lime or calcium).

urea White, crystallizable substance, a double amide or compound of carbonic acid, from the urine, blood, and lymph. It is the chief nitrogenous constituent of the urine and is the final product of the decomposition of proteins in the body. It is the form under which the nitrogen of the body is given off. It is thought to be formed in the liver out of amino acids and other compounds of ammonia.

uremia Toxic condition from abnormal urinary constituents in the blood.

ureter The fibromuscular tube that conveys urine from the kidney to the bladder.

ureterosigmoidostomy The operation of implanting the ureter into the sigmoid flexure.

urethra Canal leading from the bladder to the exterior of the body.

uric acid Crystallizable acid, trioxypurine, from the urine of humans and animals, being one of the products of nuclein metabolism. It forms a large portion of certain calculi, or stones, and in the blood causes morbid symptoms, such as those of gout.

uricosuric drugs Drugs administered to relieve pain in gout and increase elimination of uric acid.

urinary retention Retention of urine in the bladder, often caused by a temporary loss of muscle function.

urolithiasis The formation of urinary calculi or stones; also the diseased condition associated with the presence of urinary calculi or stones.

urologic Pertaining to the urine and urinary tract; the term now includes the male and female genitourinary tract.

uropathy Any pathologic change in the urinary tract.

urticaria Hives.

uterus The womb, or organ for containing and nourishing the infant before birth.

vaccination Inoculation with a vaccine as a disease preventive.

vaccine Substance derived from the growth of bacteria and used to confer immunity against certain diseases.

vaccinia Cowpox; a disease of cattle regarded as a form of smallpox. When given to a person via vaccination, it confers a greater or lesser degree of immunity against smallpox.

vagus nerve Tenth cranial nerve, which originates in an area on the floor of the fourth ventricle, extends by small cords from the side of the medulla oblongata, and distributes to larynx, lungs, heart, esophagus, stomach, and most of the abdominal viscera. *Vagus* is a Latin word meaning "wandering." Also called pneumogastric nerve.

varicella Chickenpox; an acute contagious disease, principally of young children, marked by slight fever and an eruption of macular vesicles appearing in crops and sometimes followed by scarring.

vascular Pertaining to or full of vessels, often blood vessels.

vasoconstriction Construction or decrease in size of blood vessels.

vasodilation Dilation or enlargement of the blood vessels.

ventricle Two lower cavities or chambers of the heart; there are right and left ventricles.

venule A minute vein.

vermicular Worm-like in shape or appearance.

vertigo Dizziness, giddiness; disorder of the equilibrating sense marked by a swimming in the head; a sense of instability of apparent rotary movement of the body or of other objects.

Vincent's infection (trench mouth) Inflammation caused by mixed organisms. It was commonly seen among soldiers in the trenches, hence its name. It can involve the throat, stomach, and intestines and is communicable. Also called Vincent's angina.

viscera Internal organs, especially those of the cavities of the chest and abdomen.

viscosity Quality of being sticky or gummy

vulva The external part of the organs of generation of the female, including the labia majora, the labia minora, mons veneris, clitoris, perineum, and vestibulum vaginae.

vulvovaginitis Inflammation of the vulva and vagina, or of the vulvovaginal glands.

wheal A white or pinkish elevation or ridge on the skin, as in urticaria or after the stroke of a whip.

whiplash Inflammation and muscle spasm of the neck and upper back muscles often caused by violent movement during heavy exercise or automobile accidents; often occurs as the result of a sudden backward and forward whipping movement of the neck.

Wilms' tumor A tumor containing embryonic elements; embryoma of the kidney.

Wilson's disease (progressive lenticular disease or hepatolenticular disease) Rare disease characterized by bilateral degeneration of the corpus striatum (a subcortical mass of gray and white matter in front of the thalamus in each cerebral hemisphere) and cirrhosis of the liver with symptoms such as tremor, spastic contractures, increasing weakness and emaciation, and psychic disturbance. Also called dermatitis exfoliativa.

Index